The Art of Skin Graft

Young-Chul Jang

The Art of Skin Graft

Advanced Graft Technique

Springer

Young-Chul Jang
Hallym University
Hangang Sacred Heart Hospital
Seoul, Korea (Republic of)

ISBN 978-981-97-0016-5 ISBN 978-981-97-0017-2 (eBook)
https://doi.org/10.1007/978-981-97-0017-2

This Springer imprint is published by the registered company Springer Nature Singapore Pte Ltd.
The registered company address is: 152 Beach Road, #21-01/04 Gateway East, Singapore 189721, Singapore

Preface

Now, skin graft is not exclusive to plastic surgery but a fundamental technique required by all surgical departments, and it has a significant impact on the end results of surgery. Split-thickness skin graft , a common technique for treating traumatic injuries, causes frequent functional disorders due to contractures occurring during the healing process. Full-thickness skin graft is useful for joint contracture corrective surgery; however, its disadvantages include insufficient donor sites and poor skin survival. I wrote this book to reiterate the concept of skin graft, which has been regarded as an old, conventional surgical technique by most surgeons so far, and to highlight the advancements and usefulness of such techniques. Therefore, I majorly delineated skin graft in terms of its techniques and described the concepts of advanced skin graft methods, including aesthetics, which are often encountered in reconstructive surgery, as well as basic techniques.

I named this book *The Art of Skin Graft* for the purposes of reinterpreting skin graft, which has been one of the most popular surgical techniques, from a new perspective. Such efforts were made because it was thought that cosmetic improvements in terms of aesthetics and functionality by the addition of artistic sensibilities to conventional ideas would be of help to patients who have been suffering for a long time. This book was written with the hope of providing guidance for those who want to be surgeons, by putting together all the bedside teaching and instructions I have given as a professor to students and junior colleagues and all the experiences of hope and despair that I have felt while performing more than 10,000 surgeries.

Finally, some questions in this book remain unanswered for several clinical cases, such as those related to cell culture and artificial dermis, which have not been scientifically proven as real artificial skin. This book was written with the hope of receiving answers to such questions from young surgeons who are constantly improving their abilities and have the spirit of research.

Finally, I would like to express my heartfelt thanks to the many patients who believed in, followed, and taught me for a long time, helping overcome numerous difficult problems.

Seoul, Korea (Republic of) Young-Chul Jang

Contents

1 Split-Thickness Skin Grafting

1.1 Introduction

Split-thickness skin graft (STSG) refers to a type of widely used skin graft that comprises both the full layer of the epidermis and a part of the dermis [1–4]. This technique can be categorized into a mesh skin graft, which is mainly used to treat cases of burns or trauma, and STSG, a convenient and effective method that is typically used for skin defects and wound healing. Surgical method used for a mesh skin graft is a simple reliable effect, and the take rate is considerably high; thus, most cases are dismissed as simple operations without careful consideration regarding the operation itself [5]. However, the author would like to emphasize that a thoroughly planned operation, even for a mesh skin graft, is very effective, plays an important role in the wound healing process, and greatly affects the outcome. Moreover, owing to the fact that it considerably influences the mesh pattern scars that inevitably remain, along with the need for corrective surgery for severe contractures on joints and unsightly scars on the exposure area, careful consideration and implementation of the mesh ratio, engraft mesh direction, and regions to be avoided is important [6]. In addition, in cases in which mesh skin graft is possible, shortening the wound healing process is a crucial point of the surgery [7]. Therefore, if the mesh ratio is 1:3–4 or higher, the combined use of cultured epithelial cell therapy and dermal substitute to minimize scar contracture is efficient in supplementing the dermis. Therefore, an introduction to this method will be briefly described. Please note that the introduction to this method is described in Chap. 4 "Cultured Epithelial Cell Therapy" in more detail [8–11].

STSG is the most widely performed skin grafting procedure; however, in this section, rather than introducing the basic principles or technical aspects of general STSG, a practical introduction to the components of the procedure that have a great influence on the functional and cosmetic results of surgery, such as the face and hands, will be provided. In particular, the author will discuss the considerations and operative results of facial skin graft, which remains very controversial among plastic surgeons in terms of whether or not the surgery should be performed. STSG is rarely used in most reconstructive surgery procedures owing to the frequent problems related to high contracture rate and pigmentation disorder. This work describes the author's long-accumulated methods for and results of upper and lower lid ectropion correction, which is considered one of the most difficult to achieve in terms of natural and functional recovery. Furthermore, this section will highlight the usefulness of STSG, which has not received much attention because it is dismissed as a simple operation, and provide an opportunity to expand its scope of use [12, 13].

Y.-C. Jang, *The Art of Skin Graft*, https://doi.org/10.1007/978-981-97-0017-2_1

1.2 Mesh Skin Graft

The primary purpose of a mesh skin graft is to effectively cover a large area of skin defect with a relatively smaller area of the skin. Furthermore, this method is particularly useful for rapid wound coverage because blood or fluid can be discharged through the mesh gap, thereby making the process of wound dressing easy [14]. In addition, this method has the highest engraftment rate. However, it is recommended to avoid this method for parts that are exposed to the external environment, such as the face, back of the hands, or forearms; this is because the mesh pattern scar that occurs as a result of the rapid treatment lacks a cosmetic effect. This method should also be avoided for large joints of the extremities that move considerably as well as the hands or feet, i.e., areas with a large number of joints, as the scar contracture rate is high.

In general, the mesh ratio ranges from 1:1 to 1:2 using a mesher machine (Brennen skin graft Mesher) [15].

In cases in which no expensive mesher machines are available, the skin collected with a No. 10 blade is spread flat on a hardwood or rubber board and is used conveniently by overlapping the interrupted slit incision (Fig. 1.1) [16]. The advantages of this method include easy adjustment of the mesh ratio by the operator and a less apparent mesh pattern than expected, thereby increasing the engraftment rate and ensuring the safety of this method when used for grafting [17]. However, in cases requiring wide wound coverage, such as in a patient with major burns, a mesher device is absolutely necessary owing to the fact that a ratio of 1:4 or even 1:9 may be used. If the mesh pattern ratio is >1:4, the time required for filling the mesh gap with epithelialization increases and lowers the engraftment rate. Accordingly, the author has been able to obtain satisfactory results by shortening the healing period using the sandwich technique with cultured epithelial homograft (CEH) and proceeding with stable wound healing. Owing to the fact that a cultured epithelial autograft (CEA)

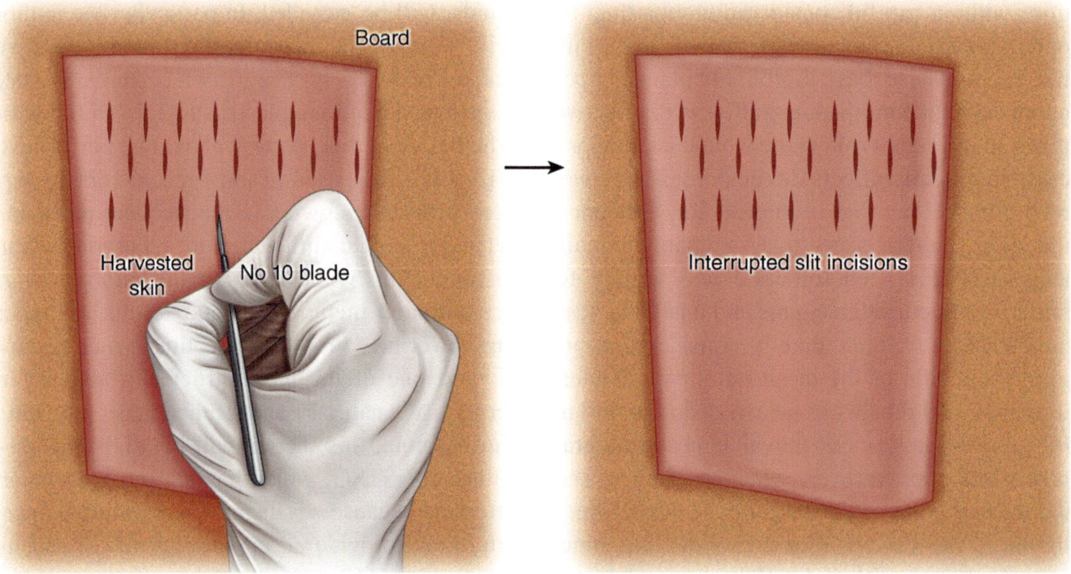

Fig. 1.1 The harvested split-thickness skin is spread flat on a hardwood or rubber board and overlapping the interrupted slit incisions with No. 10 blade to make mashed auto split-thickness skin

provides coverage using one's own cells, it provides better results than CEH in terms of increasing the engraftment rate, shortening the healing process, and replenishing small but insufficient skin [11]. This method will be described in more detail later along with a clinical case example.

Mesh skin graft is a very important and critical method used for burn management, but both plastic surgeons and patients must carefully consider this procedure and avoid using it in cases when it is not absolutely necessary. One reason for exercising this caution is to avoid wasting the sacrifice of another donor to correct the mesh-shaped deformity later. This concept will be explained in further detail in Chap. 5 (Esthetic skin grafting). Another reason is that regardless of the quality of the mesh skin graft, it will eventually undergo deformation and contracture deformation. Therefore, correction should be performed as soon as possible. Introducing a high-quality sheet graft will not only save time and money but also produce excellent results. In other words, performing a high-quality split-skin graft method can yield many benefits, such as convenience and reduction of skin consumption during future functional or cosmetic corrective surgeries. These concepts are especially important for the face and hands; therefore, the surgeons should familiarize themselves with the details given in the "STSG" section.

The surgical method and postoperative management of mesh skin graft are relatively simple. In my cases, after carefully selecting the surgical site, a protective dressing is applied using Bactigras (Smith & Nephew Medical Ltd., Hessle Road, England), a Vaseline gauze with a large mesh pattern that facilitates good fluid evacuation, followed by a saline-soaked compression gauze dressing. A stable engraftment generally begins when the dressing is opened after 3–4 days. Most meshes with a 1:2 ratio engraft well without major changes; however, the time taken for epithelialization and wound healing is delayed and skin loss is observed when the ratio exceeds 1:4. Therefore, personally using CEH in combination is considered efficient; however, its high cost remains the biggest obstacle [18]. In addition to this method, CEA, in which one's own epithelial cells are cultured and permanently engrafted in one's body, can obtain better results, but the incubation period is more than 2–3 weeks [19], and the cost is much higher than that of CEH. Thus, such unrealistic disadvantages must be overcome. In addition, the combined use of the human dermal matrix that replenishes the dermis in the joint area can also alleviate contracture deformities, which are a disadvantage of the mesh skin graft. However, the high cost of this method remains as an unresolved issue [20–22]. A clinical introduction to these techniques will be described in more detail in Chaps. 3 and 4, and only the basic cases will be briefly introduced here; rather than simply choosing a mesh graft for its generally simple, burden-free surgical method with a high engraftment rate, it is very important to make a decision after carefully considering the condition of the wound bed, the patient's general condition, the donor's general condition, the selection of areas to be avoided, and the corrective surgery that will be required in the future. The author does not consider mesh skin grafts using a mesher as an option unless it is absolutely necessary. However, in places where bleeding control is not easy, such as axilla, shoulder, and knee joints with larger and frequent movements, a No. 10 blade mesh technique is used to adjust the interval of the interrupted slit incision in place of using a mesher. The advantage of this method is that there is no need for an expensive mesher, it is fast, and the degree and width of the mesh can be arbitrarily adjusted as desired. In addition, the No. 11 blade can be selectively used if necessary as part of the graft [23]. Furthermore, the deformity caused by the mesh pattern is less than expected; thus, it is recommended to distinguish between a mesh skin graft in which a mesher is used to graft for wide area coverage and adjusting the appropriate mesh rate by simply using a slit incision. In cases when the range is not particularly wide, it is recommended to use the manual mesh method, if applicable.

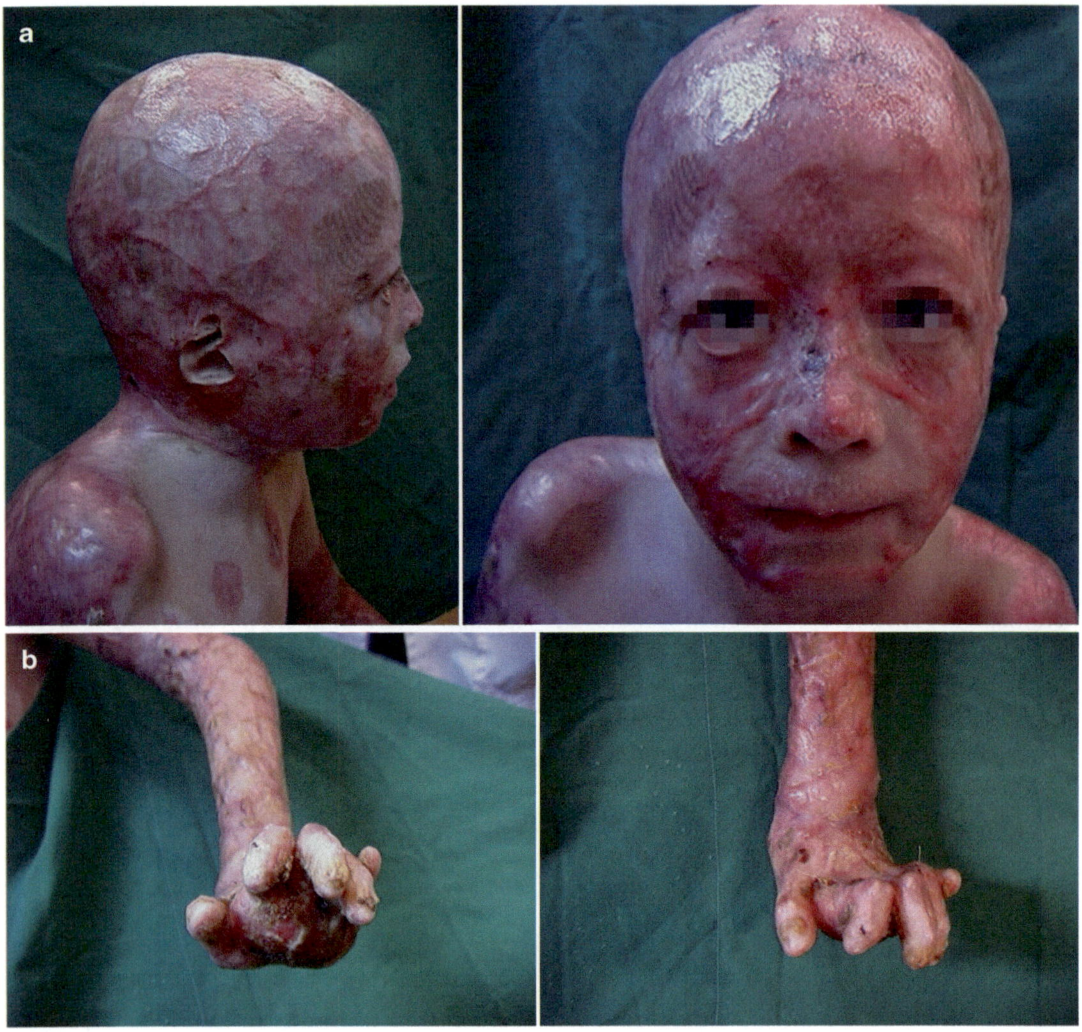

Fig. 1.2 (**a**) The problem of the skin graft by displaying a visible mesh pattern deformity on the face. (**b**) Severe scar contracture deformities were noted on the dorsum of the hand with dislocated multiple finger joints

This patient exemplifies the problem of the skin graft by displaying a visible mesh pattern deformity of the face, ectropion of both lower lids, and severe scar contracture deformities of the hands, resulting in serious functional and esthetic deformities. Because the author strongly recommends more active early management and proper skin graft selection in the acute stage, surgeons should keep this in mind (Fig. 1.2). A considerable amount of time and effort is needed to correct these problems, which thoroughly demonstrates that the use of a mesh skin graft is contraindicated for the face and hands.

This image depicts a comparison of CEH in an experimental study for rapid healing of wide-mesh grafts, showing a difference in healing time. This figure shows how CEH can effectively epithelialize a large gap in a mesh skin graft and aid in wound healing.

A 42-year-old male patient suffered a flame burn on his right lower leg. (a) Ten days after the procedure, debridement and a 1:3 mesh skin graft

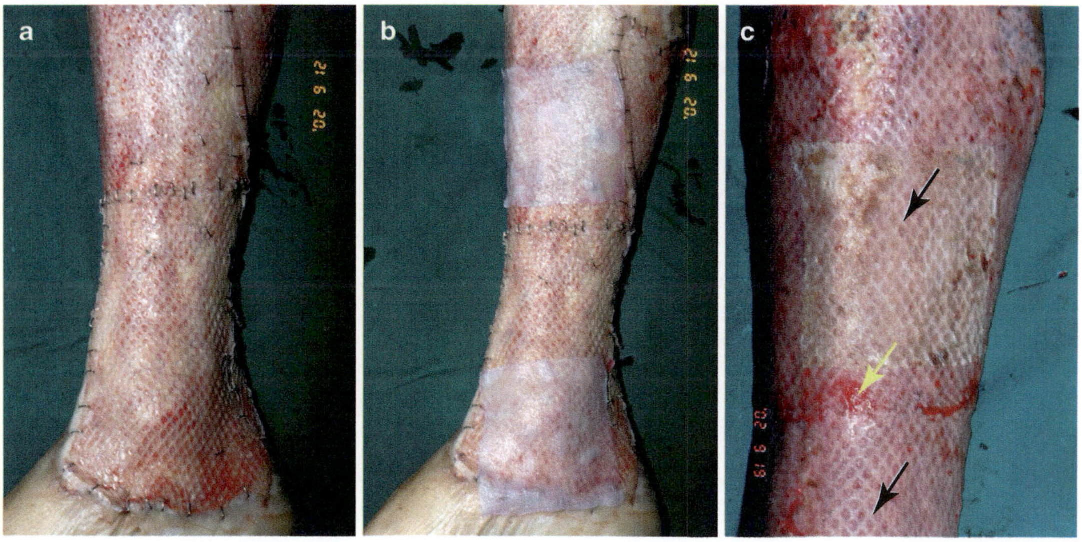

Fig. 1.3 (**a**) 10 days after operation, debridement and 1:3 meshed skin graft was performed. (**b**) Three sheets of CEH were applied on the anterior tibial area. (**c**) After 1 week, well rapid epithelialization was noted on the CEH application site (black arrow) and comparison to the CEH gap site (yellow arrow)

were performed, and (b) three sheets of CEH were applied experimentally on the anterior tibial area. (c) After 1 week, rapid epithelialization was observed on the CEH application site (black arrow) in comparison to the CEH gap site, which remained unhealed (yellow arrow) (Fig. 1.3).

The healing pattern also showed that the epithelialization between the meshes is much more stable, and the contracture progress is less developed, showing a significant difference in the healing process.

This patient was involved in a traffic accident that resulted in an above-knee joint amputation, and the raw surface was left open for more than 2 months, delaying wound healing. We applied a human dermal matrix with a 1:4 mesh skin graft. Shown on figure 1.4, you can see the differnces between the two divided areas, the area that is indicated with black arrow is where CEH was applied shows greater density epithelialization.

In comparison to the area (marked in yellow arrow), where CEH was accidentally removed after one day, shows significant difference in healing progress.

Figure 1.5 shows a reconstructive surgery that was performed to correct a severe scar contracture in a 6-year-old female patient. A 1:6 wide-mesh

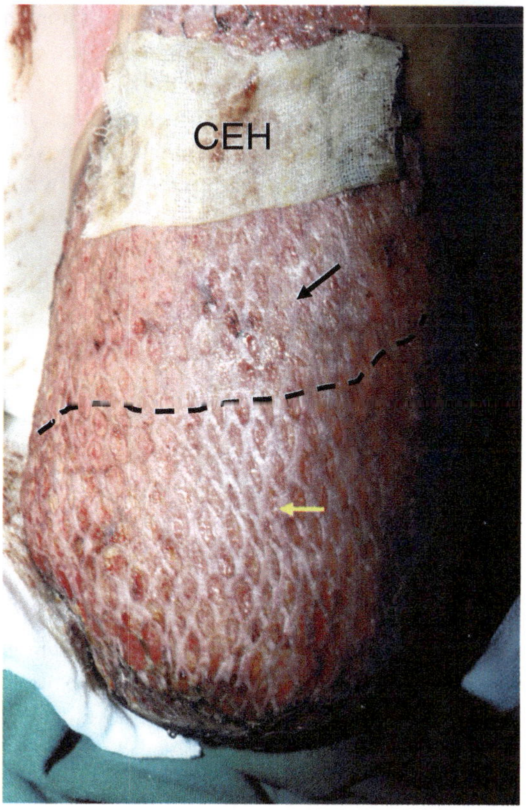

Fig. 1.4 Human dermal matrix with 1:4 mesh skin graft and covered with experimental CEH (above the dashed line). Note the different healing pattern on upper and lower parts

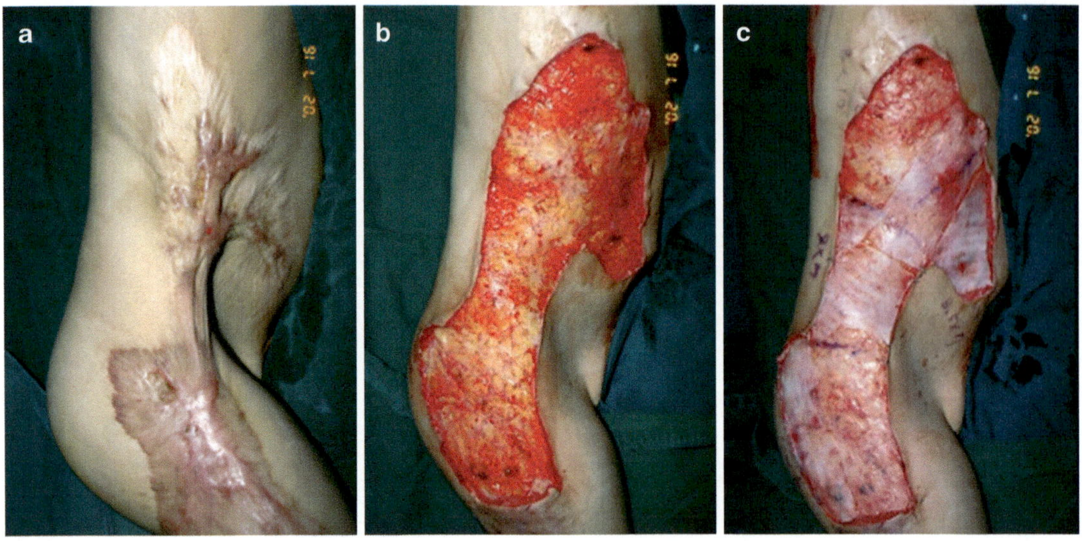

Fig. 1.5 (**a**) Severe linear scar contracture line observed with functional disturbance. (**b**) Incisional and excisional full release. (**c**) The human dermal matrix with 1:6 meshed skin graft was performed for dermal volume replacement, and CEA was covered on the top for rapid meshed gap fill with epithelialization

skin graft was performed after preparing a human dermal matrix to replenish the dermal layer, and CEA culture grafts were prepared 2 weeks in advance. At 6 and 12 days after the operation, the CEA petrolatum gauze was completely removed, and the entire mesh gap was epithelialized without difficulty.

Six days after the operation, epithelialization developed rapidly with a stable wound healing process. (b) Twelve days after the operation, the CEA petrolatum gauze and the engrafted mesh skin were completely removed, and the mesh gaps were completely covered with the patient's own epithelial cells (Fig. 1.6).

These above clinical studies have shown that the cultured epithelial graft is a very effective wound healing process and less scarring even with a 1:6 large mesh ratio [24]. However, the production cost of human dermal matrix and CEA was very high and required 2 weeks, which is a major drawback and remains an unresolved problem. Therefore, the author has developed a cell spray technique to reduce the production cost and time of CEA culture.

A 47-year-old man suffered flame burns on his left shoulder and back. Escharectomy was performed on day 17 of the incident, and a 1:4 mesh skin graft was introduced, followed by the application of three bottles of cell suspension with a fibrin sealant using tissomat cell spray (duproject spray). The three bottles were prepared 2 weeks before escharectomy (Fig. 1.7). Five days after the operation, the lower part of the operation site started healing and successfully retained the engrafted mesh skin on the shoulder area. One week after the operation, epithelialization markedly increased, and mesh gaps were almost healed. Ten days after the operation, the graft was taken completely, and the wound on the mesh gaps had healed (Fig. 1.8). This technique was observed to have a quick culture time, usually 2 weeks, short waiting time of no more than two weeks, which cuts the cost of producing the sheets. This spray technique is very effective on difficult-to-reach wound areas such as dimensional body parts like the axilla, shoulder, upper arm, and larger surface areas.

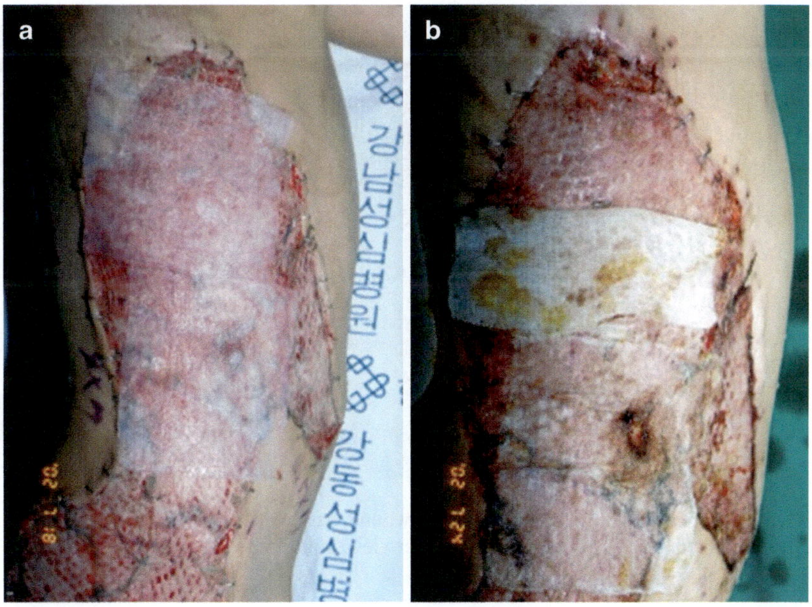

Fig. 1.6 (**a**) 6 days after the operation, the epithelialization was developed very rapidly with stable wound healing process. (**b**) 12 days after surgery, the CEA petrolatum gauze was peeled off and noted engrafted meshed skin was 100% graft take rate

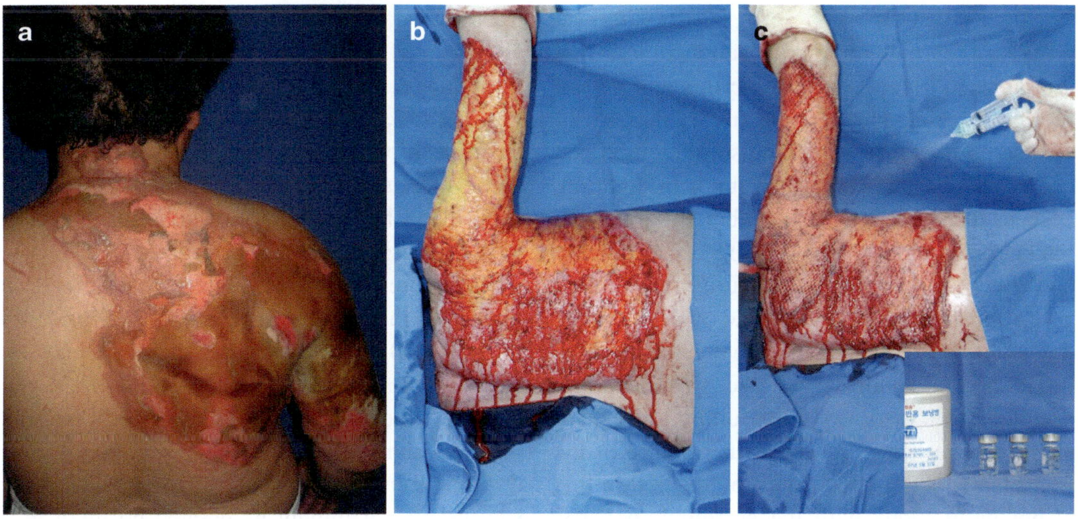

Fig. 1.7 (**a**) This man suffered flame burn on the right shoulder and back area. (**b**) Escharectomy was performed on burn day 17. (**c**) 1:4 meshed skin graft was performed, and three bottles of cell suspension with fibrin sealant were applied

As a plastic surgeon, I personally do not prefer mesh skin grafts, but since they are essential for the management of major burns or extensive wounds, methods using CEH, CEA, and cell spray techniques that are quick and also facilitate wound healing were briefly introduced in this chapter, especially cell spray technique was observed to have a quick culture time, usually 2 weeks, with none usage of the sheets that are high in cost. This will be described in detail in Chap. 4 Cultured Epithelial Cell Therapy.

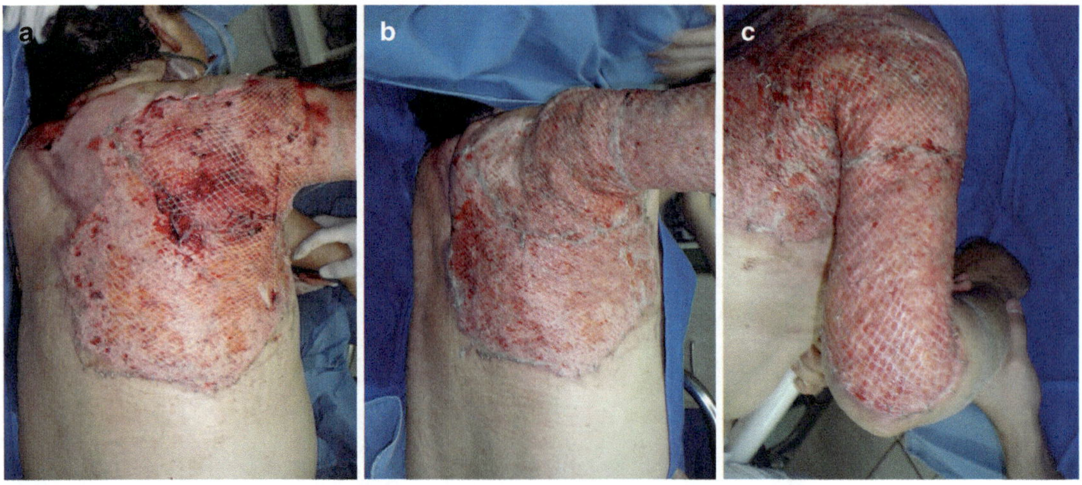

Fig. 1.8 (**a**) Postoperative day 5, operation wound was opened. (**b**) One week after the operation, marked epithelialization was noted. (**c**) Postoperative day 10 after view, 100% graft take rate was shown

1.3 Split-Thickness Skin Graft

STSG is a representative skin graft technique that grafts the full layer of the epidermis and part of the dermis using a hand or electric dermatome or skin-sampling knife. This is a useful method that can cover a wide area of a wound. In addition, because the skin engraftment is better than a full-thickness skin graft (FTSG), STSG can quickly and effectively cover and treat burns or trauma. It is the most frequently used and widely known method owing to the fact that it can be easily used in all cases of small wound size by collecting a sample with a razor or Blair/Humby knives, for slightly larger sites. However, the texture of the transplanted site is poor, with pigmentation that is not harmonious with the surrounding tissue and is prone to contracture deformation leaving large pigmentation lesions with rough, irregular hypertrophic scars on the donor site, indicating that STSGs lead to functional and cosmetic damages. Moreover, as compared with FTSG the secondary contracture of the engrafted skin surface is observed after engraftment, consequently affecting the surrounding tissues, and scar contracture deformities become unavoidable. However, if more systematic management of graft thickness, appropriate engraft timing, bleeding control, and postoperative dressing are ensured, more satisfactory functional and cosmetic effects can be achieved while managing acute hand burns; moreover, subsequent reconstructive surgery may not be required.

Therefore, the author prefers an intermediate thickness that does not exceed 0.25–0.3 mm (10–12/1000 inches) for most skin thicknesses. Recently, prevention of unsightly scars of the donor site has garnered a considerable degree of interest; thus, the author focused on an accurate excessive doner collection is avoided from the selected doner site, keeping it thinnly as possibe no more than 0.3 mm in thickness (12/1000 inches).

In the case of the author, a thickness of up to 0.38–0.5 mm (15–20/1000 inches), thick STSG can be used in cases in which a high-quality texture of the skin is considered, such as for the correction of the upper and lower lid ectropion or scar contracture correction around the nose, mouth, and eye regions. It is rarely used in my case except for special purpose of reconstruction. Considering donor site morbidity, severe or mild hypertrophic scarring or unsightly and rough scars may apparently remain according to difference of individual tendency of scarring. I highly recommend when it is possible that surgeons should aim to harvest skin from donor areas that are less visible to the patient such as the buttock and the back, instead of selecting donor areas that are much more visible such as the upper and inner thighs. Recently, with the development of an artificial dermis, a method has been developed to minimize graft construction by supplementing the thickness of the dermis. Collecting an ultra-thin 0.12–0.2 mm (5–8/1000 inches) donor skin and using an artificial dermis, it provides medium or thick STSG effect. It has now become possible to avoid donor site morbidity and scar formation to some extent. This method can be particularly useful for children who are prone to hypertrophic scarring or for older adults who do not have good skin donor sites because of their very thin aging skin. However, the considerable economic burden is a major disadvantage. As such, STSG has a great effect on the construction of the surgical site, pigmentation, and the texture of the skin, depending on the thickness of the dermal layer harvest to be collected. Recently, surgeons have shown a proclivity to avoid leaving scars on the patient's body if possible. Thus, donor site morbidity must be considered more importantly. In accordance, the thickness of the skin to be collected, donor site, area, and shape must be carefully considered, and to obtain a graft of an accurate size and a constant thickness, hand skills using a dermatome or various knives must be acquired through ceaseless efforts.

1.3.1 Donor Site Skin Collection Method

Although manual hand drum Padgett dermatomes were used in the past, these dermatomes were difficult and complicated to operate, and there are risks of explosion from the adhesive used to adhere to the skin surface and the ether solution used to dissolve it [25]. Therefore, it is now rarely used. Sometimes the author uses this instrument when necessary for esthetic skin grafts that require the desired shape and exact thickness [26–28]. Lately, a mechanical dermatome is generally used, an electrical or pneumatic-type driving method that is driven by N_2O gas. The author personally prefers using the pneumatic type owing to its good strength and sturdiness. The size of the skin collected is 2.5, 5, 7.5, or up to 10 centimeters wide at its widest, and the length is determined by the state of the donor. There is also a wide-type dermatome with a width of >10 cm; however, it is not easy to obtain the desired uniform thickness and exact area. The difficulty of handling this instrument can cause irregular pieces of skin and sometimes shortened donor skin piece. Although it is used in the management of major burns, its usage is not commonly recommended.

For the collection of split-thickness skin, when possible, the assistant should pull in the same direction as the dermatome, in the up and down direction rather than side to side. The tension control must not be too strong nor too weak, to maintain evenly distributed tension force, and the collector should collect slowly at a constant speed by adjusting the angle of the blade, pressing force, and side-to-side balance in the direction in which the dermatome is collected.

In particular, in curved areas including the buttocks, the progress speed should be reduced while controlling the balance level between the side-to-side movement, considering and checking for the full estimate width throughout. Commonly donor skin is removed from visible areas such as lateral thigh regions to be time efficient; however, scars and hyperpigmentations from these areas can have an negative psychophysical trauma on the patient because of its unsightly look. Dermatome hand skills require much effort to obtain the desired location, size, and thickness, so the author hopes that this skill can be achieved through persistent practice. Meanwhile, when selecting donor site locations,

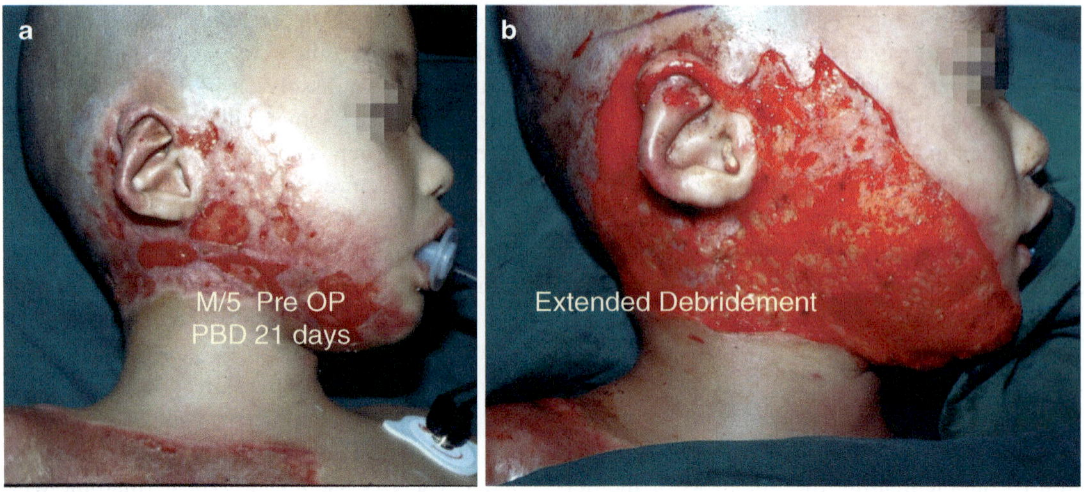

Fig. 1.9 (**a**) Unstable granulation tissue and incomplete epithelialization were noted post-burn day 21. (**b**) The incompletely healed wound bed was debrided with total removal of the granulation tissue and dirty epithelialized area to make single-sheet scalp skin graft

areas that are conspicuously exposed should be avoided to be considerate of the patients, so that the patient can later wear short sleeve tops and bottoms. Acquisition of the dermatome technique is a very important factor in the success or failure in the later part, Chap. 5 Esthetic Skin Graft ("Dermabrasion and dermal resurfacing over-grafting technique"), and the author hopes that hard and consistent efforts will be undertaken toward achieving these skills.

1.3.2 Donor Harvesting on Specific Regions

Scalp donor site is a region where one can obtain skin grafts that are of particular importance for the face of severe burn patients. However, it is very difficult to obtain a large piece of skin graft from a hard and three-dimensionally round head, thereby requiring a special manipulation.

One tip of the maximal size of skin harvesting method is to inject normal saline solution into the loose areolar space of the scalp using an 18–21-gauge needle and a 50-cc syringe on both sides of the flat, parietal area and on both sides of the round, rigid frontal and occipital area. Once the space is inflated and the area is smoothed and flattened out, a wider slice of single sheet of the skin can be sampled. Large amounts of saline (up to 200 cc) can be injected for both children and adults, as the saline is absorbed eventually without problems. The thickness of the skin graft should not exceed 0.25 mm (10/1000 inches) for children and 0.3 mm (12/1000 inches) for adults to allow safe collection without damaging the hair follicle. This is the thickness in which the skin graft can be collected without postoperative alopecia, even after a second sampling, if necessary [29–31].

Furthermore, single-sheet scalp skin grafts produce esthetically pleasing results. In this case, a single-sheet scalp skin graft was used to demonstrate how an esthetic outcome can be obtained (Fig. 1.9). The scalp skin color matches the facial skin color, and there is no donor site morbidity. The harvested thickness and length were 0.254 mm and 9.5 × 20 cm, respectively, and a saline injection was administered to the loose areolar space. The author prefers scalp skin selec-

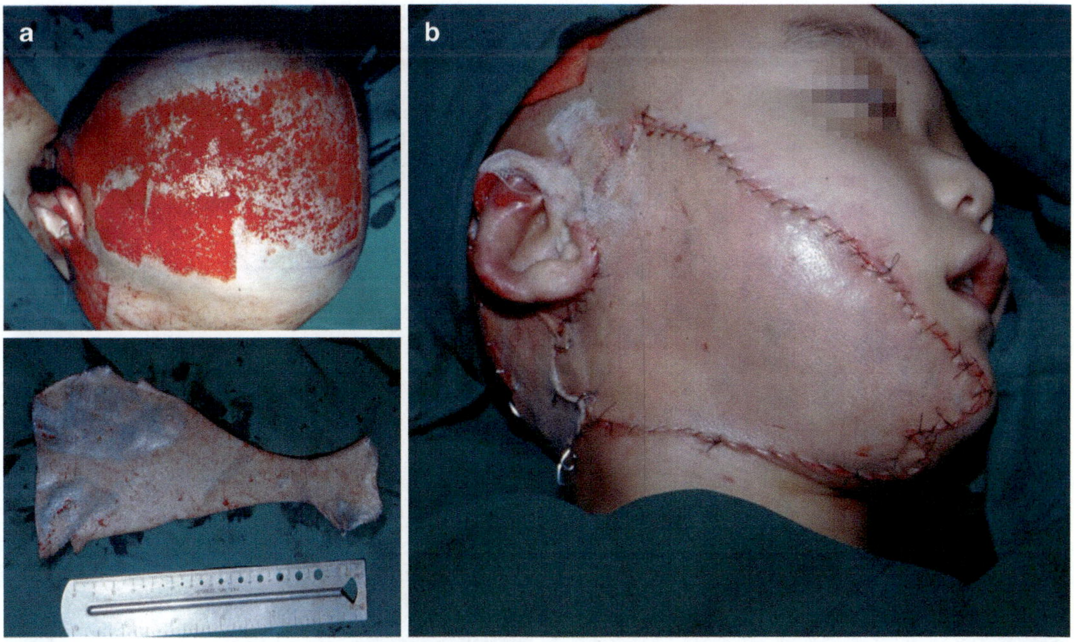

Fig. 1.10 (**a**) The harvested thickness and length were 0.254 mm and 9.5 x 20 cm. (**b**) Single-sheet graft was observed to maximize esthetic outcome without unsightly seam line

tion with a good color match to the face and can make large single sheets using the above scalp injection technique. A single-sheet graft was observed to maximize the esthetic outcome while avoiding unsightly seam lines (Fig. 1.10). Good color matching and good skin texture were observed 2 and 4 years after surgery. Ten years after the operation, there was no disfigurement of the face despite rapid growth. This patient did not undergo corrective surgery and refused additional surgery even after 16 years of adulthood. Note the whitish discoloration on the engrafted boundary due to reflected light, but this minor color mismatch was no longer an esthetic problem for him (Fig. 1.11).

When grafting on the face, recommendation point may divide the esthetic unit which's common sense in plastic surgeons. However, in the author's experience, dividing the esthetic unit is ineffective during the acute phase, so I would strongly advise using a large, single sheet of scalp-donor skin as soon as possible (Fig. 1.12).

When scalp-donor skin is unavailable, skin donor can be obtained from body areas such as the chest; however, if the patient is skinny with apparent sternum and ribs, the skin donor can be infused with IV to inflate the surrounding tissues, smoothing and flattening the area for the collection.

In the abdomen, it is difficult to obtain tension from pulling the tissue tightly side to side; however, if the tension is adequately maintained with the cooperation of assistants, it is possible to obtain a large single sheet of skin graft from this area, easier and larger than one would assume.

If the donor site skin is not properly harvested, (a) you can harvest the anterior chest area with a normal saline injection to flatten the irregular donor sites (black arrow). The abdominal area is also a good donor if well-cooperative supporters apply side to side even tension pressure (yellow arrow) (b). These harvested skin sections were taken from the anterior chest and abdomen and measured 10 × 23 cm each. The thickness was 0.2 mm for the full-face reconstruction with dermabrasion and dermal resurfacing techniques (Fig. 1.13). Note the clinical procedure in Chap. 5: Esthetic Skin Graft (Figs. 1.24, 1.25, 1.26, and 1.27).

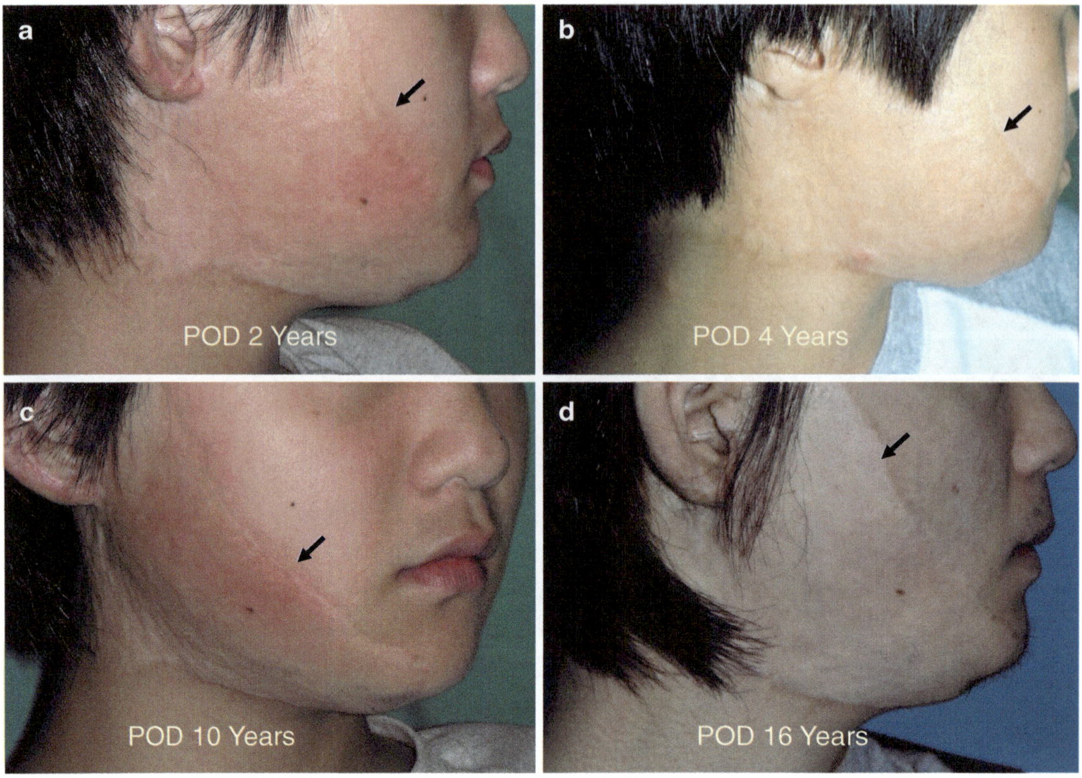

Fig. 1.11 (**a**, **b**) Postoperative view 2 and 4 years after. Focus on the very good color matching and good skin texture. (**c**) Postoperative 10 years after, there was no disfigurement of the face according to rapid growing age. (**d**) Postoperative 16 years after view

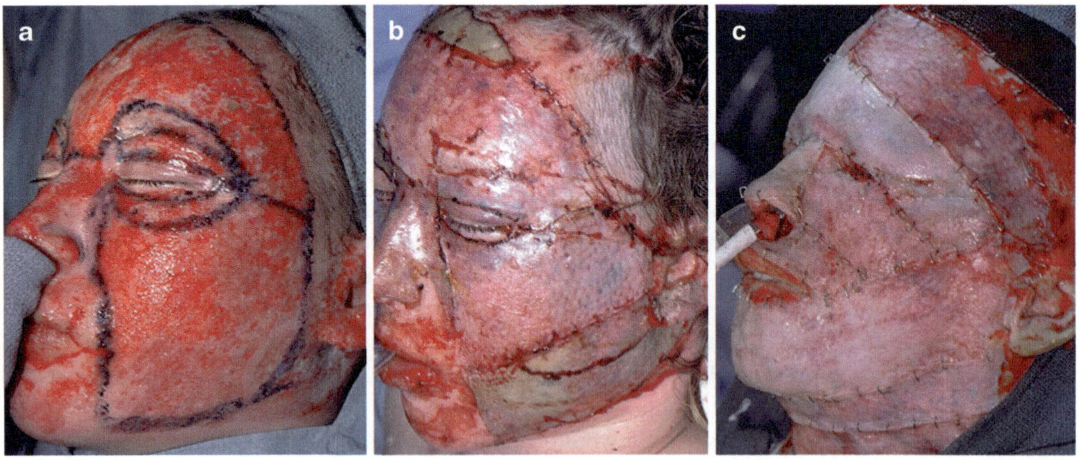

Fig. 1.12 (**a**, **b**) Grafting was performed by dividing esthetic unit on face. (**c**) Dividing esthetic unit is not meaningful in the acute phase in my experiences

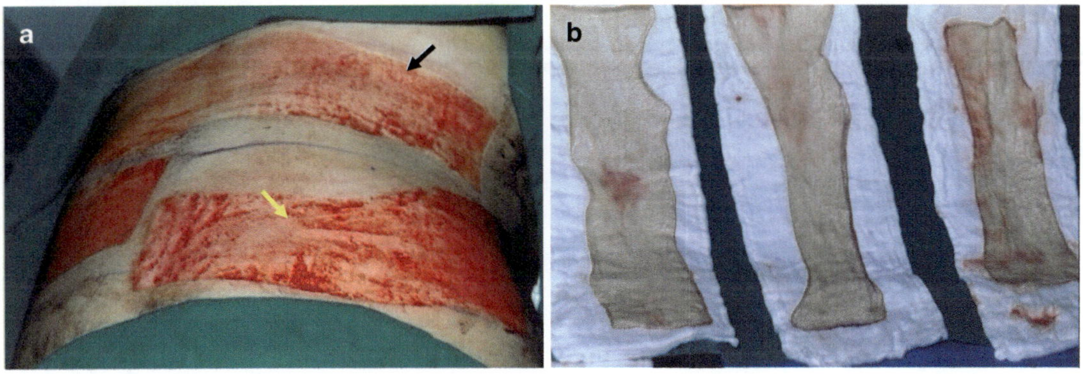

Fig. 1.13 (**a**) Anterior chest and abdomen area are also good donor sites, if using normal saline injection which flatten the irregular donor sites (black arrow). The abdomen is also a good donor if assistants cooperate well (yellow arrow). (**b**) Note three big single sheets measured 10 cm × 23 cm each; thickness was 8/1000 inch (0.2 mm) Note the clinical process on Chap. 5 Esthetic Skin Graft at (Figs. 1.24, 1.25, 1.26, and 1.27)

1.4 General Consideration of Skin Grafts

1.4.1 Conditions for Successful Skin Graft Procedure

Owing to the fact that most factors affecting a successful skin transplantation are related to local issues rather than systematic causes, efforts should be undertaken to frequently check and solve problems that are easily overlooked.

1.4.2 General Condition of the Patient

1.4.2.1 Children and Old Age

- Children: cooperation of treatment, thin skin, nutrition, tendency of hypertrophic scarring.
- Old age: mental status, nutrition, thin skin, cooperation of treatment.
- Obtaining a sufficient graft area in children and old ages is difficult owing to issues related to treatment cooperation and skin thickness. Furthermore, children are prone to hypertrophic scars; it is important to consider the thickness of the graft when selecting donor sites and donor skin.

1.4.2.2 Condition of the Recipient Site

- Inadequate escharectomy is a major cause for concern when performing early excision and early graft; furthermore, tangential excision is performed while observing the pinpoint bleeding pattern. Therefore, if necrotic tissue remains in the wound bed, it can cause graft failure. The surgeon needs to acquire a considerable amount of experience to determine the escharectomy level, accurately remove the necrotic tissue, and create an environment in which the graft can affix to the healthy wound bed. Some surgeons believe that the fat layers interfere with the skin graft taken; however, the author believes that these layers aid the healing process. Therefore preservation of fat layers is highly recommended.
- After the necrotic tissue or eschar is removed, a healthy granulation tissue bed should be formed on the wound bed.
- Infection control: check for infection with *Staphylococcus*, *Streptococcus*, methicillin-resistant *Staphylococcus aureus (MRSA)*, *Pseudomonas*, etc., among others, in particular.
- Immobilization.

  Splint, tie overdressing, and K-wire.

  By immobilizing the engrafted skin using a punched-out silicone sheet (Mepitel™), the engraft skin itself can be fixed and safely protected until it has taken.
- Operation site and position of the graft site.

  The take rate of the skin graft may vary depending on the posture or position maintained by the patient. In particular, the face, neck, groin, buttocks, armpits, and back are places where it is difficult to maintain posture during engraftment. Using a splint or vacuum assistant (VAC) system allows for a more convenient and safe management.

1.4.3 Factors Causing Graft Failure

1.4.3.1 Wound Bed Environment

There are higher chances of graft failures when escharetomy is perforemed too early for deep second- or third-degree burns, when deep burns are present, and when viable and nonviable tissues are difficult to distinguish and an inappropriate resection is performed.

1.4.3.2 Fluid Collection (Hematoma, Seroma)

Graft loss is most often caused by hematoma. The main causes of graft loss are inadequate escharectomy and bleeding control. The main postoperative cause is the insufficient immobilization and protection of the operative site. Therefore, it is necessary for the surgeon to be skilled and provide systematic management for bleeding control in the operation field. In most cases, the author only uses epinephrine injection for bleeding control and does not use electrocauterization or tourniquets. Although this method is not easily acceptable, it critically affects the success or failure of the operation and thus will be introduced in further detail in Chap. 2.

1.4.3.3 Infection

Graft loss due to systemic infection caused by wound sepsis is currently rare, and the most common cause is local pathogens.

Most of the criteria for infection are obtained by performing local bacterial culture and strain culture, but it cannot be said that the results of these cultures are accurate. The surgeon's judgment is more important. The early excision and early grafting before bacterial colonization forms results in a higher graft take rate.

1.4.3.4 Immobilization

Restricting the movement of the graft site has a very important effect on the graft take. Therefore, it is important to maintain immobilization until the graft is taken. Appropriate measures include using a splint or Surgifix®, tie-over dressing, and the VAC system to restrict movement for a certain period of time in the face, neck, waist, large joints, and hips [32, 33].

In this section, rather than discussing STSG anew, as it is quite common, the author will introduce STSG in acute facial burn management, which still has many controversies, and ectropion correction, which always becomes controversial in cases of facial reconstructive surgery.

1.5 Management of Facial Burn

In this chapter, the author will describe the importance of the decision making and time management for surgeries, to reduce reconstructive surgeries later on.

Followings are the main issues regarding facial burn treatments:

- Debates include the availability and timing of surgery for acute burns.
- Selection of partial- or full-thickness grafts for the upper and lower eyelids in reconstructive surgery of ectropion.
- Selection of skin grafting method for reconstruction of the surrounding tissue of the eyes, nose, mouth, ears, and so forth of the face.

1.5.1 Management of Acute Facial Burn

Early treatment of facial burns is very important and has the greatest influence on the patient's life. In other words, appropriate response to the initial treatment has a profound effect on not only the patient's functional recovery but also their mental suffering and social life [34–36]. Therefore, treatment that is professional and conducive to wound healing should be prioritized. In general, when treating patients with severe burns that endanger their lives, the best efforts should be focused on saving the patients' lives first. However, if facial burns are present and the initial treatment is not appropriate, serious problems may occur subsequently [37, 38]. Therefore, a cooperative treatment system that treats burns with systematic

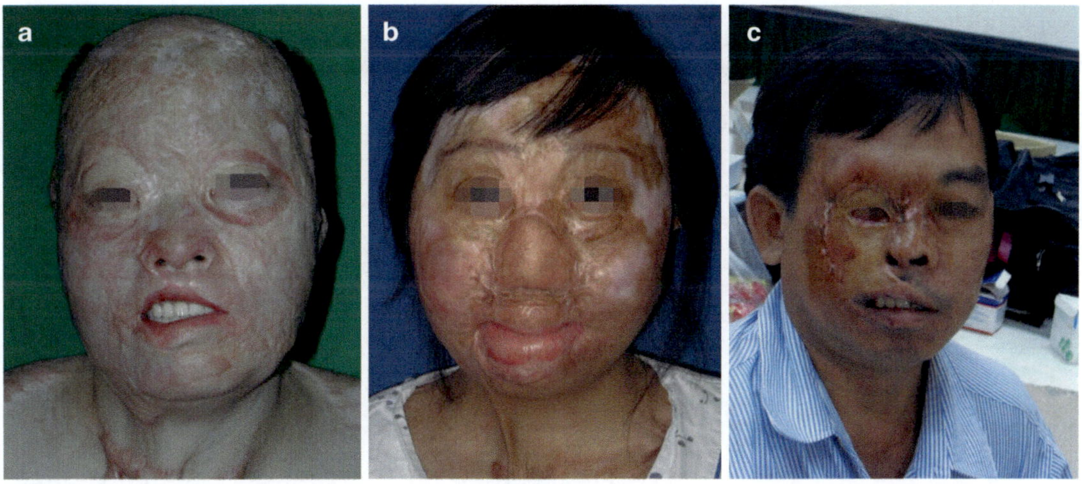

Fig. 1.14 These patients are well shown on how many difficult and serious deformities remained and they need multitudinous corrective surgeries

treatment as well as plastic surgery is essential [39]. Considering this, establishing an intimate cooperation system with specialized departments, such as plastic surgery, respiratory internal medicine, ophthalmology, otolaryngology, and orthopedic surgery, for the treatment of patients with severe burns is a very important task in the future.

These patients' cases demonstrate the critical importance of initial proper wound management in acute facial burns.

A 33-year-old woman suffered a flame burn and was treated at another department. Three years after the burn incident, she received conventional wound dressing for more than a month, a partial patch and mesh skin graft were applied to the unhealed sites. One year after the burn incident, she received FTSG to correct both upper and lower ectropion. Notice the unnatural appearance and undercorrection of both upper and lower eyelid ectropion.

A 21-year-old woman suffered a flame burn, had a total burn surface area (TBSA) of 70%, and underwent over 15 operations. This patient had an improper skin graft on the dorsum of the nose and perioral area as well as undercorrected ectropion of both lower lids. This female patient underwent reconstructive surgery on her right face three times. Note the undercorrection and disfigurement of the upper lip and nose as well as the upper and lower lid ectropion.

These patients clearly demonstrate the importance of proper initial management of burned faces and the number of corrective surgeries (Fig. 1.14).

Generally, because of the face's good blood circulation, thin skin, and good elasticity, it is easy to think that the face will respond well to burn treatment and heal well without severe scars. But for severe facial burns, meticulous management must be undertaken to avoid future facial deformity. In cases with female patients with good skin elasticity, male bearded areas, infants, children, or those with a family history of hypertrophic scarring, severe hypertrophic scarring often develops after approximately 3–6 months of burn healing. Regular periodic follow-ups and skin care programs are recommended for at least 3–6 months or over 1 year [40].

For mild second-degree burns caused by general fire or hot water, frequent usage of (once or twice per day) mask pack with a cold compress effect, a moist gauze, or a Burn Shield (Hillegom, Netherlands) is used. After the swelling and pain subside within 2–3 days, use a dressing material that can promote epithelialization. At this time, one must be careful to remove the exudate by popping the blisters if possible, but try to obtain the effect of a biological dressing by preserving the separated epidermis as much as possible. If the separate epidermis is removed, it is better to

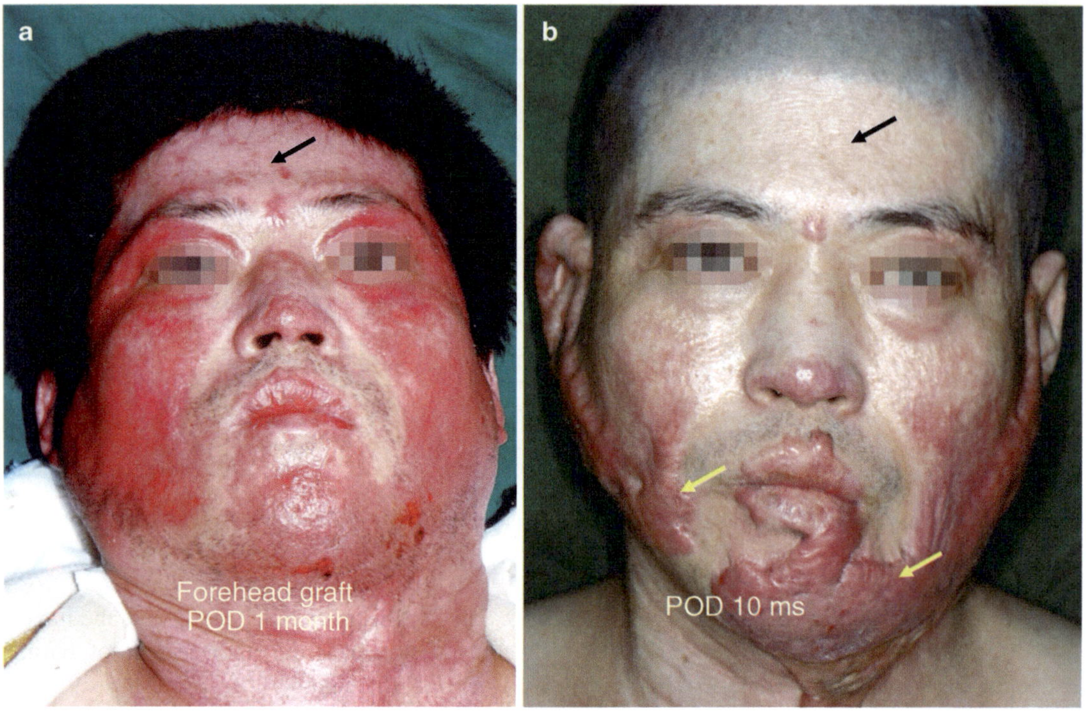

Fig. 1.15 (**a**) Postoperative 1 month view, engrafted forehead with scalp skin noted good graft taken and compared with conservative managed sites; the redness developed with mild elevated hypertrophic scarring on both the upper and lower bearded areas. (**b**) Postoperative 10 months after, severe hypertrophic scar developed on bearded area (yellow arrows)

use a cell therapy such as CEH that can replace the epidermis, to accelerate epithelialization, and shorten the treatment period. Second-degree burns with deep burns require a more careful treatment and judgment.

Most of the second-degree burns of superficial or mild thickness can be healed within 2 weeks. After healing, the pores become slightly deeper and wider than normal, and there is a hint of rough skin discoloration or hyperpigmentation. These findings start to appear gradually after approximately 3 months, and in the case of sensitive skin or children, a bright red rash and weak hypertrophic scars may be observed. Therefore, it is recommended to continue meticulous skin care for at least 3 months and, if necessary, to use laser treatment or a medical skin care unit to minimize the redness [41]. The patient should also be educated regarding the avoidance of exposure to ultraviolet light. However, even with medium-grade second-degree burns, if a male's beard area is not treated appropriately, it may develop into a surprisingly serious hypertrophic scar. This is a well-shown case mentioned.

A 42-year-old male patient suffered a flame burn with a TBSA of 30%. A scalp-donor STSG was performed on day 19 of the burn on the forehead only because the other facial sites were almost healed. (a) One month after surgery, the engrafted forehead and other sites healed into mild, elevated, and developing hypertrophic scarring on both the upper and lower bearded areas. (b) Ten months after, engrafted forehead area had good color match and texture (black arrow), but a severe hypertrophic scar developed in the bearded area (yellow arrows). Decision of time management of the surgery is very important to avoid hypertrophic scarring sites, which is presented here on the bearded areas, cheeks, and mentum

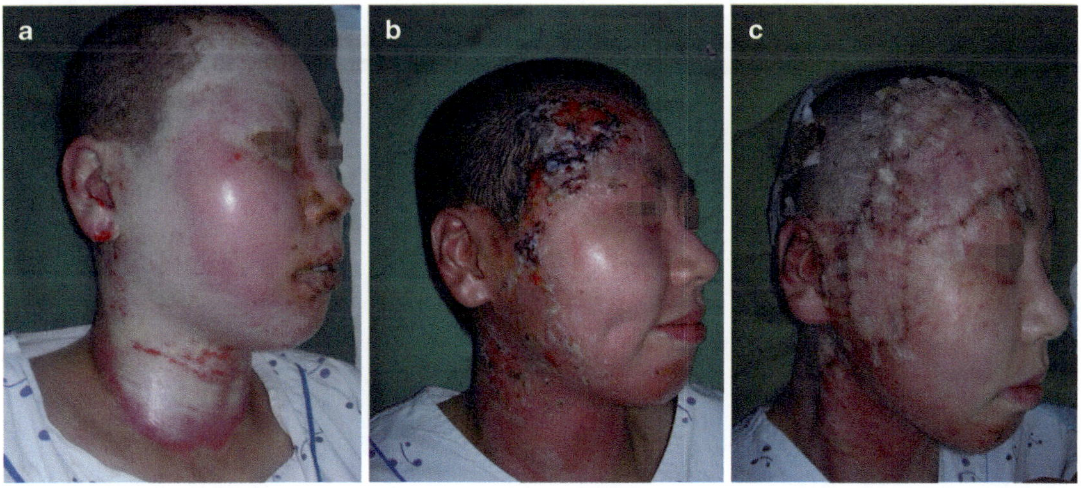

Fig. 1.16 (**a**) Deep second-degree burn on the forehead, cheek, and neck areas, (**b**, **c**) Post-burn 4 weeks, 12/1000-inch thickness scalp skin graft was performed on the forehead and right temple area

areas (Fig. 1.15). It is always important to ensure the patient is aware of the possibility of the development of hypertrophic scarring and to provide continuous management.

More than 2 weeks of treatment is required in most cases of deep second-degree burn, and in some cases, over 4 weeks is commonly needed. Controversies surrounding the variable treatment method and window is often misssed by confusion of deciding the extension area of the surgery.

A 28-year-old female patient was injured by an air balloon gas explosion on the right side of the face, resulting in a deep second-degree burn on the forehead, cheek, and neck. Four weeks after the burn incident, dirty granulation tissue remained in the unhealed wound. On the forehead and right temple area, a 0.3-mm-thick scalp skin graft was performed. However, conservative wound dressing had already healed the right cheek and neck (Fig. 1.16). Six months after the burn incident, a hypertrophic scar developed gradually. One year later, the hypertrophic scar markedly developed, and flap surgery using tissue expander method was performed. Two years after the operation, a marginal hypertrophic scar had developed on the tissue expander flap surgery margin. Observe and compare the forehead, temple, and right cheek (black arrows), which had received an earlier skin graft and conservative wound dressing. This case demonstrated the importance of early excision and skin grafting on the burned face, which resulted in a significantly different end result and necessitated considerable effort (Fig. 1.17).

In the author's case, clinical findings based on the depth of the burn are the most important criterion; however, if there are no signs of healing process after >2–3 weeks, a skin graft using scalp skin as a donor is performed.

A 36-year-old male patient suffered a flame burn with deep second-degree burns. Two weeks after the burn incident, an early excision and scalp skin graft with 0.3-mm-thick scalp skin were performed. Note the excluded area on the brow area to preserve the hair follicles. Four months after surgery, excellent results were observed with no hypertrophic scarring and well-preserved eyebrows (Figs. 1.18 and 1.19).

On day 16 after the burn incident, a 42-year-old patient underwent a scalp-donor skin graft. One year after the burn incident, the forehead and left cheek showed excellent results with good color matching and texture, and the engrafted seam line was not visible. However, in the mustache area, a hypertrophic scar developed, which was healed with early epithelialization (Fig. 1.20).

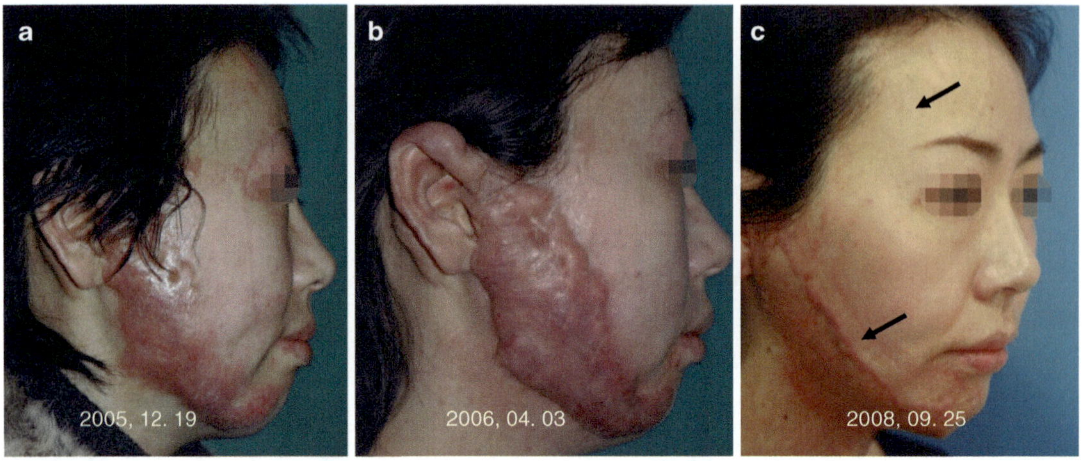

Fig. 1.17 (**a**, **b**) Post-burn 6 months and 1 year after view, hypertrophic scarring developed on the previously conservative treatment area. (**c**) Postoperative 2 years later view, note and compare forehead, cheek, and right mentum (black arrows) which received early scalp skin graft and conservative wound dressing on the right mentum

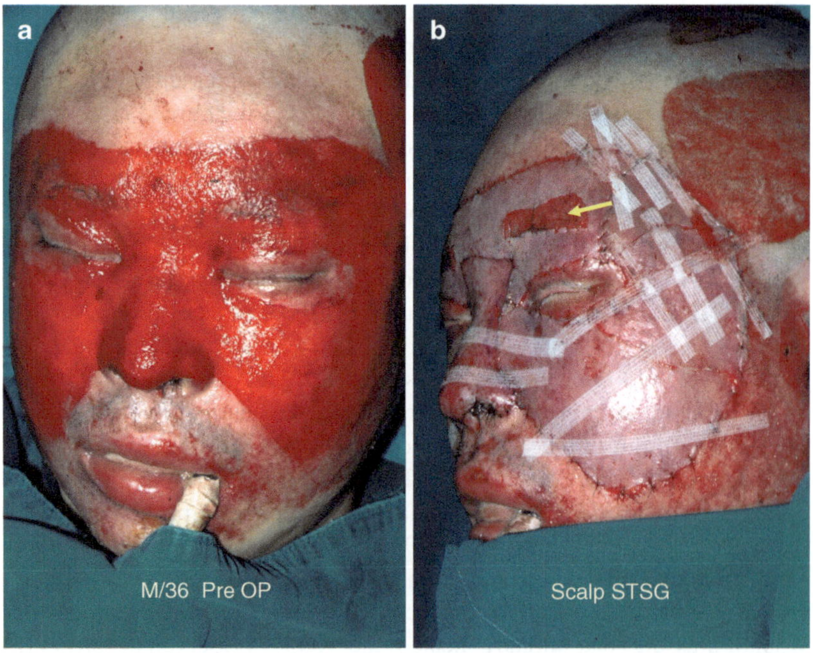

Fig. 1.18 (**a**) Early excision and scalp skin graft was performed post-burn 2 weeks with 12/1000-inch thickness scalp skin. (**b**) Note the excluded area on eyebrow area to preserve hair follicles (yellow arrow)

These cases demonstrated that scalp-donor skin achieved excellent esthetic results, which is the author's preferred donor skin for acute facial burn management.

In the author's case, even for severe flame burns, explosive burns, or even third-degree burns caused by chemical burns, the time of surgery is set at 3 weeks to ensure a chance of preservation of even a little viable tissue; however, in the absence of any signs of wound healing process, a skin graft is performed as soon as possible. The STSG was set as the base surgical method for acute facial burns, and as an important donor site, scalp skin thickness should not exceed 0.3 mm (0.25 mm for children), but if the scalp skin is not available, one may use the usual donor skin. Recently, the author prefers to use a large single-sheet graft than smaller esthetic units in acute burn stage (Figs. 1.7, 1.8, 1.21). The use of artificial dermis, which has recently been

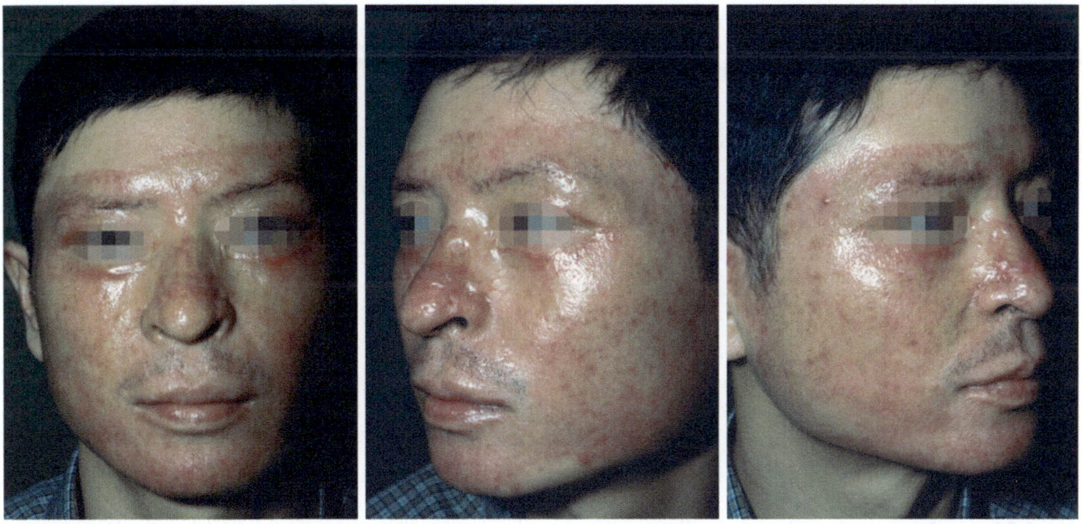

Fig. 1.19 Postoperative 4 months later, excellent result was observed with no hypertrophic scarring and well-preserved eyebrow hairs

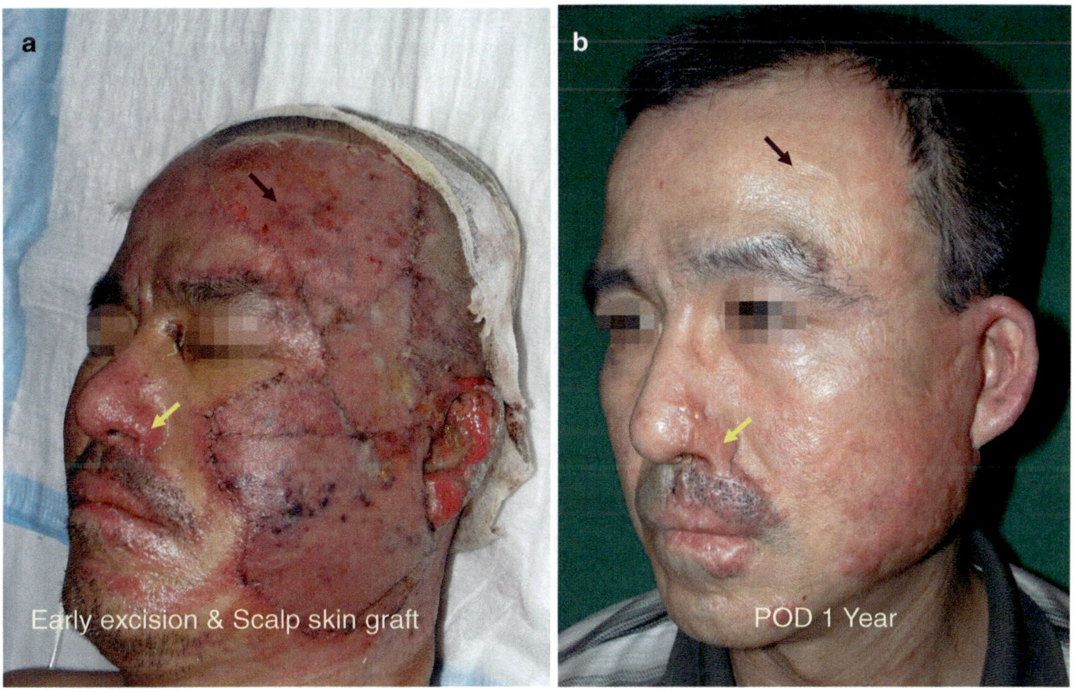

Fig. 1.20 (**a**) Post-burn day 16, 0.3-mm-thickness scalp skin graft was performed. (**b**) Post-burn 1 year later view, the forehead and left cheek area was noted excellent outcome with good color matching and texture (black arrow). Left alar and mustache area noted hypertrophic scar development in which this area was healed with early epithelialization (yellow arrows)

increasing, is not used in the facial area unless serious defects are present owing to third-degree burns. This is because the wound healing process of the facial area is very fast and has good resilience. This area is also thin, and thick scars caused by the artificial dermis leave an unnatural scar bed for reconstructive surgery and are not preferred because of the heavy cost.

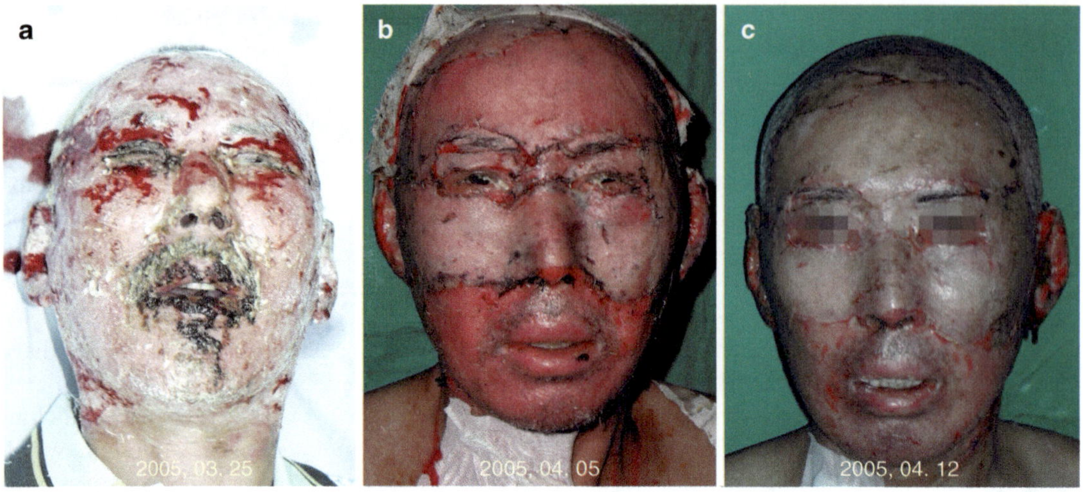

Fig. 1.21 (**a**) Post-burn day 17, early excision and early skin graft were performed with scalp skin. (**b**) Postoperative 7 days, engrafted upper, lower lid area and forehead grafts were successfully taken. (**c**) Postoperative 2 weeks after, mild ectropion had developed both lower lids

Areas to pay attention to when performing STSG are the upper and lower eyelids, eyebrows, places with a great distribution of hair follicles such as beard areas in men, and areas of cartilage such as the ears and the nose. To reduce the risk of chondritis in the ear or the nose cartilage area, timely STSG is important to prevent partial or total loss caused by chondritis; if there is an edematous and inflammatory change or sign of infections, surgery must be performed within 3 weeks.

A 53-year-old male patient suffered flame burns on his full face with deep second- and third-degree burns. Seventeen days after the burn incident, an early excision and early graft were performed using scalp skin. Seven days after surgery, the upper and lower lids, as well as the forehead area, were found to be completely grafted. Two weeks after the operation, mild ectropion had developed on the upper and lower lids. In addition, ear burns must be grafted early to prevent suppurative chondritis and ear loss (Fig. 1.21).

A 21-year-old male patient was attacked with strong sulfuric acid on the right side of his face. Eight days after the burn incident, an escharectomy was performed, and the wound was covered with a fresh cadaver allograft to preserve viable tissue and promote wound healing. After 2 weeks, the allograft was removed, and an AlloDerm® skin graft with a thickness of 0.15 mm was performed on the entire ear, right cheek, and neck. In this case, scalp skin was not used because the scalp was also injured caused by the chemical burn. Fifty-five days after the burn incident, note the well-preserved shape of the ear and the good healing on the right cheek and neck, with no scar contracture. In this case, even a strong-acid chemical injury should be treated with proper wound management and early skin graft to achieve a higher-quality outcome. I strongly recommend these wound management techniques for the treatment of chemical attack burns in order to prevent severe disfigurement deformities, which is a serious social issue in many Asian countries (Figs. 1.22 and 1.23).

In the eyebrow or beard areas, hair follicles are preserved as much as possible by refraining from grafting; however, in some cases, severe hypertrophic scarring on the mustache or beard progresses (Fig. 1.18), and the frequent occurrence of folliculitis makes the treatment difficult. Therefore, individual opinions may differ regarding the need for skin grafting, but the author's personal opinion is to place greater emphasis on the preservation of men's natural beards or eyebrows if possible. In addition, to reduce the frequency of hypertrophic scars and folliculitis in the early stages after burn treatment by refraining from skin grafting, efforts are made to obtain good results by using a combination of auxiliary therapies such as laser, pressure garment, silicone gel sheet, and steroid therapies. However, it is difficult to establish a definitive

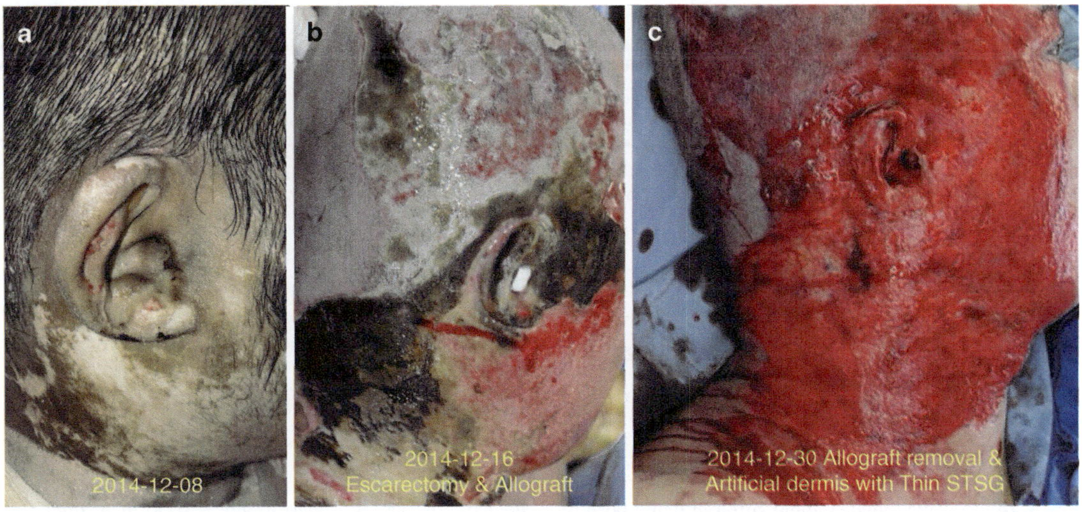

Fig. 1.22 (**a**) Patient was attacked sulfuric acid on the right face, (**b**) post-burn day 8 escharectomy and covered with flesh cadaver skin. (**c**) After 2 weeks, allograft was removed and AlloDerm with 6/1000-inch thickness skin graft was performed including the total ear, right cheek, and neck area

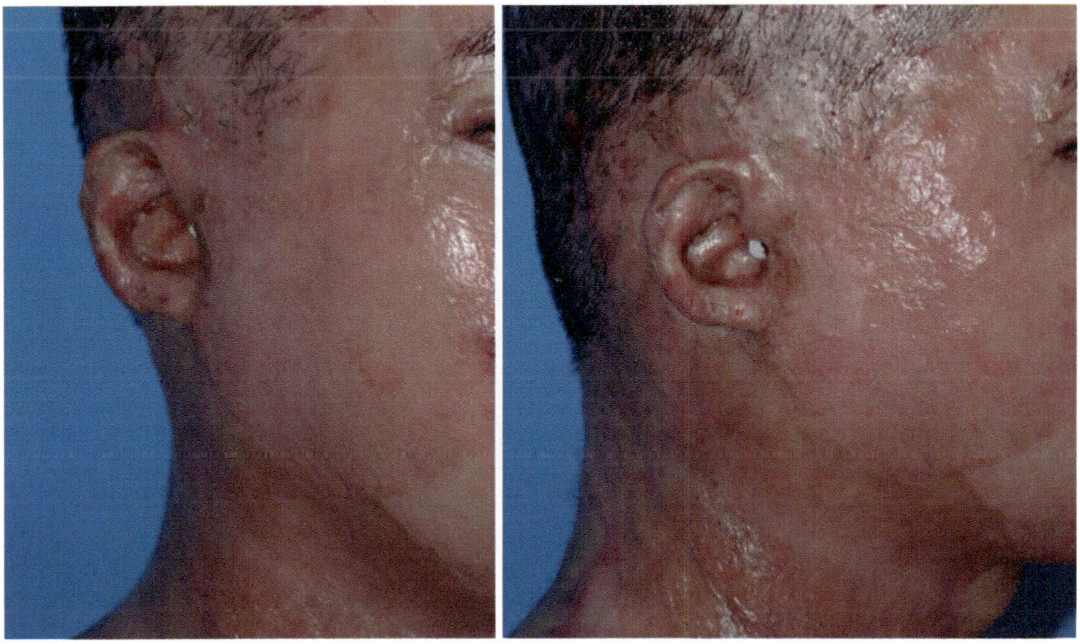

Fig. 1.23 Post-burn 55 days after, note the well-preserved total ear shape and good healing state on the right cheek and neck area

guideline because of the frequent development of hypertrophic scarring and consistent folliculitis, both of which are hard to resolve because it all depends on the individual patient.

In the case of upper and lower eyelids, the skin is the thinnest and heals well; thus, if possible, cell therapy CEH is used to induce natural healing. However, in the case of loss of the entire eyelid skin layer, 0.2 mm-thick STSG or 0.25 mm scalp skin is performed, and where possible, if a larger sufficient skin graft area is secured, more natural and good color matching can be obtained.

A 55-year-old female patient suffered flame burns on her face. Twelve days after the burn

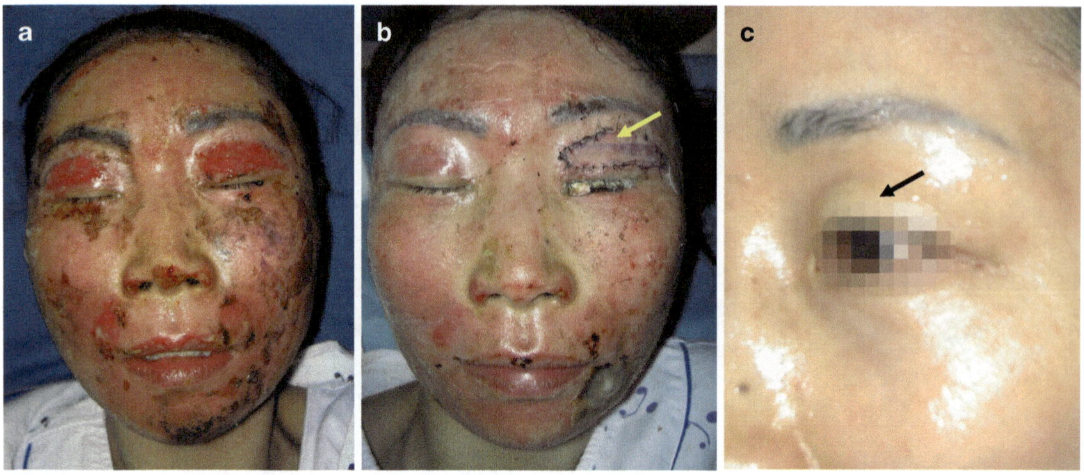

Fig. 1.24 (**a**) This female patient suffered flame burn on the face. Post-burn day 12, the raw surface was noted on both upper lids. (**b**) Post-burn day 14, right side had healed, engraft was performed 8/1000-inch thickness from the scalp skin (yellow arrow). (**c**) Postoperative 5 months later view (black arrow)

incident, a raw surface was observed on both upper lids. Fourteen days after the burn incident, the right side had healed, so engrafting was performed using 0.2-mm-thick scalp skin on the left upper lid only. Five months after the operation, a natural texture and color matching were observed, with no ectropion (Fig. 1.24).

The reason why symptomatic conservative treatment is still preferred over surgery in facial burn injuries is because it is difficult to judge the depth and extent of the burn at the initial stage of the burn as well as hesitations of not wanting to remove any of the living tissue. In addition, people refrain from undergoing surgeries for facial burn injuries because of the concern that the difference in color and texture between the engrafted skin surface and the surrounding tissue will be prominent [40]. However, rapid early wound coverage has the advantage of minimizing infection and inflammation, shortening the treatment period, and replenishing the skin surface due to burns close to the actual original surface. It also has the advantage of preventing the progression of contracture and reducing the probability of hypertrophic scarring. In particular, the scalp skin graft, which the author prefers, has the advantage of having no donor site morbidity and can obtain a very good cosmetic effect with good skin color match. Please note that some of the cases introduced above include facial burn caused by flame burn, 10 months after scalp skin graft was performed on the forehead (Fig. 1.15) As time passes, hypertrophic scarring develops in the cheek and mentum, showing that the timing of the decision for skin graft and engraft area are very important. Good color matching of the forehead shows the cosmetic effect of the scalp skin graft. Such cosmetic effects can also be seen in Figs. 1.17 and 1.19, where the maximized cosmetic effects are apparent in very good color matching of the scalp skin graft and the surrounding tissue. Nonetheless, in some cases, the remarkable results of the areas, regardless of whether graft was performed, show how important the selection of the graft area as well as the timing of the graft is, indicating the importance of the surgeon's experience and judgment ability. Consequently, in acute facial burn management,

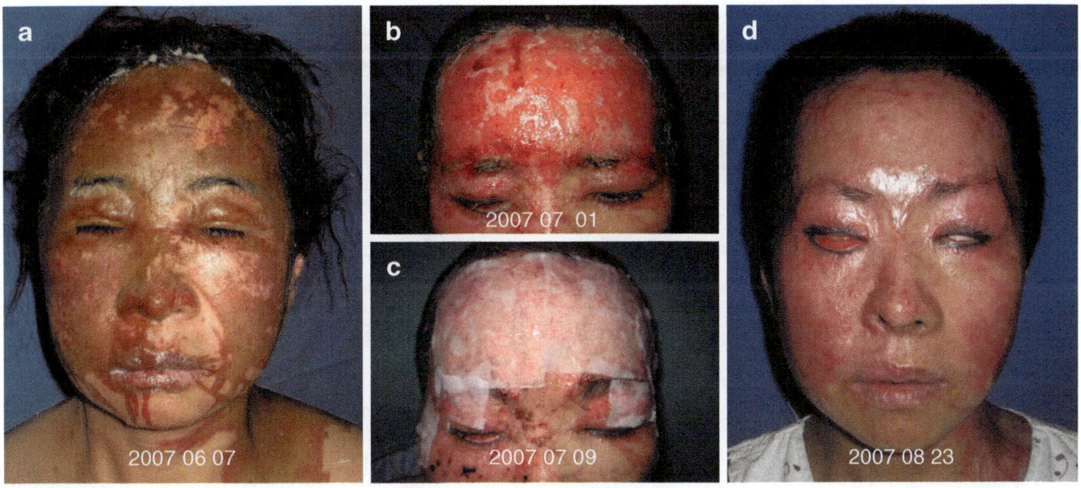

Fig. 1.25 (**a**) Patient suffered strong acid attack. (**b**) Post-burn day 30, full-thickness skin defect was noted on the forehead. (**c**) 12/1000-inch scalp skin graft. (**d**) Postoperative 1.5 months, forehead and upper lid noted excellent outcome, but lower lid area developed ectropion

the author strongly recommends scalp skin as the first choice for donor skin of a facial skin graft and would like to emphasize the importance of careful decision and experience regarding the timing and area of the graft.

This 48-year-old female patient demonstrated the importance of early proper management and early graft despite a strong-acid attack, which is the most difficult wound management and leaves serious sequela on all facial structures. Thirty days after the burn incident, a full-thickness skin defect was observed on the forehead. A 0.3-mm-thick scalp skin graft was performed on the forehead and upper lids. At 1.5 months after the surgery, excellent outcomes were observed on the forehead and upper lids, but the lower lids developed ectropion, which had quickly healed without the use of a skin graft. This means that an early graft decision is critical in facial burn management (Fig. 1.25). Eight months after the surgery, both lower lid ectropions were corrected with a 0.4-mm medium-thickness graft. Note the natural, engrafted color and texture of the forehead as well as the repositioned lower lid ectropion (yellow arrows). The lower lids adapted naturally three years after the ectropion surgery, with no recurrence of ectropion. Although most surgeons recommend FTSG to correct lower lid ectropion, the author prefers medium-thickness STSG because the skin of oriental people is darker and has a more visible graft margin than that of Caucasians. Moreover, in Asians, full-thickness skin may have a more obvious color mismatch compared with the surrounding burned skin. Another reason, according to the author, is that eyeball contact with the lower lid is critical for functional recovery, epiphora prevention, and the recurrence of unnatural appearance of mild lower lid ectropion caused by undercorrection with full-thickness skin. Note that the lower lids were naturally attached to the eyeball surface. In addition, I performed corrective esthetic surgery with double-opposing Z-plasty or dermabrasion and a dermal overgraft on the engrafted lower lid area. This technique will be described in more detail in Chap. 5. Note the small-sized image; unfortunately, many women in Asian countries have been subjected to a strong-chemical attack and have been denied proper initial chemical burn management (Fig. 1.26).

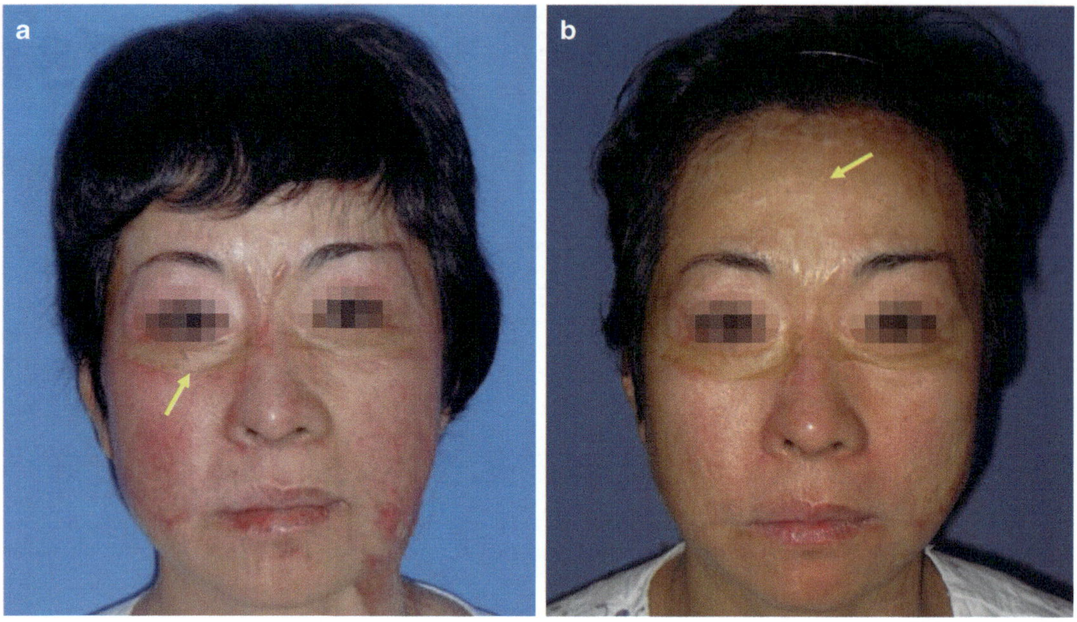

Fig. 1.26 (**a**) Postoperative 8 months later, both lower lid ectropion were corrected with 15/1000-inch medium-thickness graft. Note the natural forehead engrafted color and texture and repositioned lower lid ectropion (yellow arrows). (**b**) Postoperative ectropion surgery 3 years after view, naturally adapted lower lids without recurrence ectropion. Note the lower lid margins were naturally in contact to the eyeball surface

1.6 STSG for Reconstructive Surgery of the Burned Face

In general, reconstructive STSG is not popular especially in the facial reconstruction of burned face. The reason for this is the fact that the pigmentation of the engrafted STSG uses darker donor skin such as from the thigh or back rather than the bright skin of the face. This may be due to the preconceived notion that STSG results in functional and cosmetic losses because of the tendency toward hyperpigmentation disorder, which is a disadvantage of STSG itself, and the high contracture rate due to thin skin thickness [42]. However, the author suggests that it can be a very useful surgical method for esthetic and functional recovery if the ultra-thin, medium, or thick split thickness is used well by adjusting the skin thickness. In particular, for hypertrophic scar correction around the eye, nose, mouth, and mentum area, very similar scar release effects can be obtained without using full-thickness skin.

Mild lower lid marginal ectropion can be corrected with intermediate-thickness STSG; (a) The incisional release was performed at the incision line marking (yellow dashed line) on the lower margin of the contracted lower lid area to preserve the natural thin lower lid skin. (b) The contracted scar was undermined meticulously on the cheek area for reposition of scar retracted lower lid skin and make dart incision to secure of maximal engrafted surface. (c) A 0.4-mm medium-thickness graft was performed with tie-over dressing. Note that no slit incisions were made to prevent hematoma formation and obtain a better esthetic outcome (Fig. 1.27).

By sequentially using the dermabrasion and dermal resurfacing with thin graft introduced in Chap. 5, the cosmetic effect of skin texture improvement and correction of color mismatching can be maximized.

Here, a new concept and indication for facial reconstruction of STSG techniques will be introduced. The author, in particular, performed full release and STSG of the wide scar contracture of the dorsal side of the nose, lower lid, cheek, and perioral area using 0.4–0.5 mm medium or thick split thickness obtaining a similar release effect

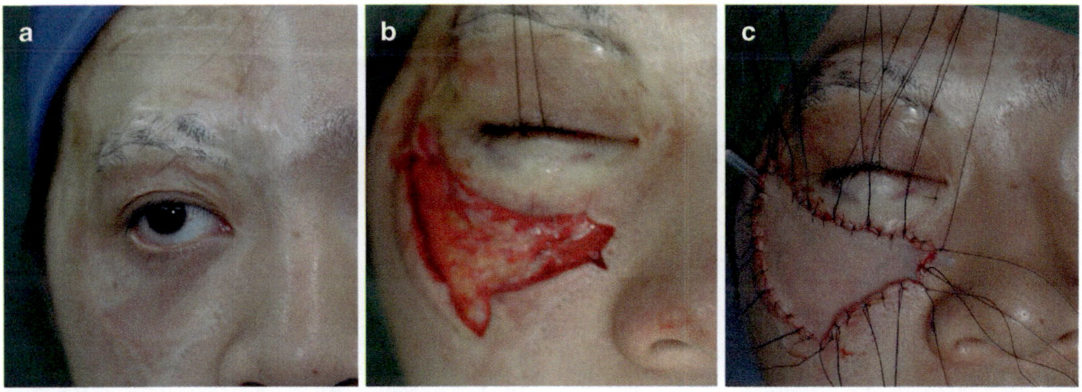

Fig. 1.27 (**a**) Scar contracture were noted on right forehead, eyebrow, and cheek with mild lower lid ectropion. (**b**) Full release scar bed with dart incision for maximal engrafted surface area. (**c**) 15/1000-inch medium-thickness STSG was performed with tie-over dressing

as FTSG around the contracture deformities of the tissue surrounding the eye, nose, and mouth.

Medium or thick STSG is very useful for reconstructive burned face. A 0.45 mm (18/1000 inch) STSG was performed on both upper and lower lids, dorsum of the nose, and upper lip area as a precondition of reconstructive surgery for burned face. Note the effective correction of the upper and lower lid ectropion, dorsum of the nose, and upper lip area. In this state, we can have a plan for both alar and philtrum reconstruction with cartilage composite graft and final dermabrasion and dermal overgraft with resurfacing of the full face. This is a very useful method as a preconditioning process to obtain the final cosmetic effect later on. The point of this method is to collect healthy skin wherever possible regardless of the color match of the donor site and to perform full release and overcorrection of the contracture around the eye, nose, and mouth without consideration of color matching.

Intermediate or thick STSG is very useful for reconstructive burned face. (a) A 43-year-old male patient underwent reconstructive surgery of his entire face. (b) A 0.45-mm-thick (18/1000 inch) STSG was performed on both upper and lower lids, the dorsum of the nose, and the upper lip area as a precondition of reconstructive surgery for the burned face. (c) Note the effective correction of the upper and lower lid ectropion, the dorsum of the nose, and the upper lip area. In this state, we can plan both alar and philtrum reconstruction with cartilage composite grafts as well as final dermabrasion and dermal overgraft (resurfacing) on the entire face (Fig. 1.28).

This 21-year-old female patient suffered a flame burn on her full face. Scar contracture was observed in the perioral area with limited mouth opening and a contracted band on the lower lip and mouth corner area. To correct the surrounding mouth area, a release preconditioning procedure is required before the correction of the three-dimensional anatomy of the lip area (Fig. 1.29). A 0.4-mm medium-thickness STSG was performed with full release scar bands and no scar excision. Three days after the surgery, the engrafted skin was almost completely removed without any difficulties. Six months after the surgery, the perioral contracture bands were released, and the patient had a more natural position. Minor deformities that remain can be corrected with minor corrective surgery, such as the variable Z-plasty technique. The author prefers medium or thick STSG as a preconditioning reconstructive facial surgery because of its ease of use, high take rate, and effective correction of severe deformities. Furthermore, this site can achieve more effective results than FTSG sites (Fig. 1.30).

The author does not use full-thickness skin for facial reconstruction other than neck reconstruction

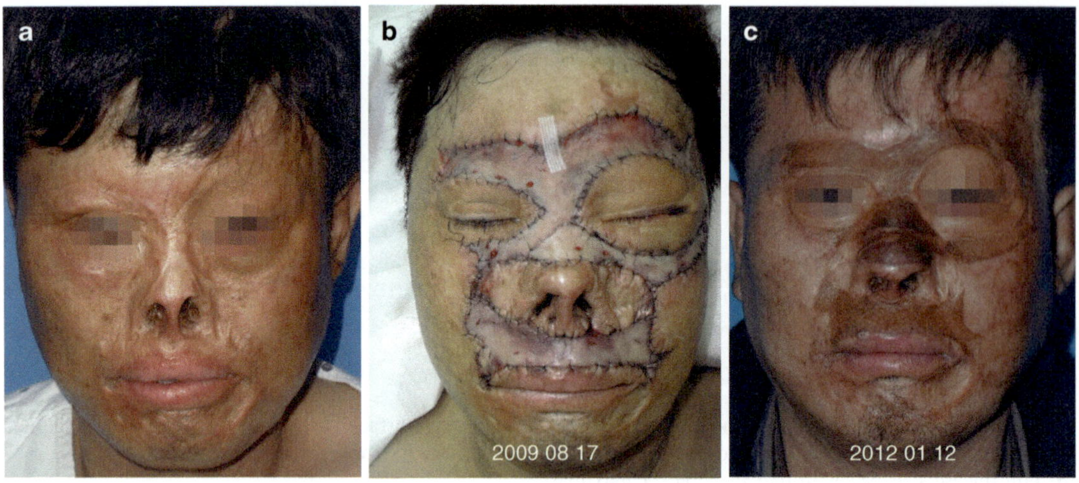

Fig. 1.28 (**a**) Preoperative view of reconstructive burned face. (**b**) 18/1000-inch thick STSG was performed on both upper and lower lid, dorsum of the nose, and upper lip. (**c**) Note the effective correction of the upper and lower lid ectropion, dorsum of the nose, and upper lip area

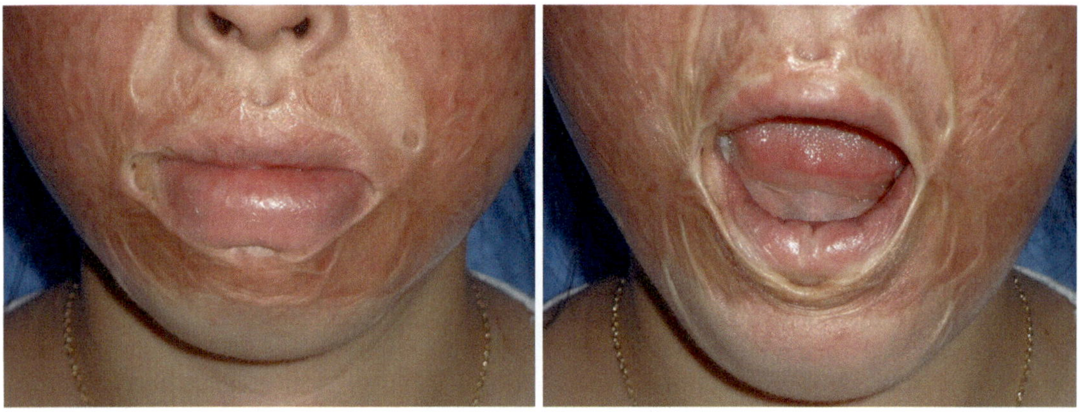

Fig. 1.29 The perioral area was noted scar contracture and limited mouth opening with contracted band on the lower lip and mouth corner area

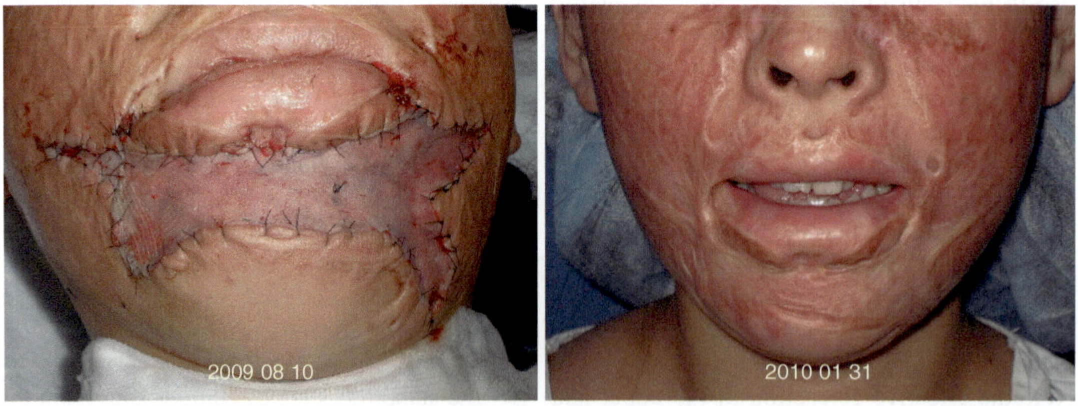

Fig. 1.30 (**a**) Postoperative 3 days after view. (**b**) Postoperative 6 months later view, the perioral contracture bands were released and back to more natural position to minor corrective surgery with minor local flaps

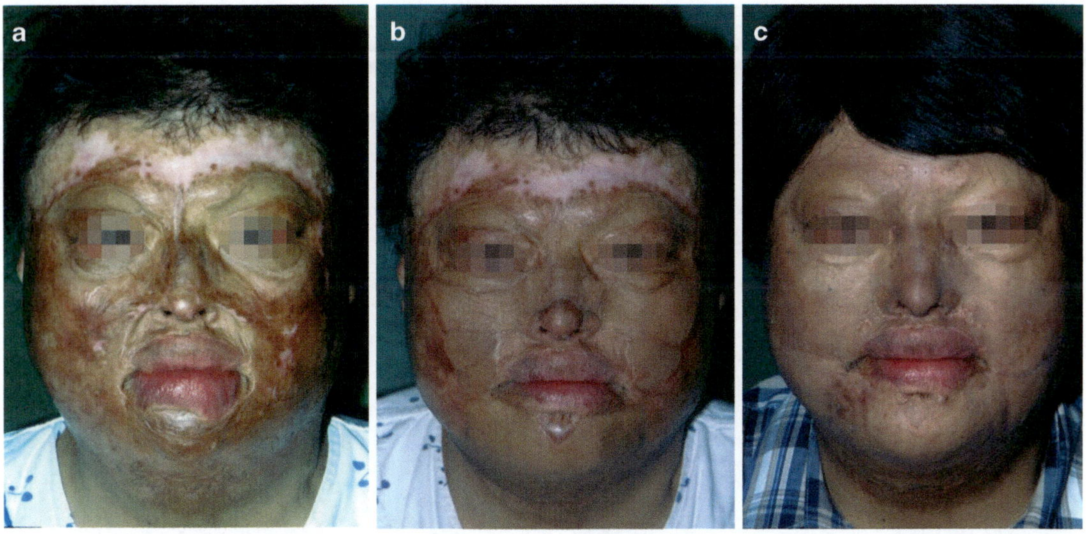

Fig. 1.31 (**a**) Preoperative view, he received several operations for correction of both upper and lower lid during 20 years. (**b**) The initial operation was performed on both lower lid, dorsum of nose, both cheeks, and upper lip. Second corrective surgery was performed on lower lip and mentum with thick STSG, anterior neck area with FTSG. (**c**) 10 months after the surgery with full-face dermal resurfacing result has shown excellent outcome

because the thin thickness, texture, and color of the facial area are not harmonious, and the effect of dermal overgraft proposed by the author in Chap. 5 is reduced. In the following section, the author will briefly introduce a series of procedures for correcting severe burn scar contracture in the facial area, providing further details later on.

This reconstruction of the face area using STSG will be fully explained in detail in Chap. 5.

This patient suffered flame burns 20 years ago. Over the course of 2 years, I performed total preconditioning of facial reconstruction. The initial operation was performed on both lower lid and ectropion deformities, the dorsum of the nose, both cheeks, and the upper lip area with a thick STSG (20/1000 inch, 0.5 mm thickness). A second corrective surgery was performed on the lower lip and mentum using thick STSG and on the anterior neck area using FTSG for a more natural position of the cervico-mental angle. The dermal overgraft technique is the final surgery; these procedures must correct all deformities, and the surgeon must wait until the operation sites have fully matured. Full-face dermabrasion and dermal overgraft were planned for the correction of the pigmented lesion on the forehead and previous operation sites on both lower lids, the nose, both cheeks, the mentum, and the anterior neck. (c) Full-face dermabrasion and dermal resurfacing procedures improved the overall outcome 10 months after the surgery (Fig. 1.31).

1.7 Reconstruction of Upper and Lower Lid Ectropion

The author's experiences and concepts described above also apply to correction of upper and lower lid ectropion; the author will introduce his clinical experiences and results regarding the many controversies surrounding whether STSG or FTSG should be performed and the problem of frequent relapse [43, 44].

Until now, FTSG has been a common method for correcting ectropion in the upper, lower, and surrounding area of the eyes [45]. However, frequently encountered results of FTSG include an unnatural appearance, color mismatch, and insufficient ectropion correction of open and closed eyes due to the differences in skin thickness. For most donor skin, thin postauricular skin with a thin and good color match with the face is most commonly used. If the graft area is large or the conditions of the donor site are unfavorable, the inner upper arm or the upper clavicle area skin

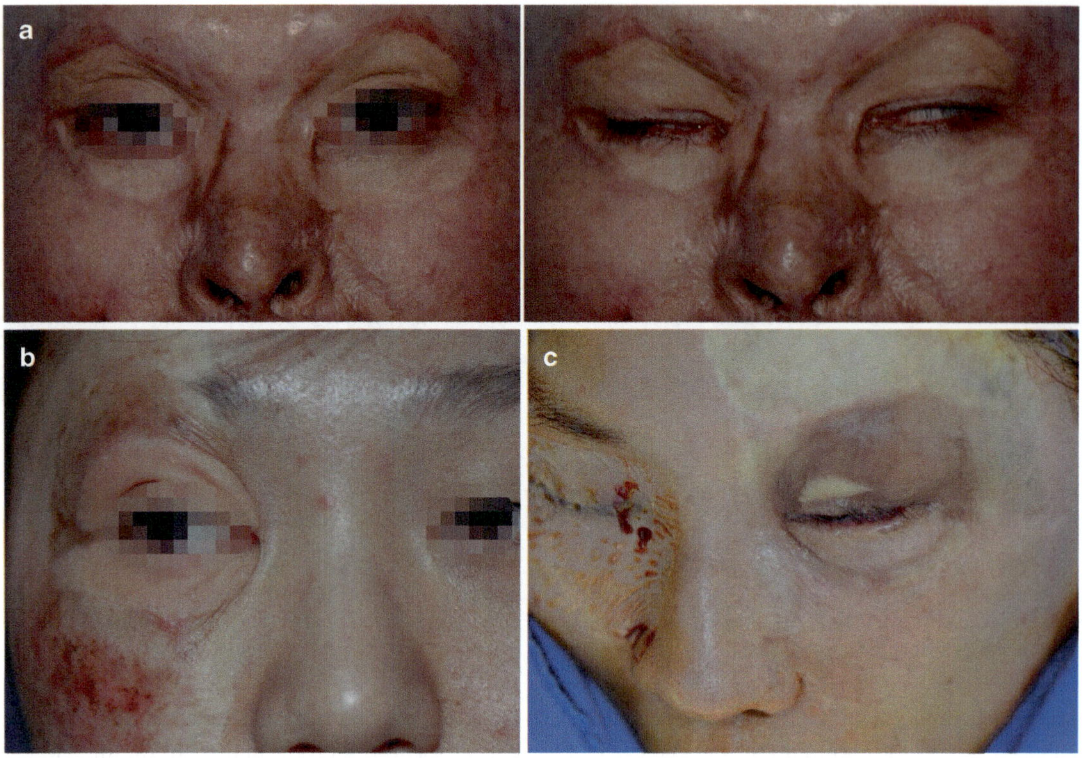

Fig. 1.32 (**a**) FTSG on the upper and lower lid, problems noted: unnatural skin texture, color mismatch, and double fold line. Undercorrected ectropion was shown in closed eye view. (**b**) Unnatural skin texture and thick double fold line noted compared with surrounding burned and opposite normal side. (**c**) Whitish small engrafted FTSG was noted with incomplete undercorrection of ectropion

may be used as well [46, 47]. Despite this, most functional and desirable cosmetic effects are not achieved because of the unnatural skin texture, color, and difference of thickness, in particular, many problems are presented regarding the correction of the existing upper lid ectropion.

This patient received FTSG on the upper and lower lids. The donor skin was obtained from the upper inner arm using dermal shaving to reduce graft thickness. The following conspicuous problems were observed: unnatural skin texture, color mismatch, a double-fold line on the upper lid, and both lower lids had undercorrected ectropion. In another case, thick skin texture, color mismatch, an unnatural appearance, and a double fold were observed compared with the surrounding areas burned and unburned. A small, whitish FTSG on the left upper lid of the ectropion was also observed. These serious issues are more common is Asians than in Caucasians (Fig. 1.32).

Burnt pigmentation is almost always noticeably unnatural in color and mismatching its surrounding skin. Usage of FTSG results in much more noticeable in color and texture [48]. The skin of the eyelids are the thinnest, and postauricular skin donor is commonly and often used to perform surgeries on the eyelids. However when the patient is of Asian background, the author recommends thick STSG, as it is difficult to achieve a natural look of double fold of the upper lid on Asian patients.

A 35-year-old female had received FTSG on the upper and lower lids. Unnatural double folds and skin texture were observed. A double-fold operation was performed for esthetic purposes. Five days after the surgery, the double fold was noted to be thicker and unnatural in appearance. Six months after the surgery, the right side was incompletely folded and the left fold had a thick appearance. Therefore, the author does not prefer

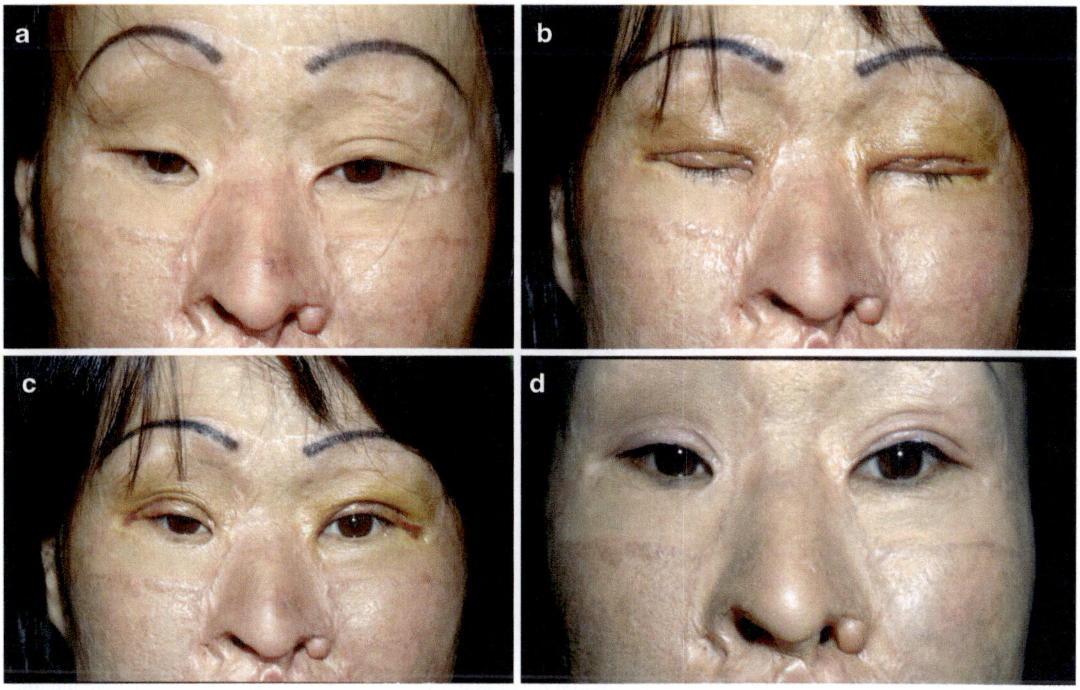

Fig. 1.33 (**a**) This patient received FTSG in the past on the upper and lower lids to the correction of ectropion. (**b**, **c**) Double-fold operation, postoperative 5 days, close and open eye view. (**d**) postoperative 6 months view, the right side was incompletely folded and left side had a too thick appearance

FTSG, especially for the upper lid correction of ectropion (Fig. 1.33).

There has been controversy on many discussions on the usage of FTSG for the correction of ectropion. Till now, FTSG has been used as a common method for correcting ectropion in the upper and lower eyelids. This 33-year-old patient suffered a flame burn; he had previously received FTSG for correcting the upper and lower lids. However, he has undercorrected ectropion and postoperative disfigurement. We planned a corrective double-fold operation and eyebrow reconstruction. Note the thick and unnatural appearance of the double fold after operation (Fig. 1.34).

This image shows the preoperative view of corrective eyebrow reconstruction and lower lid marginal ectropion. Three months later, the double-fold line had almost flattened. It means that the FTSG skin is an improperly formed double fold and has an unnatural double-fold appearance; often these folds tend to release and flatten in near time. FTSG tends to have better results on Caucasian patients. Single-hair transplantation was performed for eyebrow reconstruction, and undercorrected lower lid ectropion was observed. He received a 0.5-mm-thick STSG to correct the recurrent mild lower lid margin ectropion. Three months after the surgery, the ectropion was corrected, but unnatural step deformities were noted due to different engrafted skin thickness. In this case, the incisional release point must begin about 1 cm lower from the lower lid margin to correct recurrence of mild ectropion (yellow arrow). It means that when correcting lower lid ectropion, we must select the proper skin graft and perform enough release during correction to prevent recurrence (Fig. 1.35).

Seven months after the ectropion surgery, the double fold did not have a well-formed natural appearance (yellow arrow) because of the thick form FTSG. The prominent step deformities (black arrow) on the corrected ectropion with thick STSG were caused by the difference in thickness between the past-engrafted FTSG with advanced flap and thick STSG. Five years after the surgery, the lid margin was corrected to a

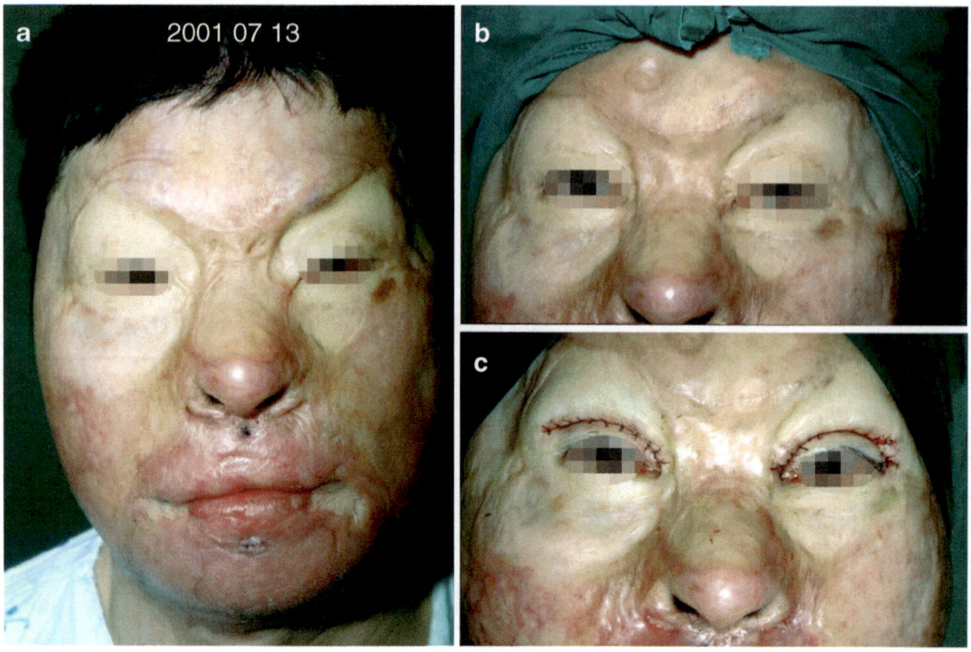

Fig. 1.34 (**a**, **b**) Preoperative view, he received FTSG on upper and lower lid for corrective surgery. (**c**) Note the thick and unnatural appearance of double fold after surgery

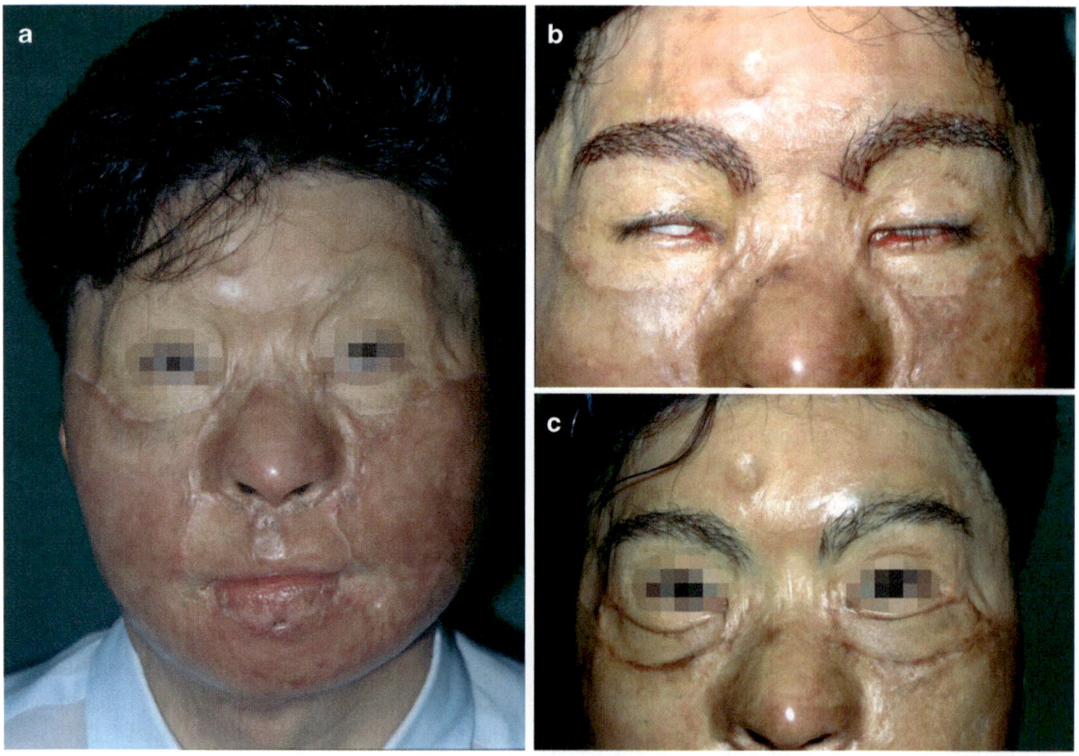

Fig. 1.35 (**a**) Preoperative view of eyebrow reconstruction. (**b**) The single-hair transplantation was performed for eyebrow reconstruction and noted undercorrected lower lid margin ectropion. (**c**) He received 20/1000-inch thickness STSG for correction of lid margin ectropion. Postoperative 3 months later view

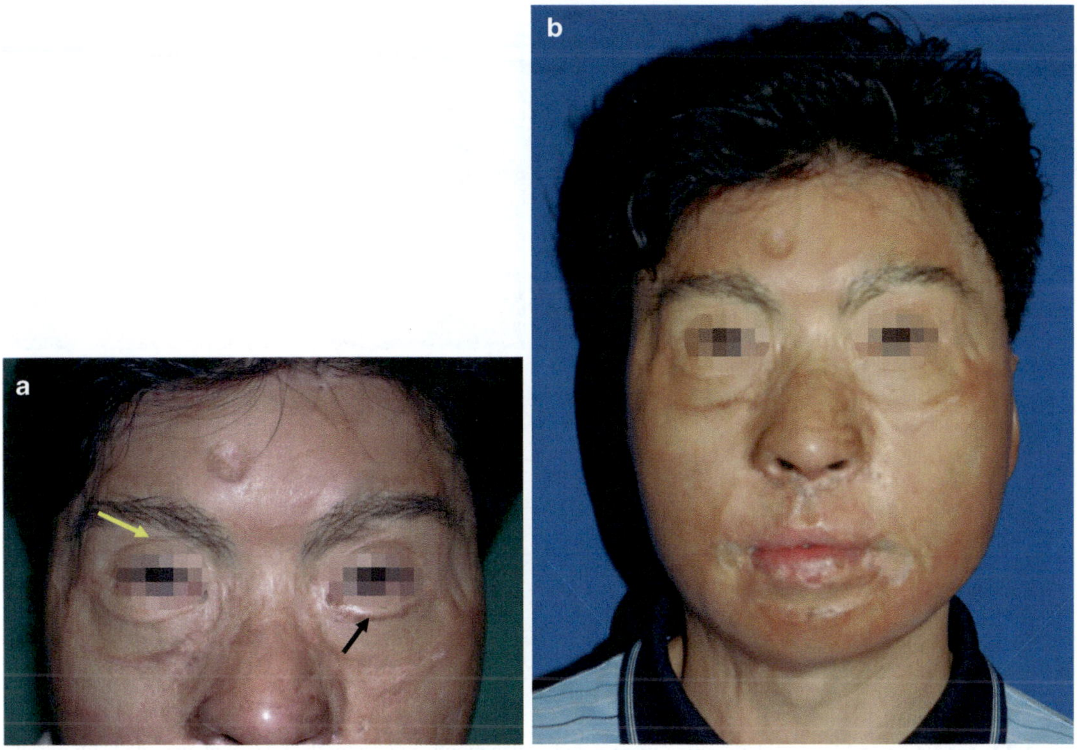

Fig. 1.36 (**a**) Postoperative 7 months view, double fold was flattened and did not have a natural appearance (yellow arrow). Note the corrected ectropion with eyeball contact. (**b**) Postoperative 5 years after, the lid margin was corrected to more natural position. Note the more natural appearance with single-hair transplantation of eyebrow reconstruction and philtrum reconstruction with triangular fossa from the ear cartilage

more natural position. Note the single-hair transplantation for eyebrow reconstruction and philtrum reconstruction with triangular fossa from the ear cartilage (Fig. 1.36).

For correction of lower lid ectropion, FTSG is performed on case-by-case basis compared with the upper lid, but it is also still difficult to obtain natural results because of skin color mismatch, texture difference, and insufficient graft surface, as a result of recurrent marginal lid ectropion which is hard to correct.

Therefore, the author has set fixed standard proposition implements of 0.4–0.5 mm medium or thick STSG for corrective surgery on the lower and upper eyelids.

1. An incision line should be made at least 0.5–1 cm below or above the lid margin, and it should be stressed that the incision line should not be attached directly under the lid margin. The author sometimes holds the incision line with a width of 2 cm or more when the contracture is severe, depending on the degree of ectropion (Fig. 1.37b). This is because, in many cases, epiphora symptoms caused by the insufficient contact of the lower lid surface with the eyeball, an important problem that is easily overlooked, are often not alleviated. As such, sufficient release space must be secured for the lid to make good contact with the eyeball. The width of the incision crosses the lateral canthus line in the medial canthus area and forms a fish mouth shape cut at the tip (refer Fig. 1.40b). The release should be done not only in the left and right direction but also vertically (Fig. 1.37), because the orbicularis oculi muscle is distributed in a concentric circle around the eyes, so it is key that full release happens both vertically and horizontally.

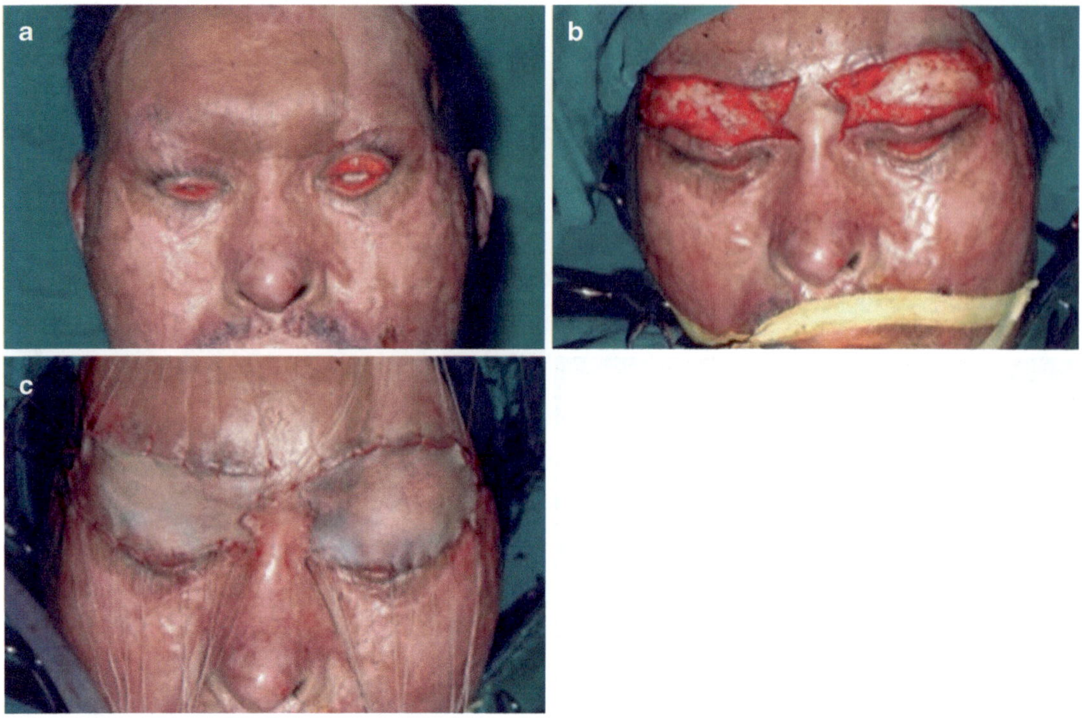

Fig. 1.37 (**a**) Upper and lower lid ectropion were noted after the conservative dressing on flame-burned face. (**b**) Full release of upper lid was performed with meticulous preservation of orbicularis oculi muscle and made cut off fish mouth pattern for the release of encircle oculi muscle. (**c**) 0.4 mm (16/1000 inches) thickness thick STSG was performed with tie-over dressing

2. Dissection should be performed while preserving the orbicularis oculi muscle. If possible, allow a very thin full release on both the upper and lower sides so that the lid margin is in good contact with the eyeball. When dissection is performed, do not be so concerned with the necrosis of the very thin dissected flap because lid skin blood supply is very plentiful and soft.
3. The graft is 0.4–0.5 mm depending on the release state, and the graft in the upper lid is thinner than the lower lid by 0.5 mm.
4. If the upper and lower lids are being performed at the same time, tarsorrhaphy must be applied for graft immobilization. In general, the graft is secured using a tie-over dressing rather than compressive dressing (Fig. 1.46b).
5. The dressing is opened on day 4 postoperatively, and saline-soaked dressing is applied up to day 7, when the tarsorrhaphy is removed.
6. Upper- and lower-step deformities due to the thickness difference in STSG can be corrected using multiple modified double-opposing Z-plasties, which acquire better cosmetic results (Fig. 1.43).

Severe ectropion was noted after the conservative management of flame burn. Full surgical release of upper lid was performed while carefully preserving the orbicularis oculi muscle. The release processing was performed in all directions with full length of oculi muscle and made cut off fish mouth pattern for the release of encircle oculi muscle. A 0.4-mm medium-thickness STSG was performed along with tie-over dressing.

Postoperative 1.5 months and 4 months: 15 months later, an open and closed eye view revealed a more natural upper lid appearance and color matching with the surrounding burned scar, although the skin was harvested from the darker buttock donor. The lower lid ectropion correction

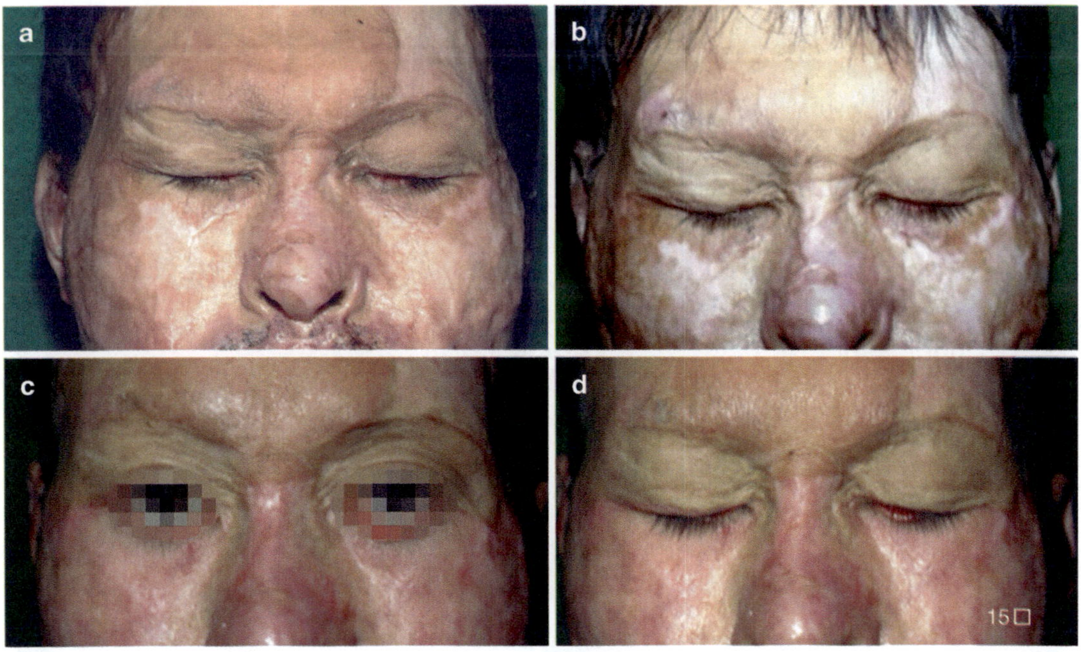

Fig. 1.38 (**a**) Postoperative 1.5 moths, (**b**) 4 months view. (**c**, **d**) 15 months later, open and closed eye views

was not performed because of the patient's financial strains (Figs. 1.37 and 1.38).

A 53-year-old female patient suffered a flame burn. Three months after the incident, immature hypertrophic scarring was observed on the entire face, and developed upper and lower lid ectropion. A 0.4-mm medium-thickness STSG was performed on both lower lid ectropion. Three months after the surgery, undercorrection was observed. Two years after the surgery, the ectropion was much improved compared to the mature surrounding scar tissue, as a result of STSG procedure. In this case, wide, medium-thickness STSG was shown to be much more effective for corrective ectropion surgery (Fig. 1.39).

A 23-year-old patient suffered a strong-acid attack and underwent multiple operations for the correction of the entire face. Preoperatively, mild upper and lower lid ectropion, defects in both alar nasi, and previous engrafted scars were observed on the mid and upper face. (b) The lower lid ectropion was corrected with full release tarsorrhaphy. Left alar composite graft was performed to correct the alar nasi. Note the full length of orbicularis oculi muscle released on lower lid and fish mouth shape release. The dart incision performed on both the medial and lateral canthal areas results in the incisional release of the entire range of orbicularis oculi muscle distribution and the fish mouth pattern (Fig. 1.40).

One year after the surgery, upper eyelid marginal ectropion was corrected with medium-thickness STSG. Four days after the surgery, the engrafted skin was completely taken. Note the corrected alar nasi and eyebrow reconstruction with composite graft and single-hair transplantation (Fig. 1.41).

One month after the surgery, more natural eyeball lid contact was observed in the upper lid region. Double-opposing Z-plasty was performed on the left lower lid, and laser therapy was given for scar management of the upper face (Fig. 1.42).

(a) The engrafted step deformities on the lower lid area could be corrected with modified double-opposing Z-plasty. (b) One year later, final procedure of full-face dermabrasion and dermal overgraft were performed for the correction of conspicuous engrafted margin on the upper and midface (Fig. 1.43).

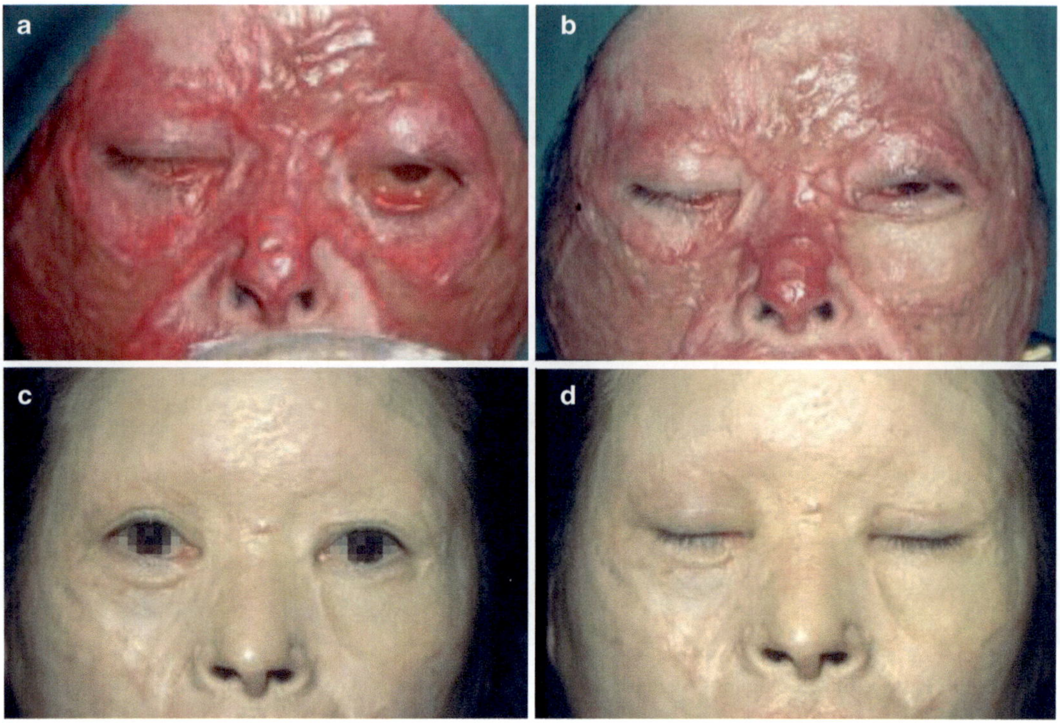

Fig. 1.39 (**a**) Noted upper and lower lid ectropion. 0.4-mm-thick STSG underwent on both lower lid ectropion. (**b**) Three months after the surgery, still undercorrected ectropion was noted. (**c, d**) Postoperative 2 years after STSG procedure shows great improvements on lid ectropion, with scars integrating with surrounding matured tissues

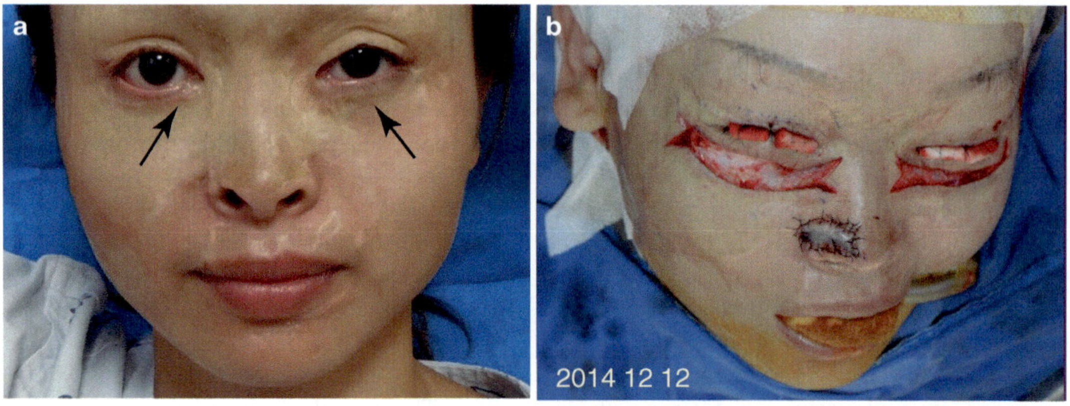

Fig. 1.40 (**a**) In preoperative view, mild upper and lower lid ectropion (black arrows) both alar nasi defect and previous engrafted scars were noted on the mid and upper face. (**b**) Full release with tarsorrhaphy and left alar composite graft for the correction of alar nasi defect

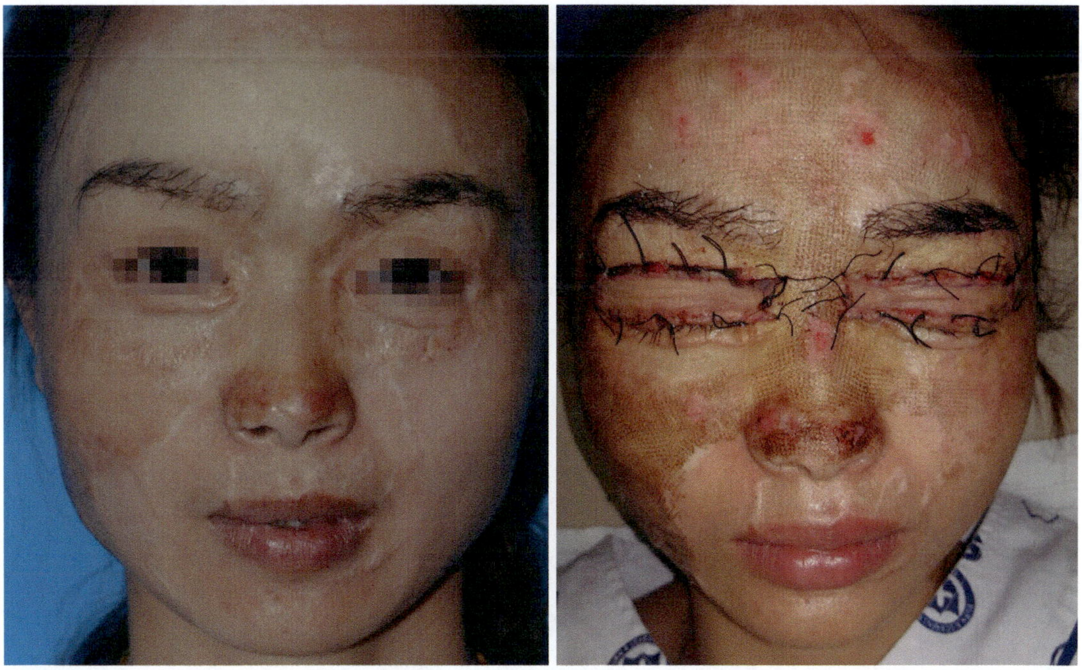

Fig. 1.41 Postoperative 1 year after, upper lid marginal ectropion was corrected and postoperative 4 days after view

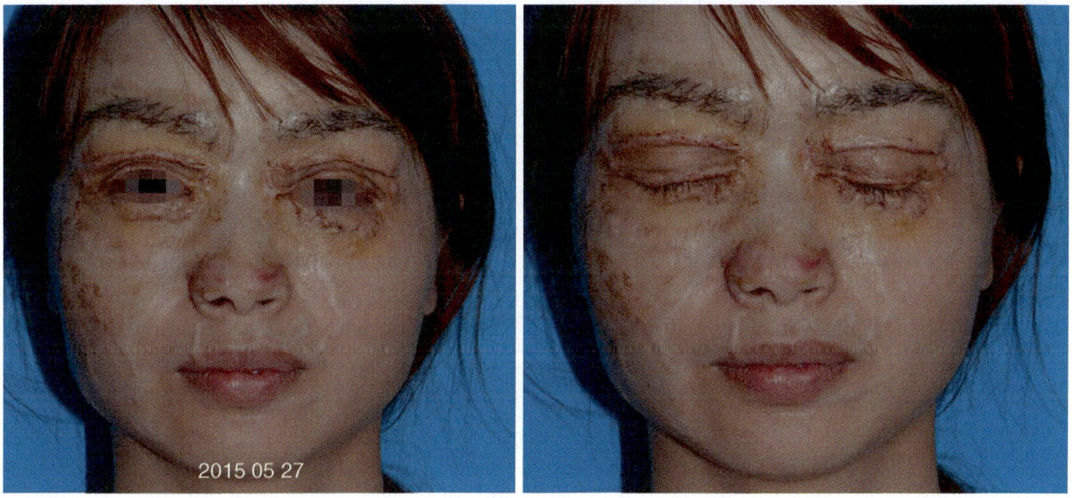

Fig. 1.42 Postoperative 1 month view, more natural eyeball contact was noted. Double-opposing Z plasty underwent on left lower lid and Fraxel laser therapy received for scar management on the upper face

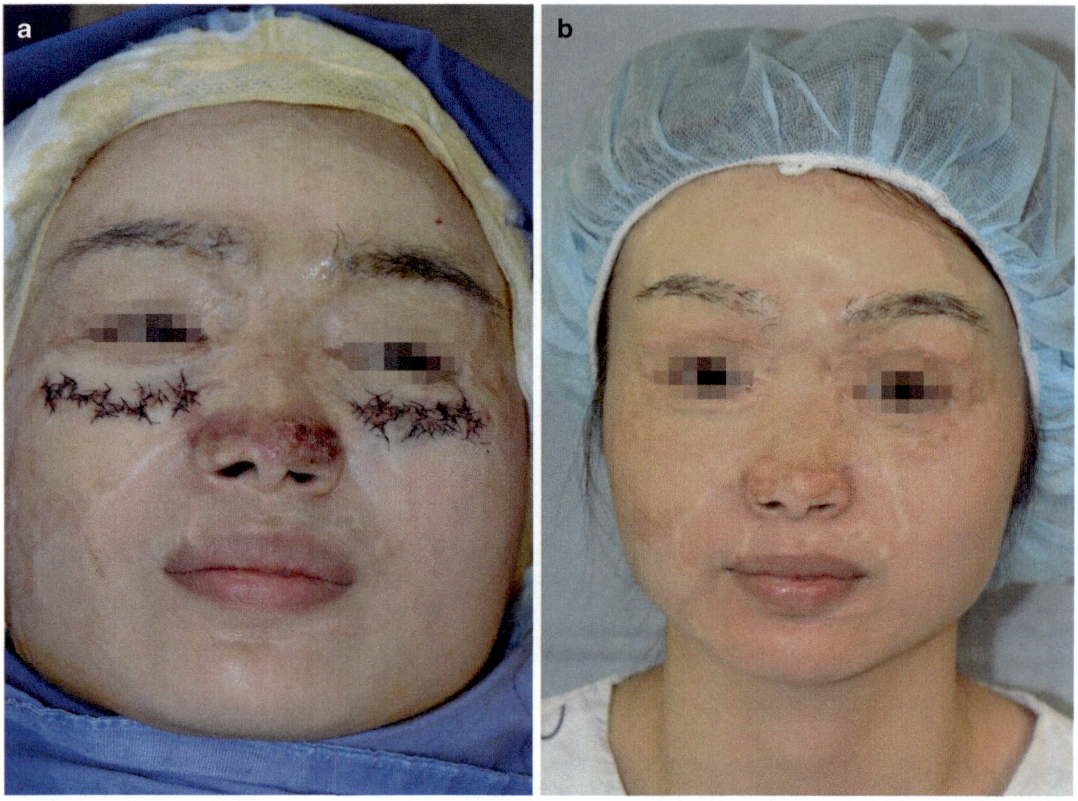

Fig. 1.43 (**a**) Step deformities on the lower lid area could be corrected with modified double-opposing Z-plasty. (**b**) 1 year after, receiving full face dermabrasion and dermal resurfacing procedure

Dermabrasion was performed on the upper- and midfacial areas, which included the upper and lower lid engrafted areas as well as the alar composite graft area to maximize the esthetic skin graft effect. Thin skin with a thickness of 6/1000 inches (0.15 mm) was used to resurface the area (Figs. 1.44 and 1.45).

Two weeks after the surgery, the engrafted skin was completely taken resulting in noticeable improvements on the skin texture as well as on the engrafted margin and burn-scarred areas. In this case, the upper and lower lid engrafted margins and both alar nasi composite graft areas had more inconspicuous effect with a natural appearance.

Figures 1.40, 1.41, 1.42, 1.43, 1.44, and 1.45 demonstrated the reconstruction of a facial defect, where esthetic skin graft was performed. This case suggests that the STSG method could be a new alternative method to facial reconstructive surgery (refer Chap. 5 Esthetic Skin Graft).

A 27-year-old male patient suffered a chemical burn on his right face; severe upper and lower lid ectropion with total loss of upper and lower lid margins were observed. Upper and lower ectropion were corrected with 0.5-mm-thick STSG with tarsorrhaphy. One year later, a medium-thickness STSG was performed on the mid and lower cheek areas for the correction of unsightly scarring (yellow arrow). Twenty-two months after the surgery, an irregular surface was visible on the upper lid margin, with total loss of eyelashes (Fig. 1.46). Six years after the surgery, the engrafted thick STSGs adapted naturally without recurrence of ectropion in both open and closed eye views. The upper and lower lid margins were well reconstructed with a good cosmetic outcome despite a total loss of lid margin and eyelashes (Fig. 1.47).

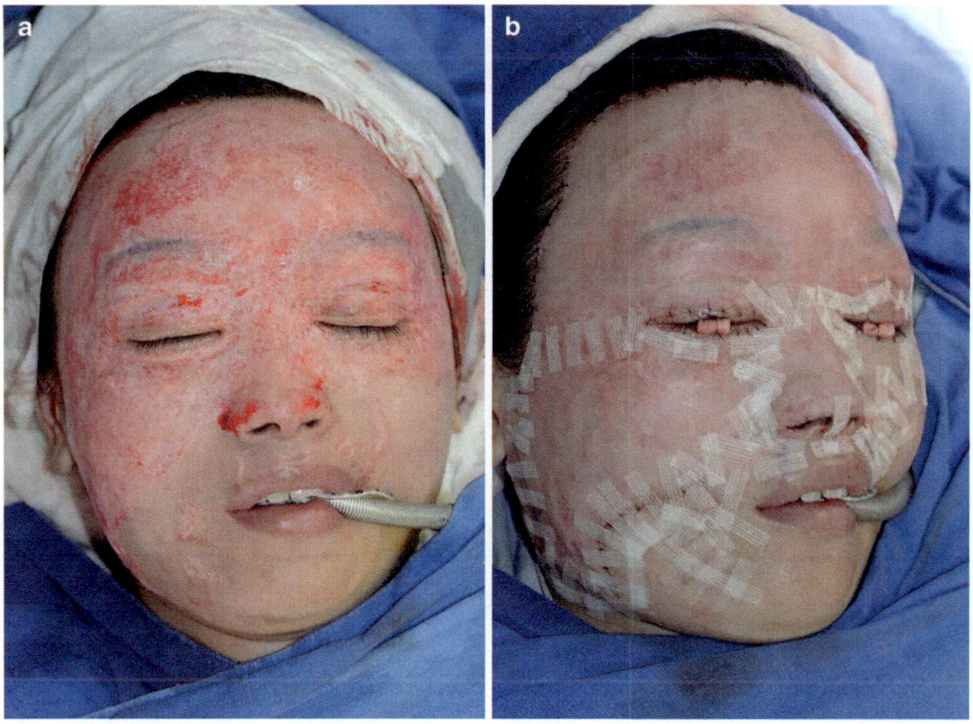

Fig. 1.44 (**a**) Dermabrasion was performed on mid and upper face. (**b**) Esthetic skin graft using thin skin with a thickness of 0.15 mm is performed to cover and resurface the area

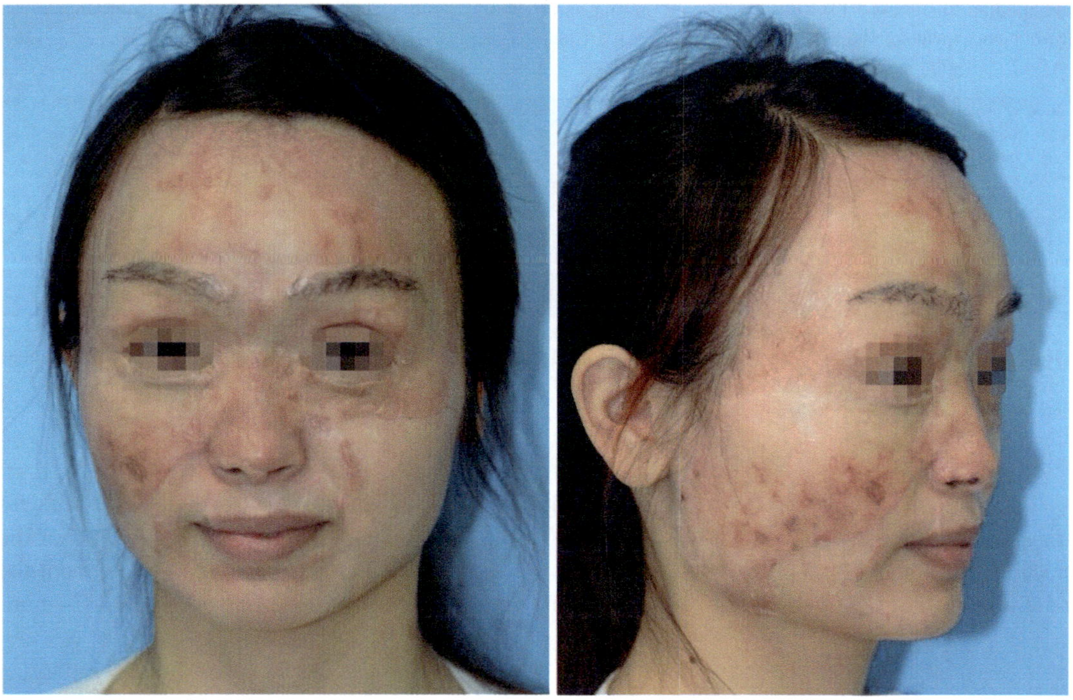

Fig. 1.45 Postoperative 2 weeks after view, the engrafted skin was completely taken and noticeable improvement on the skin texture and conspicuous graft margin

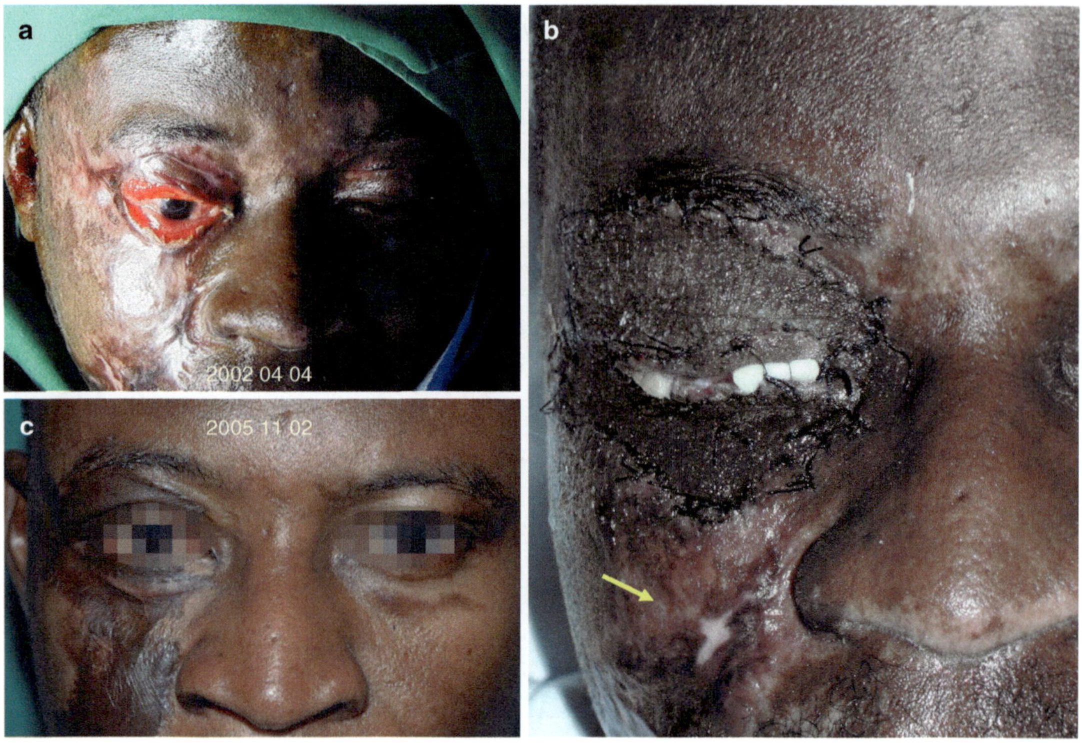

Fig. 1.46 (**a**) Severe upper and lower lid ectropion and total loss of eyelid margin. (**b**) Ectropion was corrected with thick 20/1000-inch STSG. One year after an intermediate-thickness STSG was performed on mid and lower cheek areas for the correction of unsightly scarring (yellow arrow). (**c**) Postoperative 22 months later, still irregular surface remained on the upper lid margin with total loss of eyelashes. But note the upper and lower lid contact with eyeball without functional disturbance

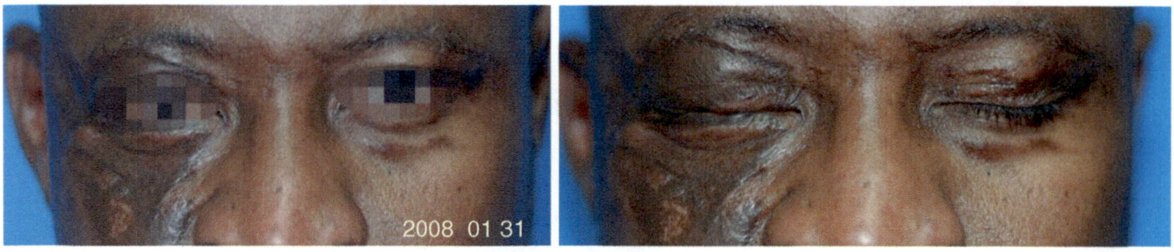

Fig. 1.47 Postoperative 6 years later view, engrafted thick STSG was adapted naturally without recurrence of ectropion in both open and closed eye views. Especially upper lid margin was well reconstructed with adequate functional and cosmetic outcome

This patient suffered a strong-acid attack on the face, resulting in right eyeball loss, scar contracture, a retracted upper lip, total loss of the right alar cartilage, and shrinking of the dorsum of the nose and the tip. Artificial eye ball was inserted on right, a full rotational release of the lower-cheek flap was performed to augment the nose tip, followed by a full release and 0.4-mm-

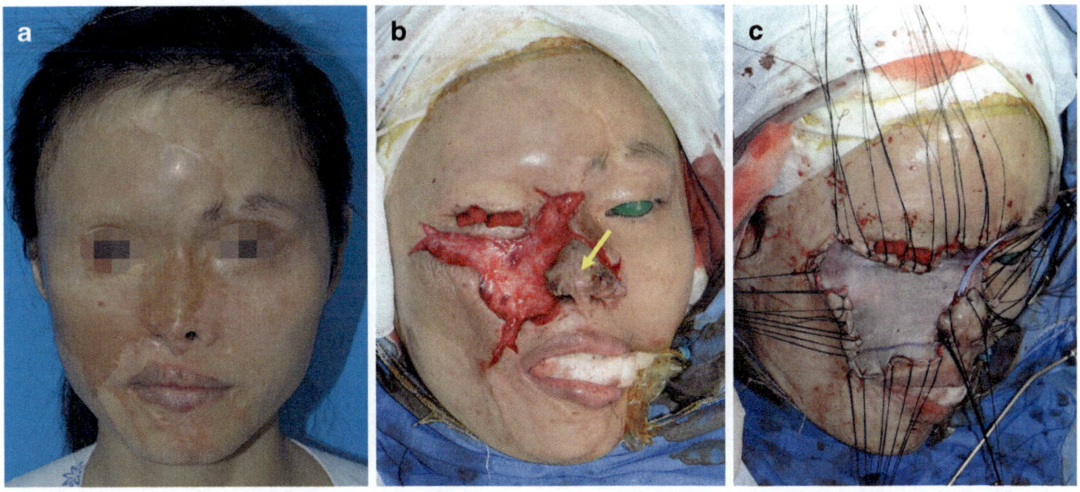

Fig. 1.48 (**a**) The right artificial eyeball provoking difficulty in eye closure; the hardened scar contracture noted retracted upper lip, total loss of right alar cartilage, dorsum of the nose and nose tip. (**b, c**) Initial full rotational release of lower cheek flap to augment the nose tip (yellow arrow) and release of 0.4-mm-thick STSG was performed

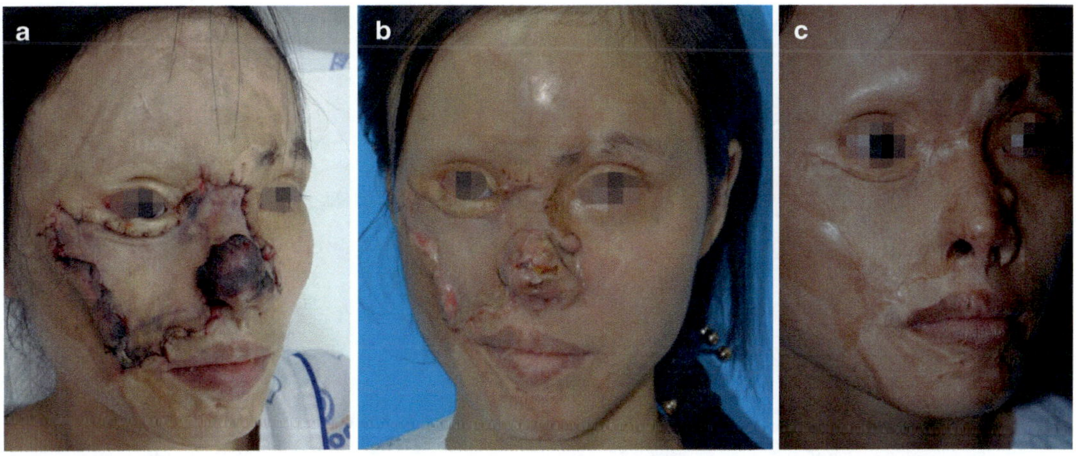

Fig. 1.49 (**a**) Postoperative 6 days after, the engrafted skin was completely taken. (**b**) Postoperative 18 days after the rotated local flap survived without any tissue loss. (**c**) Postoperative 10 months after, markedly improved skin texture on the right cheek and nose tip augmented

thick STSG to correct lower lid ectropion with tarsorrhaphy and tie-over dressing (Fig. 1.48). Six days after the surgery, the engrafted skin was completely taken. Eighteen days after the surgery, the rotated local flap recovered without tissue loss. Ten months after the surgery, the skin texture on the right cheek and augmented nose tip had notably improved (Fig. 1.49). The author planned to correct the ectropion and reshape the nose tip and alar area. A thick STSG was performed on the left upper and lower lids, right upper lid, and cheek simultaneously. FTSG with

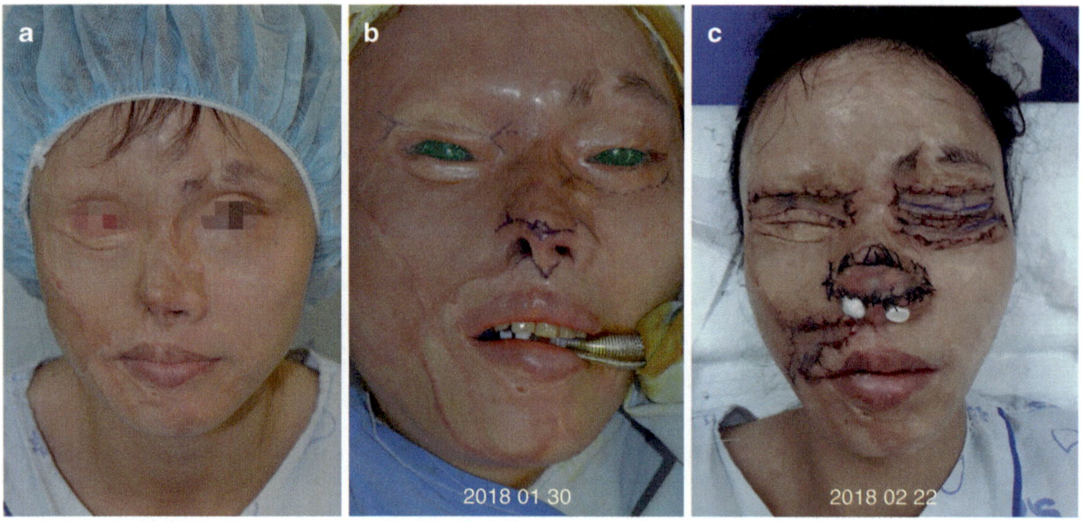

Fig. 1.50 (**a**) Postoperative 10 months after view and preoperative view of second operation. (**b**) Correction of the ectropion and reshaping of the nose tip and alar area. (**c**) 23 days after the operation, all engrafted skins were taken without difficulty

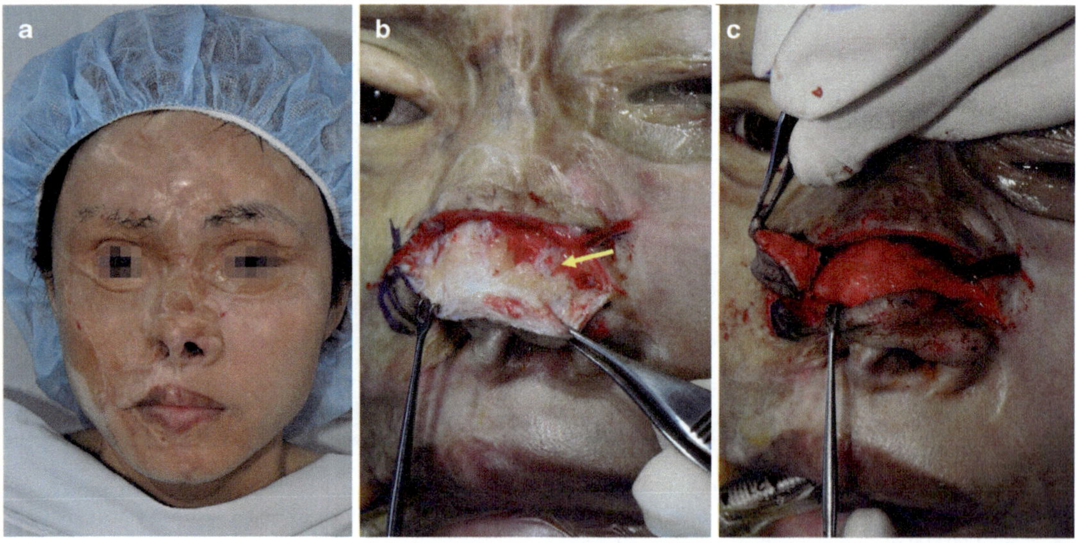

Fig. 1.51 (**a**) Preoperative view of final third Re-FTSG with fat composite graft repeated for nose tip augmentation. (**b**) Intra-operative view, note the well preserved fat layer from pervious FTSG with fat graft. (**c**) Intra-operative view, during the final third Re-FTSG

composite fat graft was performed on the nose tip and alar augmentation (Fig. 1.50). Eight months after the surgery, a second FTSG with fat composite graft was performed for additional nose tip augmentation. (b) Note the well-preserved fat layer (yellow arrow), which was the first engrafted FTSG with composite fat graft. It is an important finding in FTSG with composite fat graft, generating effective augmentation. (c) Full release of the nose tip and columella area, second engraftment was performed on the previous FTSG site (Fig. 1.51).

In the original postoperative view, an artificial eyeball, upper and lower lid ectropion, right ala,

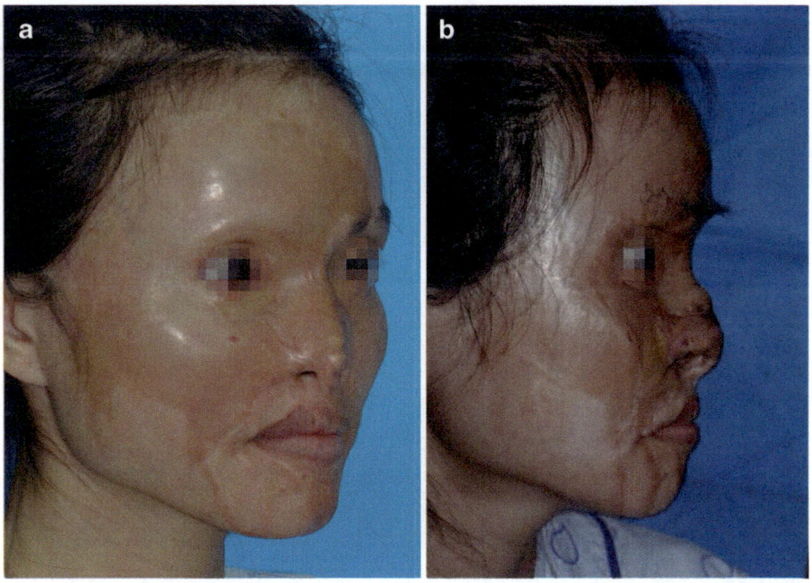

Fig. 1.52 (**a**) Original preoperative view. (**b**) Postoperative 1 year 8 months view, marked improvement on upper and lower lid ectropion and improved facial contour and nose tip with nostril

and nose tip defect were observed. At 1 year and 8 months postoperatively, marked improvement on the upper and lower lid ectropion, facial contour, augmented nose tip, and nostril was observed. The next operation will be a right alar reconstruction with an ear cartilage composite graft (Fig. 1.52).

Although there is still much left to debate regarding the pros and cons of FTSG and STSG, from my experience, thick STSG can achieve more natural and even characteristic results than FTSG, especially in Asian patients. The most common reason for the recurrence of ectropion is holding the incision line too close to the lid margin causing mild undercorrection of ectropion. Overcorrection of skin graft must cover the full area of oculi muscle.

1.8 STSG for Acute Burned Hand

In the acute burn stage, as in the facial area, the hands also require a high-quality STSG as well as quick and accurate wound management [49]. Burn management of the hand and graft timing are very important, but it is not easy to judge and perform an escharectomy or appropriate debridement in this area, because of numerous joints and tendons, covered in thin skin that is supple [50–52]. The usage of mesh grafts, which allows for much easier and convenient wound management, is contraindicated because they are accompanied by serious functional disorders as well as cosmetic deformity. To achieve high-quality results on hands, it should have first priority [53]. The author believes that applying the concept of early excision and graft more actively than the facial region and performing a single-sheet STSG can yield greater benefits in terms of functional and esthetic results and that a thickness of 0.25–0.3 mm (10–12/1000 inches) is appropriate. More experience is surely needed for burned hand management; the author recommends that debridement should be carried out in no more than 2 or at least 3 weeks and that skin grafting be actively performed even at a deep second-degree burn based on the need and circumstances [50]. This is because, if possible, it is helpful to replenish the area and amount of skin lost by burns, even a little. First, the wound healing process and contracture progress more rapidly as time progresses (starting 2 weeks in, according to my clinical experience); approximately 3 weeks after, the engrafted skin is smaller than the area of the actual lost skin, and there is a possibility that the contracture process

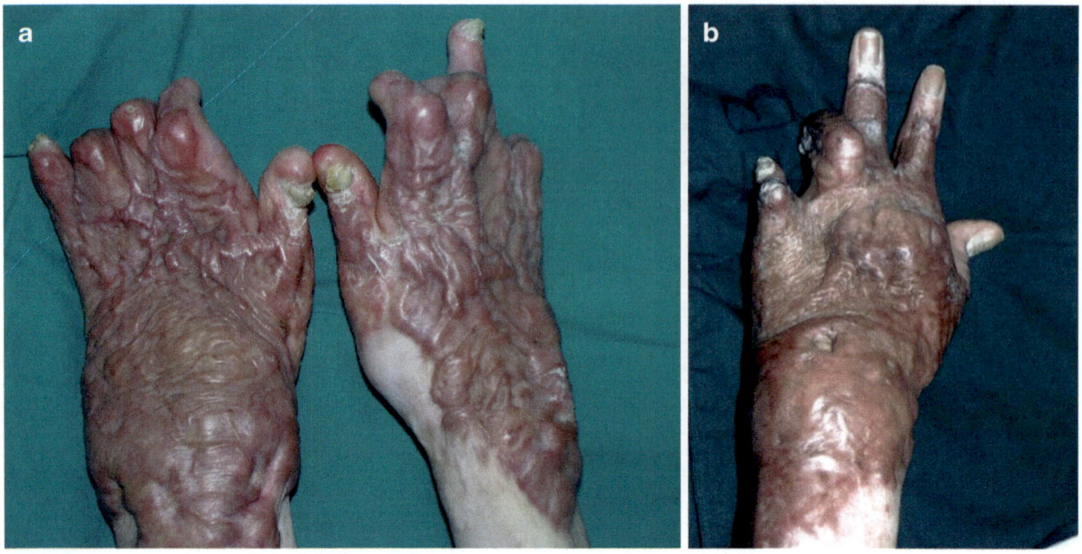

Fig. 1.53 (**a**) This patient received mesh skin graft on post-burn day after 40 days. (**b**) This patient was also treated with partial mesh skin graft 3 years ago

will rapidly become more severe. Secondly, a healthy granulation bed provides a good environment for skin intake. But overgrowth of granulation tissue is thought to have detrimental effects on the healing process due to scarring. For this reason, performing the graft in the shortest time possible in optimal environment is recommended. Thirdly, early wound coverage has many advantages as it reduces the inflammatory reaction and edematous period. This early mobilization aides faster recovery in tissue and hand function [54, 55].

The next example shows how mesh skin graft of the hand is contraindicated by displaying the severe functional and esthetic disorder brought on by the missed timing of earlier graft with a conservative wound dressing for more than 3 weeks and performing a meshed skin graft.

(a) This patient received a mesh skin graft 40 days after the burn incident. One year after the surgery, severe hypertrophic scar contracture with a cicatricial syndactyly was observed. (b) This patient was also treated with a partial mesh skin graft 3 years ago. In these cases, there is a clear distinction between early proper management and early sheet graft compared to mesh skin graft (Fig. 1.53).

(a) Severe volar displacement and extensor deformities were observed on the 17-year-old scar contracture of the left hand because of an improper skin graft at the time of acute burn management. (b) Severely dislocated fingers and cicatricial hypertrophic scarring on the metacarpophalangeal joint area were observed. Figure 1.54 shows deformities that progressed after missing the crucial timing of the skin graft, when natural wound healing without proper wound coverages occurs, severe hypertrophic and scar contracture develops. The following is a case where a sheet type STSG was performed only on the dorsum of the hand and not extending up to the fingers, causing severe dislocation and tendon adhesion of the finger joints later on (a). This case shows results of insufficient mesh graft performance as the maximum area could not be secured due to the failure of maintenance of engrafted hand's first position (b) (Fig. 1.55).

These cases are examples where a skin graft was performed with the fist position well maintained, with early excision and graft on day 16. It can be seen that hand function was well maintained without reconstructive surgery (Fig. 1.56).

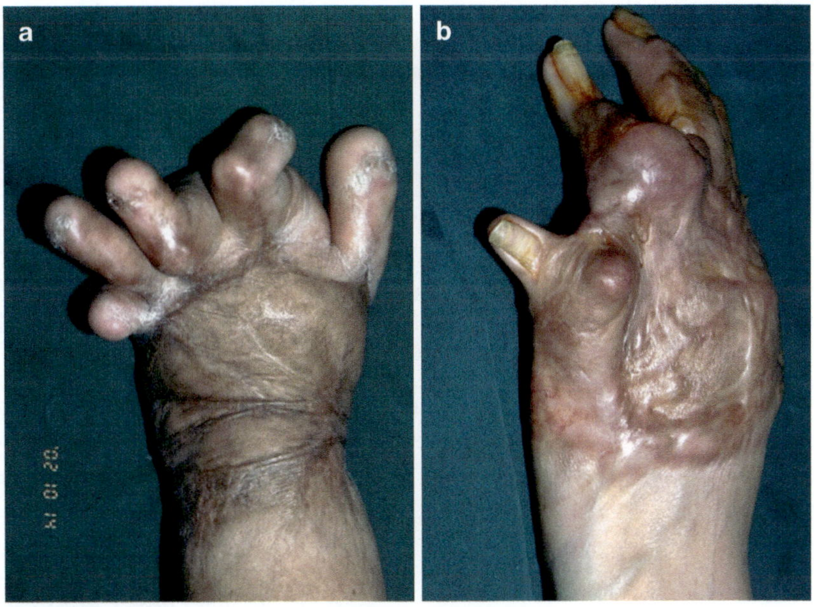

Fig. 1.54 (**a**) Left hand with long-term severe contracture was observed with volar displacements and severe extensor deformities. (**b**) Severe dislocated fingers were observed and cicatricial hypertrophic scarring on the MCP joint area

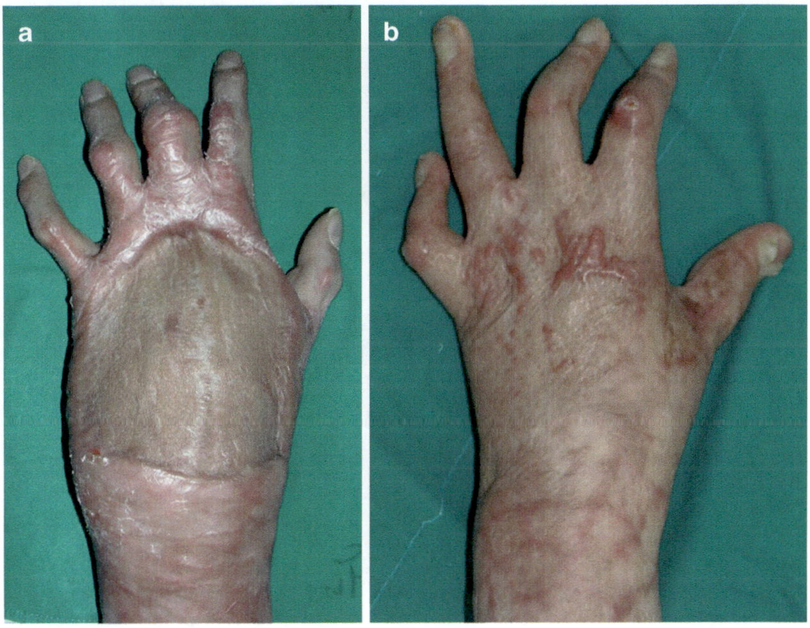

Fig. 1.55 (**a**) Unfavorable result observed even after a sheet graft and (**b**) delayed meshed skin graft in acute state

A 16-year-old female patient suffered a deep second-degree scalding burn on the left dorsum of the hand and wrist. On post-burn day 15, a 12/1000-inch STSG was performed on the dorsum of the hand only, and the wrist area had already undergone epithelialization. At 1-year post-burn, there were no scar deformities on the dorsum of the hand. Two years after the surgery, an excellent esthetic result was observed on the dorsum of the hand, except for the wrist area, which had healed spontaneously without a skin graft (yellow arrow) (Fig. 1.57).

If the entire hand has third-degree burns or if the proper wound management time is exceeded,

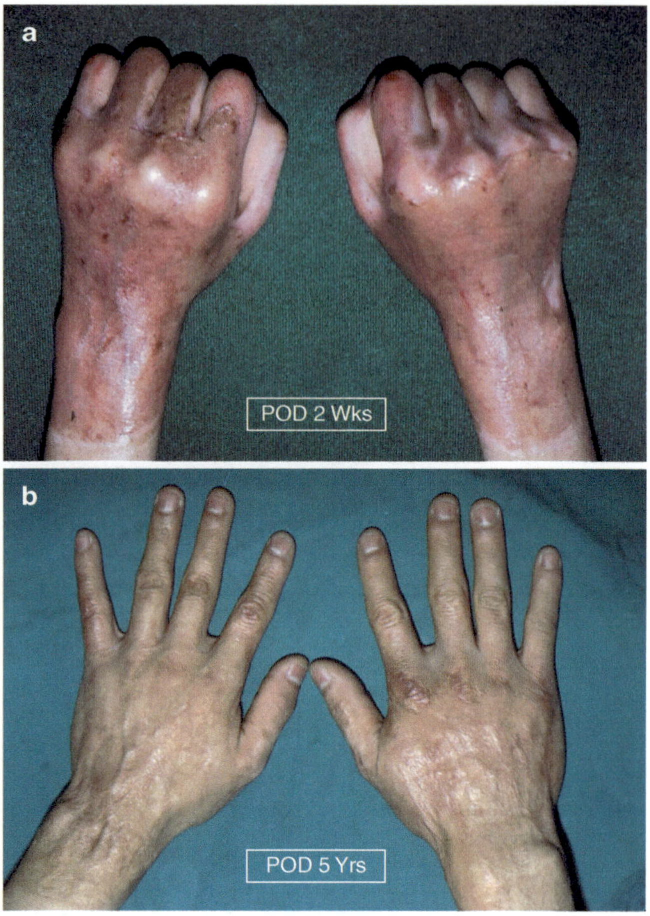

Fig. 1.56 (**a**) Post-burn day 16, the patient received 0.25-mm-thickness thin STSG according to early management of hand burn plan. (**b**) Postoperative 5 years later, he had no functional disturbance and no additional corrective surgery

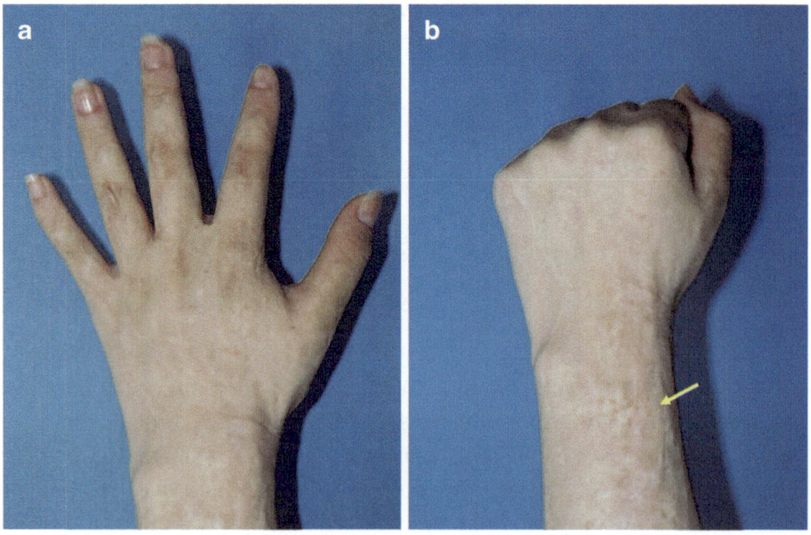

Fig. 1.57 (**a**) Post-burn day 15, 0.3-mm intermediate-thickness STSG was performed on the dorsum of the hand only, post-burn day 1 year after view. (**b**) Postoperative 2 years after view, excellent esthetic result was noted on the dorsum of the hand except for the wrist area (yellow arrow)

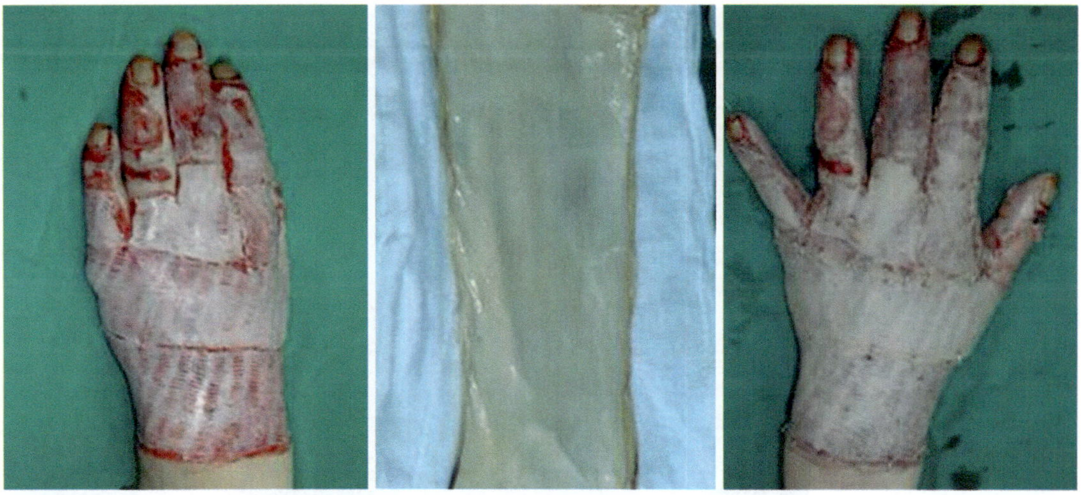

Fig. 1.58 Post-burn day 18, human dermal matrix graft with 8/1000-inch single-sheet autograft was performed

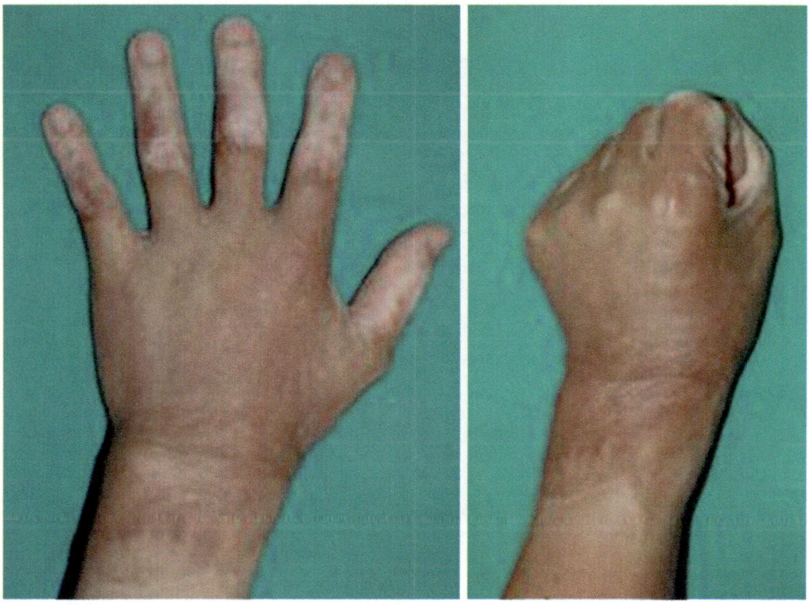

Fig. 1.59 Postoperative 1.5 years after view, excellent result was noted

a human dermal matrix could be used to reinforce the dermal layer, producing better-than-expected results and eliminating the need for subsequent reconstructive surgery [56–58]. As a result, the high cost of the dermal matrix could be offset.

This patient was injured with a deep second-degree flame burn. On post-burn day 18, a human dermal matrix graft with an 8/1000-inch single-sheet autograft was performed. At 1.5 years post-operatively, an excellent result was noted without any functional disturbance or scar contracture. In this case, early excision and early grafting with a dermal substitute system combined with surgery result in a high-quality outcome (Figs. 1.58 and 1.59).

The following shows excellent results of the final dermal overgraft after early excision and

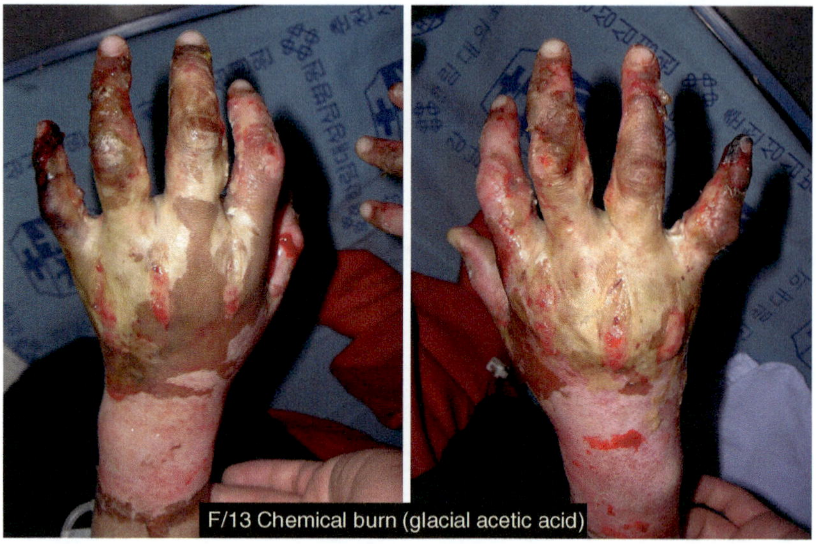

Fig. 1.60 Glacial acetic acid chemical burn on both hands. Note the emergency escharotomy

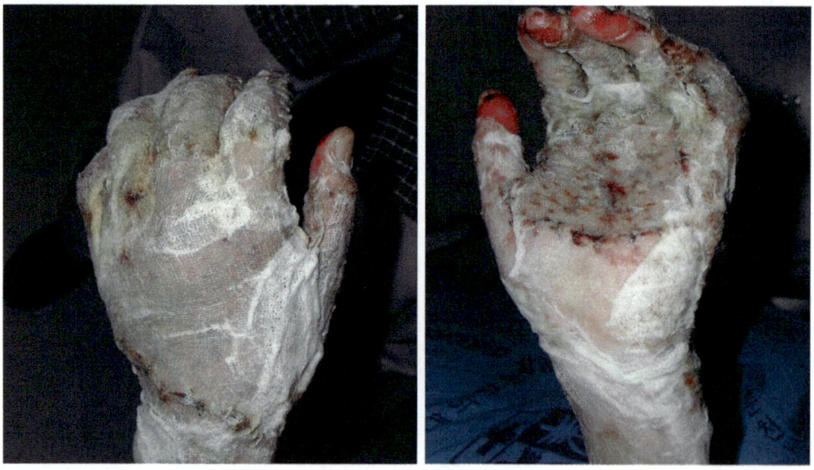

Fig. 1.61 Post-burn day 17, escharectomy and human dermal matrix with 0.15-mm thin autograft

early graft were performed on a third-degree chemical burn.

A 13-year-old female patient sustained glacial acetic acid chemical burns on both hands. Emergency escharotomy was performed to prevent compartment syndrome and to salvage her fingers. On post-burn day 17, escharectomy and human dermal matrix with 0.15-mm-thick thin autograft were performed (Figs. 1.60 and 1.61). Dermabrasion and dermal resurfacing were performed to obtain a more esthetic result. Five years after the burn incident, we obtained excellent functional and esthetic results. Chemical burns always present many problematic setbacks. Early graft and appropriate wound management are a must when available (Figs. 1.62, 1.63, and 1.64).

Most important key point for acute hand burn injury is the timing of the operation, and the concepts as well as the technique of early excision.

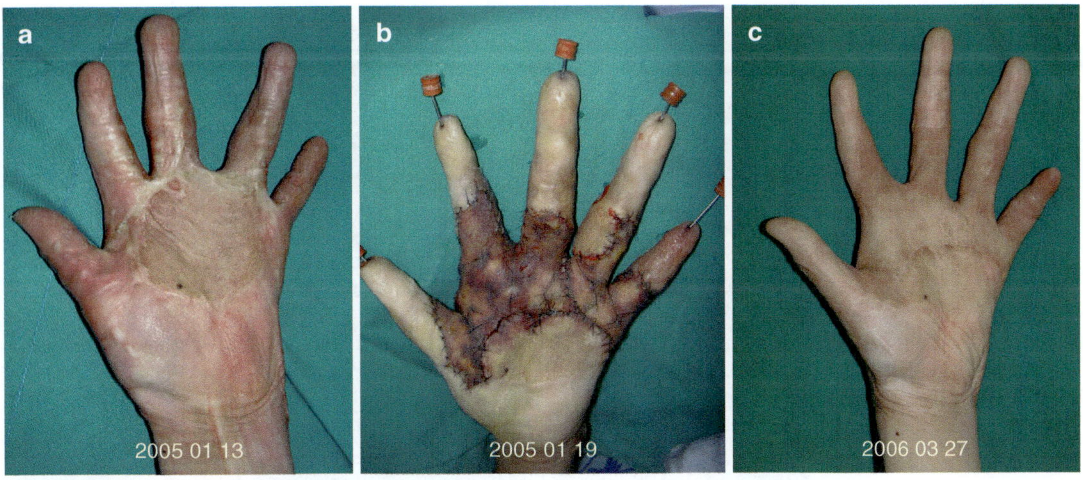

Fig. 1.62 (**a**) Human dermal matrix system engraftment 1 year later, release, and FTSG were performed on both palms. (**b**) Six days after operation. (**c**) Postoperative 1.2 years view

Fig. 1.63 At 3.5 years postoperatively, excellent results were noted on both palms

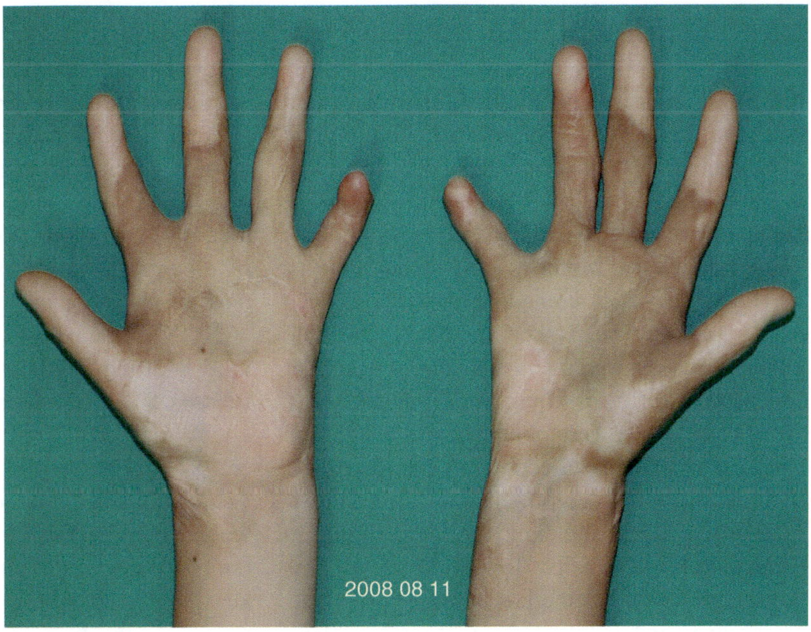

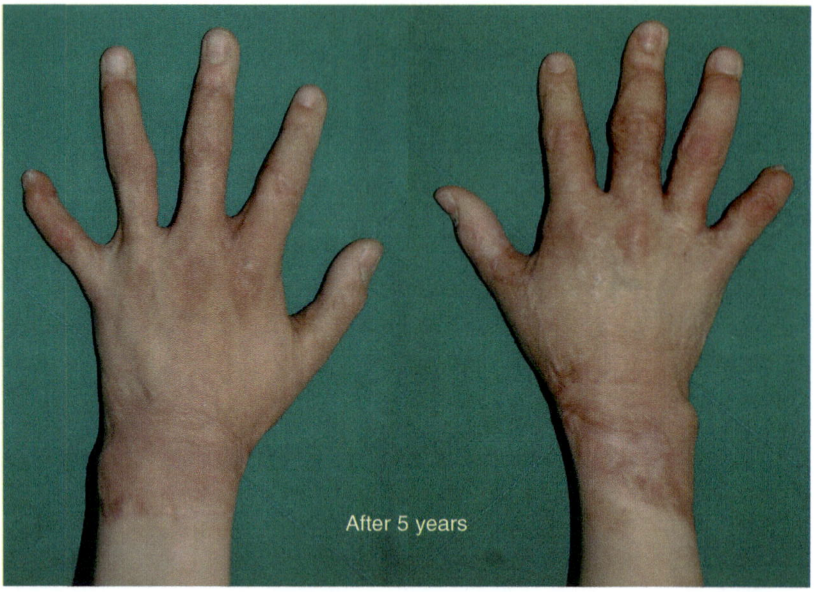

Fig. 1.64 Post-burn day 5 years after view, we obtained excellent results showing adequate function and esthetics on the dorsum of the hand with one-stage early operation with dermal matrix

1.9 Conclusion

Mesh skin graft is very effective for wide wound coverage, but it is not comparable with general STSG in terms of cosmetic and functional aspects. The author has introduced a technique that uses cultural epithelial cell therapy to enable rapid and effective wound healing in major burns. CEH can be used immediately when needed using a prefabricated sheet graft. In addition, clinical trials showed that a ratio of 1:4 or higher was very effective in filling a high mesh space; significant results were obtained, albeit the high cost. CEA is a more effective method than CEH in terms of replenishing the lacking skin by permanently covering the empty space of the mesh using cultured auto cells. However, there are disadvantages to this method: it takes over 2 weeks to produce and the high cost. To relief these issues, a cell suspension technique is developed by the author in order to shorten the manufacturing time while covering a wider area, resulting in more sustainable outcome. Another way to relieve severe scar contracture due to mesh grafts is to alleviate the severe contracture deformities of the major joint area by using human dermal matrix systems that can perform a single-step operation in combination. However, the methods mentioned above still face financial strain and are time-consuming processes that often result in ineffective outcomes.

STSG remains the most widely known and used grafting method worldwide. The author focuses STSG on face and hand skin graft to obtain successful graft results compared to general STSG.

Accompanied by the basic principles of wound bed condition, bleed control, and infection prevention, the author emphasizes that the key point is fix the operation time within 2–3 weeks for the face and hands, with his recommended usage of scalp skin for the facial region, which resulted in excellent color and texture match. With regard to the hands, more timely operation decisions and maintenance of postoperative engrafted fist position are of key importance. It is also very important in hand STSG to replenish the dermal layer, if possible. If financial means are present, author recommends using a combination of human dermal matrix and STSG. In general, STSG of the face is rarely used in reconstructive surgery, but for the scar contracture release of the eyes, nose, and mouth region, where full thickness skin donor clavicle, inner arm or postauricular areas is a often used. The author prefers to perform medium or thick STSG to create a preconditioning state and to preserve donor. In the correction of ectropion, commonly and most often FTSG is used routinely, which centers the controversy of "why" FTSG is so accepted and most used on facial reconstruction. With more clinical experience and result achievement, the author suggests thick STSG is more effective than FTSG, especially on upper lid ectropion of Asian patients. For the lower lid, FTSG of the postauricular and upper inner arm donor is used rarely. Common errors in ectropion surgery are inadequate release and skin graft. The author always uses thick STSG to overcome this problem by releasing the incision line from medial to lateral canthal area and fish mouth shape cut to increase the vertical width of the skin defect. Finally, refer Chap. 3–5, where various techniques are introduced to describe in further detail.

References

1. Kinner MA, Daly WL. Skin transplantation. Crit Care Nurs Clin North Am. 1992;4(2):173–8.
2. Kirsner RS, Falanga V, Eaglstein WH. The biology of skin grafts. Skin grafts as pharmacologic agents. Arch Dermatol. 1993;129(4):481–3.
3. Koljonen V. Techniques of skin grafting. Duodecim. 2011;127(20):2139–47. [PubMed].
4. Braza ME, Fahrenkopf MP. Split-thickness skin grafts. In: StatPearls. Treasure Island, FL: StatPearls Publishing; 2022.
5. Lyons JL, Kagan RJ. The true meshing ratio of skin graft meshers. J Burn Care Res. 2014;35(3):257–60. [PubMed].
6. Capek L, Flynn C, Molitor M, Chong S, Henys P. Graft orientation influences meshing ratio. Burns. 2018;44(6):1439–45. [PubMed].
7. Sakamoto M, Morimoto N, Inoie M, Takahagi M, Ogino S, Jinno C, Suzuki S. Cultured human epidermis combined with meshed skin autografts accelerates epithelialization and granulation tissue formation in a rat model. Ann Plast Surg. 2017;78(6):651–8.
8. Oshima H, Inoue H, Matsuzaki K, Tanabe M, Kumagai N. Permanent restoration of human skin treated with cultured epithelium grafting—wound healing by stem cell based tissue engineering. Hum Cell. 2002;15(3):118–28.
9. Yanaga H, Udoh Y, Yamauchi T, Yamamoto M, Kiyokawa K, Inoue Y, Tai Y. Cryopreserved cultured epidermal allografts achieved early closure of wounds and reduced scar formation in deep partial-thickness burn wounds (DDB) and split-thickness skin donor sites of pediatric patients. Burns. 2001;27(7):689–98.
10. Schiozer WA, Gemperli R, Mühlbauer W, Munhoz AM, Ferreira MC. An outcome analysis and long-term viability of cryopreserved cultured epidermal allografts: assessment of the conservation of transplantable human skin allografts. Acta Cir Bras. 2013;28(12):824–32.
11. Yanaga H, Udoh Y, Yamamoto M, Yoshii S, Mori S, Yamauchi T, Kiyokawa K, Koga M, Yanaga K. Cryopreserved cultured epithelial allografts for pediatric deep partial dermal burns: early wound closure and suppression of scarring. Regen Ther. 2017;6:74–82.
12. Adams DC, Ramsey ML. Grafts in dermatologic surgery: review and update on full- and split-thickness skin grafts, free cartilage grafts, and composite grafts. Dermatol Surg. 2005;31(8 Pt 2):1055–67.
13. Hazani R, Whitney R, Wilhelmi BJ. Optimizing aesthetic results in skin grafting. Am Surg. 2012;78(2):151–4.
14. Taghizadeh R, Gilbert PM. Comparison of commonly used mesher types in burns surgery revisited. Burns. 2008;34(1):109–10.
15. Vandeput J, Nelissen M, Tanner JC, Boswick J. A review of skin meshers. Burns. 1995;21(5):364–70.
16. Yanai A, Hiraga Y. Method for preparing meshed skin grafts without using skin-graft meshers. Plast Reconstr Surg. 1991;88(3):524–6.
17. Sinha M. Meshing small skin grafts manually: a simple, quick, and effective method using discard-A-pad. Ann Plast Surg. 2005;55(4):433–4.
18. Compton CC, Hickerson W, Nadire K, Press W. Acceleration of skin regeneration from cultured epithelial autografts by transplantation to homograft dermis. J Burn Care Rehabil. 1993;14(6):653–62.
19. Sood R, Roggy D, Zieger M, Balledux J, Chaudhari S, Koumanis DJ, Mir HS, Cohen A, Knipe C, Gabehart K, Coleman JJ. Cultured epithelial autografts for coverage of large burn wounds in eighty-eight patients: the Indiana University experience. J Burn Care Res. 2010;31(4):559–68.
20. Sheridan R. Closure of the excised burn wound: autografts, semipermanent skin substitutes, and permanent skin substitutes. Clin Plast Surg. 2009;36(4):643–51.

21. Oravcová D, Koller J. Currently available skin substitutes. Cas Lek Cesk. 2014;153(1):7–12.
22. Haddad AG, Giatsidis G, Orgill DP, Halvorson EG. Skin substitutes and bioscaffolds: temporary and permanent coverage. Clin Plast Surg. 2017;44(3):627–34.
23. Ferguson MW, O'Kane S. Mesh skin grafting. E R Pope PMID: 2405566.
24. Matsuzaki K, Kumagai N, Fukushi S, Ohshima H, Tanabe M, Ishida H. Cultured epithelial autografting on meshed skin graft scars: evaluation of skin elasticity. J Burn Care Rehabil Sep-Oct. 1995;16(5):496–502.
25. Ameer F, Singh AK, Kumar S. Evolution of instruments for harvest of the skin grafts. Indian J Plast Surg. 2013;46(1):28–35.
26. Ogawa R, Hyakusoku H, Ono S. Useful tips for successful skin grafting. J Nippon Med Sch. 2007;74(6):386–92.
27. Cohen AA, Har-Shai L, Ad-El D, Shay T. "POMELO PROJECT" —a simple and low cost simulator for harvesting skin graft by plastic surgery residents. Burns. 2020;46(7):1681–5.
28. Egro FM, Saliu OT, Zhu X, Corcos AC, Ziembicki JA. Dermatome-induced lacerations: an unspoken problem in burn surgery. J Surg Res. 2020;245:45–50.
29. Weyandt GH, Bauer B, Berens N, Hamm H, Broecker EB. Split-skin grafting from the scalp: the hidden advantage. Dermatol Surg. 2009;35(12):1873–9.
30. Croley JAA, Hirshburg JM, Wagner RF Jr. Clinical Pearl: advantages of the scalp as a split-thickness skin graft donor site. Cutis. 2019;103(6):369–70.
31. Oh SJ. A systematic review of the scalp donor site for split-thickness skin grafting. Arch Plast Surg. 2020;47(6):528–34.
32. Chou PR, Wu SH, Hsieh MC, Huang SH. Retrospective study on the clinical superiority of the vacuum-assisted closure system with a silicon-based dressing over the conventional tie-over Bolster technique in skin graft fixation. Medicina (Kaunas). 2019;55(12):781.
33. Bern R, Serror K, Alvo R, Chaouat M, Mimoun M, Schmidt M, Boccara D. Original and modified technique of tie-over dressing: method and application in burn patients. Burns. 2018;44(5):1357–60.
34. Friedstat JS, Klein MB. Acute management of facial burns. Clin Plast Surg. 2009;36(4):653–60.
35. Kalinova KI, Raycheva RD, Petrova N, Uchikov PA. Acute management of deep facial burns. Folia Med (Plovdiv). 2021;63(6):847–57.
36. Abubakar ML, Ibrahim A. Management of facial burns: an update. Curr Opin Otolaryngol Head Neck Surg. 2021;29(4):299–303.
37. Hammer R, Molembi B, Morgenegg M, Mottet L. Management of patients with facial burns. Soins. 2021;66(859):52–4.
38. Zhu XX, Hu DH, Chen B, Han JT, Dong VL, Jia CY, Yao QJ. Clinical management of deep facial burn. Zhonghua Shao Shang Za Zhi. 2006;22(1):19–22.
39. Zhang G, Sun Y, Yan R. Management of deep facial burn with early postburn debridement and delayed skin grafting. Zhonghua Shao Shang Za Zhi. 2001;17(6):327–9.
40. Ahrenholz DH, Clayton MC, Solem LD. Burns and wound management. Otolaryngol Clin North Am. 1995;28(5):1039–55.
41. Griffin JE, Johnson DL. Management of the maxillofacial burn patient: current therapy. J Oral Maxillofac Surg. 2005;63(2):247–52.
42. Philp L, Umraw N, Cartotto R. Late outcomes after grafting of the severely burned face: a quality improvement initiative. J Burn Care Res. 2012;33(1):46–56.
43. Klett A, Rebane R. Reconstructions after periorbital burn injuries. Klin Monbl Augenheilkd. 2013;230(1):23–7.
44. Keilani C, De Faria A, Baus A, Delbarre M, Schaal JV, Froussart-Maille F, Bey E, Duhamel P. Eyelid chemical burns: a multidisciplinary and challenging approach. Ann Burns Fire Disasters. 2021;34(4):312–8.
45. Tost F, Kempin R. Post-surgical management of split-thickness skin grafts in oculoplastic surgery. Klin Monbl Augenheilkd. 2015;232(1):27–32.
46. Bouguila J, Ho Quoc C, Viard R, Brun A, Voulliaume D, Comparin JP, Foyatier JL. Management of eyelid burns. J Fr Ophtalmol. 2011;34(9):655–62.
47. Greenhalgh DG, Hinchcliff K, Sen S, Palmieri TL. A ten-year experience with pediatric face grafts. J Burn Care Res. 2013;34(5):576–84.
48. Tost F. Periocular surgery and the impact of split-thickness skin grafts. Klin Monbl Augenheilkd. 2011;228(1):35–40.
49. Goodwin CW, Maguire MS, McManus WF, Pruitt BA Jr. Prospective study of burn wound excision of the hands. J Trauma Jun. 1983;23(6):510–7.
50. Richards WT, Vergara E, Dalaly DG, Coady-Fariborzian L, Mozingo DW. Acute surgical management of hand burns. J Hand Surg Am. 2014;39(10):2075–85.
51. Pan BS, Vu AT, Yakuboff KP. Management of the acutely burned hand. J Hand Surg Am. 2015;40(7):1477–84. quiz 1485.
52. Mosier MJ, Gibran NS. Surgical excision of the burn wound. Clin Plast Surg. 2009;36(4):617–25.
53. Soni A, Pham TN, Ko JH. Acute management of hand burns. Hand Clin. 2017;33(2):229–36.
54. Dargan D, Kazzazi D, Limnatitou D, Cochrane E, Stubbington Y, Shokrollahi K, Ralston D. Acute management of thermal hand burns in adults: a 10-year review of the literature. Ann Plast Surg. 2021;86(5):517–31.
55. Choi M, Armstrong MB, Panthaki ZJ. Pediatric hand burns: thermal, electrical, chemical. J Craniofac Surg. 2009;20(4):1045–8.
56. Shang F, Hou Q. Effects of allogenic acellular dermal matrix combined with autologous razor-thin graft on hand appearance and function of patients with extensive burn combined with deep hand burn. Int Wound J. 2021;18(3):279–86.
57. Robinson EP, Chhabra AB. Hand chemical burns. J Hand Surg Am. 2015;40(3):605–12.
58. Lou RB, Hickerson WL. The use of skin substitutes in hand burns. Hand Clin. 2009;25(4):497–509.

Full-Thickness Skin Grafting

2

2.1 Introduction

In wide range of skin grafting techniques, full-thickness skin graft (FTSG) represents primary graft technique that is crucial in esthetic enhancements and functional recovery of patients. FTSG also has the following disadvantages: longer surgery duration, limited selection of donor site, graft size, and a lower graft take rate than STSG.

In this chapter, I would like to introduce how to overcome these disadvantages and concomitantly resolve patients' functional and esthetic problems, by studying and developing advanced techniques, particularly for reconstruction of the head and neck as well as the upper and lower extremities. Based on my recently published journal "Skin-fat composite grafts for reconstructing large full-thickness skin defects." I will be introducing in depth: explaining surgical techniques, outlining wider implications and advantages of dermal overgrafting based on clinical experiences on dermabrasion and dermal over grafting, supported with findings on various clinical trials [1]. FTSG with composite fat graft will be discussed futher with an innovative approach.

Examples of rare long-term follow-up results over 10 or 20 years after pediatric FTSG will be encountered further in the chapter.

2.2 Full-Thickness Skin Grafting

Full-thickness skin grafting (FTSG) is a grafting technique that involves the entire dermis, including the epidermis. FTSG procedure results in better skin texture than that is observed after STSG maintaining the original skin color and elasticity of the donor site, causing less contracture on the engrafted skin [2, 3]. FTSG is ideal in surgeries for reconstruction of the joint area, thereby improving the skin color and texture for esthetic benefits [4–6]. However, the available range of the donor sites is limited to both sides of the groin, inner side of the upper arms, or both sides of the small area of the postauricular skin. Skin graft take rate of FTSG is lower than that of STSG. Hematoma and fluid collection can be prevented with various methods with compressive or tie-over dressing technique [7, 8]. For FTSG especially in children, the availability of the donor site for matching skin texture and color must be considered in great care to match the recipient site. Consider the availability of a donor site, sparing of a donor site for the next surgery, and matching of the donor site skin texture and color with those of the recipient site. In the cases of hand and foot burns in children, great efforts must be made to completely repair one affected hand using a graft from one side of donor site on the basis of factors such as whether burns are on

Y.-C. Jang, *The Art of Skin Graft*, https://doi.org/10.1007/978-981-97-0017-2_2

the dorsal or flexor area or both, which fingers are burned, or whether the wrist is affected. This is because for growing children, donor sites are only limited to the two sites: the right and left inguinal regions; thus, if a surgery is planned, surgeons should make a sustained effort to resolve all problems in a one-stage surgery [9–12].

The optimal way of achieving surgical success and avoiding supplemental surgeries is by combining several techniques to obtain a perfect skin graft take rate without losing any of the grafted skin [13–16]. In this chapter, a new surgical technique will be introduced that ensures excellent clinical outcomes and reduces surgery duration. I would like to suggest on the basis of my experiences, the preconceived notions of basic techniques of FTSG. To ensure this, each of the FTSG stereotypes mentioned below has been discussed with additional suggestions on the basis of my experience to date.

First, let us consider the stereotypes regarding the preconceptions about FTSG.

Some queries based on the preconceptions about FTSG are mentioned below:

1. Should the dermal shaving of full-thickness skin be performed as thin as possible to help increase the graft take rate?
2. Does the full-thickness skin graft floor space have to fit enough to the defect size as soon as possible to prevent late contracture of the grafted margin?
3. Is it true that facing a graft to the graft seam line affects the linea contracture and increases the incidence of contracture with unsatisfactory outcomes?
4. Do we have to make slit incisions on the engrafted full-thickness skin to *self-evacuate* blood clot and prevent hematoma and fluid collection?
5. Can full-thickness skin grafts with composite subcutaneous fat survive and be completely accepted?

In response to the first question, I believe the answer is "no." Based on my clinical experience, I have not performed dermal shaving since 2013. On the contrary, I attach dense areolar fat lobules directly beneath the dermis. (a) One larger soft fat lobule (white arrow) and another small dense lobule (black arrow) were noted in the harvested inguinal full-thickness skin. The dense fat lobule layer is attached to the full-thickness skin as a composite fat graft. (b) However, these two types of fat lobule layers are sometimes difficult to distinguish depending on the individual; therefore, surgeons should be able to differentiate them; the ability to do so depends on the surgeon's experience with such cases (Fig. 2.1), which results in better outcomes in terms of increased graft take rate and fast postoperative graft remodeling [17, 18]. In general, most surgeons believe that the incidence rate of skin graft failure is high and post-grafting esthetic enhancements decline due to bulky unsightly appearance of the grafted skin, even if the graft is accepted. However, personally, I have not experienced any case of complete skin graft failure or substantial bulky appearance. This might be because of the high number of fat lobules that promote angiogenesis and bleed control as well as prevention of hematoma formation. The soft fat tissue might block the empty space in the severed blood vessels in the wound bed, thus controlling the bleeding easily. Recently, some studies have suggested that fat and endothelial cells share the same mesodermal origin embryologically, the former might be somewhat involved in angiogenesis and the graft acceptance [19–21]. Future studies should investigate this relationship between fat cells and endothelial cell of blood vessel involvement.

I ensure marginal full release of 2 or 3 cm underneath the scar wound margin tension free to prevent bulkiness without marginal contracture, due to this method the result have been smooth.

Regarding the second question, most surgeons believe that, if possible, sufficient supplementary full-thickness skin can reduce postoperative scar contracture of the engrafted skin with good results [22]. Generally, postop-

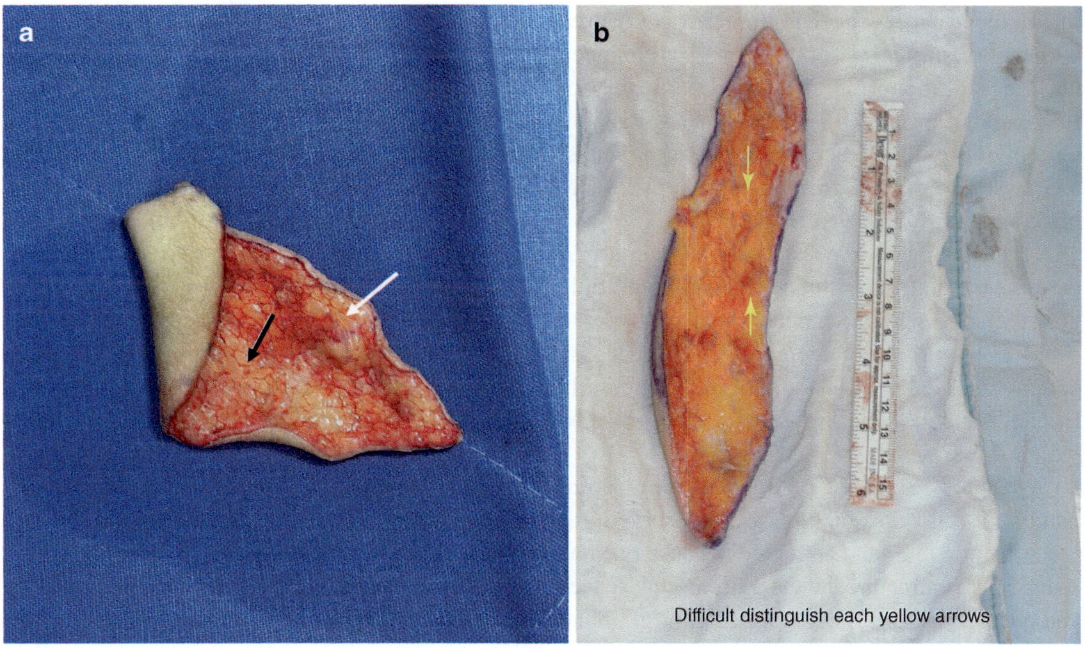

Fig. 2.1 (**a**) One larger soft fat lobule (white arrow) and another small dense lobule (black arrow) were noted in the harvested inguinal full-thickness skin in a child. (**b**) Note the maximal size 7 × 23 cm in an adult. But this two types of fat lobule layers are sometimes difficult to distinguish depending on the individual

erative scar contracture is more common and severe in STSG when the engrafted skin is not enough in size or thinner in skin thickness, wherein engrafted skin has significant contracture; but, in FTSG, remodeling occurs in the entire engrafted skin bed as the graft matures; thus, the contracture incidence is lower or well adapted. In general, it is believed that when FTSG is performed, sufficient graft amount is necessary to avoid contracture. However, considering the long-term outcomes of FTSG in children, it can be noted that the engrafted skin grows along the original skin and expands through rearrangement, despite an insufficient graft amount. The long-term (>10 years) follow-up results reported in this part are not commonly observed around the globe.

(a) In my early days as a surgeon (15 years ago), I used the conventional dermal shaving method to perform full-thickness engraftment; (b) postoperative 1 year after view; (c) and (d) postoperative 2 and 3 years after view. Even after 2 years, there was no contracture or deformity in this growing child; (e) and (f) postoperative 10- and 23-year view (Fig. 2.33). It is necessary to conduct further studies on the remodeling process of full-thickness skin [23]. Nevertheless, based on my clinical experience and the long-term follow-up results of the children, the engrafted skin is well adjusted without any special alterations; moreover, there were only few cases of reoperation because of contracture. Furthermore, in my experience, a slightly insufficient graft amount in FTSG results in mild tension that compresses the wound beds, which enhances bleed control and reduces hematoma complications, increasing graft take rate.

The size of the excised skin defect size was 5.5 × 10 cm. The size of the harvested donor skin size was 4.5 × 13 cm, in elliptical shape (note the attached fat layer). The defect was covered with mild stretching controlled by balanced tension and anchoring aided with elasticity of full-thickness skin. (b) For even compression, a tie-over dressing was used. (c) After 3 weeks, a completely grafted area with no skin loss or hematoma was observed (Fig. 2.2).

Regarding the third question, in my opinion, if possible the graft area should not feature multiple grafts in one operation field when possible to avoid poor surgical outcomes. This is because contraction begins at the seam line, particularly in hand surgery, grafting should be performed with a single sheet.

When the results of both hands were compared, the following findings were observed: (a) less effect on left hand appeared because of linea seam line contracture in the interdigital spaces and palm areas. (b) The texture of the right hand was more natural and tighter in elasticity. By using a single sheet of FTSG, no contracted seam line in the interdigital space or the palm area was observed (Fig. 2.3). This is an important factor that is often missed by general surgeons while especially performing hand surgery.

Regarding the fourth question, most surgeons tend to make multiple slit incisions on the STSG to increase its graft take rate and prevent hematomas and fluid collections. This pratice of multiple slit incisions is also applied in FTSG, or silastic drains are made in regions that are at risk of hematomas or silastic drains or small portable suction instruments are used. In my opinion, such incisions leave tiny unsightly scars, compromising the esthetic effect of the graft, and should be reserved only for cases with high bleeding tendency or less effective bleed control sites. One of the common questions may follow what if a hematoma occurs? My answer is just simple: in such cases, the problem should be resolved by making slit incisions at that time of finding the hematoma and daily application of saline-soaked gauze dressing following an open operation wound.

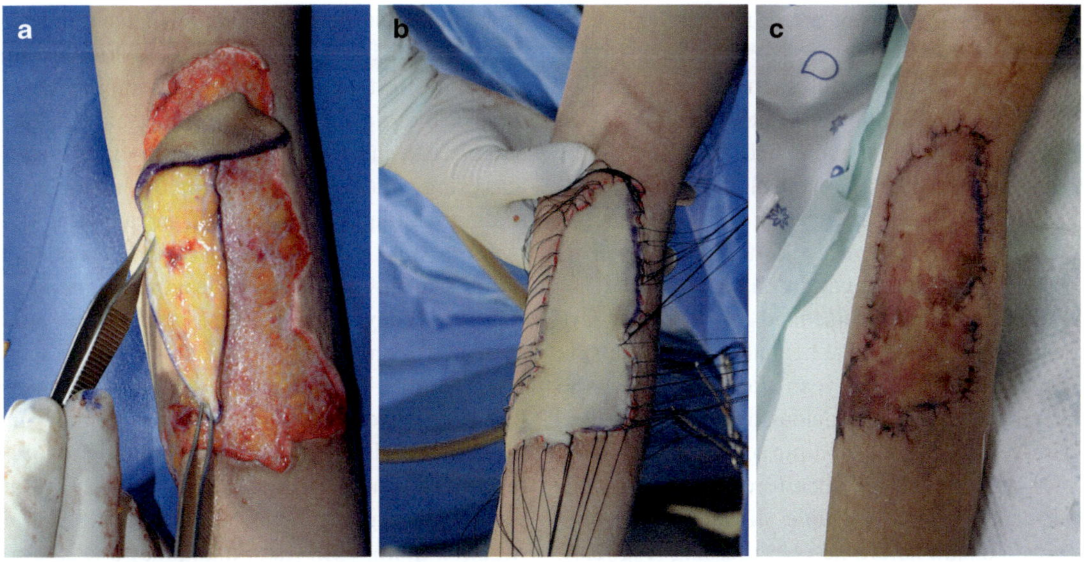

Fig. 2.2 (**a**) The excised skin defect size was measured 5.5 × 10 cm and the harvested donor skin size was measured elliptical in shape 4.5 × 13 cm (note the attached fat layer). The defect was covered with mild tension according to balanced tension anchoring to all direction. (**b**) Tie-over dressing was performed for even compression. (**c**) Postoperative view 3 weeks after, complete graft was taken

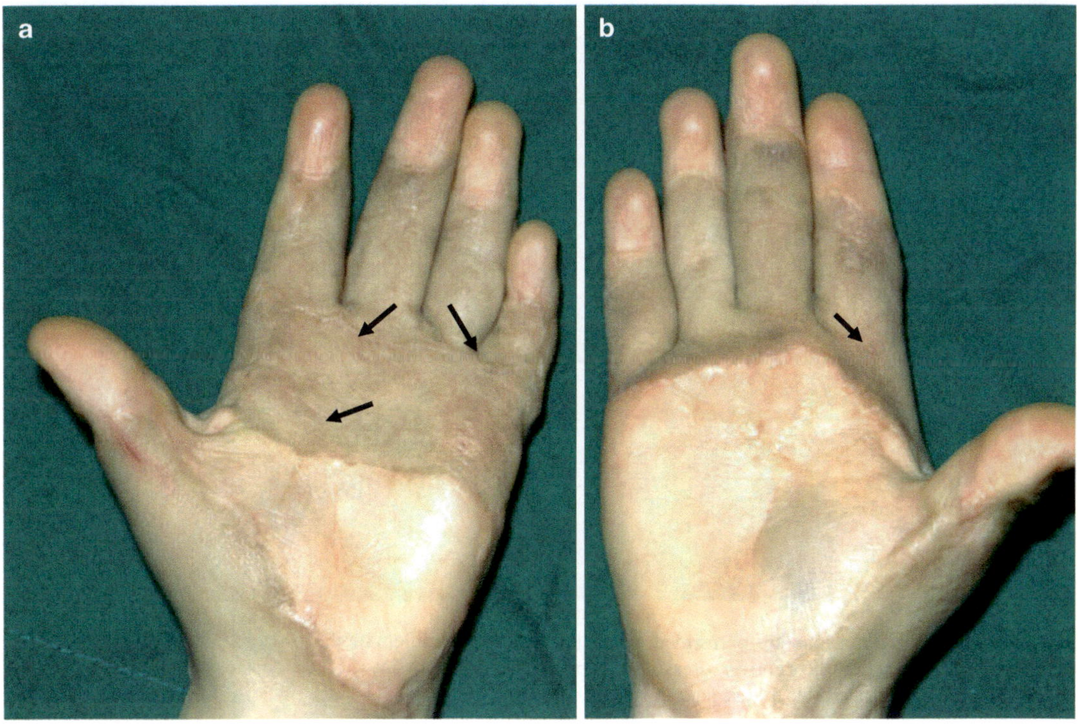

Fig. 2.3 (**a**) Less effect due to linea seam line contracture on the left interdigital and palm side (black arrows). (**b**) Compare the end result (**a**) and (**b**). Right is more natural and has elastic texture. Note the single-sheet FTSG without seam line in the right palm (black arrow)

The author does not prefer making a slit incision before applying a tie-over dressing, except for special circumstances such as high bleeding tendency or difficult bleed control sites. (a) When tie-over dressing is open, and if hematoma is observed, multiple incision slits are made followed with daily application of saline-soaked dressing (black arrow). If the hematoma is observed during tie-over dressing removal, I prefer a twice-daily saline-soaked gauze compressive dressing to evacuate the hematoma until the skin is recovered. (b) One year after the surgery, no skin problem on the previous hematoma site was observed, except for multiple scars at slit-incision sites (yellow arrow). Therefore, the author does not make habitual multiple slit incisions on the engrafted skin before tie-over dressing (Fig. 2.4). Although this problem might appear difficult to understand, the ability to comprehend and resolve such complications comes with experience and constant effort, to overcome this complication. I control the bleeding by performing an effective surgery causing fewer injuries, fast wound coverage using engrafting skin for rapid bleed control, sealing the tiny bleeding points, and applying tie-over dressing. As an additional remark, I routinely performed tie-over dressing leaving on for periods of 5–6 days. This increases the take rate and prevent hematoma.

Regarding the fifth question, previously there has been reports of clinical experimental surgery that used similar technique but only involving much smaller FTSG region [24–27]. But almost all surgeons believed that the full size of inguinal donor skin (maximal about 8 × 25 cm) with subcutaneous fat composite graft will have

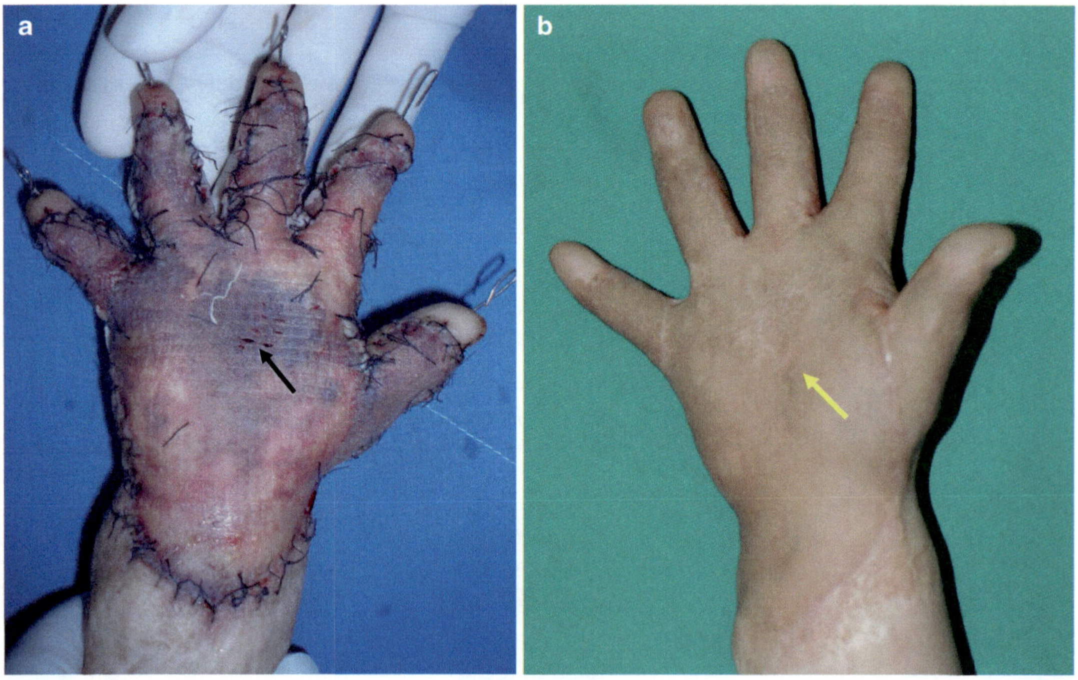

Fig. 2.4 (**a**) The slit incisions are performed, when the hematoma is found after the tie-over dressing is open (black arrow). (**b**) Postoperative 1 year later, note there is no skin problem on the previous hematoma site except for multiple scars at slit incision sites (yellow arrow)

a higher failure take rate, so they do not attempt to use larger size. However, the author actively applied full size skin grafts from inguinal donor sites in order to improve surgical outcomes, and the results have been published recently. More effective and systemized graft techniques will be introduced, which involve a wider range of functional and esthetic benefits of full-thickness skin grafts.

Changing our perception about FTSG, which has been habitually performed as mentioned above, improving the technique through new approaches will help us achieve the desirable grafting outcomes. I earnestly hope that the information presented in this book will move us closer to our ultimate goal of ensuring excellent patient outcomes and believe that persistent and fresh attempts as well as sincere efforts are necessary to enhance a surgeon's competence.

2.3 A Guide to Obtain Excellent FTSG Outcomes (Based on My Basic Preparation and Skills)

2.3.1 Bleed Control

The success or failure in achieving bleed control depends on the surgical technique, which is a crucial and fundamental factor in all types of surgery that significantly affects surgical outcomes and is a key factor influencing surgical success, particularly in FTSG [28]. My consideration regarding skin grafting and reconstructive burn plastic surgery for which my response tends to be negative execution. These include the following: (1) no bleed control with electrocauterization; (2) no use of tourniquet instrument during surgeries involving the hands, feet, and upper and lower extremities [29, 30]; and (3) no slit incision on the engrafted skin during operation to prevent hematoma. The features mentioned above of my surgical style are the results of consistent attempts and training myself. The reason I avoid using the methods mentioned in points 1 and 2 can be attributed to my unique bleed control method, which will be discussed in the following section.

2.3.1.1 Bleed Control Technique

Mentioned above bleed control technique is relatively simple, the fact that not many surgeons are confident enough to perform it makes it difficult. Many surgeons doubt the ability of epinephrine injections to control the bleeding from shallow regions [31–33]. This is possible because the subdermal plexus supplies the blood to the entire dermal layer through an intradermal perforator; hence, substantial bleeding should be controlled directly at the intradermal level. In other words, since the blood is supplied via blood connection within the dermis through other sites of subdermal perforator, bleed control in the subdermal plexus is not effective (Fig. 2.5). The epinephrine dilution ratio is recommended to not exceed high concentration of 1:100,000 in the small operation field, but the dilution ratio range can increase from 1:200,000 to 1:400,000 or more if the surgical site is wide as like chest or breast area. Sufficient diluted epinephrine-soaked gauze should also be prepared, and the absorbent compress dressing should be applied to the surgical site on the occurrence of bleeding [34, 35]. In the occasional incidence of arterial bleeding, electrocauterization is avoided, instead fine mosquito clamps are used to stop the bleeding of arterioles; this is followed by the injection of a small amount of epinephrine solution to coat the surrounding area. If the bleeding continues on releasing the clamps after approximately 5 minutes, the area is tied with a silk hand tie or surgical tie. The reason behind no use of electrocauterization and electric surgical knife is to avoid multiple points of artificial burns on flesh tissue, but the primary purpose is to avoid

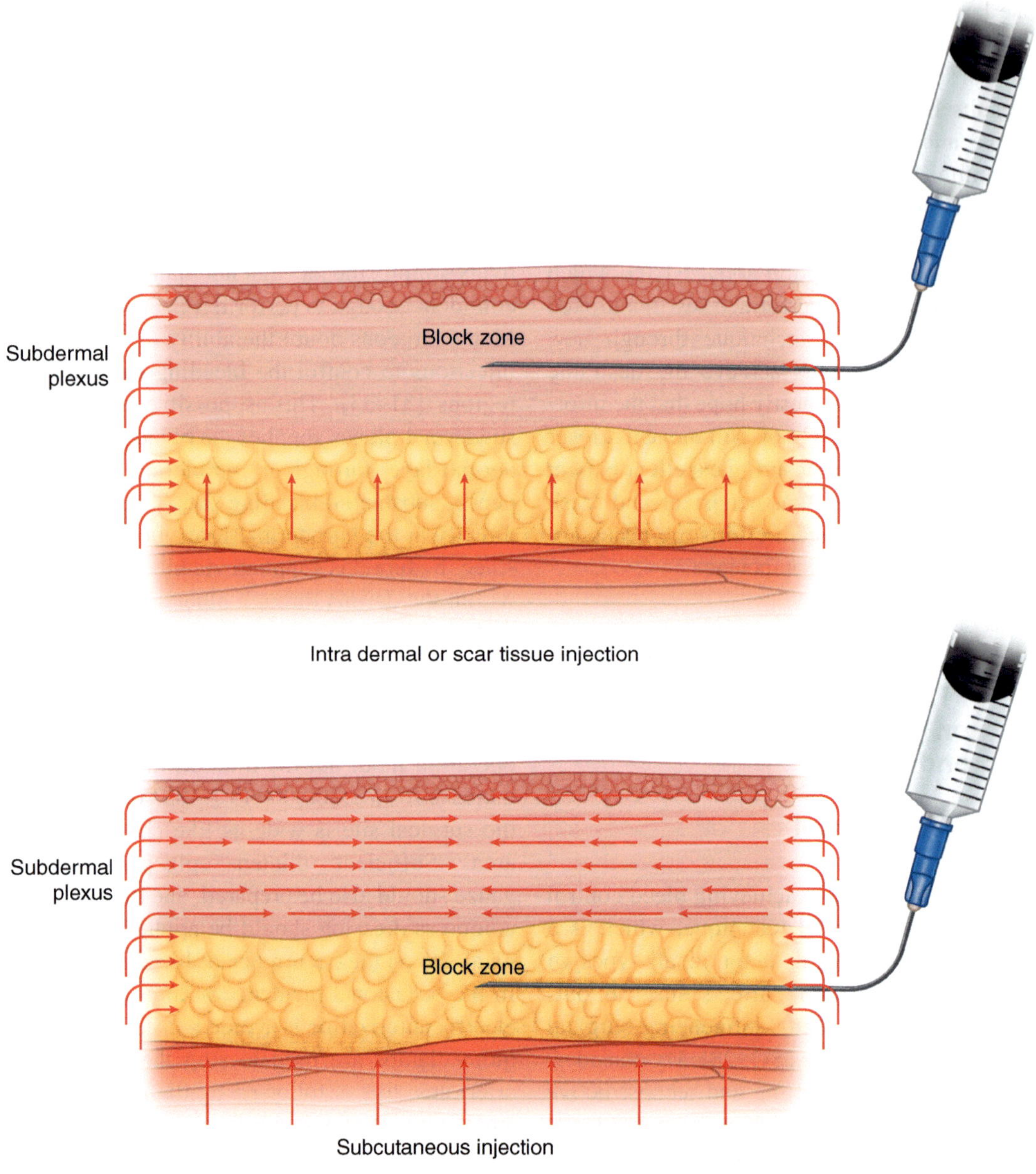

Fig. 2.5 The key point technique is to almost bend the needle at the right angle (white arrow) and place it alongside the parallel injection region. Injection is administered deeply in the intradermal or intrascar tissues, not at the subcutaneous level, and deep enough to reach end of the injection site, then slowly tapered backward with film injection to confirm the observation of a whitish hard wheal elevation (red dashed line). This action is repeated from one injection site to the next with the direction changing in a fan out-fashion (arrow marking pen)

increasing surgery duration. A clean and fast surgery is crucial for surgical success, particularly in case of FTSG. As epinephrine maximum hemostasis lasts up to 2–3 hours, and if rebound bleeing occurs and to avoid using additional epinephrine, I try keep the surgery duration short. In the case of difficult surgeries such as hand surgery with severe contracture where the palm and multiple fingers are involved, I rarely operate over 3 hours with tie-over dressing included. This excludes the time of donor site repair. The following reasons are mentioned below:

1. To save time that is wasted in the unnecessary use of electrocauterization and tourniquet setting time.
2. To decrease the time spent in dissection for which an electric surgical knife is used because it requires bleed control with cauterization for every bleeding point.
3. Avoid suturing multiple pieces, try to keep the sheet as larger whole piece, especially in hand surgery.
4. To save time through engraft suture using tie-over dressing which is possible while simultaneously performing marginal graft skin suture and compressive tie dressing on an operation wound.

By taking the factors mentioned above into consideration, the surgery can be completed within a short duration. During my 20 years of experience as a hand surgeon, I have not used tourniquets or rubber bands in the surgery of the hands and fingers of children or adults, except in the earlier period. In several thousand cases of finger and hand surgeries performed by me so far, the bleeding was controlled using epinephrine injections, and there have been only two cases of an unfortunate loss of fingers. These two incidences were not due to epinephrine injections; hence, we should overcome the stereotyped preconceptions.

Epinephrine injection, particularly into the fingers, requires experience and skills of the injector, an attempt should be made carefully, and the administration range should be increased gradually. The key feature of a local epinephrine injection is that it must be forced into the intradermal or intrascar tissue and not merely the subcutaneous or subdermal tissue. Therefore, sufficient pressure must be applied during the injection so that a whitish hard, raised wheal appears on the skin; this ensures the effective control of bleeding due to a perforator of the subdermal plexus [36–38].

A suggestion related to the injection technique would be to keep the needle in parallel with the surface of the surgical site and insert into the skin to the end of the intradermal layer, without exceeding it. The trick is to make a wheal through a forced injection while slowly performing the withdrawal tapering. An interlocking syringe is useful for this purpose.

Injectional bleed control with epinephrine is one of the most important techniques described in this book. The key point technique is to almost bend the needle at the right angle (white arrow) and place it alongside the parallel injection region. Injection is administered deeply in the intradermal or intrascar tissues, not at the subcutaneous level, and deep enough to reach the end of the injection site, and then slowly tapered backward with film injection to confirm the observation of a whitish hard wheal elevation (red dashed line). This action is repeated from one injection site to the next with the direction changing in a fan-out fashion (arrow marking pen) (Figs. 2.5 and 2.6).

Generally, a 23- or 24-G needle is suitable in the scope of small lesions, whereas a 24-G needle or spinal needle can be used in the scope of larger lesions. Thus, if bleed control is effectively possible, electrocauterization or tourniquets are unnec-

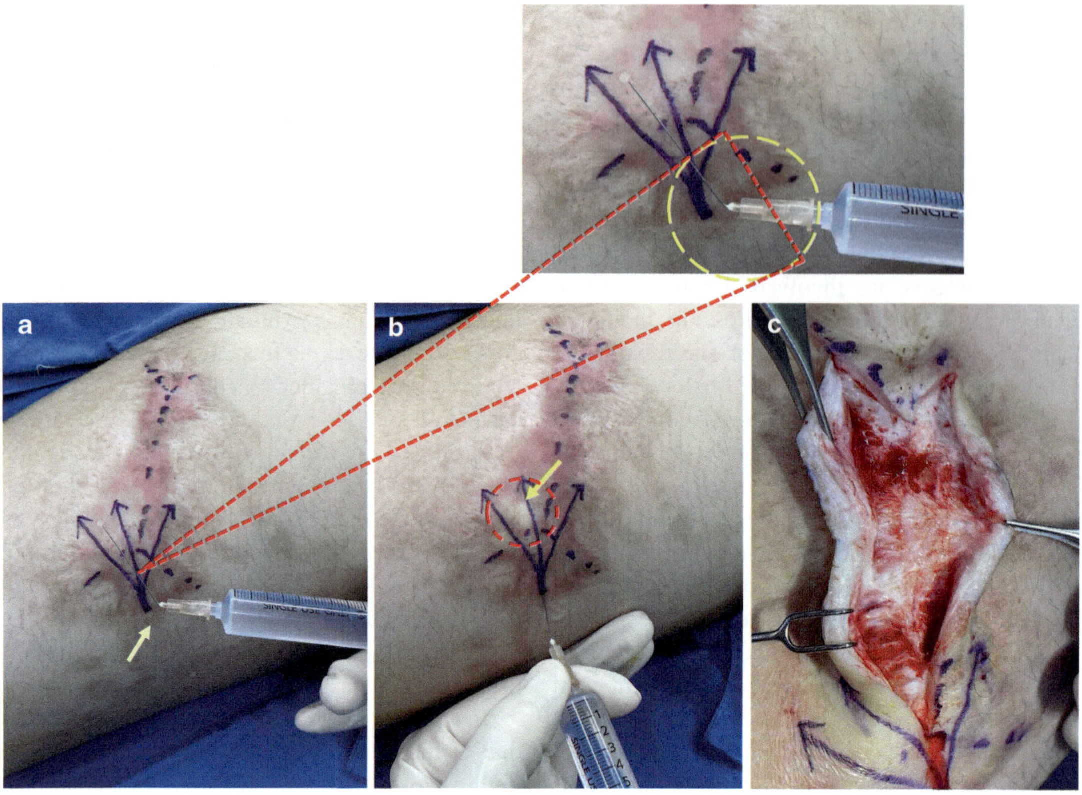

Fig. 2.6 (**a**) Bend the needle of the starting point almost at the right angle (white arrow) and place the needle alongside the parallel injection region. (**b**) Injection is performed deeply intradermally or at the intrascar tissue not at the subcutaneous level and deep to reach and slowly taper backward with film injection to confirm an observation of whitish hard wheal elevation (red dashed line and yellow arrow). (**c**) Intraoperative view, excellent bleed control was observed with simple epinephrine injection only

essary; hence, the chances of avoiding a multiple slit incision above described in Sect. 2.3.1.1 (3) effectively reduce operation time.

Therefore, the shortcut to obtain a high-quality skin graft involves injection-related bleed control and familiarity with the procedure. Owing to prolonged history of clinical practice, most hand surgeons still tend to restrict the use of epinephrine injection to the hands and feet, including fingers and toes. However, if the surgery is performed while adhering to the injection level mentioned above, epinephrine flows out mostly during the procedure because the incision and dissection levels match the injection point, which reduces the risk of perturbed blood supply. In the early stages of learning the skill, it is a good practice to make only simple attempts at incisions and not forcibly perform slit incisions as skin loss due to hematomas is an undesirable outcome. With increased experience and hand adjustment gained through the gradual reduction of the number of times, slit incisions according to effective bleed control are performed, the surgeons will be able to ensure clean and excellent surgical outcomes without any skin loss.

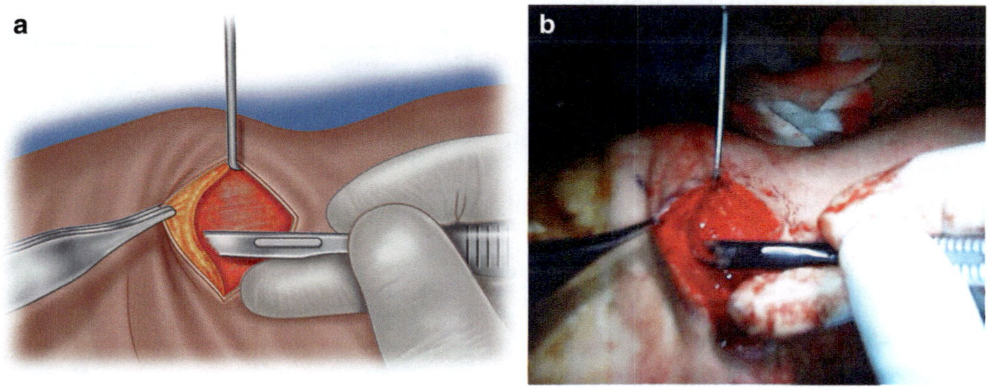

Fig. 2.7 The diagram shows using a No. 10 or 15 blade edge lay down shaving tissue not cut or direct incision. This scalpel dissection may be performed on the same level of epinephrine injected level

All the surgical cases introduced in this book that I have lead, only epinephrine injections were used to control bleeding and not used electrocauterization or tourniquets.

2.3.2 Dissection Technique

My dissection technique is one of the key factors involved in bleed control technique; dissecting scissors such as Metzenbaum, Steven's scissors, and sharp iris scissors as well as electric surgical knife are avoided, except for surgical blades Nos. 10 and 15. This is because the use of scissors usually leads to a deeper dissection than intended. The movement of the inner blade and the outer blade of the scissor can mangle the skin tissue in between, which can also rise chances of directly cutting a vessel, leading to severe tissue injuries. The key consideration for scalpel dissection is to perform a beveled sharp angled dissection using the edge of a knife and try to avoid direct incision and straight cut with the scalpel. The point of dissection technique is also a very important skill. The key point is to perform a dissection with a scalpel instead of a cut or direct incision manner; it is recommended to perform a dissection with No. 10- or 15 blade laid down diagonally for slicing tissue. This scalpel dissection can be made at the same layer level as the epinephrine injection (Fig. 2.7). The advantage of such dissection is that because the injection site is almost at the same level as the intended dissection site, the injected epinephrine solution effectively controls bleeding and released; thus, a local injection into the fingers is also possible and safer. Other advantages include: reduced surgery duration and efficient scar release; the surgeons do not need to worry about the exposure of the tendon, joint capsule, or the bone, which is a significant concern for hand surgeons. This topic is important in reconstructive burn surgery and will be covered in another chapter, and how it helped me to resolve and avoid complications in most hand reconstruction surgeries using only a simple skin graft, without the need for performing flap surgeries including local, reverse, or free flaps. These bleed control and dissection technique are resolving problems with simple skin graft without any other flap surgery on all of my burnt hand reconstruction.

2.3.3 Donor Selection and Repair

Because of the limitation of donor site selection, it is essential to plan well in advance regarding the efficient use of the limited donor skin. First, the following questions should be considered:

1. Is the affected site a joint area or does it require FTSG?
2. Are either sides affected or only a single side?
3. Is the patient a child or an adult?
4. If a region requires functional FTSG, has the donor site already been used or was it lost due to a burn?

To perform a successful, one-time pediatric hand reconstruction warrants more careful planning. An efficient FTSG is crucial for joint recovery; therefore, surgeons must keep in mind to be familiar with both fundamental and high-level FTSG techniques. It is difficult to harvest sufficient full-thickness skin in children as the donor site is limited to only two sites in the inguinal region. Therefore, I have always tried to resolve all problems in a single surgery for pediatric patients whenever possible, the results will be subsequently discussed in detail. Because functional joint recovery for pediatric patients is of a great importance, the preparatory process and technology associated with FTSGs have been also discussed.

I prefer to harvest a graft from the inguinal donor site in an elliptical shape such that the incision line does not cross over the image line of the superior iliac spine. The engrafted recipient site should be inconspicuous if possible; the skin color darkens closer to the inner thigh, and the thickness of the skin graft should match that of the recipient site of thickness as the skin at the upper border is thinner than that of the lower border.

The territory of donor skin collection does not extend beyond the superior iliac spine (red dashed circle). Surgeons must understand the characteristics of donor skin thickness, such as upper thinner and lower thicker, as well as color,

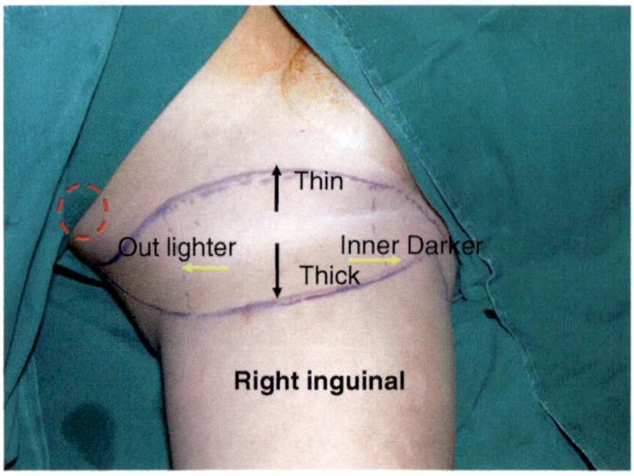

Fig. 2.8 The territory of donor skin collection does not extend beyond the superior iliac spine (red dashed circle). Take note, this should be maximum collectable donor skin size in children

such as outer lighter and inner darker. Usually, the maximum width of the donor skin is 5 cm in children and 7 cm in adults; these sizes have fewer complications with direct primary closure. However, a donor skin length of over 20 cm can be taken from the outer lateral thigh to the inner thigh in case of adults. This figure shows the maximum collectible territory of donor skin in children (Fig. 2.8). Dissecting scissors are recommended, if possible, for harvesting a graft by separating the tissues between the small dense subcutaneous fat layer and the fat layer with larger fat lobules underneath it. These two layers are more distinct in children than in adults (Fig. 2.1). In donor sites' suture scar, long and wide scars might be unsightly and cause psychological stress, particularly in children and young women; hence, wounds should be repaired by adjusting the heights of the sewing points in the dermal layers of varying thicknesses. For example, the inguinal skin is thin on the abdominal side and thick on the thigh side; therefore, when performing wound elevation, the height of the subdermal suture site should be raised by at least 1–2 cm to adjust the heights of the upper and lower layers in order to achieve an esthetic effect without the later appearance of disruption and wide donor-wound scars (Fig. 2.9).

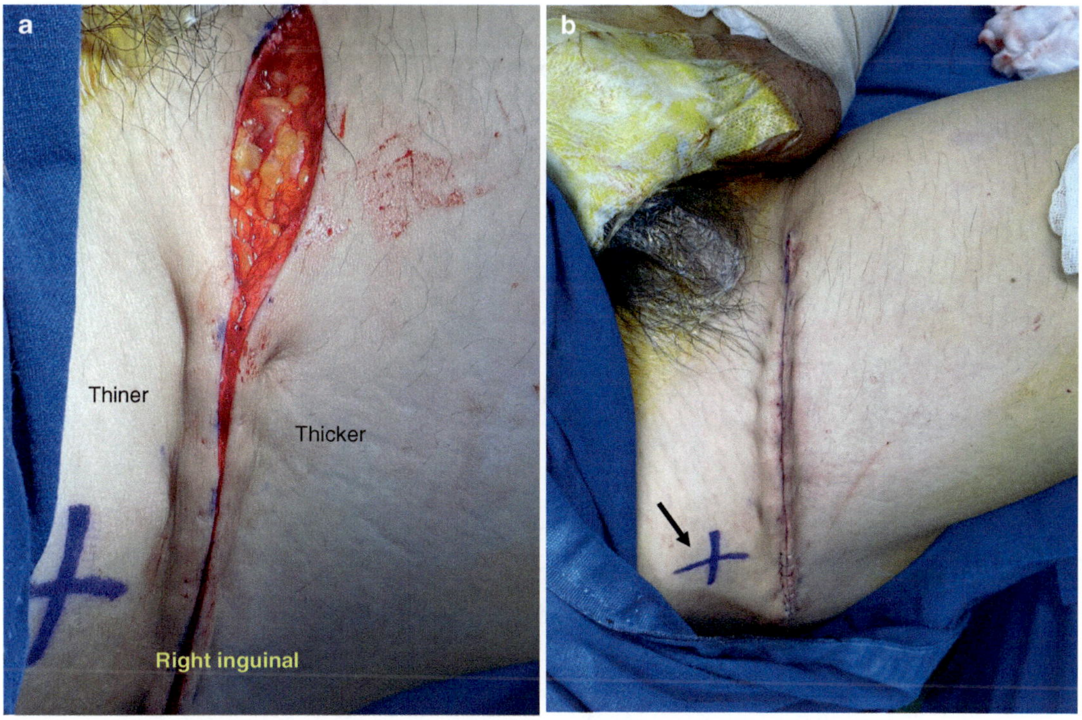

Fig. 2.9 (**a**) Donor wounds should be repaired by adjusting the heights of the sewing points in the dermal layers of varying thicknesses. (**b**) The extent of elevated wound suture is at least over 1 or 2 cm or more. Abdominal side skin is thinner, deeper, and more elevated to the opposite thicker upper thigh side skin. This will give a better result at the end. GV marking (black arrow) is superior iliac spine location

2.3.4 Full-Thickness Skin Engraft Technique

Full-thickness skin is thick and soft, unless wound bed bleeding is controlled, it is prone to hematomas; however, detecting a hematoma through the thick skin is challenging. Because of this possibility and concerns regarding this situation, many surgeons tend to open earlier the tie-over dressing within 2–3 days, or slit incisions are made on the engrafted skin to determine whether there is a hematoma or not. Therefore the wound margin mentioned above (Fig. 2.10) of wound bed bleed control is a crucial point to determine the success of the surgery with best results.

In many cases, bleeding is not controlled easily at the graft margin; hence, I use the following engrafting suture techniques to overcome this problem. For tie-over sutures, the surgeon should start operating at the engraft skin margin from the inner side to the outer side and make a knot, sliding it toward the outer side to achieve a pulling effect so that the graft margin is firmly tightened and slightly elevated. In cases of suspected bleeding, when stitching the engrafted skin margin to the wound margin, an extra stitch is sewn under the wound margin, to aid bleed control. (Fig. 2.10). A tip to reduce the wound margin tension is to free the wound margin from the scar bed if possible and stitch the wound bed

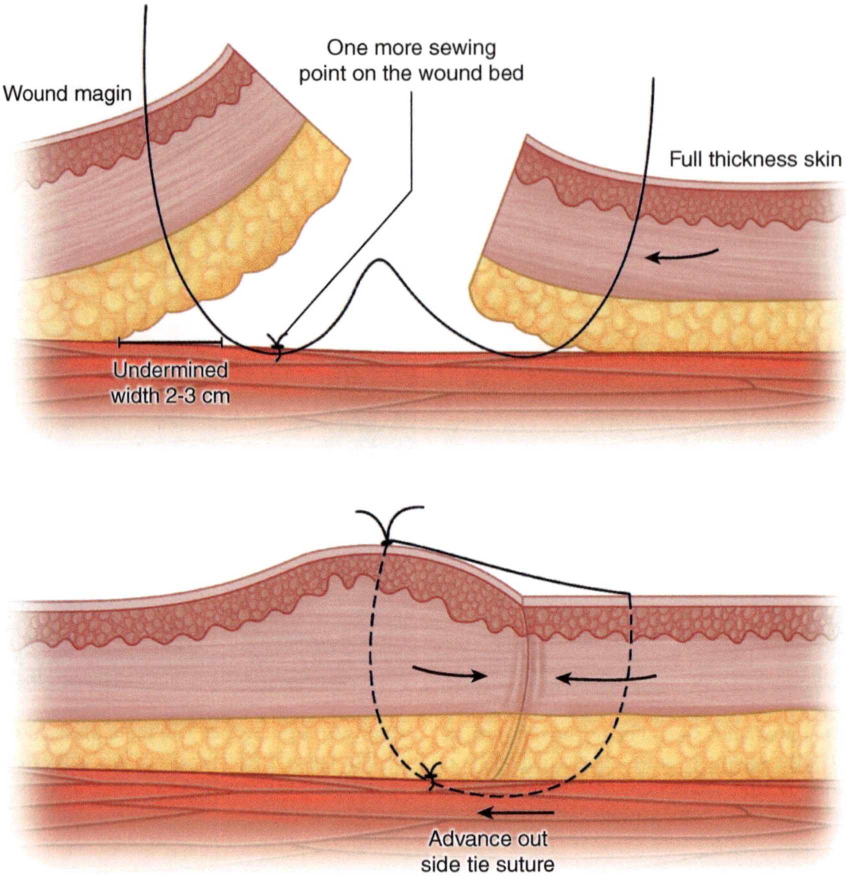

Fig. 2.10 In conjunction with tie-over suturing, this procedure allows bleed control effectively from the graft margin, and occasionally performed sewing fixation at the wound bed allows a wider engrafting floor space, leading to wound effective maturation, which reduces the chances of marginal wound contracture

approximately 2–3 cm inside the undermined bed to ensure a wider engrafting floor space.

In conjunction with tie-over suturing (contributes to reducing operation duration), this procedure allows effective control of bleeding from the graft margin, and occasionally performed sewing fixation at the wound bed allows a wider engrafting floor space, leading to wound maturation, reducing the chances of marginal wound contracture (Fig. 2.10).

Full-thickness skin engraft techniques must stick to this principle, with initial sutures placed on the engrafted skin's edge and working outward to the wound margin. I normally perform dissections with 2–3 cm extra in advance to inner side wound margin and later on the way one more secure suture at wound bed (yellow arrow) and next wound margin suture perform because common bleeding points are frequently located on the wound margin. (engrafted skin margin start—next undermined wound bed one anchoring suture—final outside of wound margin and suture tie) (Figs. 2.10, 2.11).

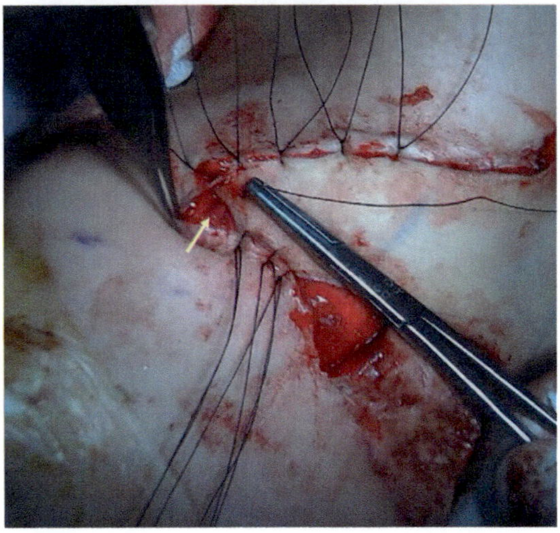

Fig. 2.11 Start initial suture on the edge of engraft skin to the outside of the wound margin (engraft skin margin start to undermined wound bed one anchoring suture to outside of wound margin and tie)

When possible I avoid making a long straight suture line, instead, I occasionally make fish-mouth cuts to break up the straight line to irregular zigzag broken line, to lessen the recontracture. This is crucial for preventing delayed postoperative scar contracture and should be confirmed on the basis of long-term follow-up results in addition to previous experiences.

To prevent postoperative recontracture, create a zigzag flap to break the long straight line (multiple arrows). Note the clean operation field; I did not use a tourniquet or an electric surgical knife, and cauterization was performed using only epinephrine injection for bleed control (Fig. 2.12).

As full-thickness skin is elastic and resilient, it can retract and anchor to a triangular space created with a slit (dart) incision. In the author's experience with long-term follow-up results, there were no signs of recontracture or disfigurement, especially in children (Fig. 2.13).

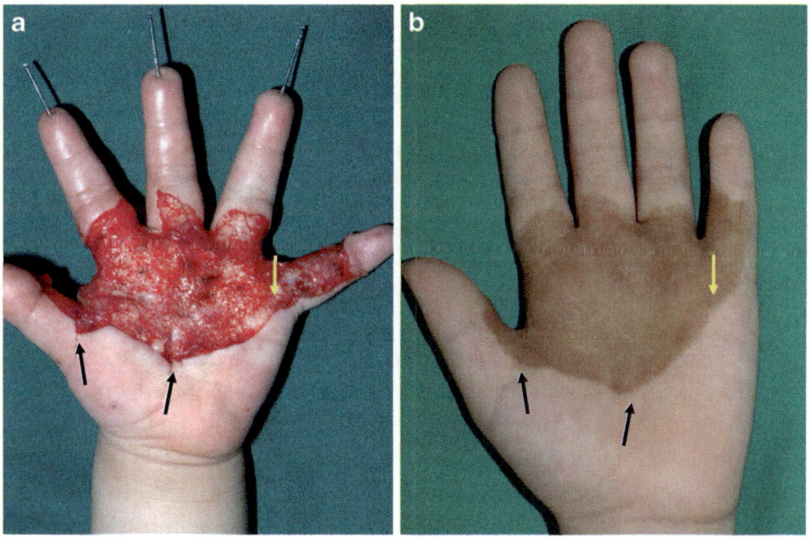

Fig. 2.12 (**a**) Making zigzag flap to break the long straight line to prevent postoperative recontracture (multiple arrows). Note the effective bleed control with only epinephrine injection. (**b**) Compare results with 5 years after the surgery

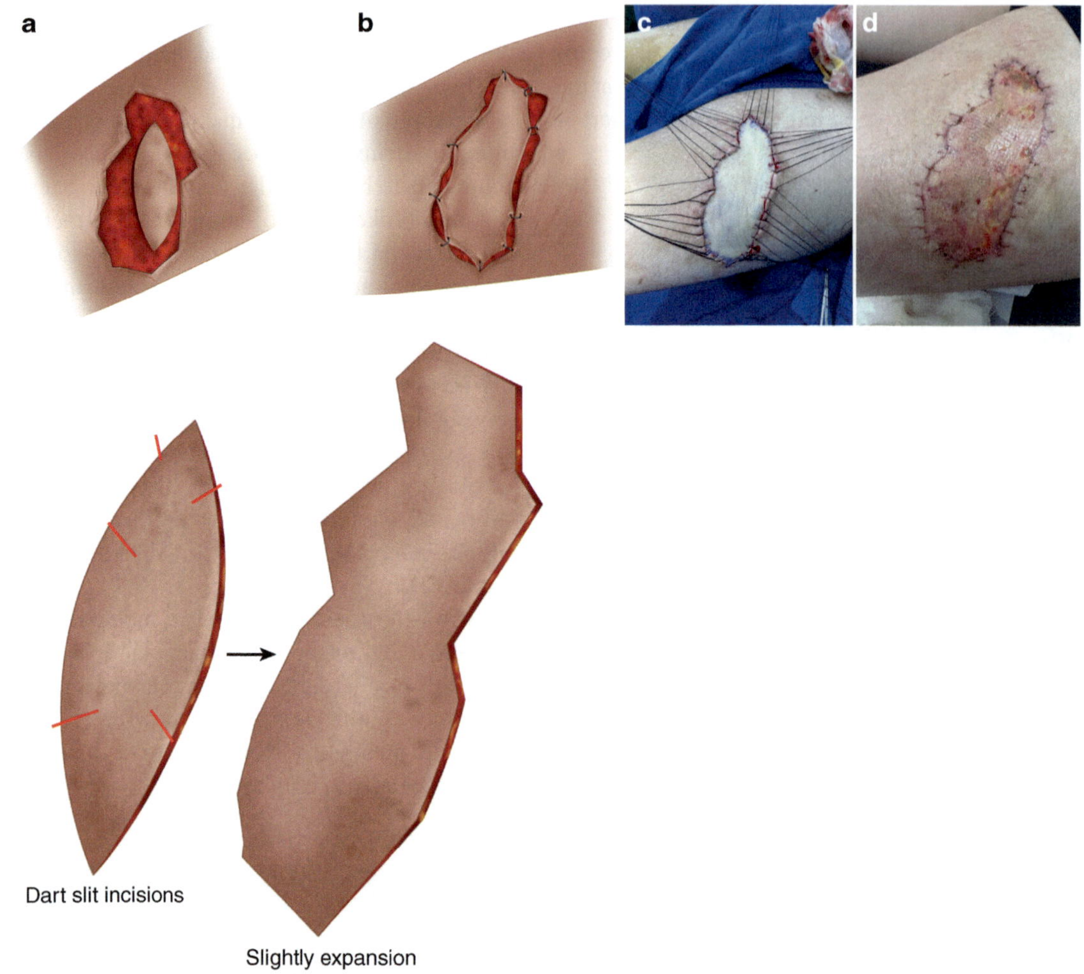

Fig. 2.13 (**a**) Full-thickness skin is elastic and resilient; (**b**) it can retract and anchor to the triangular space created with slit cut. (**c**, **d**) In author's experience of long-term follow-up result, there were no recontracture and disfigurement especially in children. Because full-thickness skin is elastic and resilient, it can retract and anchor to a triangular space created with a slit (dart) incision. In the author's experience with long-term follow-up results, there was no any recontracture or disfigurement, especially in children

This technique is a very important procedure to prevent postoperative scar contracture. Therefore, with increasing experiences, you have to consistently check the long-term follow-up results while learning to master the precise skill and developing discernment.

2.3.5 Soft Tissue Inserted K-Wire Fixation Technique

I developed this unique immobilization technique for long time. In this technique, a K-wire is inserted into the soft tissue (not the phalangeal bone itself) horizontally alongside the fingertip to the direction of the palm, manually by hand not a hand drill instrument. The main point of this technique, the five fingers should be in maximally hyperextended position, maintaining the thumb and little finger at the maximal abduction position. A K-wire is inserted deeply though from the tip of the thumb to hypothenar, and another from tip of the little finger to hyperthenar.

This technique is important and useful, especially for children. Note the direction of each finger and maintain maximum extension of the fingers and expansion of the engrafted skin surface. The K-wire must be inserted deeply into the bottom of the palm (dashed arrows).

The insertion technique begins at the fingertip and is forcefully inserted alongside the soft tissue of the fingers; occasionally, the K-wire passes through the flexor tendon, but tendon injury is rare.

When the K-wire reaches the MP joint area, the procedure may be paused because of the bump of the volar plate; at this point, recline the finger, smoothly cross over the volar plate, and continue to the bottom of the palm (red dashed circles).

Note: Twenty years ago, I used to perform dermal shaving procedure on the full-thickness donor skin and slit incisions, not routine tie-over dressings.

This is performed to prevent hematoma by maintaining the maximal engraft space and making an immobilization fixation. The K-wire can be easily removed by pulling it out by hand approximately 2 or 3 weeks after grafting, which provides adequate time for the engrafted skin to be taken. This K-wire insertion technique has several advantages such as reduced possibilities of injuries due to bone drilling, no adverse effects, and ease of removal. Therefore, this method is useful for finger and hand immobilization in children who are unwilling to cooperate as well as in adults who have severe flexor deformities or articular joint dislocation. Leave the wire in adult hands for a little longer after the graft is accepted. This can facilitate the prevention of joint recontractures or dislocation. However, if finger contracture has progressed due to joint dislocation for an extended time, bony fixation should be performed through the joint space.

2.3.6 Tie-Over Dressing

Tie-over dressing is the last step in the surgery, which is a significant factor in determining surgical success or failure [39]. Therefore, I routinely perform tie-over suturing in cases of all FTSG but try to complete the surgery and pay full attention. This technique involves gently and evenly compressing the engrafted skin to prevent the formation of hematomas or seromas between the engrafted skin and wound bed. The role of tie-over dressing is to protect the engrafted skin by maintaining even compression state to the attachment between the graft and wound bed [8]. After completion of tie-over suturing, for the protection of the engrafted skin, it is covered with a fine mesh paste created with either petrolatum or antibiotic ointments. We can also conveniently use Bactigras™ (Smith & Nephew, England) big hole mesh gauze. Compressive dressing is performed with saline-soaked fluffy gauze, such as fine chip gauze, 4 × 4-gauze pads, and surgical pads, depending on the surgery site, which is generally prepared in advance before or during operation. I do not use cotton balls because they are too soft and dry adequately when compressed and maintain its wetness stage throughout the surgery [8, 39, 40].

The tie-over silk threads should be applied with even pressure to ensure their symmetry on either side, so that the threads reverse fan out shape. The empty spaces between the wound margin and tie-over silk thread should be tightly filled in with small pieces of gauze. Be mindful of the dead space created when the threads are pulled to close the wound margin and the wound bed. The strength of the tightness tension depends on surgeons' experience especially in cases of children's fingers the circulations of the fingers must be checked frequently for several days after [41, 42].

When the stitches are made for tie-over sutures, the positions of the thread should be placed so that they face each other directly across operative wound, for even tie-over suture. There are many concerns from many surgeons on the subject of children's hand surgery, the author believes that obtaining the knowledge and performing frequent circulation checks will result in a high graft take rate and prevent finger loss (necrosis) (Fig. 2.15).

In the case of multiple fingers of children, tie-over dressing is also useful because it maintains even compression strength, particularly in each web space.

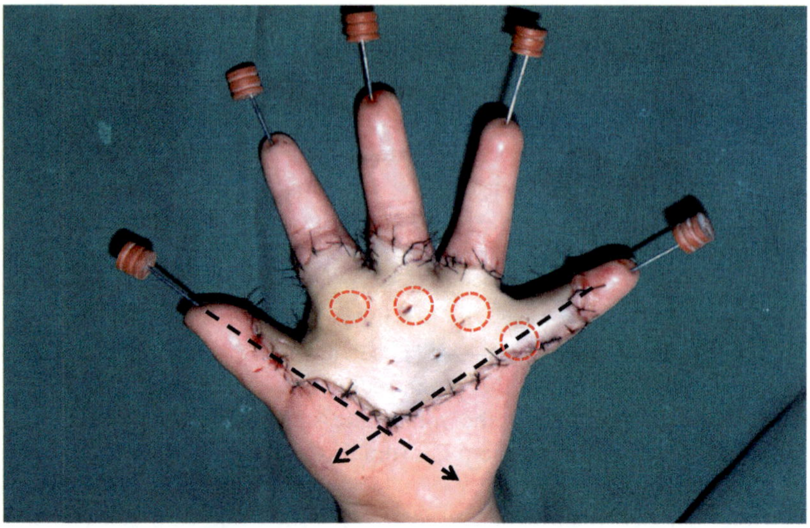

Fig. 2.14 Note the direction of each finger and keep maximal extension of fingers and expansion of engraft skin surface. The K-wire must be inserted deeply into the bottom of the palm (dashed arrows)

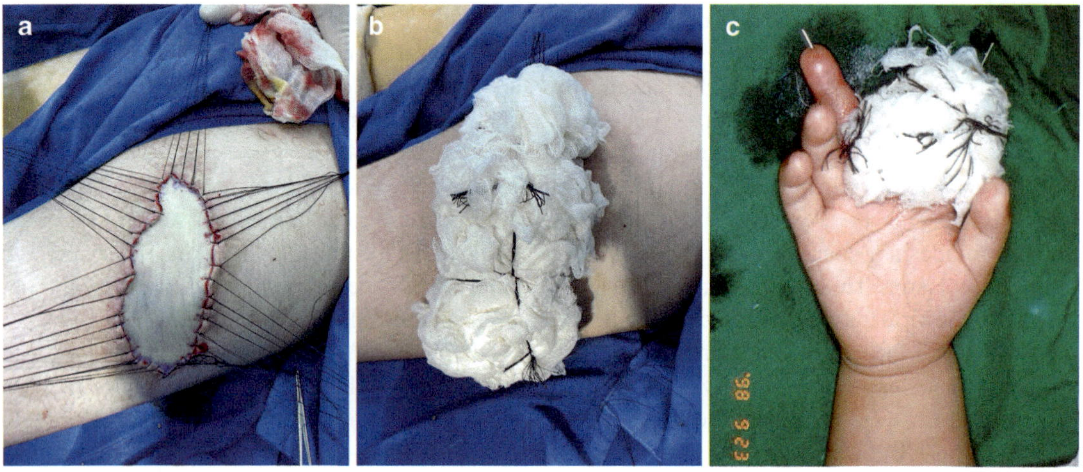

Fig. 2.15 (**a**, **b**) The positions of the thread should be placed so that they face each other directly across operative wound. (**c**) Obtaining the knowledge and performing frequent circulation checks will result in higher graft take rate and prevent finger loss

The procedure mentioned above involves simultaneous engrafting and compressive dressing, which reduces surgery duration and prevents hematomas. A summary of the entire graft technique is presented below:

1. Promptly control the bleeding with a simple epinephrine injection.
2. Save time by preserving the superficial or dense subcutaneous fat layer rather than shaving the dermal layer of skin.
3. Simultaneously perform engrafting and tie-over suturing to reduce surgery duration, leading to less complications and high-quality surgical outcomes.

Described above: 3 reasons can lead to shorten operation duration, pediatric hand surgery is complex and time consuming, I aim not to go over 3 hours.

In cases of unsuccessful FTSG surgeries, often valueable doner skin is wasted, which were harvested from very limited doner sites. Therefore these procedures must be well and meticulously prepared and be considered for any circumstances before, during, and after the surgery. One must not be ill-prepared and take repetitive attempts.

The surgical guidelines introduced here are based on my experiences and conclusions reached through considerable contemplation, various attempts, and long-term follow-ups. In addition, this book aims to bring back the main focus on technique of skin graft, which recently has been neglected and regarded solely as a routine and conventional practice for simplified needs. Therefore, I sincerely hope that this book helps to develop a solid foundation for young surgeons, which will enhance their surgical skills.

2.3.7 Postoperative Wound Dressing

A common question on the appropriate timing of the opening of the tie-over dressing is often shared among surgeons. The author normally opens the dressing 5–6 days after following surgery, except in cases of insufficient perioperative bleed control, wound's bleeding tendency, inadequate arterial bleed control, or improper tie-over dressing of the surgical site. However, although the time may vary depending on the surgeon's judgment, it is necessary to wait for at least 3 days. The reason is that the attachment surface that is pressed to some degree between the engrafted skin and wound bed needs to be stabilized so that it can endure minor trauma such as dressing and prevent formation of new hematoma. Although tie-over dressing is very accurate and quick, anxiety regarding postoperative hematoma is a factor that concerns surgeons. However, even if a hematoma is found upon wound opening, it is not too late to apply compressive soaked fluffy gauze dressing daily. This can cause anxiety in many surgeons, this can get better with practice and experiences over time. At the time of opening the dressing, a hematoma in the wound bed is difficult to detect as the skin is thick and its color has changed to purple; if there is any preliminary sign of suspected edematous and the epidermis is swollen and there is bullae formation, deep slit incisions can be made, one or two points can be stitched out at engrafted margin, so the skin can be squeezed with a cotton swab. During this process, caution must be exercised by the surgeon to avoid peeling the epidermis and maintain the dressing until the engrafted skin is taken and stabilized. In case the epidermis peels off, the exposed dermis dries up, resulting in partial skin loss, hyperpigmentation disorders, or scarring, all of which diminish the esthetic effects. Hence, dressing should be maintained until the graft completely takes. Daily dressing, if possible, should be performed; the skin color gradually changes from reddish purple to closer to whitish yellowish color tone of original skin color. Day 1 of postoperative wound opening is essential to determine the accurate treatment status. Therefore, daily observation of any postoperative changes in the skin color is beneficial. In this part, examples have been provided for full-thickness skin with subcutaneous fat composite graft, which many surgeons regard as having high chances of failure, and the survival trajectory of the entire engrafted skin has been described in detail supported with pictures.

An 11-year-old female patient underwent reconstructive surgery on the right upper chest, shoulder, and axilla areas. To prevent contracture recurrence, the three-dimensional release procedure was performed on the contracture lesion, with a triangular flap interrupted using surrounding scar tissues (white arrows) and a zigzag pattern made to a long, linea, straight-line brake. The inguinal donor skin preserved a dense subcutaneous fat layer (black arrow), and the harvested donor skin size was 4.5 × 15 cm (Fig. 2.16). Tie-over suture was performed before tie-over dressing; the tie-over dressing was removed on day 4. Because the patient complained of pain, tie-over dressing was opened 2 days earlier. However, these images provided an excellent opportunity for verifying the sequence

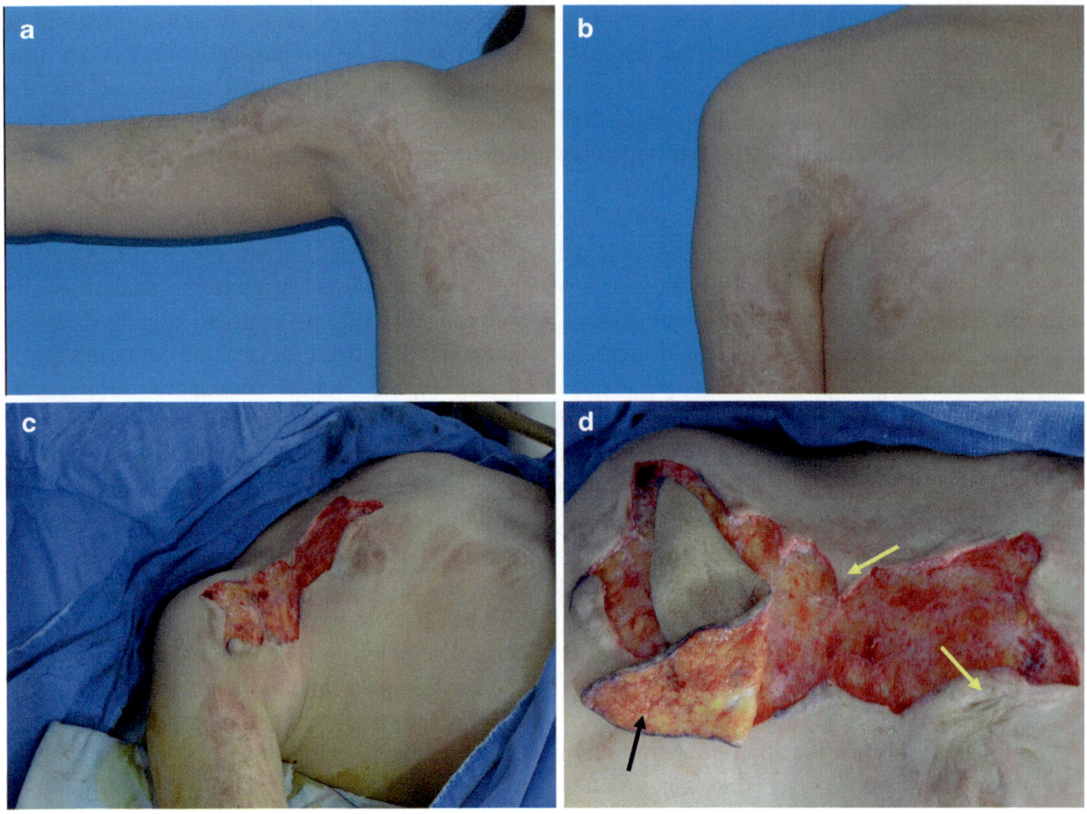

Fig. 2.16 (**a**, **b**) Preoperative view, note the scar contracture was on the right upper chest, shoulder, and axilla area. (**c**, **d**) Contractre release procedure was performed on the upper breast, chest and shoulder dimensional areas (white arrows)

of the composite fat graft taking procedure. Notice the deep purplish tinted color at the immediate opening, which appears edematous and unstable graft take process. On removal day 5, a brighter purple color was observed, but there was no significant difference. On removal day 6, the purple color changed to orange and appeared more stable in skin color. Normally the author removes the graft on day 5 or 6 because the engrafted skin becomes stable (Fig. 2.17). On tie-over dressing removal day 7, more stable engrafted skin with minor edematous appearance was observed. On removal day 14, the graft was completely removed by performing a full stitch-out (Fig. 2.18). After 40 days and 2 months from the procedure, an immature grafted marginal scar was observed, but I did not perform an ancillary procedure for postoperative scar management with the Fraxel laser because the patient was too young and refused it.

Four months after the procedure, the engrafted skin appeared more stable and supple, but a minor marginal hypertrophic scar was observed. After 2.5 years from the procedure, the engrafted skin had an increased floor space of 17 × 6 cm and was well adapted to the three-dimensional areas of the growing breast, axilla, and shoulder (Figs. 2.19 and 2.20).

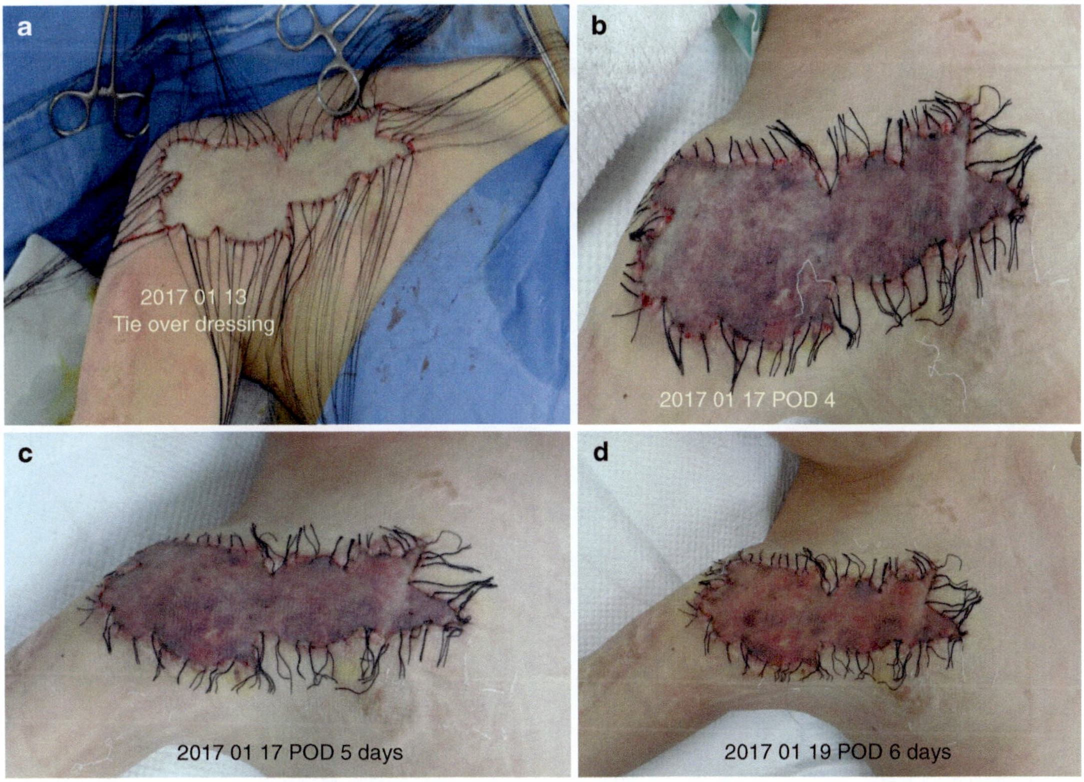

Fig. 2.17 (**a**) Finished tie-over suture before tie-over dressing; (**b**) after tie-over dressing early removal day 4. (**b**) Notice deep purplish color underneath at immediate open state looks edematous and unstable graft. (**c**) On removal day 5. (**d**) On removal day 6

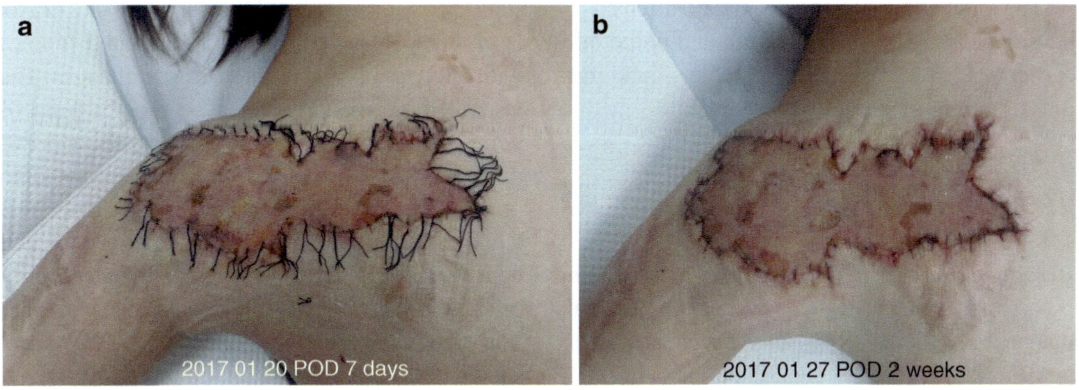

Fig. 2.18 (**a**) Tie-over dressing removal day 7, more stable engrafted skin with minor edematous appearance. (**b**) On removal day 14, graft was taken completely with full stitch-out performed

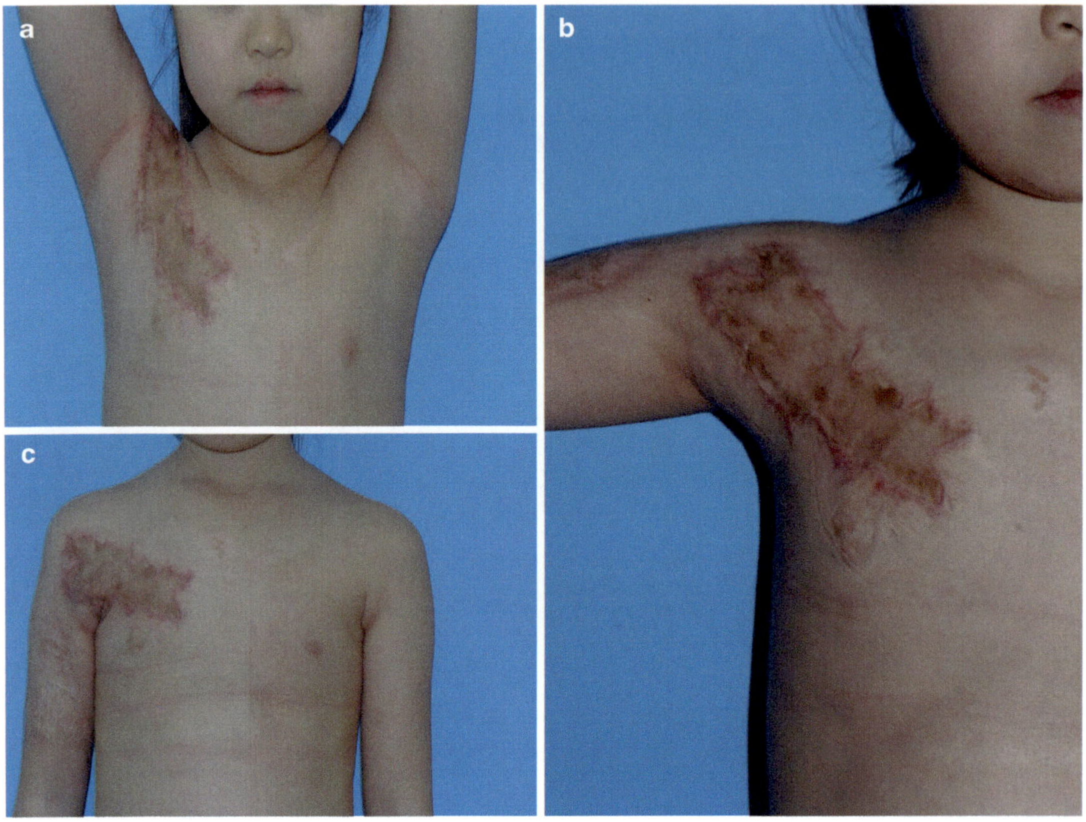

Fig. 2.19 (**a**) Postoperative 40 days later view. (**b**, **c**) 2 months later view

The stitches are typically removed after 10–14 days depending on operation site and potentially earlier or later in cases with unstable wound margins or emerging necrotic changes.

2.3.8 Postoperative Management

Regarding long-term postoperative management, proper management of the engrafted skin bed and margin is crucial to ensure excellent patient outcomes; the patients should be encouraged to continue receiving treatment. The surgical wound stabilizes after 3–4 weeks, following the Fraxel laser therapy I started at the graft margin 5–6 times with intervals of 3–4 weeks as the scar matures. The laser therapy is restarted after 2–3 months or keeps going with the aforementioned intervals, and this procedure can be applied continuously depending on scar maturation. In the initial stage, the wavelength is set to 1550 nm, pulse energy to 20 mj, and density of 6–8/MTZ; the strength is altered depending on the degree of scarring. In addition, combination of pressure garment and silicone gel sheet should be continued for at least 6 months or over to ensure satisfactory surgical outcomes.

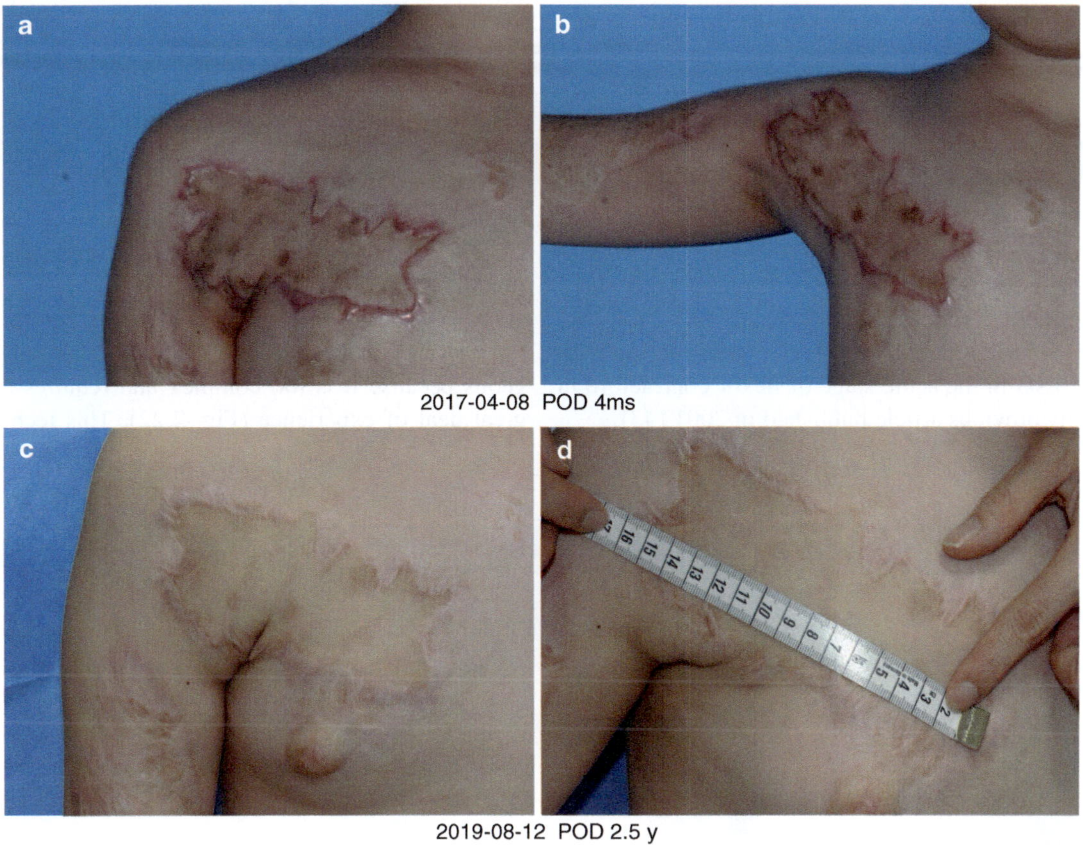

Fig. 2.20 (**a**, **b**) Postoperative 4 months after view. (**c**, **d**) Postoperative 2.5 years later view, the engrafted skin had increased floor space 17 × 6 cm and has well-adapted three-dimensional area

2.4 FTSG Presentation According to Cases

2.4.1 Pediatric Hand Reconstruction with FTSG

Examples of surgical techniques for complex and essential pediatric hand reconstruction will be discussed here. One of the common preconceptions is that most surgeons are reluctant to performing FTSGs on pediatric patients as they anticipate multiple corrective surgeries in the future as they are still growing and developing. For that reason, many surgeons recommend the surgery to take place over several years at interval of growth or when the child matures into an adult. But I believe that it is much more beneficial to perform surgeries on younger patients, earlier the better, for functional and aesthetic benefit outcomes, which are essential for the psychological health of the growing children. A surgery involving small and vulnerable fingers requires meticulous surgical skills and abundant experience, and a well-planned and detailed skin graft technique will facilitate the resolution of these issues.

2.4.2 Flexor Deformity of the Pediatric Hand

Flexor contracture is one of the most common burn deformities in children; a typical example of this is the steam burn caused by electric rice cookers in Asian countries. An average electric rice cooker produces very hot steam that can cause deep second- and third-degree burns. Example below shows burns on the flexor parts of the finger and the palm of a less than a year old child. Flexor contracture of the fingers and palm, cicatricial syndactyl, and webbing deformities are examples of common deformities in this kind of burn (Fig. 2.21).

I have reported one-stage reconstruction with FTSG in the acute stage of flexor contracture in my previous article published in 2001 [43].

This case depicts an immediate FTSG at the time of the acute injury. Extensive debridement was performed to predict the possibility of development of scar contracture on the burned hand. Immediate FTSG was performed with a single sheet to prevent scar contracture along the seam line. Two years after the operation, there was no recurrence of flexor contracture, with excellent functional recovery without any corrective surgery. However, I no longer perform this type of surgery and do not recommend it to other surgeons because it is too complex and requires a great deal of experience (Fig. 2.22). This tech-

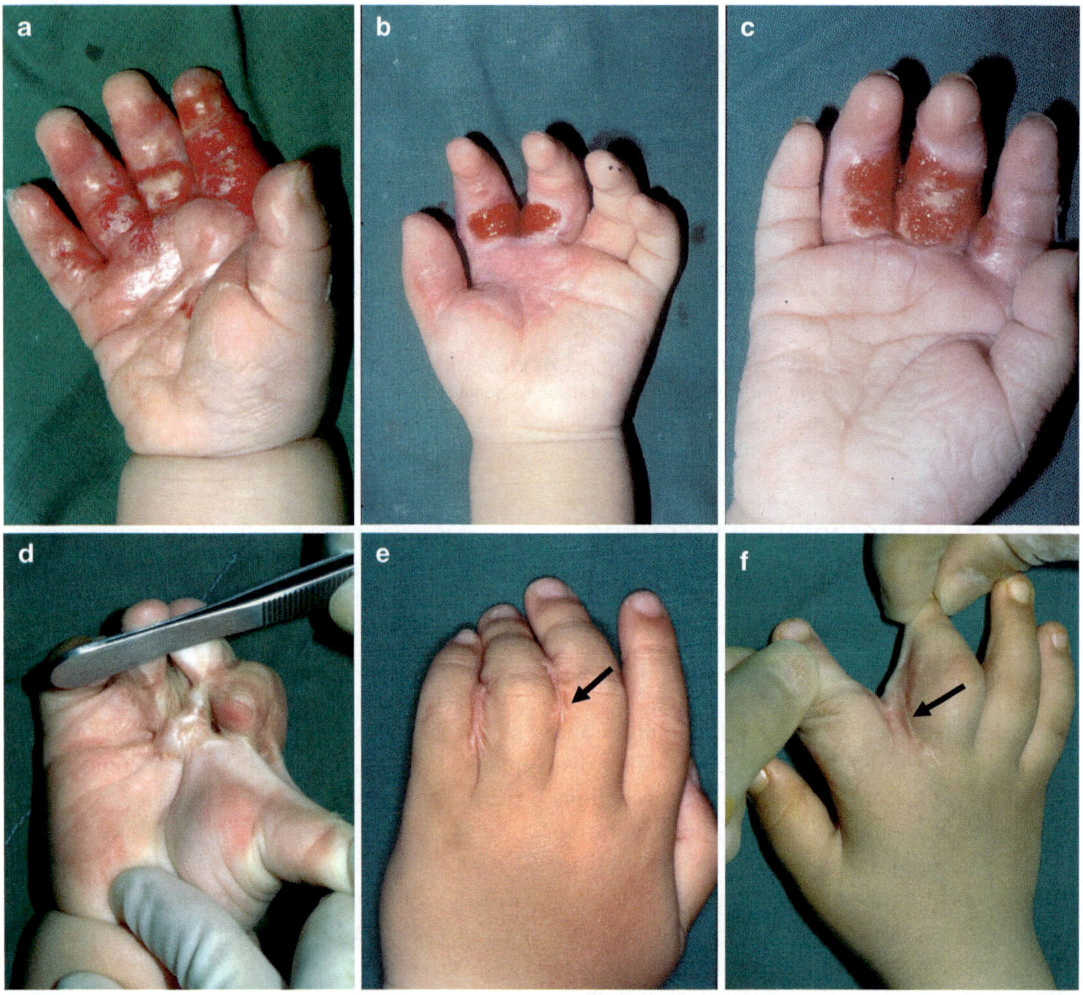

Fig. 2.21 (**a–c**) Common steam burn injury caused by electric rice cooker, note deep second- and third-degree burn. (**d**) The common deformities are shown on flexor contracture fingers and palms, (**e**) cicatricial syndactyly, and (**f**) webbing deformities (black arrows)

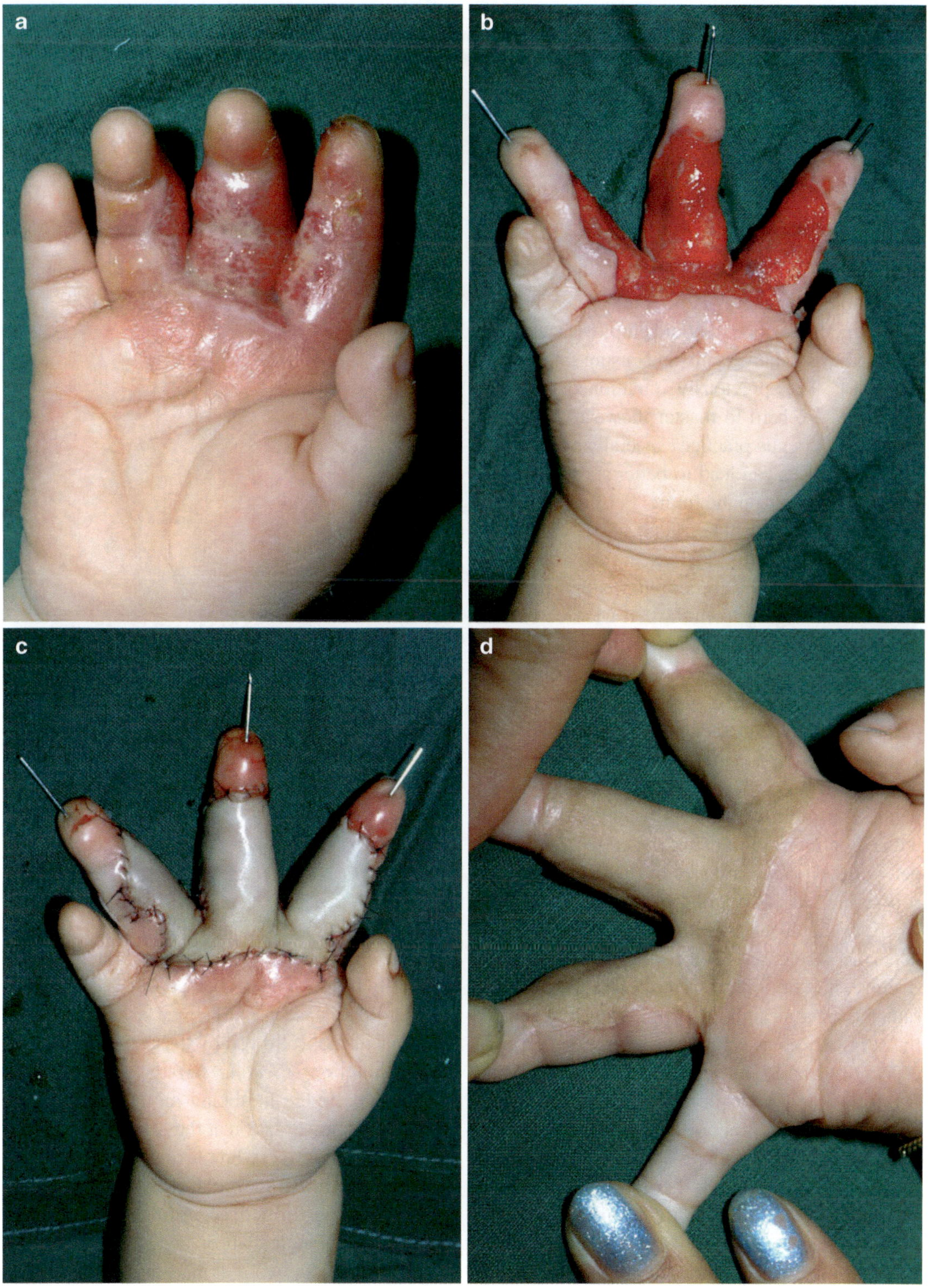

Fig. 2.22 (**a**) Common steam burn caused by steam from electric rice cooker. (**b**) Extensive debridement was performed to prevent scar contracture. (**c**) Immediate FTSG was performed with single-sheet graft. (**d**) Postoperative 2 years after view, excellent functional recover with no corrective surgery anymore

nique is no longer recommended because it is too complex and needs plentiful experience about immediate FTSG to the acute burn stage with high incidences of wastage of two important inguinal donor sites.

Some surgeons recommend early excision and FTSG [44, 45], but my opinion has changed; instead, now I recommend wound healing with conservative dressing and performing reconstruction following a sufficient review and a 1-year maturation period. This is because I later realized that a beneficial surgery should employ a technique that can be used universally and ensure satisfactory outcomes. The previously mentioned valuable techniques are hard to master; however, I believe with hard work and practice especially on children, these techniques can lead to better surgery performances and results in the future. Performing FTSG on children is especially difficult.

Consider the following case as an example. A 1-year-old toddler submerged his/her hand in the steam emerging from the electric rice cooker out of curiosity but because of immature reflex, he/she was unable to remove it, resulting in deep second- or third-degree burns in the flexor part of the hand. Surgery can be performed after 1 year following the maturation and contraction of the scarring on flexor part of the fingers and palm. The main caution as follows: dissection with a slicing motion using the edge of the scalpel while avoiding injuries to the deep artery or soft tissue. As undermine is on the same level where epinephrine injection site is, where epinephrine is released. To prevent relapse of contracture, it is important to make a zigzag pattern rather than a straight long incision line during the surgical release. Finger release technique is especially important because of the wide range of motion and multiple interphalangeal joints, as well as the high recurrence rate of flexor contracture. To prevent these deformities, a zigzag flap must be made on the interdigital crease (black arrow), and the wound margin bed must be fully released and detached with a scalpel undermining (white arrow) (Fig. 2.23).

The author developed the three-step release basic technique:

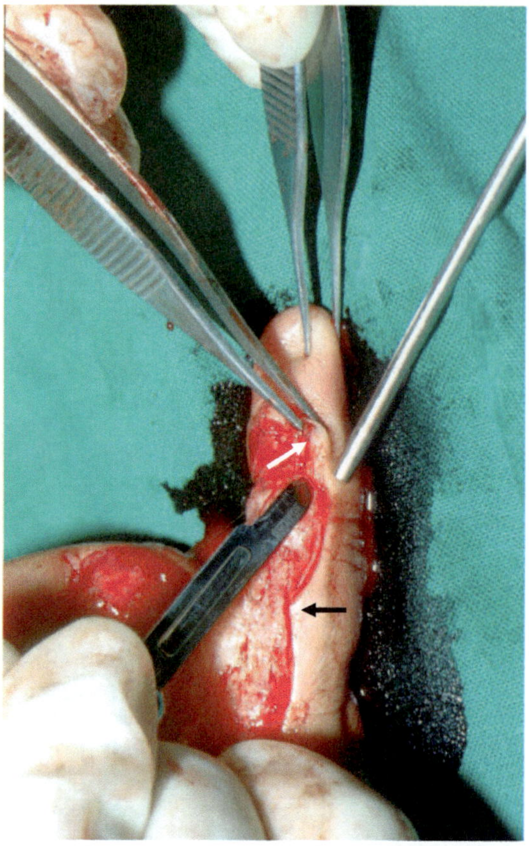

Fig. 2.23 The triangular flap (black arrow) is an important feature to prevent linea contracture, breaking the straight line. Another important key point is wound margin bed must be fully released and detached with scalpel undermining (white arrow)

On author's bleed control method, a 1:100,000 diluted epinephrine solution was injected intradermally into the intrascar tissues. *First step*: Incisional release is performed at the center of the scar tissue, followed by dissection in moving away directions. *Second step*: Scar bed release with scalpel edge in slicing motion and healthy wound bed preservation at the level of the wound bed and scar tissue (white arrow) are performed. To prevent linea scar contracture, scar tissue excision is performed according to the wound bed, and a triangle flap or zigzag line is made. *Third step*: The wound margin is released to relieve the tension on the graft margin and preserve maximum engrafting space. Remaining scar tissues in the wound bed are carefully excised and released (black arrow), but no force is required as the remaining amount of scar tissue absorbs and softens spontaneously when the surrounding tension reduces. The benefit of this technique is that it preserves healthy tissues, tendon, dorsal vein, etc. (arrows). AlloDerm (black arrow) is a useful substitute for full-thickness skin (Figs. 2.24 and 2.25).

The technique mentioned above can also be applied to flexion contracture of the fingers.

In cases where both the palm and fingers are all affected, overcorrection should be performed with full release of contracture and enough skin graft to prevent contracture particularity on the palm.

A common burn scar contracture was observed on the left hand of a 3-years-old boy after getting burnt by the hot steam produced by the electric rice cooker. When the scar contracture affects the palm, full release and overcorrection must be performed to prevent frequent recontracture of the interspace of the fingers and palm (black arrows). After 1, 2, 3, and 5 years after the procedure, there were no contracture deformities, and the interspace of the fingers and palm was well maintained (Fig. 2.26).

Reconstruction of the palm should be approached with caution as the insufficient release of contracture will lead to surgical failure in terms of both functionality and esthetics. Moreover, since the palm and fingers act as a unit, the surgery should be concluded in a single session to maintain a harmonious cooperation among them.

A 9-year-old female patient suffered a friction injury and underwent reconstructive surgery with FTSG twice in a different hospital. The fourth and fifth fingers on the right palm were severely retracted, with scarring and previously incom-

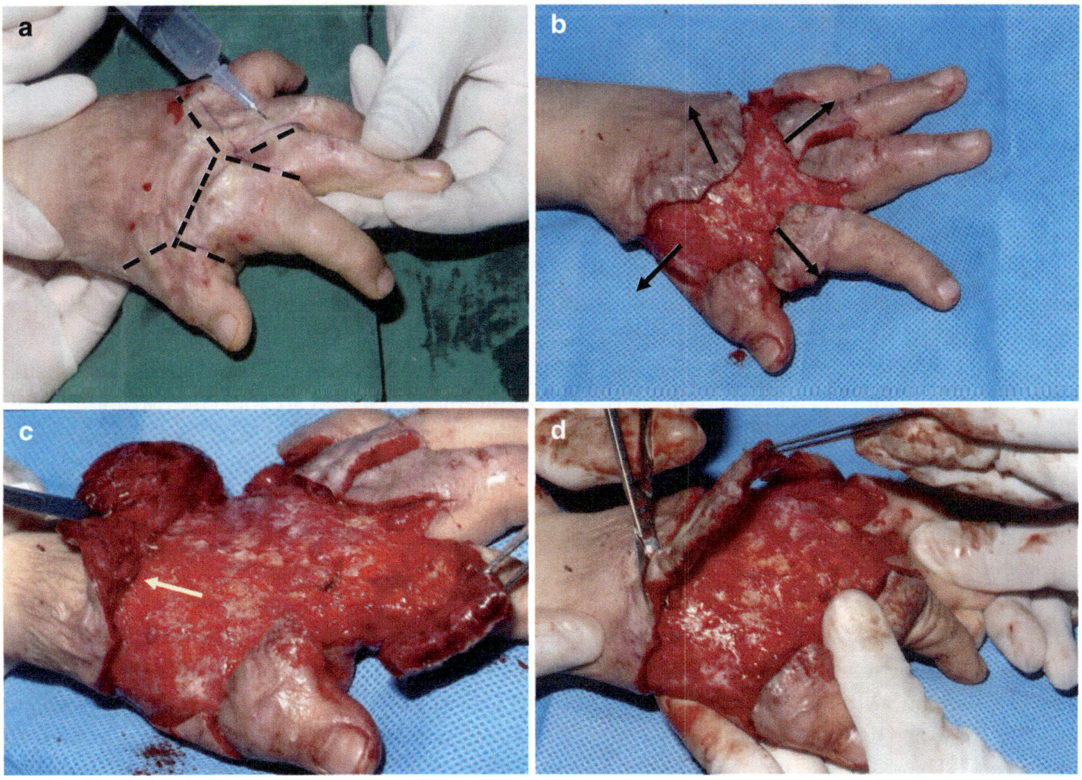

Fig. 2.24 (**a**) 1:100,000 diluted epinephrine solution injected to intradermal and intrascar tissue. (**b**) Incisional release at the center of scar tissue and dissection in centrifugal directions. (**c**) Second step, scar bed release with scalpel edge shaving action (white arrow). (**d**) Proper scar tissue excision

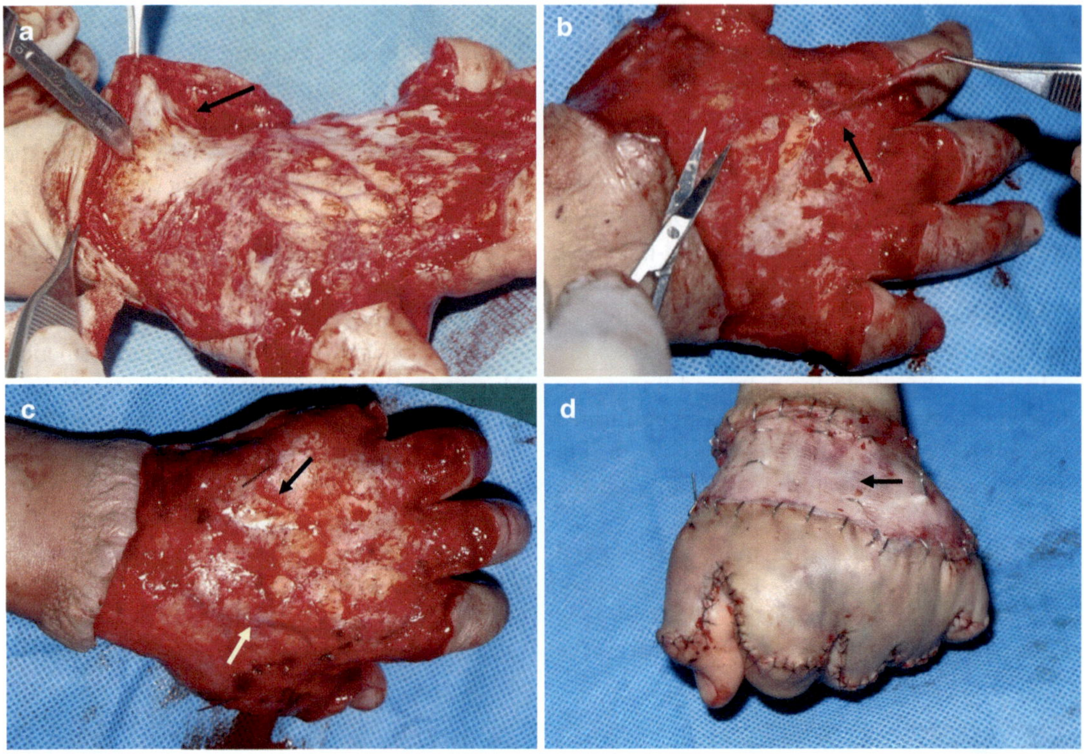

Fig. 2.25 (**a**) Third step, the wound margin release. (**b**) Remained scar tissue excised and released on the wound bed (black arrow). (**c**) Note well-preserved healthy tissues (arrows), etc. (**d**) AlloDerm® (black arrow) is a useful substitute material for full-thickness skin

plete FTSG sequelae. Note the two sites of short engrafted FTSG lesions and the undercorrected hyperthenar area. The functional disturbance of the limitation of full extension was noted in the dorsal view of the hand. As previously stated, palm scar contracture has hidden pitfalls between the interspace of fingers and the palm and also wrist areas (arrows and dashed line) (Fig. 2.27). The key step of the procedure is the full release of the fourth and fifth interdigital spaces (white arrow), followed by the construction of a triangular flap (black arrow) to prevent linea contracture and to maximize engraftment in the hyperthenar and wrist areas (two-way arrow). Two months after the operation, there was no recontracture and the third and fourth web spaces were well preserved. The skin texture and remodeled engrafted skin recovered rapidly because the operation was performed using release and FTSG with a subcutaneous composite fat graft (Fig. 2.28). Six months after the operation, the skin texture had rapidly recovered, and the fingers, palm, and wrist had naturally repositioned themselves with no functional disruption or disfigurement. One year after the operation, full recovery with regular shape and function was observed, and a double-opposing plasty was performed to correct an irregular hyperthenar mound as final esthetic surgery (Fig. 2.29).

A 3-year-old male patient sustained a scalding burn on his right hand and wrist. To save the fingers, emergency escharotomy was performed on the dorsum of the hand, and an escharotomy scar was noted (black arrow). There was severe flexor contracture throughout the palm and all fingers, including the wrist area (Fig. 2.30). Incisional and excisional release were performed from the distal phalanges to the wrist-joint area.

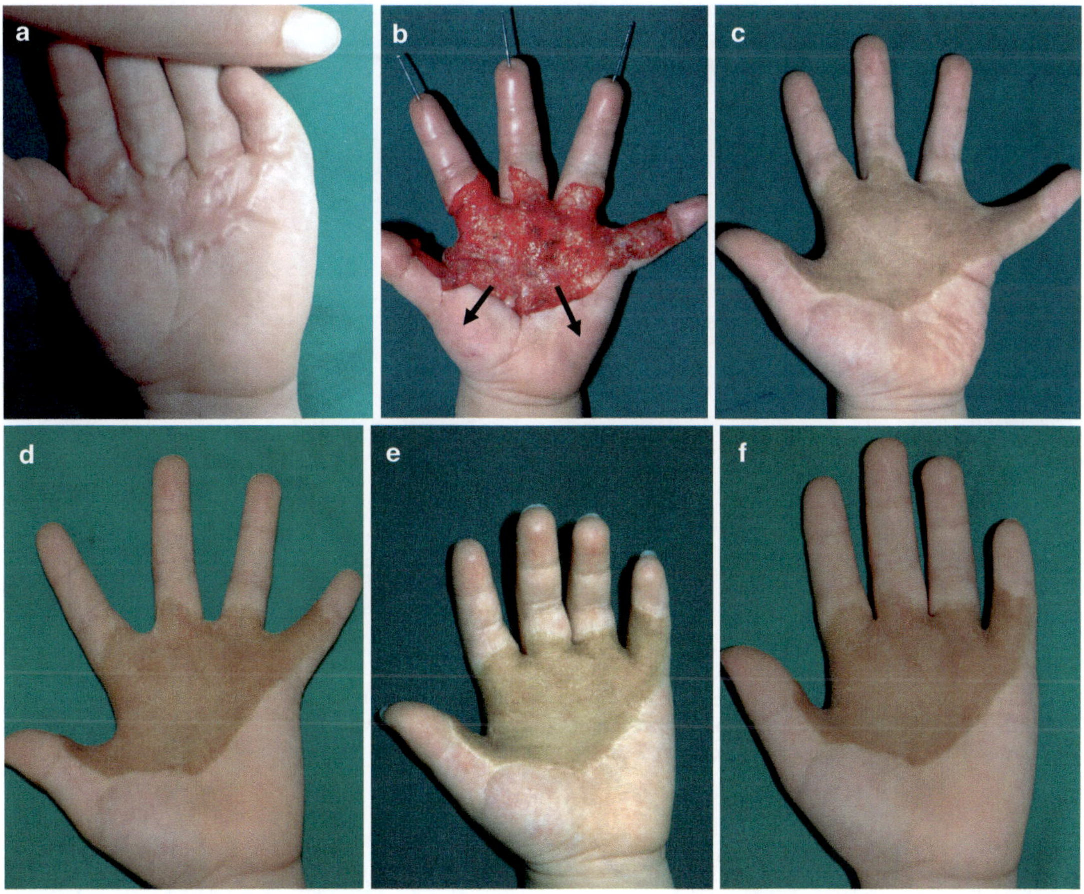

Fig. 2.26 (**a**) Typical scar contracture, after an electric rice cooker steam burn. (**b**) Full release (black arrow direction) and overcorrection. (**c**) Postoperative 1 year after, (**d**) 2 years, (**e**) 3 years, and (**f**) 5 years after view

Electrocauterization or tourniquets were not used, The bleed control was well managed, indicating that a simple epinephrine injection can effectively control bleeding. The entire hand and wrist area were treated with a single sheet of full-size FTSG. During early 2000s, conventional dermal shaving technique with a tie-over dressing was used. A slit incision (black arrow) was made to remove hematoma when the tie-over dressing was open (Fig. 2.31). All digits and the palm were fully functional 5 years after the operation. A mild contracted seam line was observed at the base of the thumb, but there was no functional disturbance (black arrow). This circumstantial evidence explains exactly why I avoid making a seam line in a graft sheet. One year after the operation, no contracture deformity on the palm, fingers, or wrist areas was observed. Full-thickness skin is very effective in fast growing children, which is why I strongly recommend an FTSG at an early age to take advantage of the concurrent growth of grafted FTSG skin and aging body growth (Fig. 2.32).

By observing long-term follow-up images, resolving functional and esthetic problems in a single surgery maximizes the advantages of FTSG. All of the techniques mentioned above can be applied in hand surgery for infants who have small-sized hands. The important point is to learn and master relevant skills for the FTSG technique to avoid unnecessary and wasted attempts.

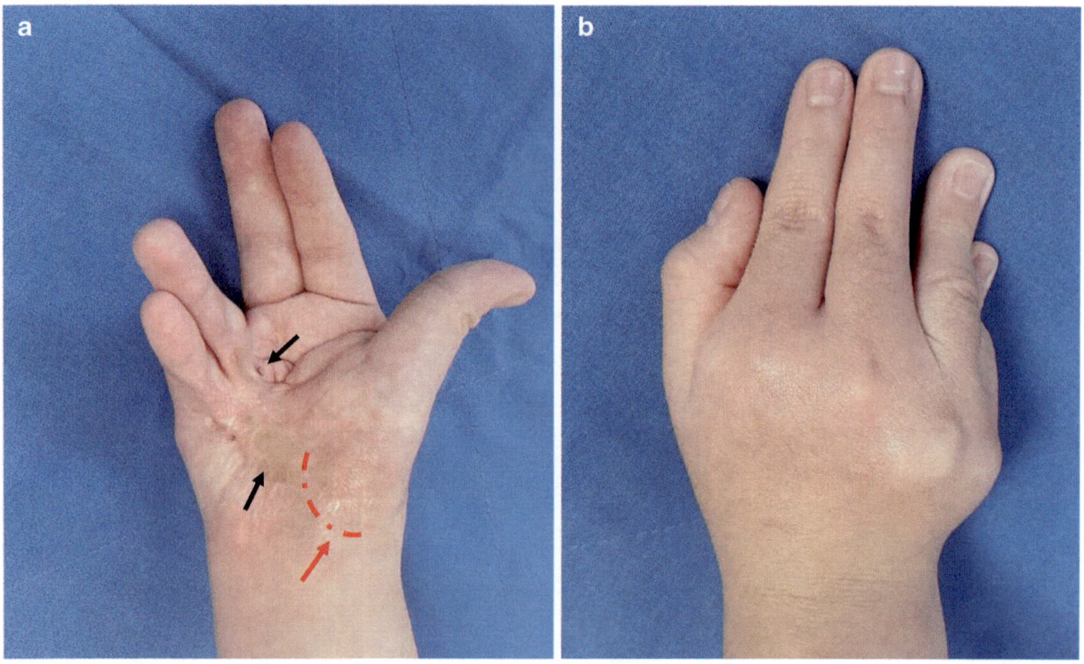

Fig. 2.27 (**a**) Severe contracture on the palm and fourth and fifth finger retraction. Note the incomplete grafted and shrunk FTSG lesion at the two sites (black arrows) and incomplete released hyperthenar area (red dashed line). (**b**) Dorsal view

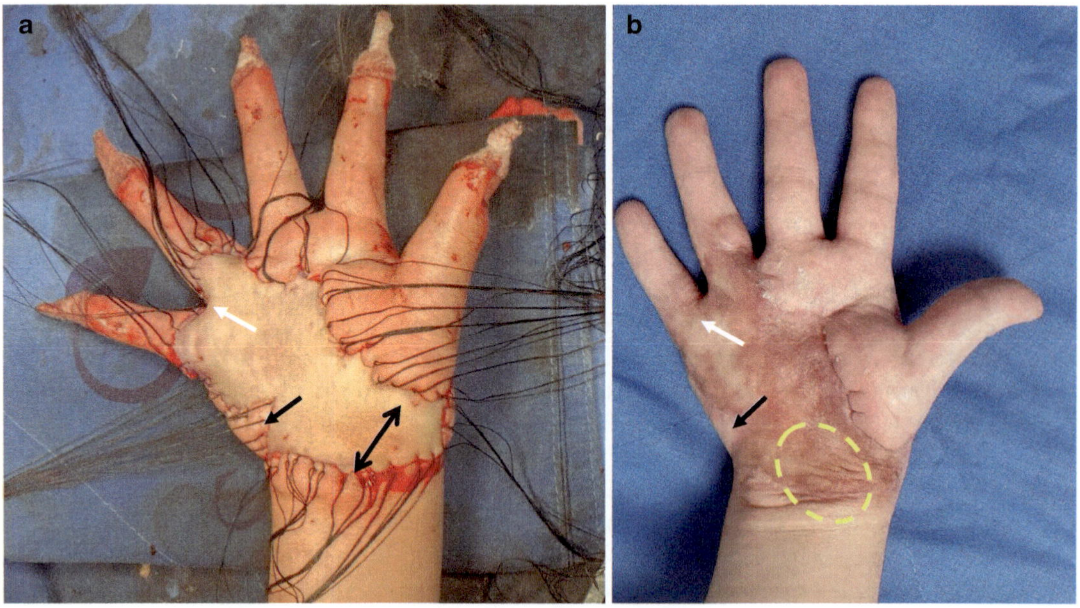

Fig. 2.28 (**a**) Complete tension-free full release was performed on fourth and fifth interdigital space (white arrow), make triangular flap (black arrow), maximal over engraft on hyperthenar and wrist area (two-way arrow). (**b**) 2 months after the operation, note the palm and well-preserved third and fourth web space (arrows and dashed yellow circle)

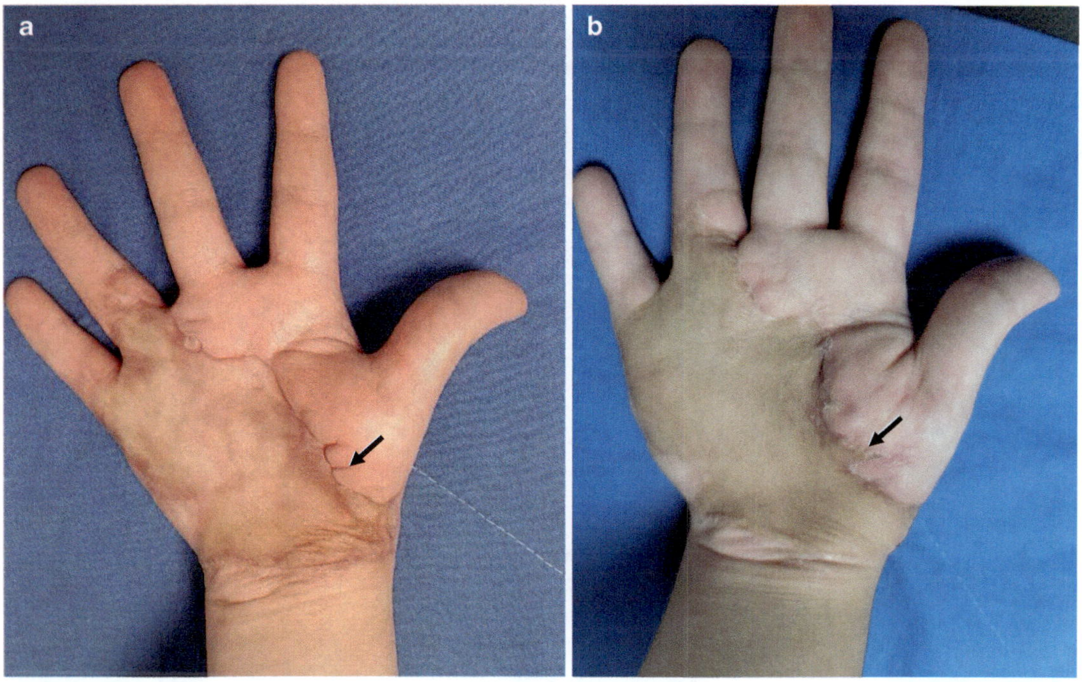

Fig. 2.29 (**a**) Postoperative 6 months later view. (**b**) 1 year after the operation, double-opposing Z-plasty was performed (black arrows)

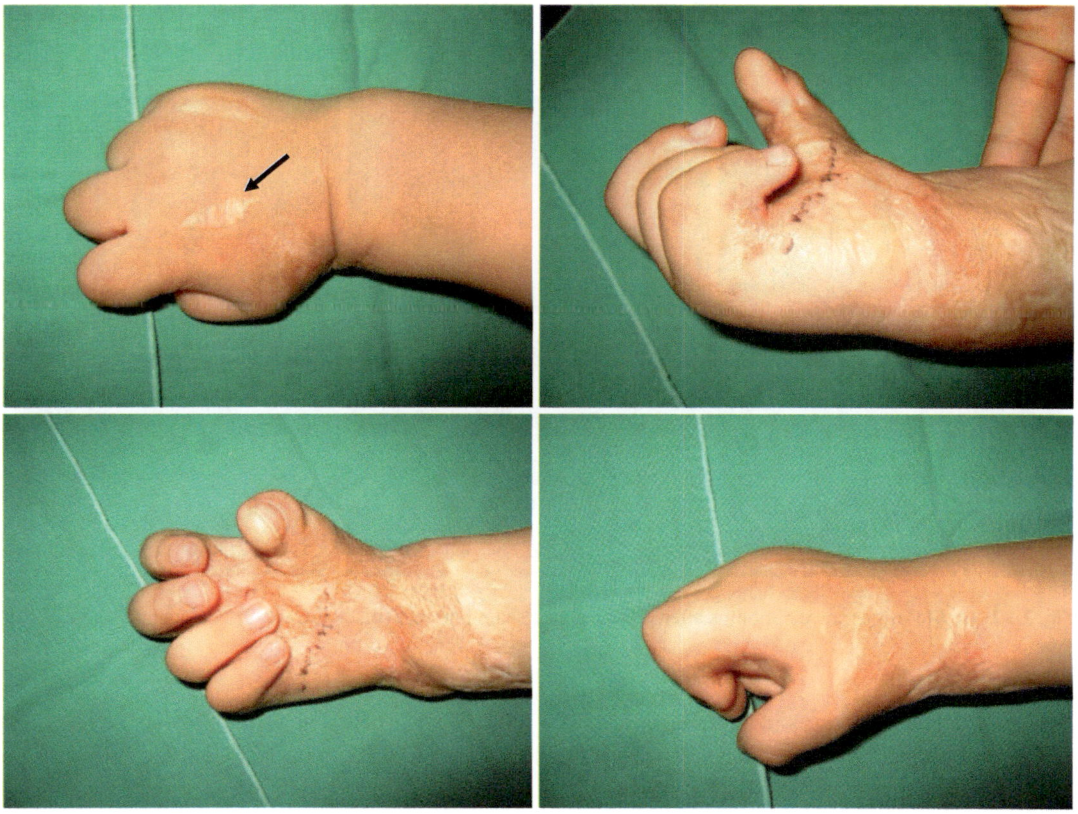

Fig. 2.30 Note the severe flexor contracture with escharotomy scar on the dorsum of the hand (black arrow)

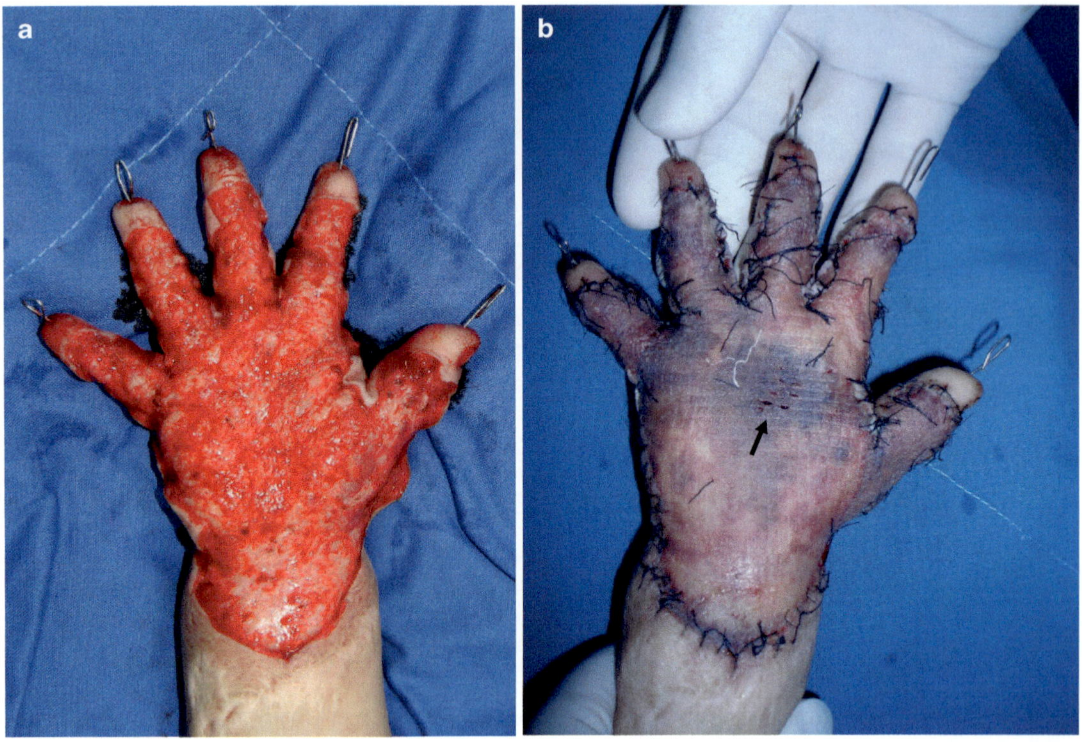

Fig. 2.31 (**a**) Incisional and excisional full release was performed. Notice good bleed control. (**b**) Single-sheet FTSG on the entire hand and wrist. Localized multiple slit incisions (black arrow) were made to remove the hematoma when the tie-over dressing is opened

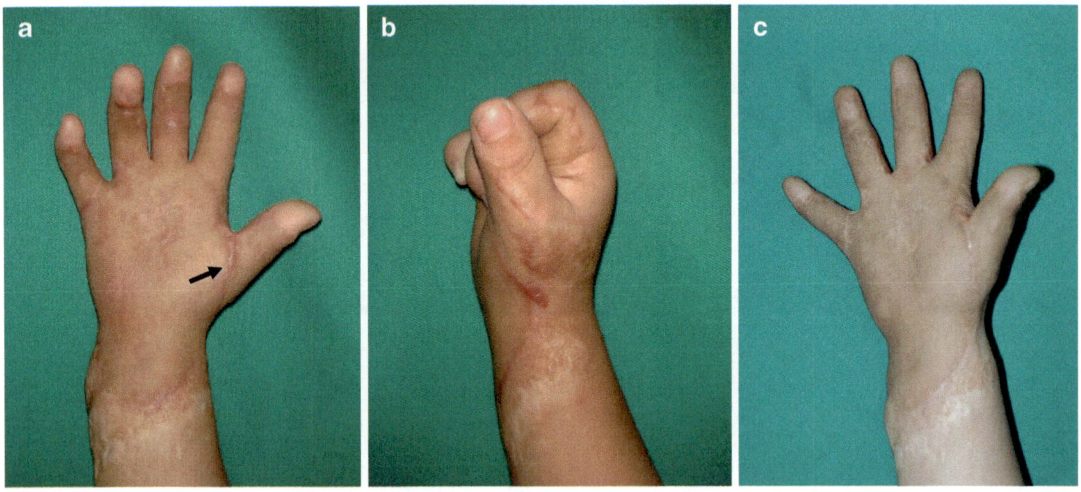

Fig. 2.32 (**a**, **b**) Postoperative 5 months after view, note the seam line scar (black arrow) (**c**) Postoperative 1 year after view

Almost all difficult cases involving the affected flexor part of pediatric hands can be resolved if the FTSG technique is performed without the use of a tourniquet instrument in a single surgery. I hope that many more surgeons acquire these skills to enhance their surgeries.

(a) A 2-year-old female patient sustained an electric rice cooker steam burn injury. (b) The following release technique was performed: full release and K-wire fixation. (c) After 40 days, the FTSG was performed as a single-sheet graft without a seam line to prevent seam line contracture. (d) After 4 months from the procedure, a good functional and esthetic result was observed, with a rapid maturation process (Fig. 2.33). After 1, 2, 3, and 4 years, the engrafted full-thickness skin was well adapted and growing. As shown in the results, early FTSG is ideal for growing children. No additional surgery was performed in this case, but if the patient wants an improved natural appearance for an esthetic result, she should undergo procedures to correct minor webbing deformities (Fig. 2.34).

(a) A 2-year-old male patient with burn caused by the steam from a rice cooker, who was operated 2 years ago, long-term follow-up, flexor contracture along with cicatricial syndactyly was noted in the second, third, and fourth fingers. The following reconstruction was performed: full release of the wound margin (white arrow) and construction of a zigzag broken line. Full release of the finger base and palm area was also performed (black arrow). It is critical to fully release the scar's wound margin in the flexor digit areas to prevent the reoccurrence of flexor deformity (Fig. 2.35). After full release, the scar bed was

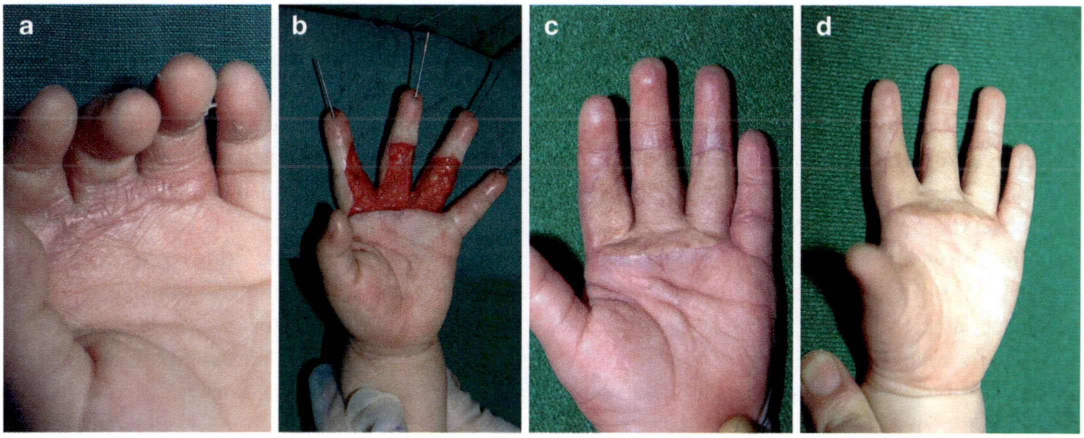

Fig. 2.33 (**a**) Electric rice cooker steam burn. (**b**) Full release and k-wire fixation, (**c**) Postoperative 40 days. (**d**) Postoperative 4 months after view

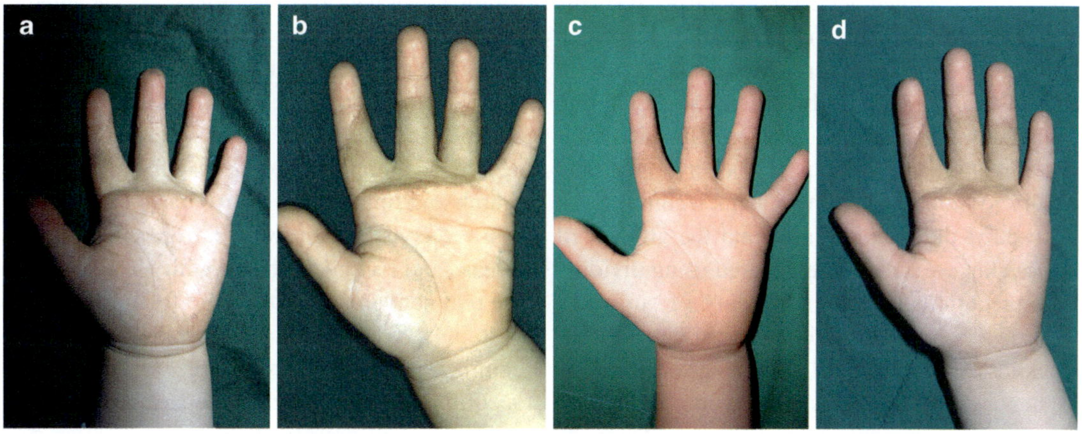

Fig. 2.34 (**a**) Postoperative 1 year, (**b**) 2 years, (**c**) 3 years, and (**d**) 4 years after view

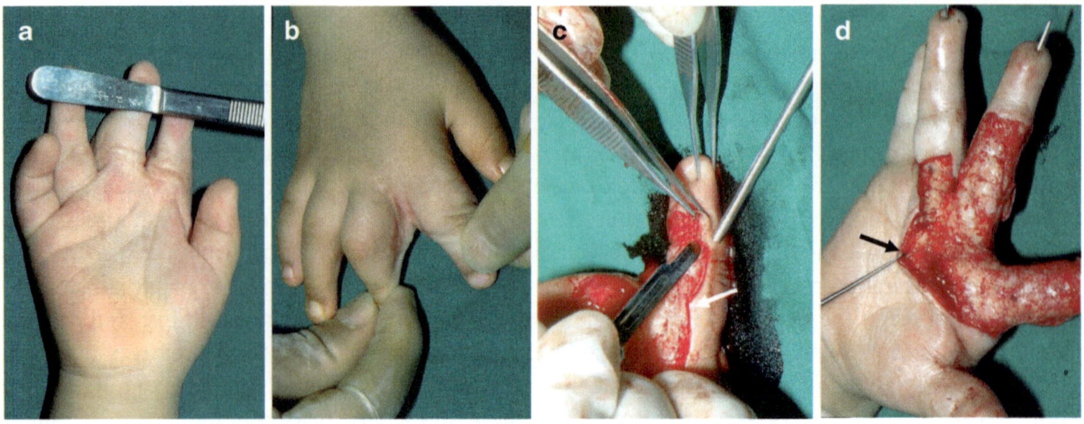

Fig. 2.35 (**a, b**) Common post-electric rice cooker steam burn injury deformity. Note second, third, and fourth fingers' flexor contracture with cicatricial syndactyly. (**c**) Full release wound margin and make broken zigzag line (white arrow). (**d**) Full release scar margin of the finger and palm (black arrow)

completely excised and FTSG was applied. Full-thickness engraftment was performed using the conventional dermal shaving method in my initial time as a surgeon (b). After 1, 2, and 3 years since the operation, no contracture or deformity was observed on this growing child. Now as an adult in his twenties, he has no signs of funtional impairment or disfigurement. This indicates that early reconstructive FTSG is a very effective solution for reconstructive surgery (Fig. 2.36).

Incase of split-thickness skin was harvested (Fig. 2.37a). from the in-step split-thickness skin on the sole of a 4-year-old boy for the simultaneous correction of mismatched skin texture and contracture deformity. Note the incompletely corrected cicatricial deformities with STSG. This image depicts a single-sheet operation technique on each of the four fingers. The tips make use of the elasticity of the full-thickness skin, beginning with the index finger and moving to the next middle finger, then to the next fourth finger, and finally to the last fifth finger. This technique can be used if the recipient area and the amount of donor skin are precisely estimated using dividing cutting points and requires plenty of surgeon's experiences. Furthermore, the elasticity of full-thickness skin with mild stretching tension may be beneficial without having to worry about contracture development. After 1–2 years from the operation, natural and functional effects were evident, and supplemental surgery was not required (Fig. 2.37).

Although this guide cannot fully introduce every technique regarding pediatric hand reconstruction, I have explained the important fundamental techniques and points in addition to the surgical outcomes and long-term follow-up results to provide a reliable reference.

Scar contracture on the dorsal side of the hand leads to extensor and flexor tendon imbalance, such as a claw hand, swan-neck, and button whole deformities, eventually dislocating the finger joints or lateral band. Therefore, in principle, correction follows the release and FTSG is a priority performed for the dorsal part, and then for the flexor part, this principle is also adapted in adult hand.

A 4-year-old boy sustained a scalding burn injury on the dorsal side of his hand. Thick hypertrophic scarring and severe contracture had developed along with extensor deformities on the thumb and fingers as well as volar plate dislocation. Reconstruction was performed with full release and FTSG combined with STSG because the recipient area was too large for full coverage with only FTSG donor skin (yellow arrow). The contracture release procedure was performed according to the author's three-step release technique. A well-preserved dorsal vein after scar release was observed (black arrow), and the fist

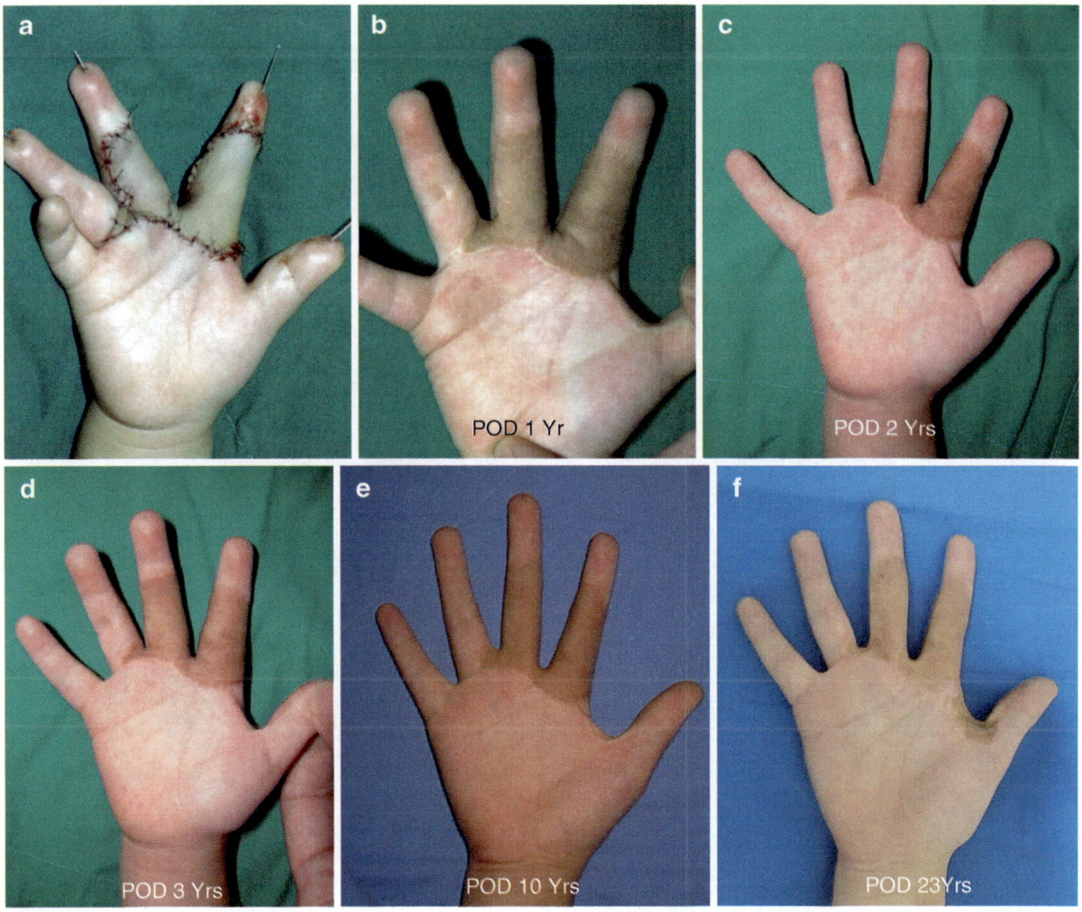

Fig. 2.36 (**a**) Intraoperative view, (**b**) postoperative 1 year after view, (**c**, **d**) postoperative 2 year and 3 years after view, (**e**, **f**) postoperative 10 years and 23 years after view

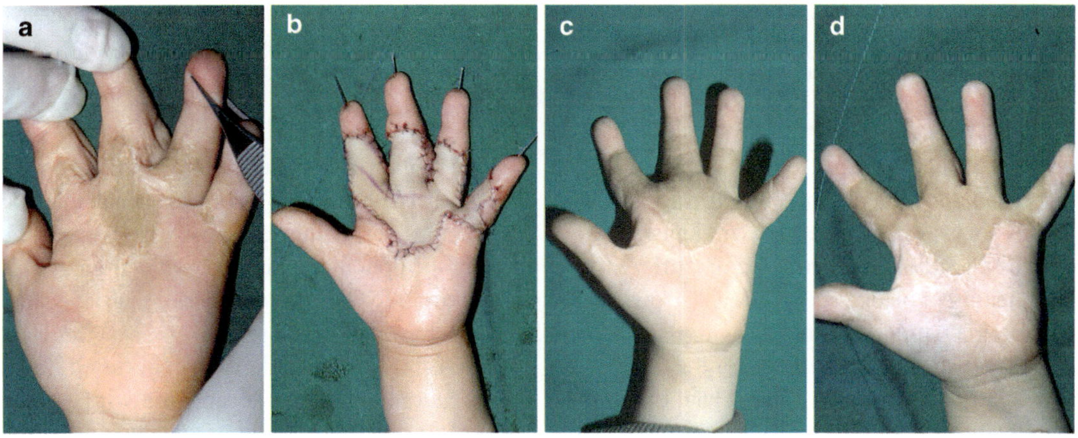

Fig. 2.37 (**a**) Note undercorrected cicatricial deformities with STSG, which are collected from in-step split-thickness skin of the sole. (**b**) Single-sheet FTSG on each individual four fingers without seam lines. (**c**, **d**) Postoperative 1 year and 2 years after view

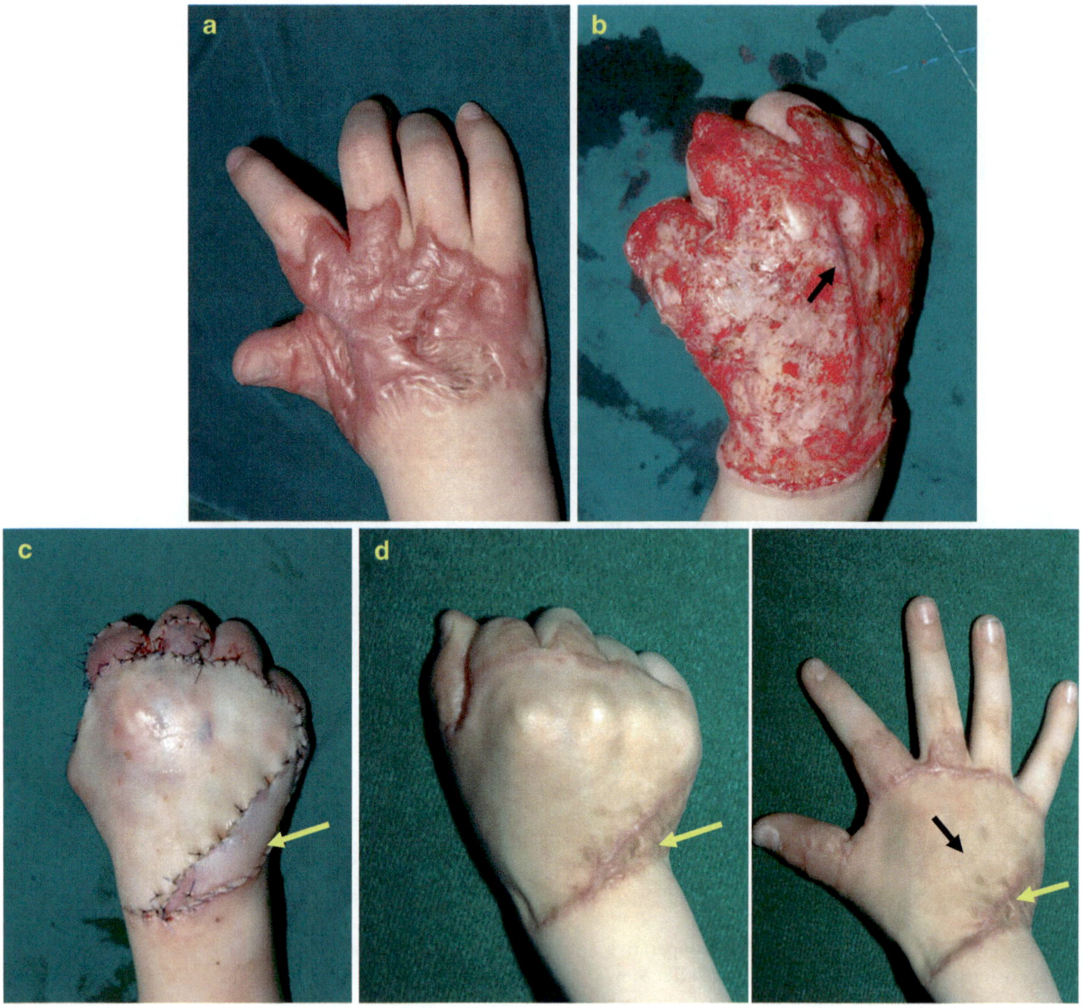

Fig. 2.38 (**a**) Preoperative view. (**b**) Excisional full release and FTSG in combination with STSG. Note well-preserved dorsal vein after scar release (black arrow) and fist position for the maximal engraft surface area. (**c**) Intraoperative view, combined skin graft was performed with FTSG and STSG (yellow arrow). (**d**) Postoperative 3months later, note the skin texture and outcome compared to FTSG with STSG (black and yellow arrows)

position in postoperative dressing is critical for preserving the maximum engraft surface. The figure shows the immediate findings after 3 months after the operation; note the difference in skin texture (black and yellow arrows) and engrafted contracture effects with FTSG and STSG (yellow arrows) (Fig. 2.38).

Pediatric burns on both hands and circumferential injuries pose the greatest challenge to hand surgeons. For pediatric burns on hands, the key point is the decision to use FTSG or not, if chosen the funtional recovery of the thumb is of great importence as it is one of metacarpophalangeal joint. However, if the required graft exceeds the area of the donor skin size, a combination of skin graft with STSG or human dermal matrix system can be considered.

(a) A 2-year-old male patient suffered flame burns, and his wound was covered with a mesh skin graft. Severe contracture developed on the dorsum of the hand along with swan-neck deformities and flexor contracture all the way down to the finger joints, resulting in cicatricial syndactyly. (b) The correction of dorsal deformities is the priority, followed by the correction of the remaining flexor deformity. An initial operation was a full release and excision of scar tissue as well as correction of the hyper-reclined MCP joints for flexor repositioning. The reclined MCP joints were corrected with manual reduction without open capsulotomy. When there is an effective full release contracture on the dorsum of the hand, manual reduction is easier without extensor tendon exposure. Nine months after the operation, the wrist and surrounding thumb area had been corrected; this point was also an important priority of the operation (Fig. 2.39). One year after correcting extensor deformity, corrective flexor deformity surgery was performed with FTSG. (a) Notice the little finger's tip (black arrow); there is no blood supply issues. (b) Notice the impaired circulation of the little finger (red arrow) after tightening the skin graft. Missed regular checks on blood circulations of the fingertips. (c) Resulted in loss of the little finger at the distal phalanx level. This is one of the two finger loss cases I have encountered. However, this was not due to an epinephrine injection. It means that the bleed control technique using an epinephrine injection is a safe procedure. Three months after the operation, the main contracture deformities were corrected with good joint movement function, but thumb movement and webbing deformities remained uncorrected (Fig. 2.40).

After 3 years, the thumb and wrist-joint areas were corrected with FTSG, but there was severe contracture and limitation of joint movement. Because the recovery of wrist and thumb function is important, FTSG skin harvested from the left abdominal skin was substituted with human dermal matrix to harvest full-thickness skin. Full release was performed; interrupted flaps were created using surrounding scar tissue (yellow arrows) and a broken zigzag line; and single-sheet FTSG was performed (Fig. 2.41). Ten years after the operation, a significant improvement in functional and esthetic characteristics was observed. Note the differences between the before (a), (b), and (c) and after (d), (e), and (f) results (Fig. 2.42).

Based on my experience, the simultaneous reconstruction of both dorsal and ventral sides is not recommended because they adversely affect each other.

Alternatively, an FTSG can be performed as the final choice of important reconstruction after a correction with artificial dermis or an STSG.

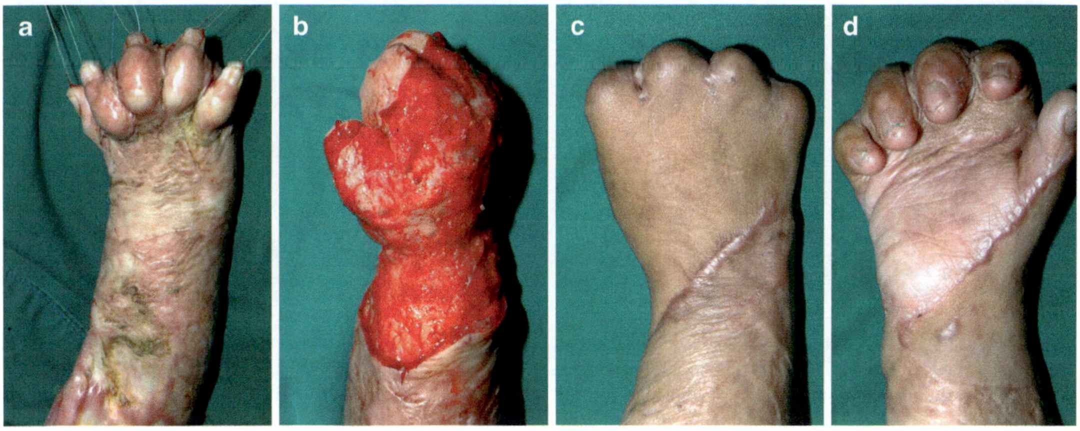

Fig. 2.39 (**a**) Preoperative view. (**b**) Intraoperative view full release and excision of scar tissue and correction of the hyper-reclined MCP joints. (**c**) Postoperative 9 months view. (**d**) Note the outcome on the wrist and surrounding thumb area

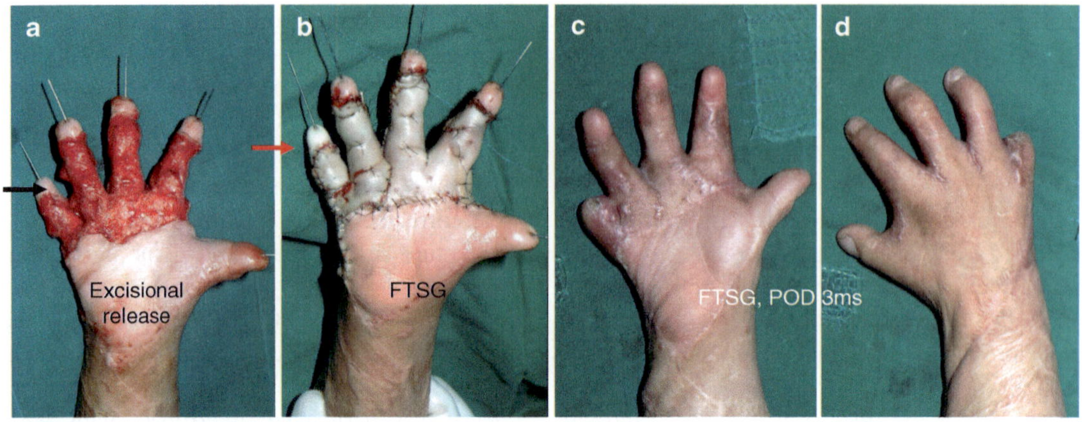

Fig. 2.40 (**a**) 1 year after, second stage of corrective surgery of flexor deformities. Notice the little fingertip (black arrow), there was no observed problem of blood supply. (**b**) Note the impaired little finger circulation (red arrow) after skin graft is finished. (**c**, **d**) Postoperative 3 months after view, incompletely undercorrected thumb and webbing deformities

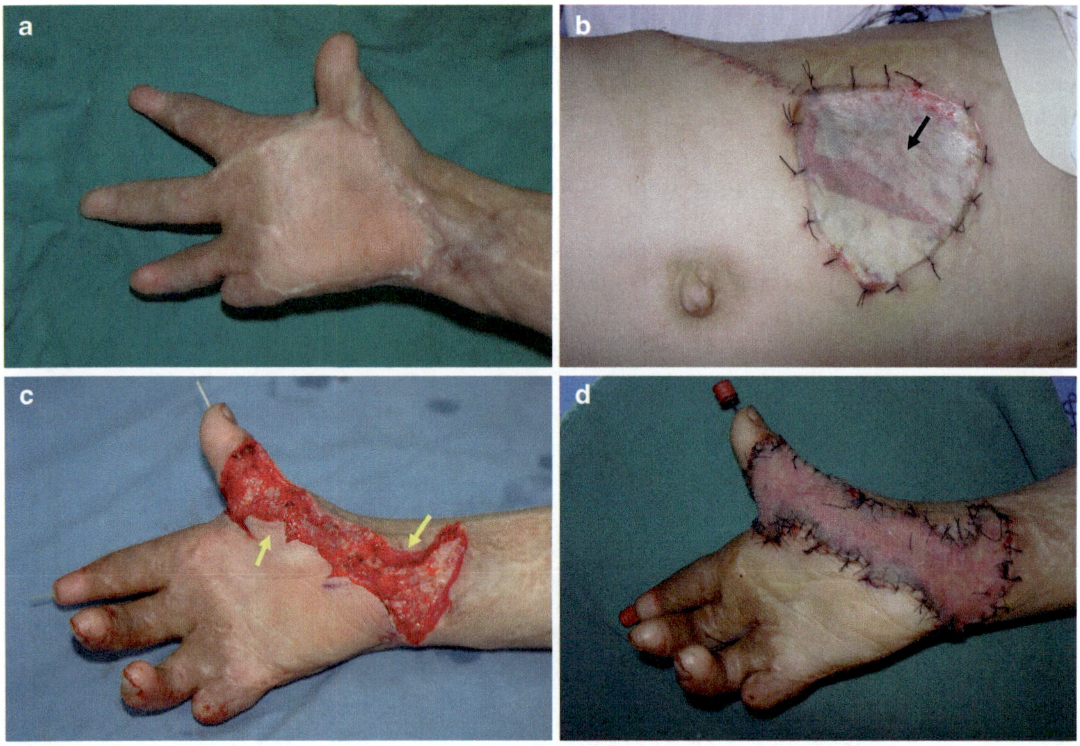

Fig. 2.41 (**a**) 3 years after the surgery, preoperative view. (**b**) Full-thickness skin was harvested on the left abdominal area. The donor skin defect was replaced with human dermal matrix (black arrow). (**c**) Interrupted flaps were made using surrounding scar tissue (yellow arrows) with broken zigzag line. (**d**) Usage of single-sheet FTSG, which was obtained from the abdomen area

Deformations in the dorsal part of the hand should be prioritized over the flexor part when treating circumferential burn deformities. However, in the cases of acute burns, the skin graft should be simultaneously applied on both parts. In case of contracture release of the dorsal

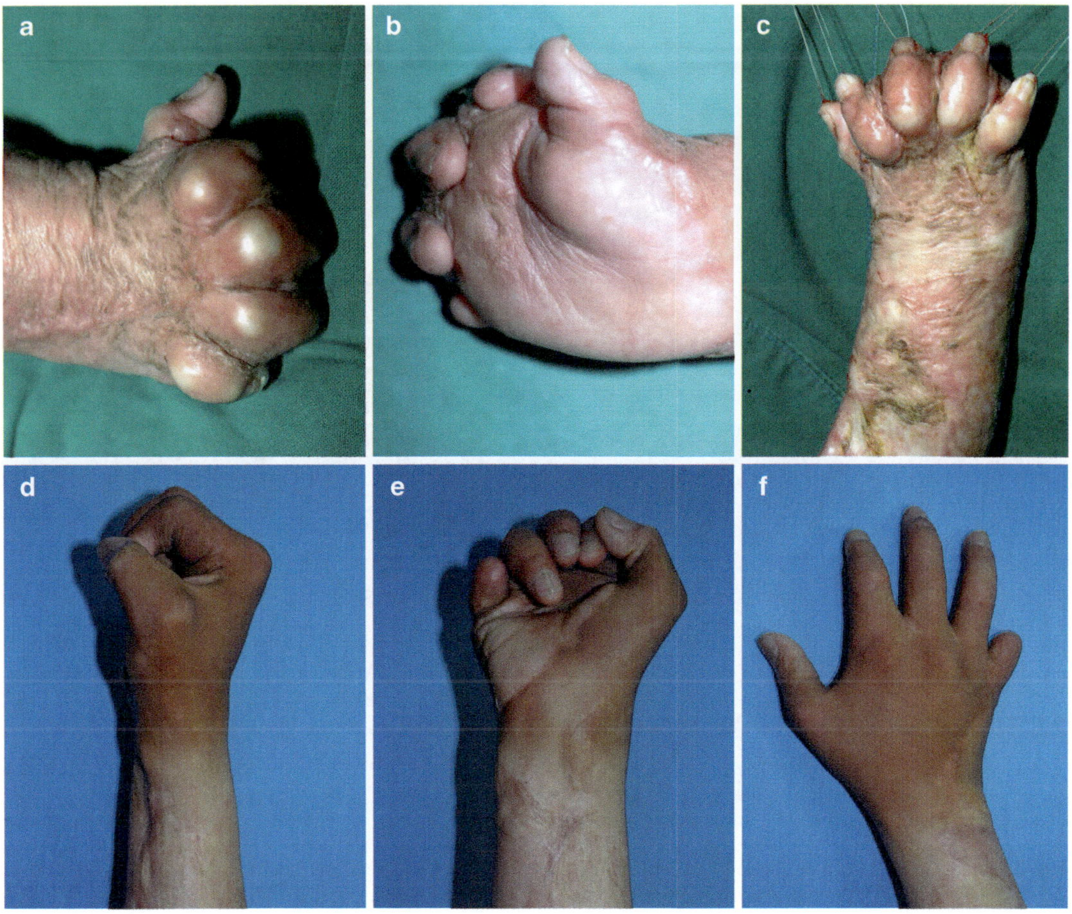

Fig. 2.42 Postoperative 10 years after view. Note the results compared before (**a**–**c**) and after (**d**–**f**) results

side of the hands, issues in the flexor part can still be resolved after dorsal side has been resolved with FTSG in a near-perfect manner and maturation of the surgical site has shown sufficient progress.

I believe that maximum surgical benefits can be obtained with minimal surgery if principles mentioned above are followed.

However, if both the flexor and extensor parts are severely deformed at the same time, simultaneous surgery should be performed on both sides.

A 2-year-old male patient sustained a scaling burn on his left hand (the encircled area). One year after an initial conservative treatment, severe extensor and flexor contracture deformities developed with interphalangeal dislocation (Fig. 2.43). On the extensor and flexor parts of the hand, a single-stage reconstructive surgery was performed using FTSG and human dermal matrix. In this rare severe case, full release on the dorsal side and third, fourth, and fifth flexor contracture releases were performed simultaneously. FTSG engraftment was performed on the flexor and extensor parts on both sides of the hand, and the wrist was engrafted with dermal matrix (Fig. 2.44). Three years after the operation, the results showed good functional recovery. This exceptional single-stage operation on both sides of flexor and extensor was performed simultaneously. Resulted in excellent outcome because of good amount of less damaged palm was left (Fig. 2.45). In this case, a simultaneous surgery is possible because the affected site is not very large, and some skin remained intact on the dorsal side. If possible, it is suggested in principle that correction is performed at different times.

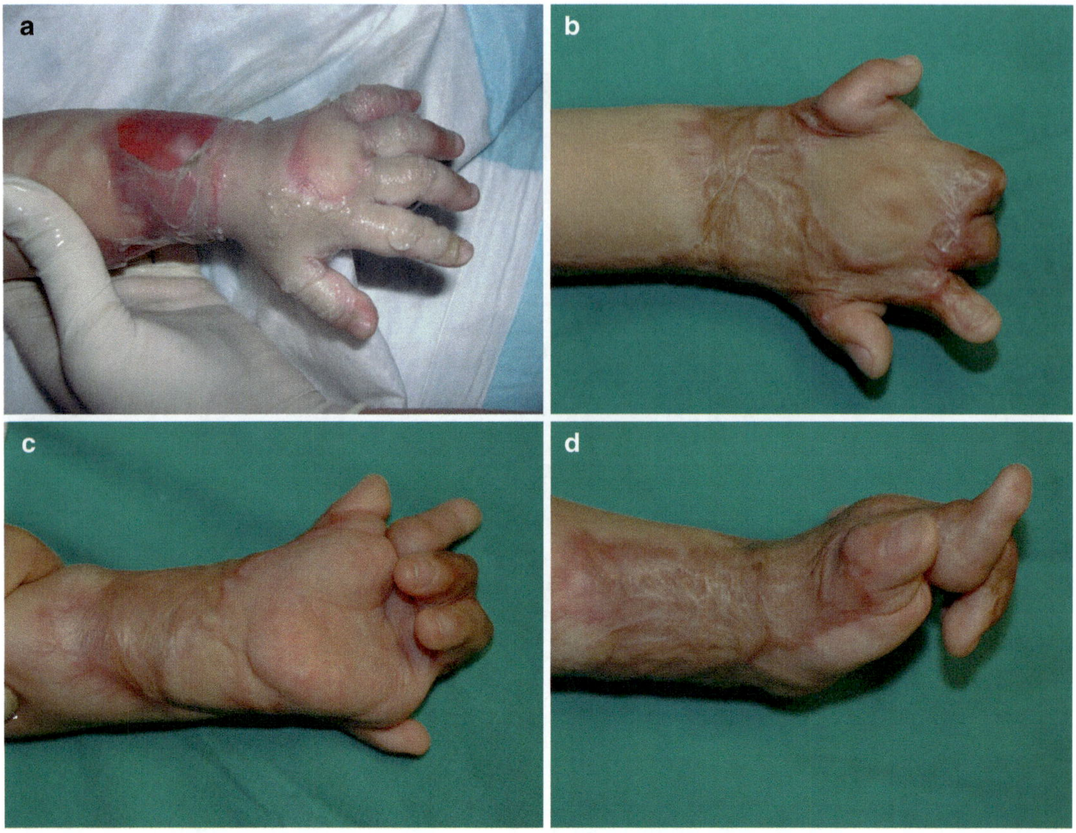

Fig. 2.43 (**a**) Scaling burn on the left hand encircling the area. (**b–d**) One year after an initial conservative treatment, severe extensor and flexor contracture deformities developed with interphalangeal dislocation

Particularly, in a case where the fingers and palm area are simultaneously involved, the following important point must be considered: no seam line single-sheet grafting and overcorrection. One of the reasons why correction is not perfect despite multiple corrective surgeries is that if there is a seam line between two fingers or between the fingers and the palm, the straight line can be the primary cause of linear contracture, and the contracture deformity can get worse with aging of the patient.

Single-sheet grafting that sufficiently covers the skin without creating a seam line is recommended for children, particularly in the flexor area.

When the operation site involves multiple fingers and the palm side, single-sheet skin graft is very effective for correction of contracture and reducing webbing deformity.

(a) In the case of the right thumb, full release and single-sheet FTSG are very effective techniques. (b) Two years after the operation, the engrafted skin developed mild contracture, but the first web space was preserved without functional disturbance. (c) In the case of the second, third, and fourth fingers, (d) a single-sheet graft and a triangular skin flap were inserted deeply into each web space to prevent webbing deformity. Three years after the operation, a well-preserved web space was observed, and additional surgery was not required. This technique may be useful in preventing webbing deformities (Fig. 2.46).

Because the growth of the engrafted skin is crucial until a pediatric patient grows up, efforts

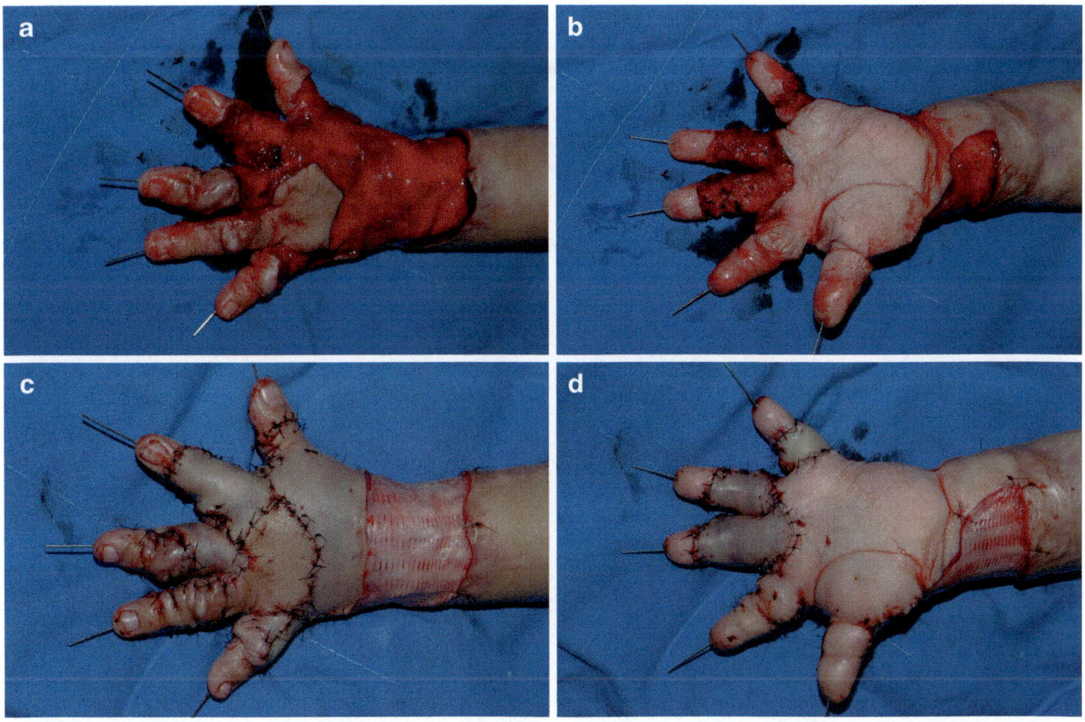

Fig. 2.44 (**a**, **b**) One-stage reconstructive surgery with FTSG and human dermal matrix on extensor and flexor part. (**c**, **d**) FTSG on the flexor and extensor of the hand and dermal matrix graft on the wrist area

should be made to reduce frequency of additional/supplemental surgeries. I have encountered mild webbing deformities in approximately less than 8% of cases during long-term follow-ups, with the main cause and effect being the dimensional difference that arises from grafting a two-dimensional skin change location into a three-dimensional space as well as skin traction that occurs due to continuous growth. Such instances can be prevented by fully releasing the webbing space during surgery and making a triangular split cuts to insert the graft into a triangle-shaped space. Although this deformity does not affect functionality, it cosmetically shortens the finger length appearance and, therefore, can be resolved using modified double-opposing Z-plasty.

Three and ten years after the operation, no functional disturbance was observed; however, the patient wanted a more natural appearance of the web spaces. So, double-opposing Z-plasty was performed on the first and third web spaces for esthetic purposes (Fig. 2.47).

I emphasize the significance of early hand reconstruction in children because the importance of FTSG is evident from the long-term follow-up images. Early skin graft in childhood shows a satisfactory skin growth without scar contracture even after 20 years; in addition to this, double-opposing Z-plasty is beneficial in maximizing the esthetic effects and resolving webbing deformities.

(a) A 3-year-old female patient underwent reconstructive surgery on the first, second, third, and fourth fingers, as well as on the dorsum of the hand to the wrist area, with a single-sheet FTSG. The results of a follow-up after 11 years are presented. Note the dark-colored skin on the inner side of the inguinal skin. I placed light-colored skin on the dorsum of the hand and moved the dark skin to a less apparent site on the forearm side for

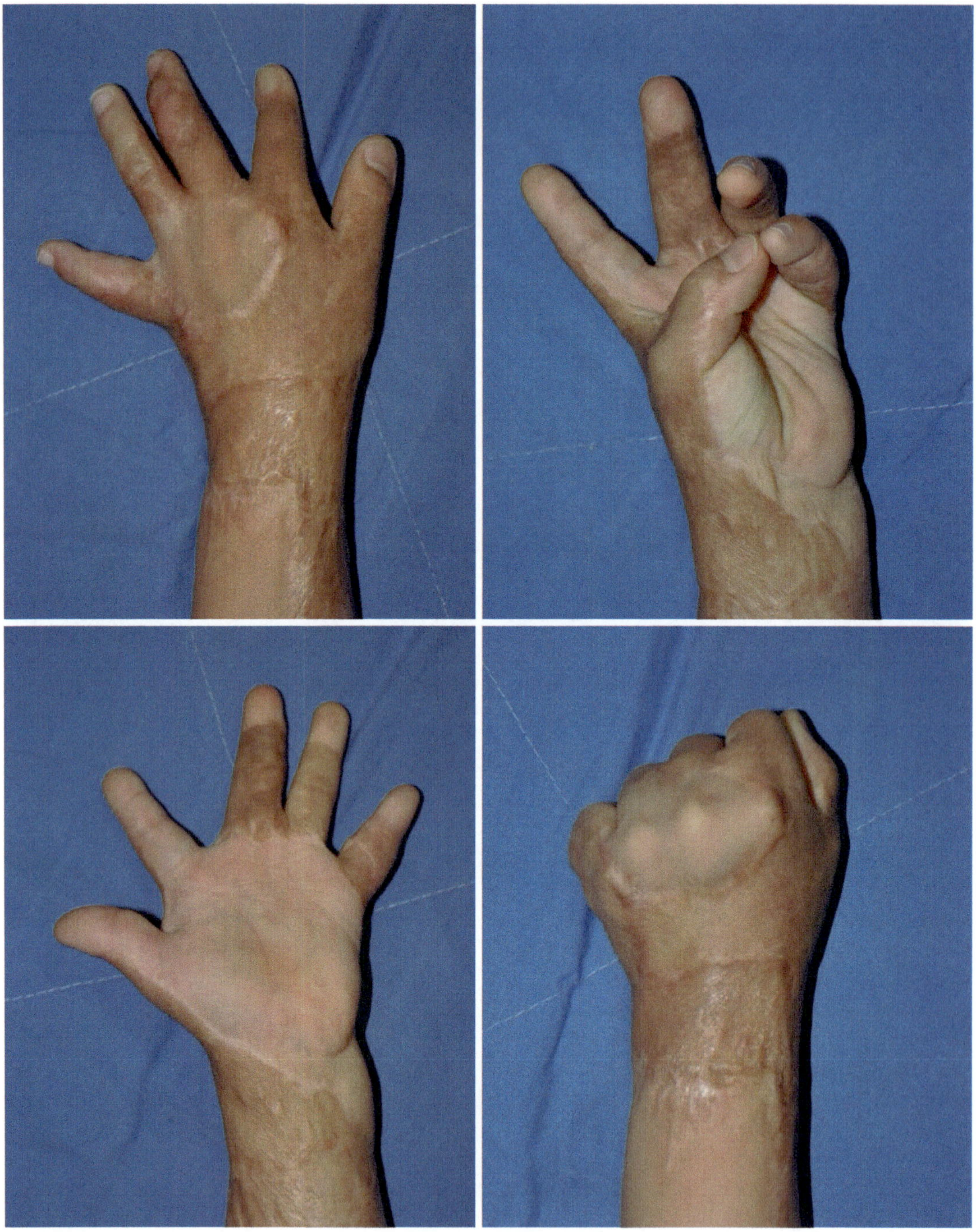

Fig. 2.45 Postoperative 3 years after view, almost functional deformities were corrected

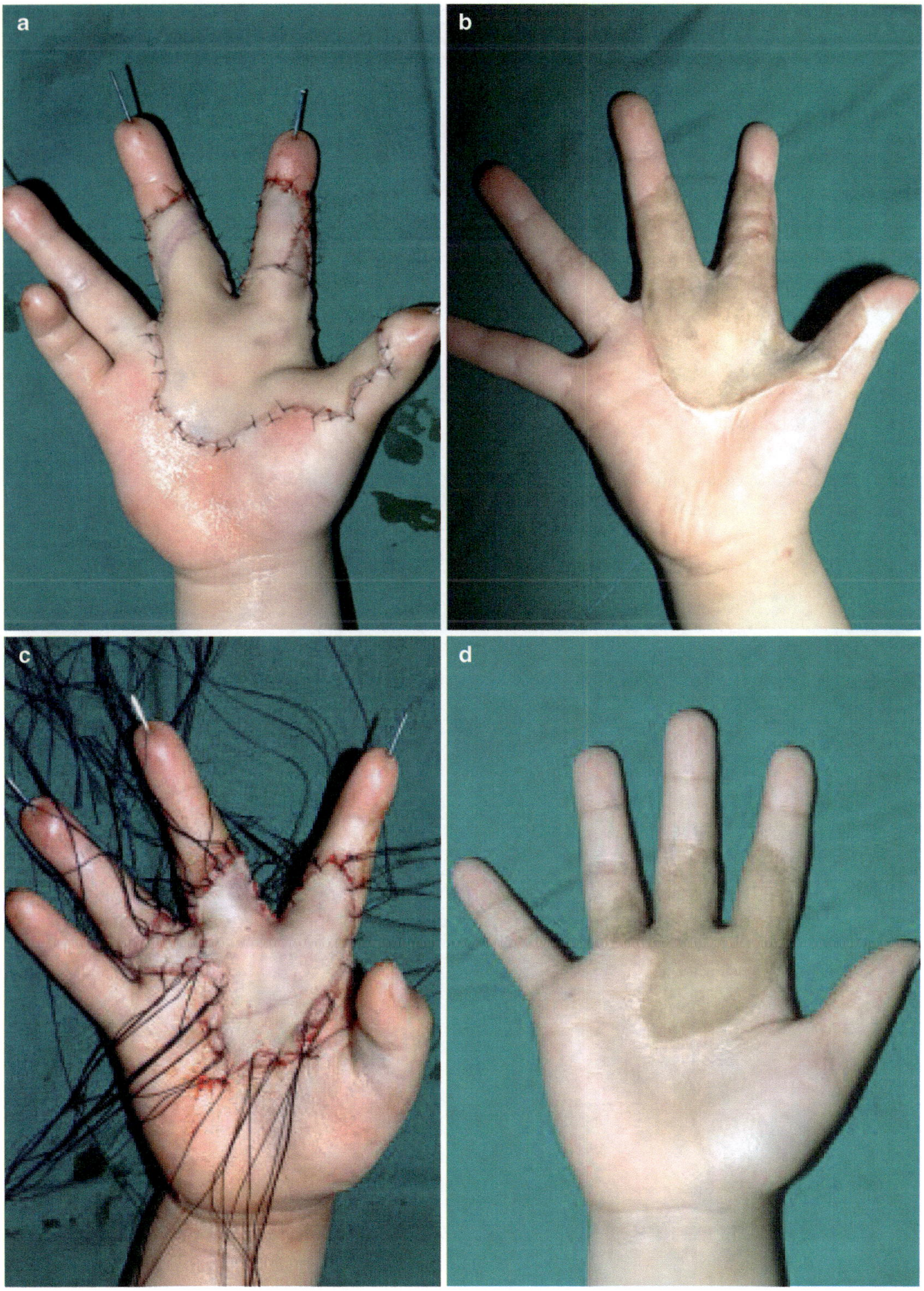

Fig. 2.46 (**a**) In case of involving the right thumb, full release and single-sheet FTSG is a very effective technique. (**b**) Postoperative 2 years after view. (**c**) In case of involvement of second, third, and forth fingers, single-sheet graft and triangle skin flap were made. (**d**) Postoperative 3 years later, well-preserved web space with no need for additional surgery

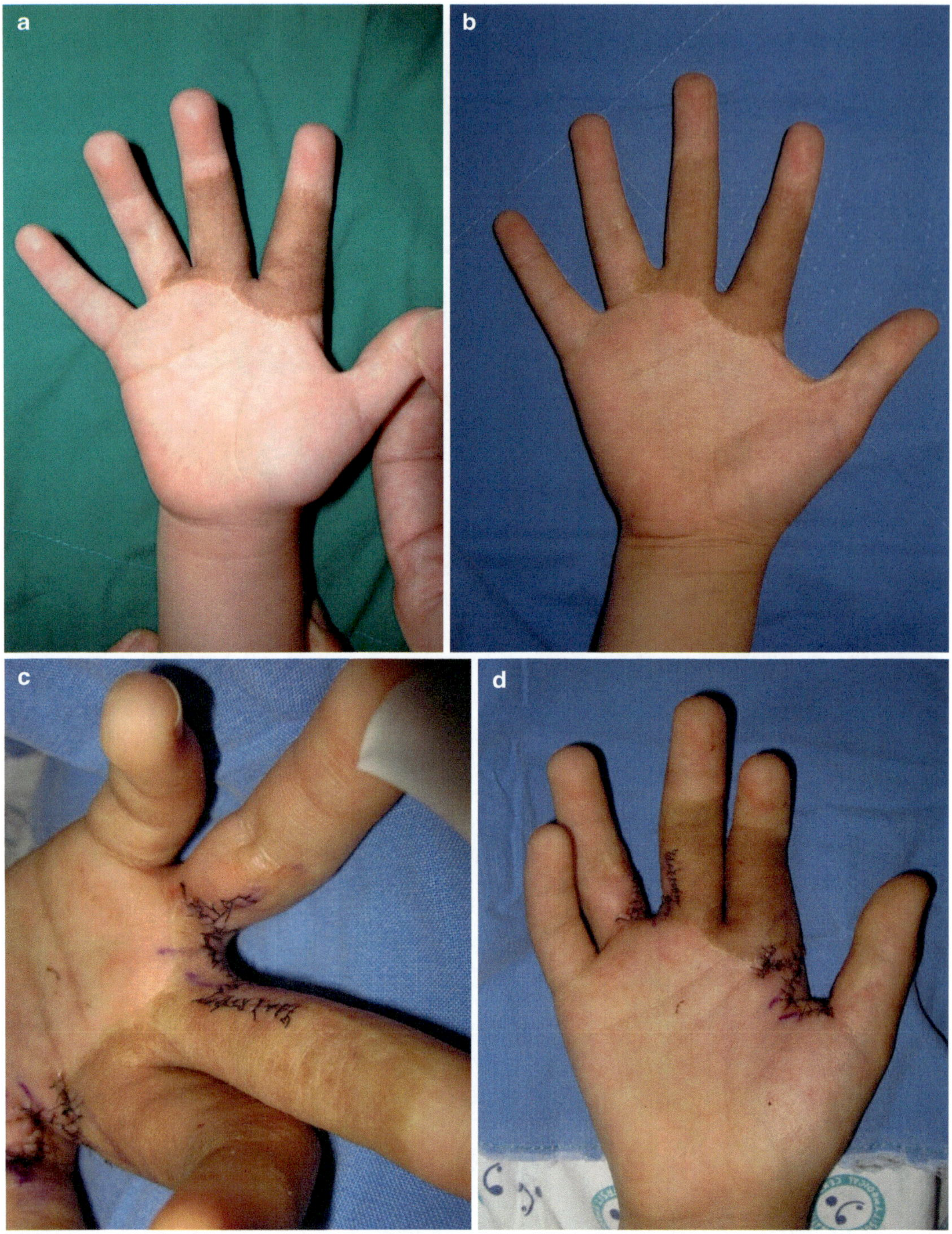

Fig. 2.47 (**a**, **b**) Postoperative 3 years and 10 years after view. (**c**, **d**) Double-opposing Z-plasty for esthetic purpose

a more natural esthetic outcome. Esthetic appeal can be a minor concern for a surgeon, but it may be of a great importance for the patient (black arrow). (b) The engrafted skin size was estimated to be 27 × 11 cm (length × width). This means that early childhood reconstructive FTSG is a huge gift, with the added advantage of the graft growing simultaneously with the body. (c) Note the long zigzag line from the little finger to the wrist in order to prevent long straight-line contracture (black arrow) (Fig. 2.48). Eleven years later, modified double-opposing Z-plasty was performed to correct minor webbing deformities. Note the natural line of web space grooves. I designed and developed the flap angles that were modified for the natural direction of the groove line (dashed yellow arrows). Three months after the operation, minor webbing deformities were corrected, and fingers appeared to be of a normal length (Fig. 2.49).

The most common errors encountered in pediatric hand reconstruction result is primarily from an insufficient amount of skin graft, the surgeon's inability to ensure the complete scar bed and marginal release, and failure of balancing between removal and preservation of an adequate amount of scar tissue.

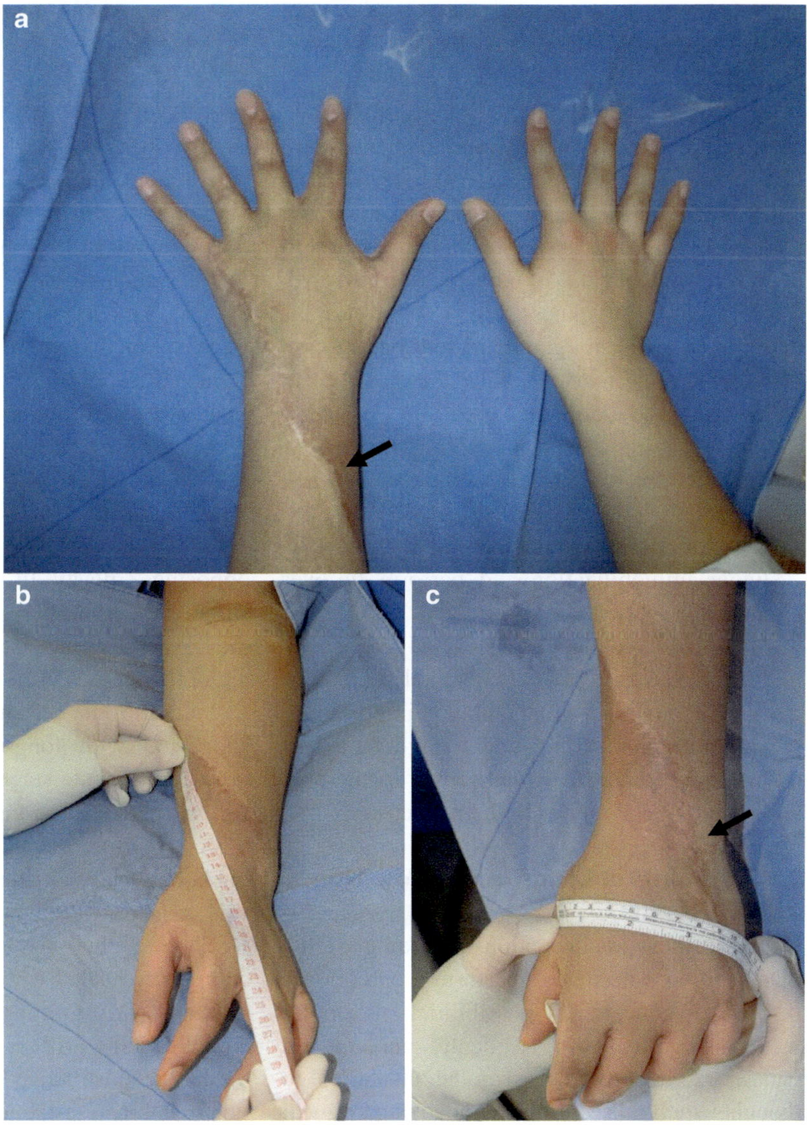

Fig. 2.48 (**a**) Reconstructive surgery on the first, second, third, and fourth fingers and dorsum of the hand to the wrist area with single-sheet FTSG. (**b**) Long-term follow-up after 11 years, engrafted skin size was estimated 27 × 11 cm. (**c**) Note the long zigzag line from the little finger to the wrist (black arrow)

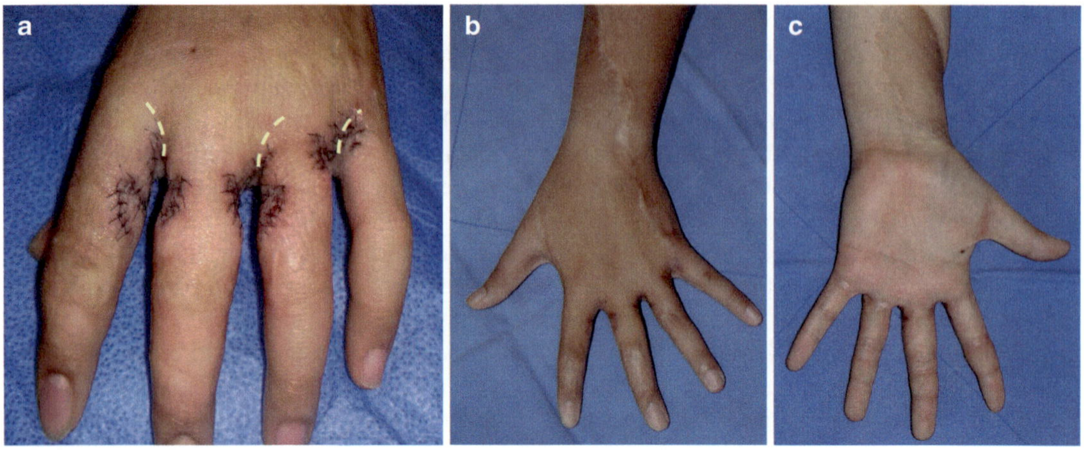

Fig. 2.49 (**a**) Long-term follow-up 11 years after, modified double-opposing Z-plasty was performed for correction of mild webbing deformities. Note the natural line of web space grooves (dashed yellow arrows). (**b**, **c**) Postoperative 3 months later, mild webbing deformities were corrected and looked more natural length of fingers

My key points of consideration in pediatric hand reconstruction are mentioned below:

1. Perform perfect early reconstruction with FTSG in a single surgery with anticipation to ensure the benefit of accompanied growth ability of full-thickness skin.
2. Perform a full marginal and scar bed release to reduce the tension (make tension-free) in the engrafted margin.
3. Avoid making a seam line within the graft, if possible, and graft using a single sheet when possible.
4. Use soft tissue k-wire fixation for pediatric finger immobilization and perform tie-over dressing.

My ultimate goal in pediatric hand reconstruction is to achieve all possible desirable outcomes in a single surgery. To that end, it is important to prepare for donor sparing, which might be essential when the pediatric patient grows up and possible additional surgeries in the future.

2.4.2.1 Points of Long-Term Follow-Up Results

Owing to their preconceptions regarding FTSG, many surgeons hesitate to perform it on children because of concerns of possibilities of supplemental surgeries with frequently encountered undesirable results. This can be attributed to thoughts such as securing the adequate surgical site is difficult—particularly, in pediatric hand burn reconstruction, obtaining successful FTSG outcomes is difficult, and patient's cooperation for treatment is not guaranteed.

Nevertheless, the long-term follow-up results of my patients reveal several advantages of FTSGs, such as the complete reconstruction achieved in >95% of patients with steam burn injuries treated after 1 or 2 years after the incident using a single surgery before the child grows up. To resolve esthetic appearances and not funtional deformities, such as simple mild webbing deformities, can easily be corrected with double-opposing Z-plasty. In particular, it shows that a surgery, the primary resolution target for which is the flexor deformity, can be successful in terms of patient outcomes in a single surgery.

I will introduce a complete sequential process, supported with long-term follow-up over 10 years, from acute stage management to the final reconstructive surgery procedure.

A 1-year-old female patient sustained a scalding burn. One week after the injury, the acute burn was treated with human dermal matrix. Three weeks after the operation, the acute wound was completely healed with no graft loss. Early excision and early grafting are very effective in the wound healing process and have a good effect on the late reconstructive surgery process with good functional and esthetic results. One year after the operation, severe scar contracture was noted on the right big toe and in step area. Excisional release and conventional FTSG were performed (Figs. 2.50 and 2.51). One and five years after the operation, no functional disfigurement was noticed, and the esthetic result was excellent. Ten years after the operation, no functional disfigurements were noticed. This excellent result proves that full-thickness skin is effective in growing children and supports the author's conviction that early childhood surgery is highly recommended (Figs. 2.52 and 2.53). (a) Peelings caused

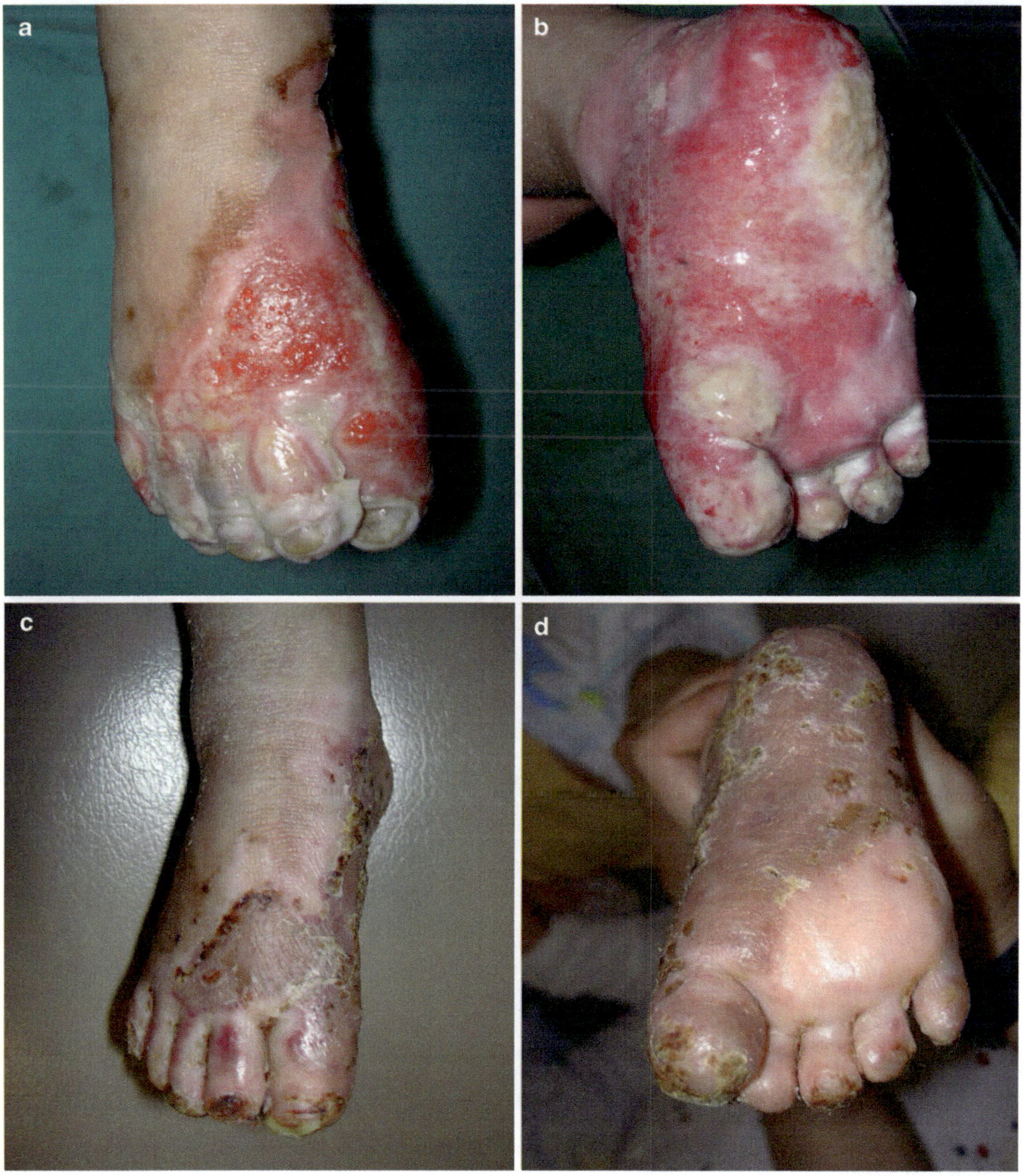

Fig. 2.50 (**a**, **b**) The acute burn management was treated with human dermal matrix 1 week after the injury. (**c**, **d**) Postoperative 3 weeks later view

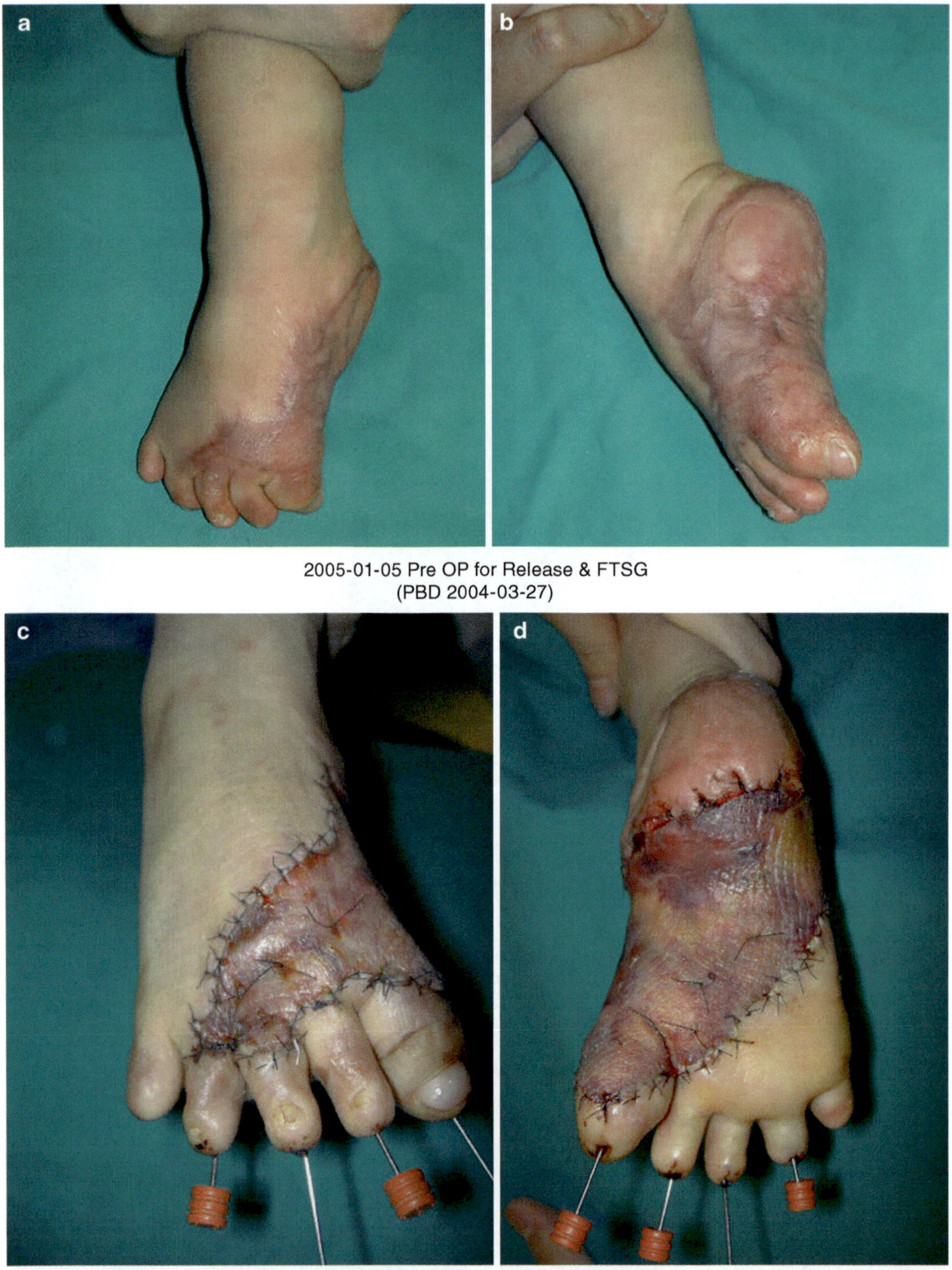

Fig. 2.51 (**a**, **b**) Postoperative 1 year after, severe scar contracture was noted on the right great toe and in-step area. (**c**, **d**) Excisional release and FTSG were performed

by abrasion, especially on the great toe and heel area. Healed at acute burned state (black arrows). After 10 years, she visited our clinic, with unstable weakening and trouble with easy exfoliating on the weight-bearing site of the heel and great toe. To correct this problem, we used an innovation idea using dermabrasion and dermal resurfacing technique for reinforcement of weight-bearing area in the sole. Preoperatively, note easy peeling of scabrous/flaking skin on the weight-bearing sole on the heel and great toe (black arrows). (b) Dermabrasion was performed using the dermal overgraft technique. (c) On the opposite side of the normal step area, a 0.5-mm-thick split-thickness skin donor site was designed (Fig. 2.54). (a) Postoperative immediate view. (b) Six months after the operation, the engrafted sole STSG skin was stabilized and well adapted to the surrounding sole skin (black arrows). (c) One year after the operation, there were no complications, and the weight-bearing sole skin was well preserved (Fig. 2.55). This technique is also very beneficial for correcting the mismatched color of the engrafted FTSG on the palm (refer to Chap. 5; Fig. 2.55).

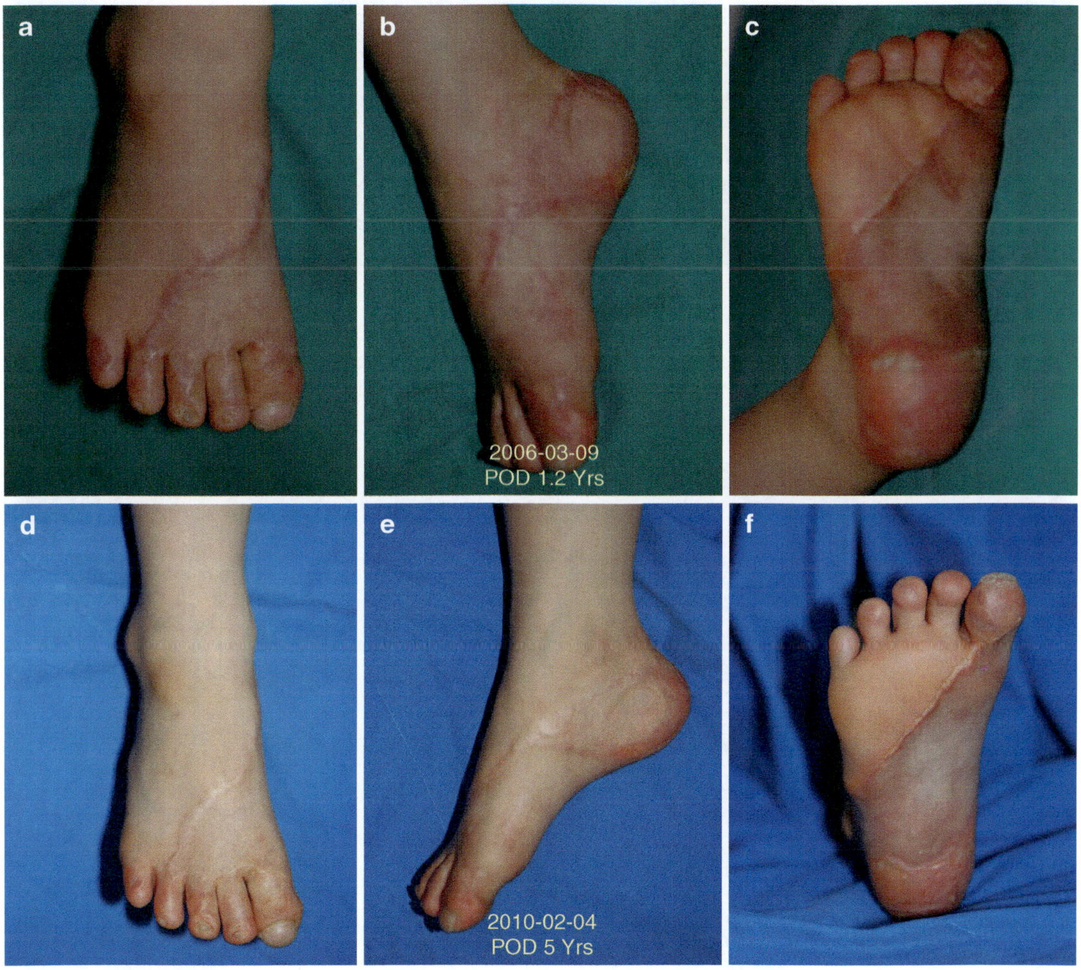

Fig. 2.52 (**a**–**c**) Postoperative 1 year after view. (**d**–**f**) Postoperative 5 years after view

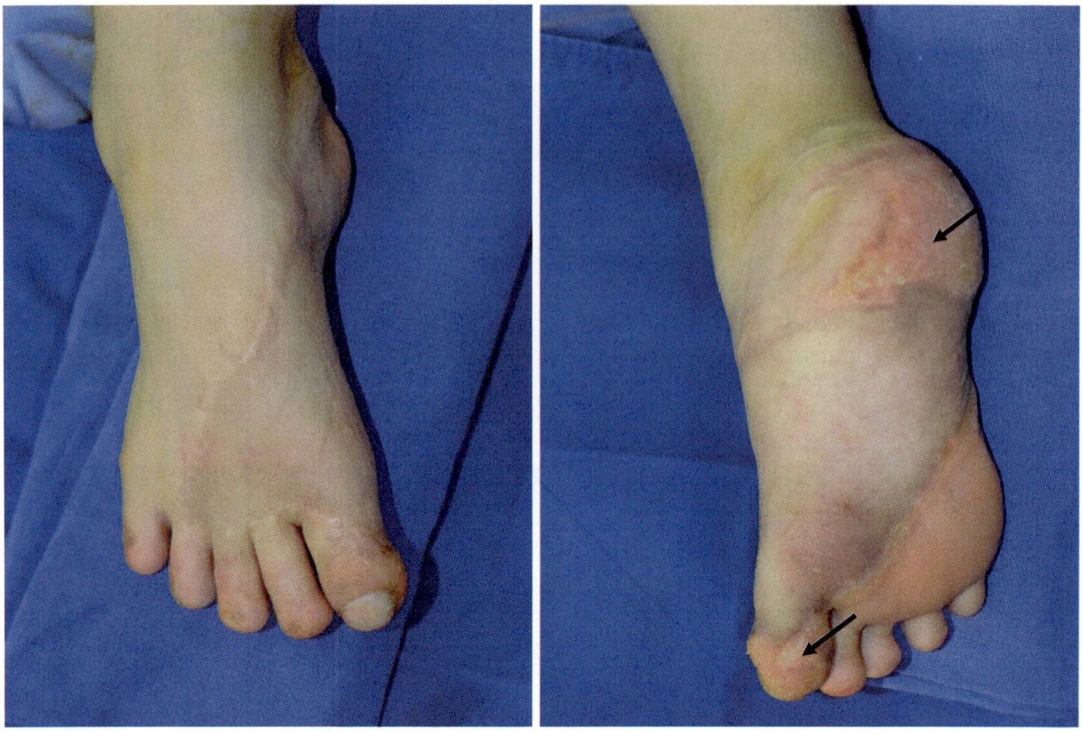

Fig. 2.53 Postoperative 10 years after, noted unstable weak troubled skin condition on heel and great toe (black arrows)

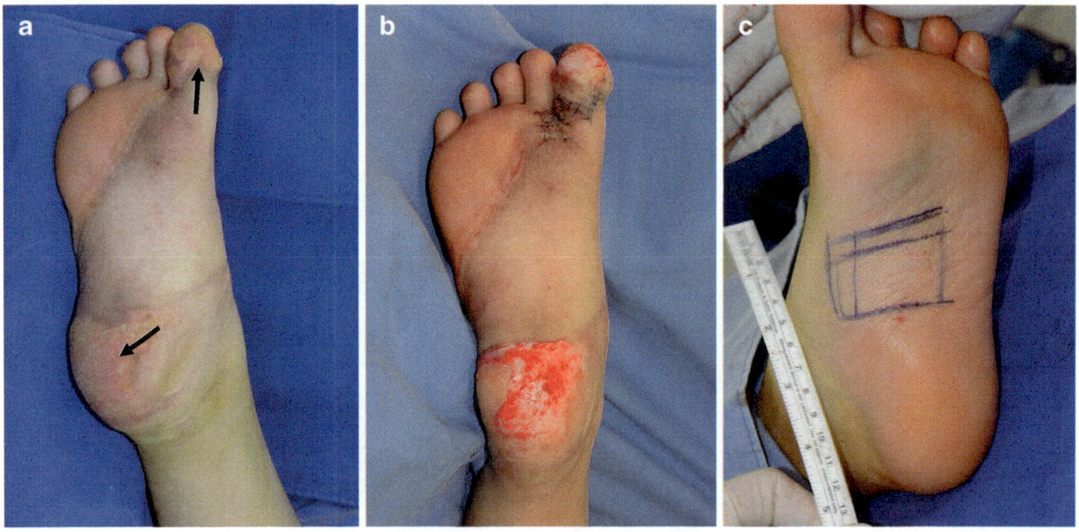

Fig. 2.54 (**a**) Preoperative view (black arrows). (**b**) Dermabrasion was performed for dermal overgraft technique. (**c**) Donor site designed view, 20/1000 inches thickness split-thickness skin

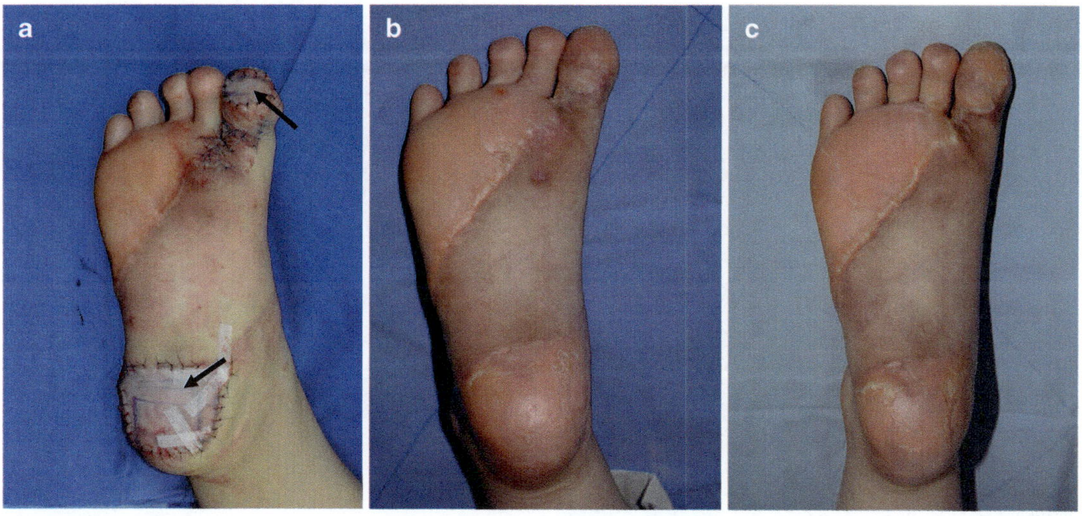

Fig. 2.55 (**a**) Dermabrasion and dermal resurfacing (black arrows). (**b**) Postoperative 6 months view (**c**) Postoperative 1 year after view, well-preserved weight-bearing sole skin

These principles also apply to different parts of the body. As mentioned earlier, FTSG effectively facilitates the acceptance and maturation of the skin through remodeling, without impeding its continuous growth, regardless of insufficient engrafted skin area or tension occurring in several directions. Furthermore, long-term follow-up results reveal that its area increases far wider than the original engrafting site, which also improves surrounding scar maturation. Hence, early reconstruction surgery with FTSG is recommended for children when possible.

Increase in the area affects remodeling of the surrounding tissues, considerably improving the progress of surrounding scar maturation in wide burn scar contracture, which can be regarded as another advantage of FTSG.

An 8-year-old female patient sustained a scalding burn resulting in wide, thick, unsightly burn scars; her main concern was related to the esthetic appearance. The center of the scar area was engrafted with full-thickness skin and a composite fat graft to relieve tension in all scar directions. Scar release was performed in a centrifugal direction, and a triangular flap was made to reduce the tension on scar tissue and maximize the release effect. Eight days after the operation, the graft was taken almost completely without any skin loss. Note there were no slit incisions made in advance to prevent the hematoma. After 3 months and 1.5 years since the operation, there was a significant increase in the engrafted skin surface, and improved thick scarring of the surrounding scars was observed (Fig. 2.56). Three and six years after the operation, the engrafted skin was substantially increased on the surface, with an estimated length of 21 cm and a width of 9.5 cm; the original engraft size increased by twofold (5 × 14 cm), and the surrounding scar tissue was noticeably improved in terms of maturation and texture (Fig. 2.57).

If necessary, I use a part of the scar tissue as a flap to rearrange the overall scar tissue. Additional desirable and flexible surgical outcomes can be obtained by undermining the adjacent scar bed release and repositioning it as a flap rather than proceeding with the surgery using the insufficient amount of skin. If the surrounding scar tissue and full-thickness skin were properly combined for release on contracted area, the remaining surrounding scar can also significantly improve the coordinated effect.

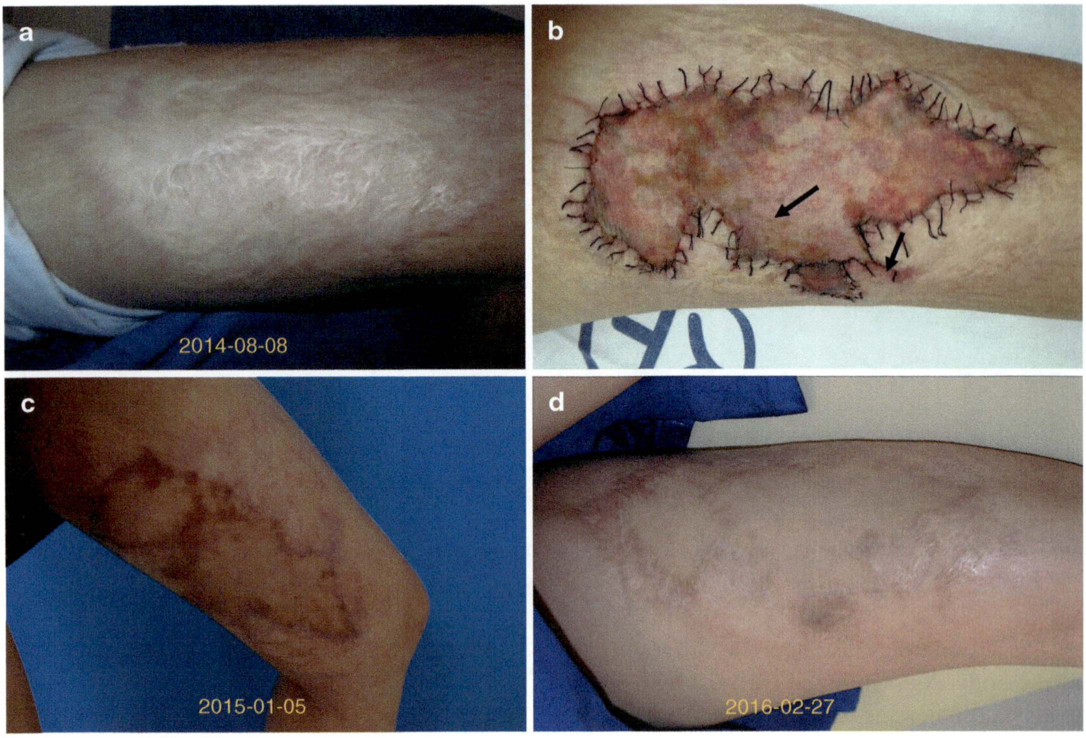

Fig. 2.56 (**a**) Preoperative view, chief complained unsightly wide burn scar, inner left thigh. (**b**) Postoperative 8 days' graft was taken completely, (**c**) 3 months after, (**d**) postoperative 1.5 years after view

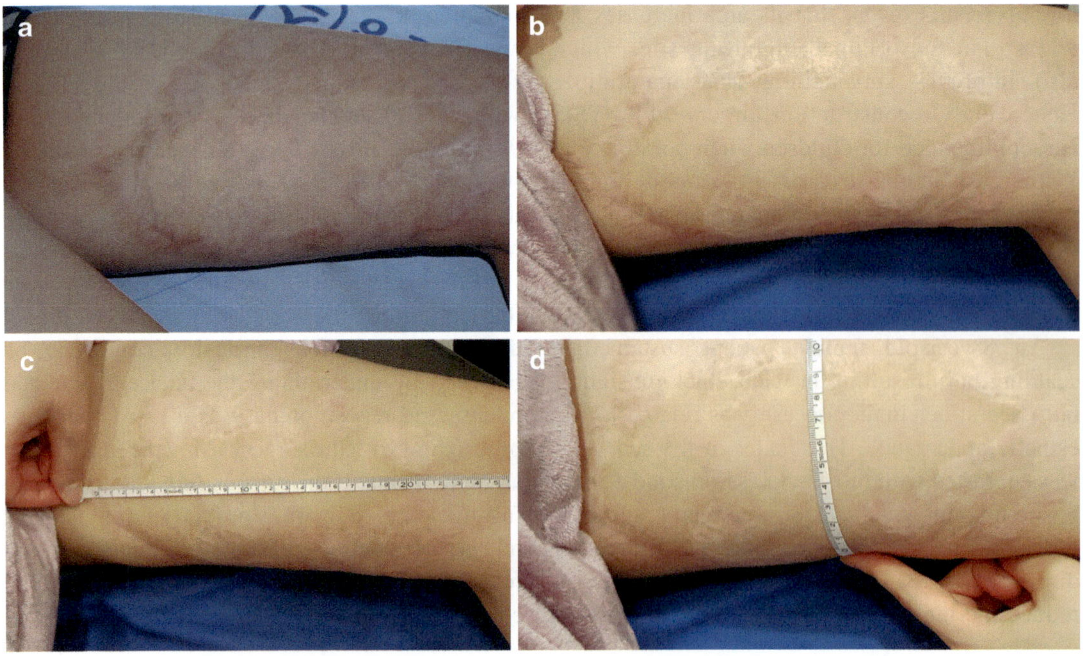

Fig. 2.57 (**a**, **b**) 3 and 6 years after the operation results. (**c**, **d**) The engrafted skin's estimated length was 21 cm and width 9.5 cm; original engraft size was 5 × 14 cm

2.4.3 Adult Hand Reconstruction

Adult hand reconstruction demands the use of techniques that require high skills of the operator who can find and resolve functional and esthetic problems simultaneously. If the skin graft technique is successful in adult reconstructive hand cases, FTSG can be performed in other areas with ease.

Main problems of adult hand reconstruction is that there is never enough donor skin, for full-thickness or split-thickness skin. One of the main reasons could be inadequate acute state management. The surgeon must consider more precise, planned, and effective acute burn management, which depends on the success or failure of late reconstructive surgery. Burns can cause various types of hand deformities, such as extensor, flexor, and circumferential deformities; buttonhole or swan-neck deformities; joint dislocations and stiffness; and bone and thin skin deformities [46, 47] (Fig. 2.58).

Most surgeons tend to resolve majority of the problems with flap surgery [48, 49]; however, I believe that skin graft can help resolve such problems using several techniques applied in children, rather than flap surgery. This can be verified through the cases of successful reconstruction of the hands that I have performed on throughout my clinical practice using 100% of skin graft without any flap surgery. When treating severe hand deformities such as those shown in the preceding cases, ordinary hand surgeons, especially young surgeons, will perform flap surgeries such as free flap, reverse flap, and local flap. However, the author believes that flap surgery has unexpected disadvantages like long operation times, unsightly disfigurement, flap bulkiness, and donor site morbidity, especially in hand reconstructive surgery (Fig. 2.59). The author does not perform flap surgery in hand reconstructive surgeries but only performs skin graft techniques.

Myself also a hand and microvascular surgeon, I only use skin graft techniques to resolve issues in hand reconstruction, which has been successful. There are hesitations from many surgeons regarding exposure of the tendon, joint capsule, or bone and resort to flap surgery first to solve such problems. I perform release and dissection without bone and tendon exposure; if these are exposed, skin grafts can be used to resolve this issue. I do not consider flap surgery as the best choice because it is time-consuming and requires extensive efforts without providing any guarantee of satisfactory outcomes and leaves unsightly scars on the area. Hand reconstruction in adults is not significantly different from the graft techniques used in children, this has been described already; however, the surgery should be performed with more focus on substantial functional recovery rather than expected graft growth. I reiterate that the key to success in hand reconstruction is to follow dissection techniques, which depend on epinephrine injection-related

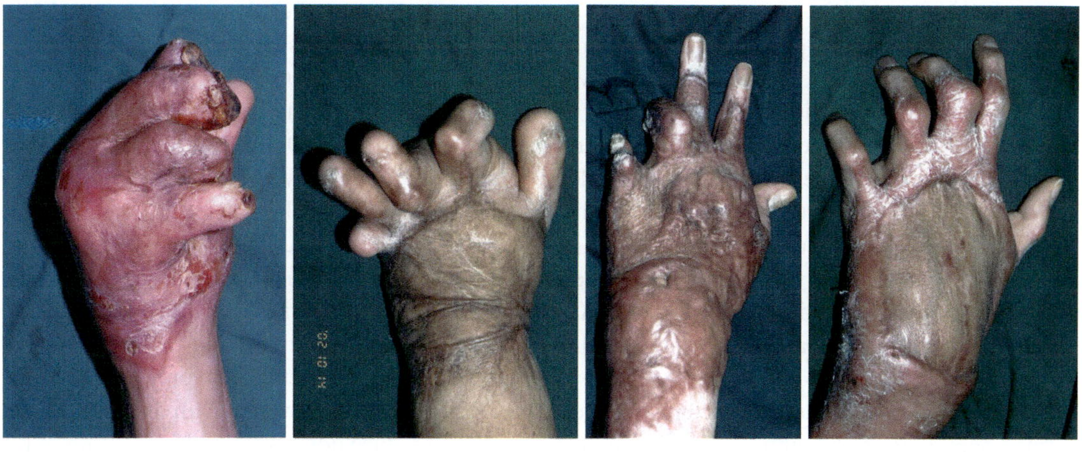

Fig. 2.58 Burned hand deformities later

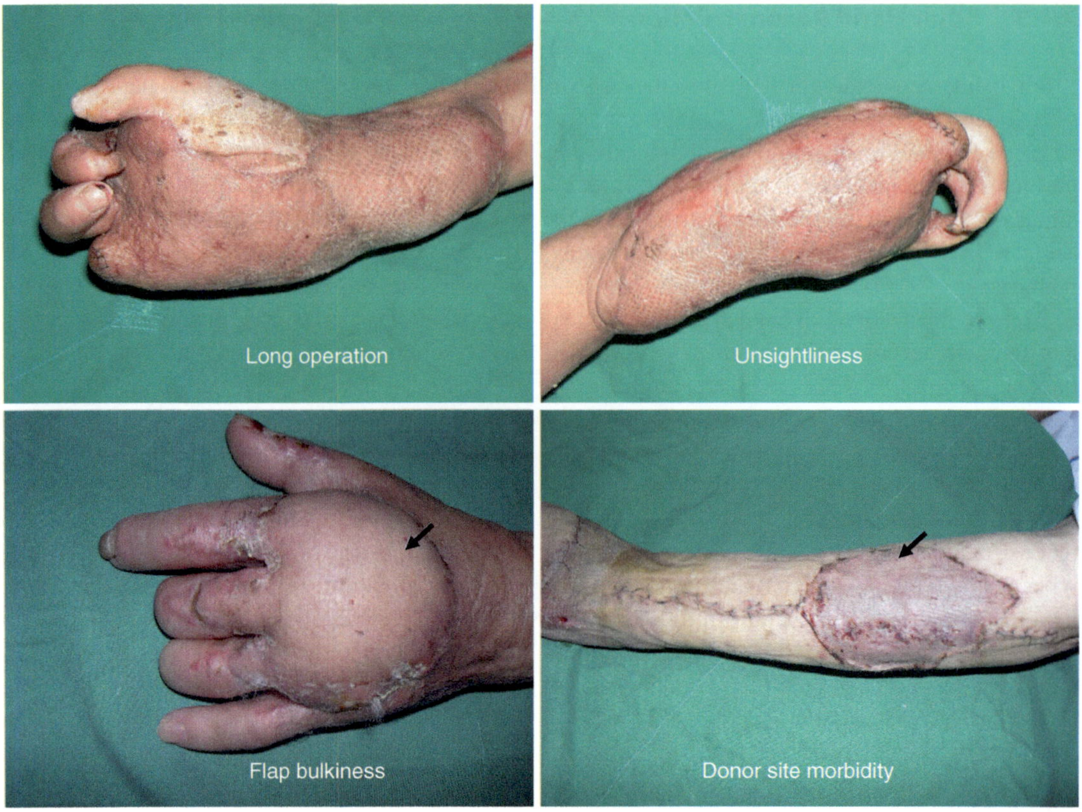

Fig. 2.59 Flap surgery brings many unexpected disadvantages

bleed control, as mentioned earlier. Although this requirement can be unfamiliar to surgeons attempting this technique for the first time and can be difficult to learn, I do believe that if all the know-hows introduced in this book are followed through with sustained effort, the desirable outcomes will be awarded.

A 39-year-old male patient suffered flame burns 20 years ago. A severe scar contracture was observed on the entire dorsum of the hand, as well as significant functional disruption, including a pinch action of the thumb with the index finger. All MCP joints were somewhat movable to some degree. This status indicates that partial hand functional recovery is likely. (a) All interdigital joints were set solid, except for the MCP joints. All dislocated volar plates had a limited range of motion.

Full release of the scar contracture was performed according to the author's own three-step release technique. The advantage of this technique is its safety and practicality for releasing tendon and joint capsule without exposure. The released scar area was covered with FTSG using the conventional dermal shaving method (dashed arrow). Note the released and repositioned point from 20 years ago, the former STSG scar bed (star mark), and the repaired MCP joint (star mark). Two years after the operation, the MCP joints have been repositioned with good function, and he can fully grasp objects (Fig. 2.60).

A 51-year-old male patient suffered a flame burn 17 years ago. On the left hand, cicatricial syndactyly and a swan-neck deformity were noted. A severe volar plate dislocation was observed on the thumb. Hyperextension and button-hole deformities were observed on the right hand (Fig. 2.61). For the left hand, we replaced abdominal full-thickness skin for corrective FTSG, and the remaining abdominal donor defect was covered with human dermal matrix to reduce donor site morbidity. Both of his inguinal donor skin had been used for the reconstruction of his right hand and for other recon-

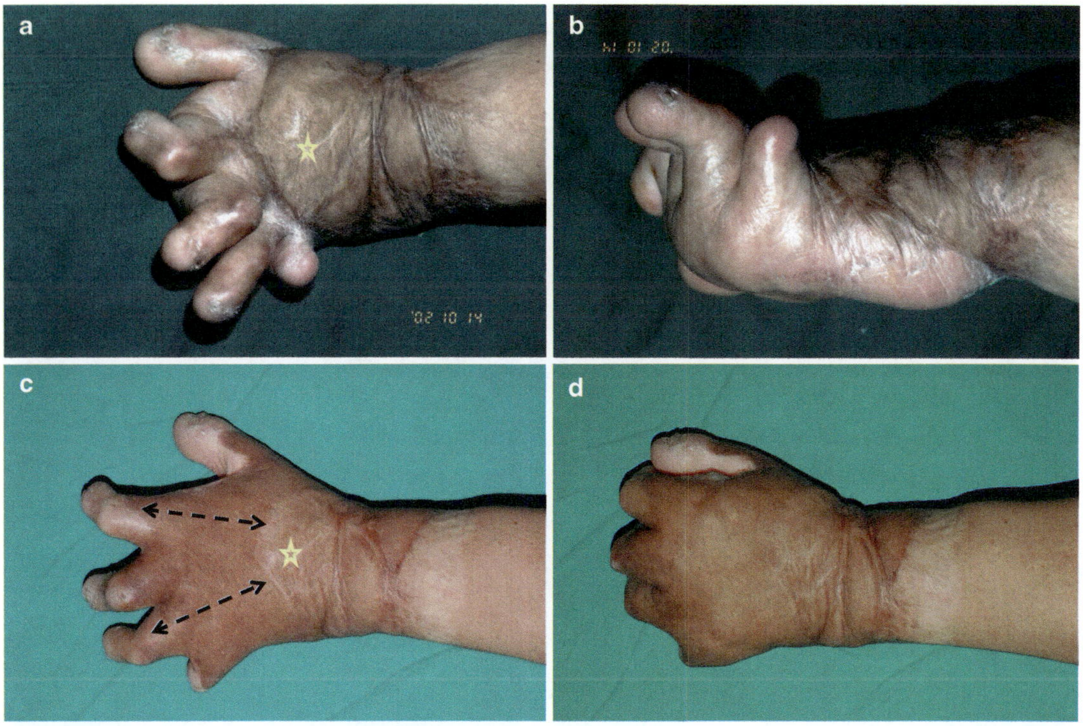

Fig. 2.60 (**a**, **b**) Preoperative view, severe hyperextensive MCP joints and severe functional disturbance. (**c**) Note the (**a**) star mark was moved backwards, (**c**) star mark (two way dashed arrows). Compared to the previous star mark from 20 years ago (**a**). (**d**) Postoperative 2 years after view, he can fully grasp objects

structive procedures in a different hospital. After full release of the dorsal cicatricial scar tissue, manual reduction of the MP joints was performed. K-wire bone fixation was performed in a right-angle position through the digital phalanges and MP joints, which were covered with full-thickness skin harvested from the left abdominal donor skin. Two weeks after the operation, the engrafted skin was removed, and the fist position was maintained with K-wire bone fixation. Two years after the operation, both hands showed esthetic and functional recovery. (a) Note the positive results in the left hand. (b) The severe scar contracture at the MCP joint of the thumb was returned with functional recovery for opposing action with the index and other fingers to pinch and catch small objects. He can grip and catch with his right hand while writing with a small object such as a pen (Figs. 2.62 and 2.63).

An important consideration for hand reconstruction in adults is that several countermeasures should always be taken to fully supplement the shortage of skin area. Therefore, combining FTSG with STSG or dermal substitute can be considered [50–52]. However, before discussing this, it should be noted that the most important point related to hand reconstruction in adults is the fact that the improper management of acute burns and trauma is prone to error, which makes management in the initial stage crucial. This issue has been covered in Chaps. 1 and 3. It should be also noted that a proper response in the initial stage will influence surgical outcomes [53, 54]. For adults who have a wider area for skin grafting, unlike children, functional recovery should be prioritized. The skin graft should be primarily geared toward the thumb, which is the most important contributor to functional recovery and has the largest range of motion, because the amount of skin on both of the inguinal donor sites is not sufficient in adults. Similar to what is observed in children, reconstruction of the dorsal side of the hands should be prioritized in adults. Its reconstruction should be performed with care to avoid lateral displacement of the extensor tendons and lateral band shortening, followed by

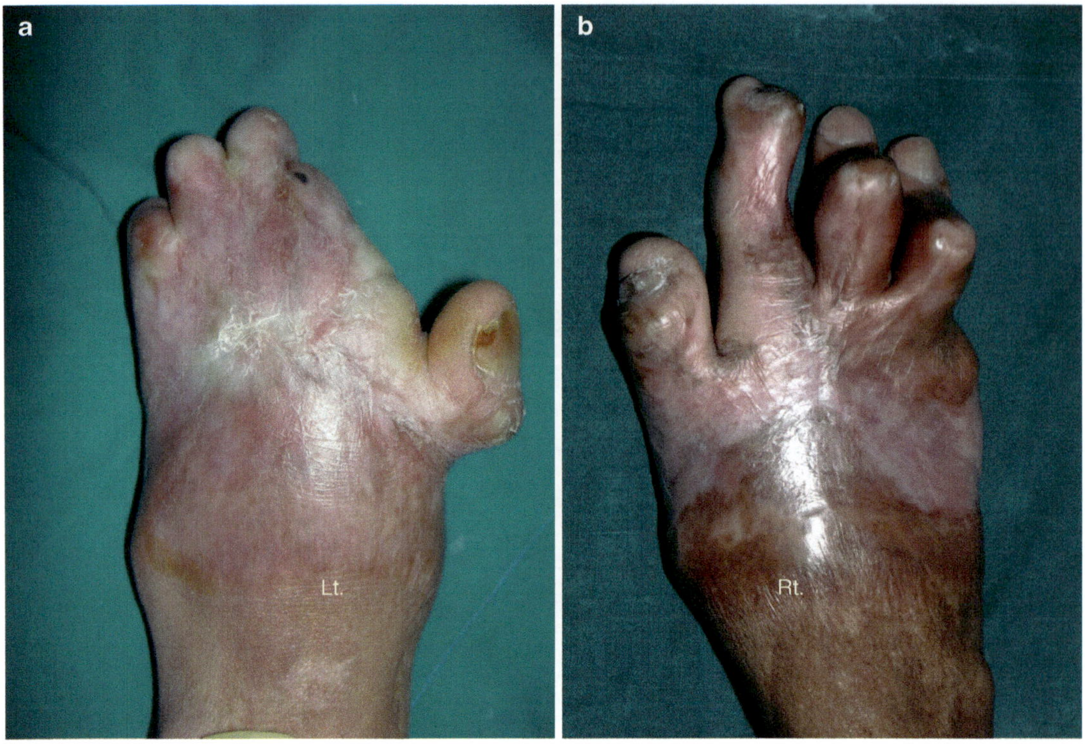

Fig. 2.61 (**a**) Cicatricial syndactyly and swan-neck deformity on the left hand. (**b**) Hyperextensive deformities and button-whole deformities on the right hand

reconstruction of the flexor area. Because skin graft is the top priority in hand reconstruction, FTSG is the key to overcome the shortage of the skin and resolve a functional recovery issue as much as possible.

A 44-year-old female patient suffered a flame burn. Severe contractures were noted on the left hand, and all fingers were dislocated. In this case, step-by-step release of each finger was performed, and afterwards manual reduction was performed carefully to prevent joint capsule exposure. After full contracture release, FTSG covered the MP joints and interphalangeal joints first and STSG was used for the lack of skin on the end of the dorsum of the hand. The tips of finger joint release begin near the joint and extend further away from the joint for a diffusely entire release rather than a localized release, which is an important tip to avoid tendon or joint capsule exposure. Six months after the operation, the hand functions were almost fully recovered only with a simple graft technique and no additional procedures. The author normally performs closed capsulotomy than open-joint capsule. Many surgeons are intrigued by this procedure, but if you first release the surrounding scar tissue of the joint area and meticulously dissect a more wider surrounding scar to soften and harden the surrounding joint scar tissue, you can release full reduction with a closed capsulotomy without tendon or joint capsule exposure (Fig. 2.64).

A 40-year-old female patient's left hand was found to be severely contracted on the dorsum of the hand, with swan-neck deformities on the fourth and fifth fingers and wrist area. Because the primary goal was to restore flexor function, an FTSG was performed to cover the proximal part of all digits, especially the thumb area with hyperabduction. Note the interdigital K-wire bone fixation on the fourth and fifth fingers (yellow arrow). The remaining defect area was covered with human dermal matrix and a thin STSG (Fig. 2.65).

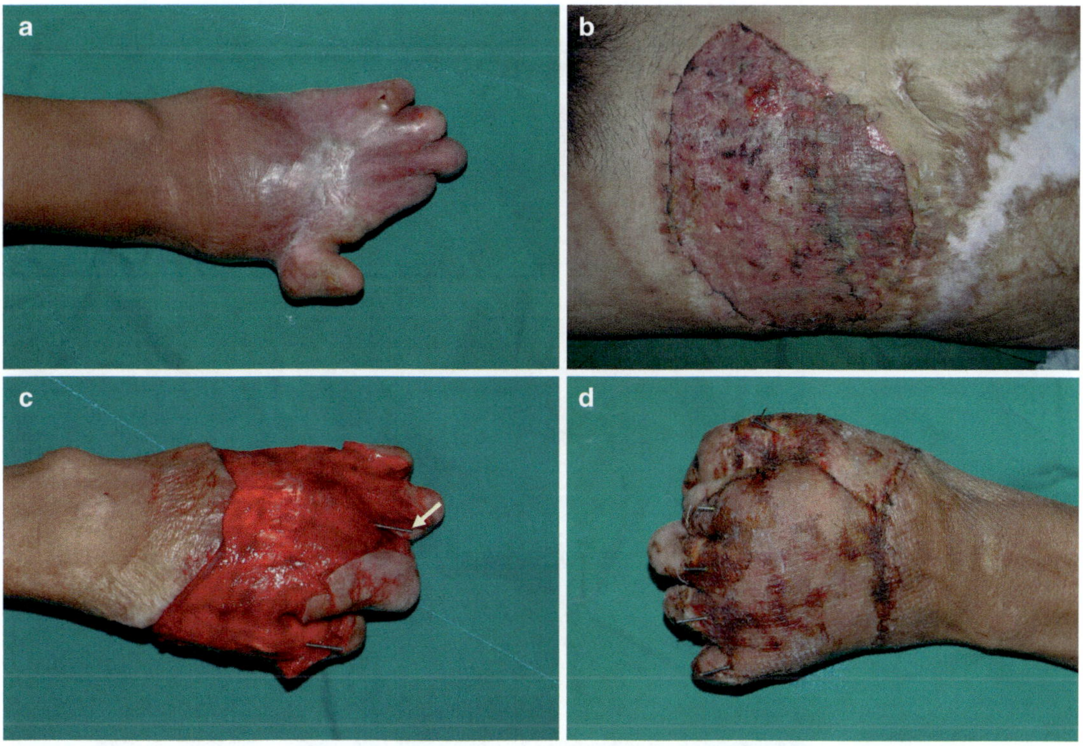

Fig. 2.62 (**a**) Preoperative view. (**b**) Abdominal full-thickness skin was replaced with reconstruction of the left hand and the donor defect was covered with human dermal matrix. (**c**) Manual reduction of MCP joints, K-wire bone fixation (yellow arrow). (**d**) Postoperative 2 weeks' view, engrafted skin was taken completely and fist position continued with K-wire bone fixation

I often use this technique because the top priority in FTSG among adults is the functional recovery; if both donor sites have already been used, skin can be harvested from the areas with sufficient amount of skin, like near the inguinal area, flank, or abdomen. The skin defect donor site can be replaced with human dermal matrix in a single surgery to resolve any esthetic problems (Fig. 2.62b).

2.4.4 FTSG on the Other Sites

In the case of FTSG for parts other than the hands as well as the wider surfaces of the upper and lower extremities, it is necessary to learn the appropriate design and release as well as engrafting techniques to ensure maximum efficiency while performing FTSG with a small amount of donor skin, which is always scarce and limited. The previously described release and grafting techniques should be applied here as well.

As described previously, the following points should be considered:

1. During grafting, do not try to force fit the engrafted skin to the shape of the skin defect. Graft the skin using the elasticity of the full-thickness skin, ensuring both vertical and horizontal tension balance of the skin elasticity are controlled carefully to enhance the graft take.
2. For scar release, do not cut out the scar in its shape in advance instead release the scar bed centrifugally from the center while making incisional release from the center to the cross or in all directions. Afterwards, it is recommended not to remove the gross scar tissue, because some scars play an important role of interpositional flap for supplement of graft tissue (Fig. 2.24).

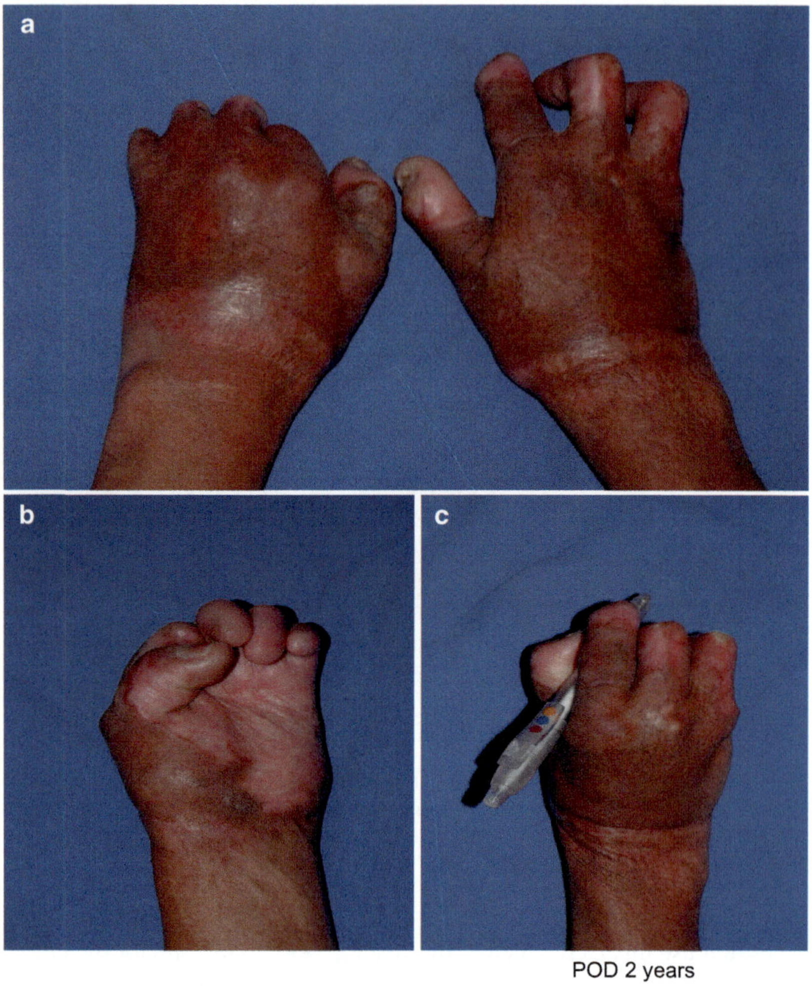

Fig. 2.63 (**a**, **b**) Postoperative 2 years after, both hands are showing esthetic and functional recovery. (**b**) Note the dislocated MCP joint of the thumb was recovered with functional recovery. (**c**) Grip and catch with ability to hold a pen to write

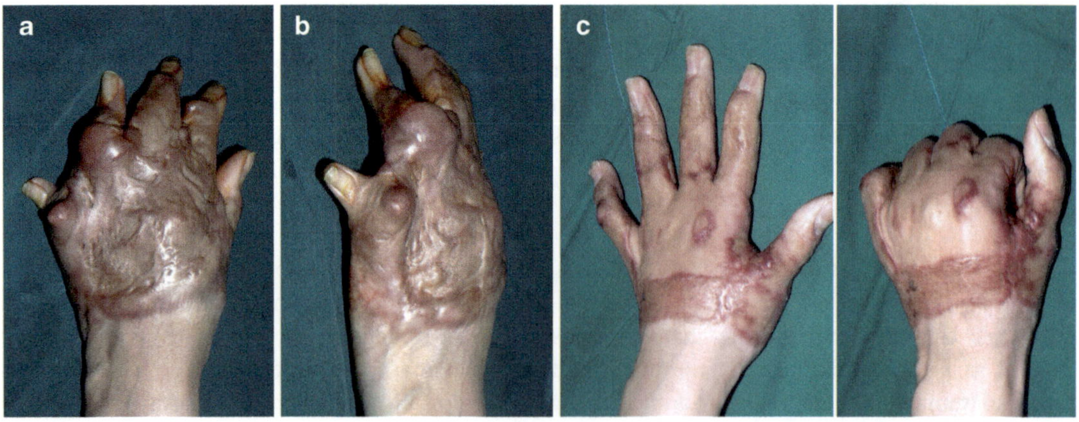

Fig. 2.64 (**a**, **b**) Preoperative view. (**c**) Postoperative 6 months later, the hand functions were almost fully recovered with just simple graft technique without any additional procedure

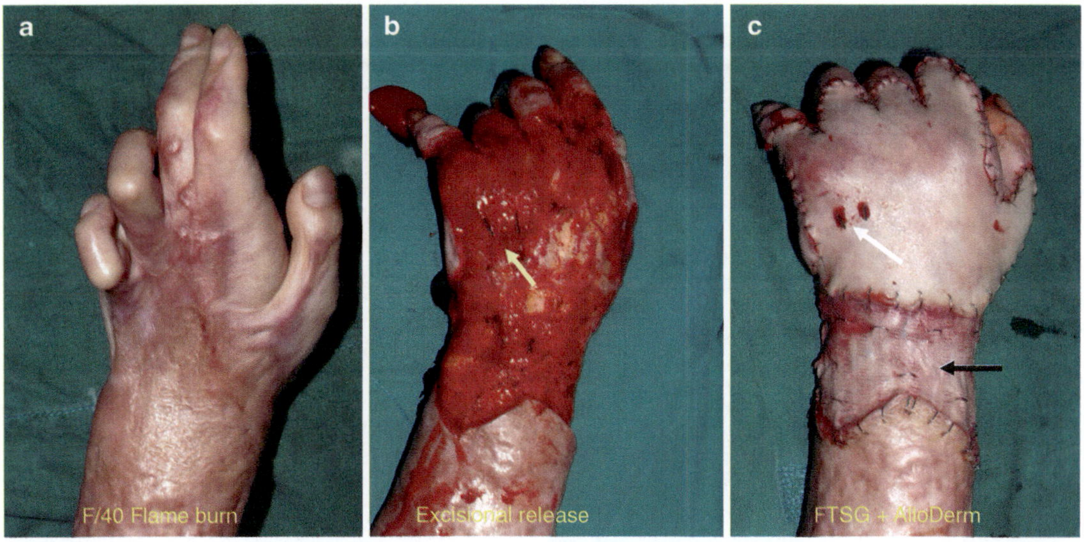

Fig. 2.65 (**a**) Preoperative view. (**b**) Note K-wire bony fixation (white arrows). (**c**) The remaining defect area was covered with human dermal matrix (black arrow)

3. If the scar margin has been released completely, make zigzag slit incisions (broken straight lines and not a long straight line) by making a fish-mouth shape or triangular flap (Fig. 2.16).
4. Remove the scar tissue so that the harvested donor skin can cover the site by controlling and adjusting the tension of full-thickness skin. If possible, leave the scar tissue in a triangular shape to act as a broken flap in a long linear line.
5. As tie-over dressing is crucial for the prevention of hematoma and improvement of the graft take rate, perform film compressive dressing using even pressure by dividing the groups of thread equally on both of the opposite sites for a balanced tension tie ups (Fig. 2.14).

The points mentioned above must be considered with great care as these regions usually require over a maximal-sized skin graft. It is impossible to release all the scar tissues. For the scar release I always perfer to start the release from the most concentrated contracture point on the scar bed, while checking the released area size containing scar tissue and determine excise or reserve the scar tissue according to possible size of harvest skin. The scar tissue sometimes can help cover the wound and release contracture; therefore, the scar tissue should not be totally excised in advance. Based on my experience, releasing tension from all the directions combats the interposition of the elasticity of full-thickness skin, which improves the quality of the surrounding scar according to maturation process. This result is maximized particularly in growing children, which is why I emphasize an early age of reconstruction with FTSG (Figs. 2.56 and 2.57).

2.4.5 FTSG with Fat Composite Graft

The advantages of FTSG include the elasticity of the engrafted skin, retention of the original color, texture of the donor site, and restoration of skin volumes to some degree [55, 56].

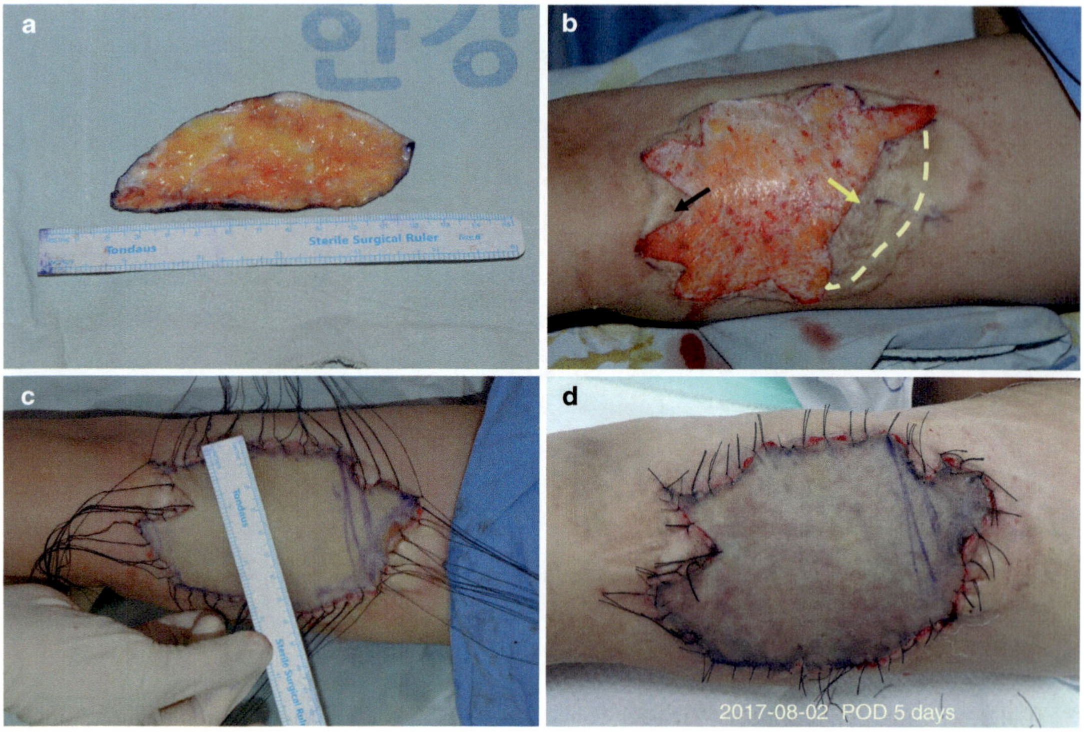

Fig. 2.66 (**a**) Note the full-thickness skin with attached subcutaneous fat layer. (**b**) The unsightly scar tissue was removed partially and note the remaining scar tissue (dashed line, yellow arrow). Note the triangular flap (black arrow). (**c**) The collected donor width was 6 cm, but its width increases to 7.5 cm after engraft. (**d**) Postoperative 5 days after tie-over dressing was opened

Since 2013, I have been refraining from dermal shaving of full-thickness donor skin, which is a conventional technique, while harvesting skin grafts containing subcutaneous fat layer for FTSG to maximize volume replacement, which is an advantage of FTSG. However, supplementing the graft with subcutaneous fat tissue has been proven to be successful with extra several advantages which are increasing graft take rate.

(a) Note the full-thickness skin with attached subcutaneous fat layer skipped conventional dermal shaving process. (b) The unsightly scar tissue was removed partially and replaced with surrounding scar tissue because the entire scar area was too difficult to entirely cover. In my case, the maximum collectible inguinal donor width is not more than 7 cm. Note the triangular flap used to prevent recontracture and relieve tension in the surrounding scar tissue (black arrow). (c) The collected donor width was 6 cm, but after engraftment, it increased to 7.5 cm. I slightly made the skin smaller for a more stable engrafted condition. (d) Postoperative 5 days after tie-over dressing was opened (Fig. 2.66). Fifteen and twenty-four days after the operation, the original engrafted width of 7.5 cm remained unchanged. Note the markedly improved triangular flap and surrounding scar tissue maturation. Therefore, using surrounding scar tissues is an important step to cover wide scars and achieve esthetic and functional recovery. Two months after the operation, the engrafted skin texture softened rapidly. Usage of subcutaneous fat composite in graft shows its advantages, which must be investigated further (Fig. 2.67).

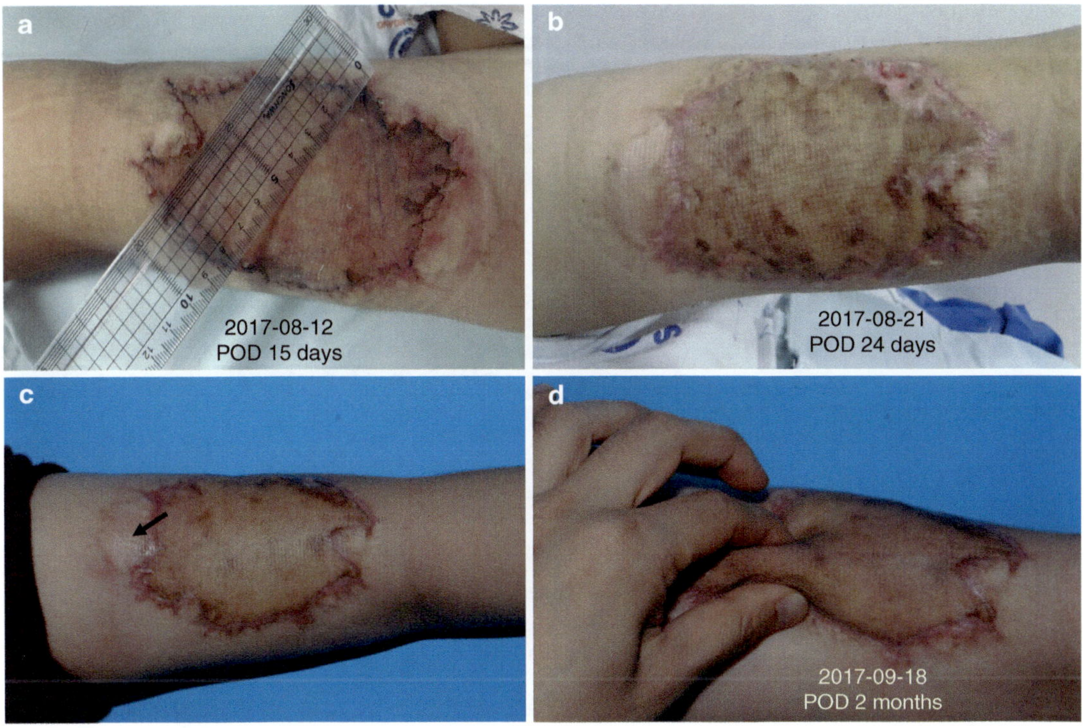

Fig. 2.67 (**a**, **b**) Postoperative 15, 24 days after, there was no change of original engrafted width 7.5 cm (**c**) Note the marked improved triangle flap itself and surrounding scar tissue maturation. (**d**) Postoperative 2 months later view, engrafted skin texture softened very quickly

As mentioned previously, composite grafts, in which the fat has not been removed, provide the following benefits for several years of long-term follow-up even after a graft is taken.

A 9-year-old female patient sustained a scaling burn at the age of 2 years. A wide scar and contracture band were noted on the right thigh and knee joint areas, including the lateral popliteal area. The harvested skin size was 5 × 18 cm which was criterion of my usual maximal size in children of inguinal area which includes subcutaneous fat layer. Incisional full release and FTSG with composite fat graft were performed on the thigh and lateral popliteal areas (Fig. 2.68). Ten days after the operation, the engrafted skin appeared to be healing well. Note the inevitable seam line that connects the main engraft skin to the small popliteal skin (yellow arrow). One year after the operation, well-adapted engrafted skin with a surrounding wide scar was noted (Fig. 2.69). (a) Seven years after the operation, there was increase in size (length 20 cm, width 7.5 cm) without a contracture band, with surrounding scar tissue softening and texture improvement according to the growing period. (b) Note the seam line and the small engrafted skin area in the lateral popliteal area. The seam line below the small engrafted skin (black arrow) was less adapted to increasing size compared with the upper big engrafted skin. This is the reason why I prefer when possible single-sheet engraft without a seam line (Fig. 2.70).

The several advantages of FTSG with fat composite graft that I have experienced are presented below:

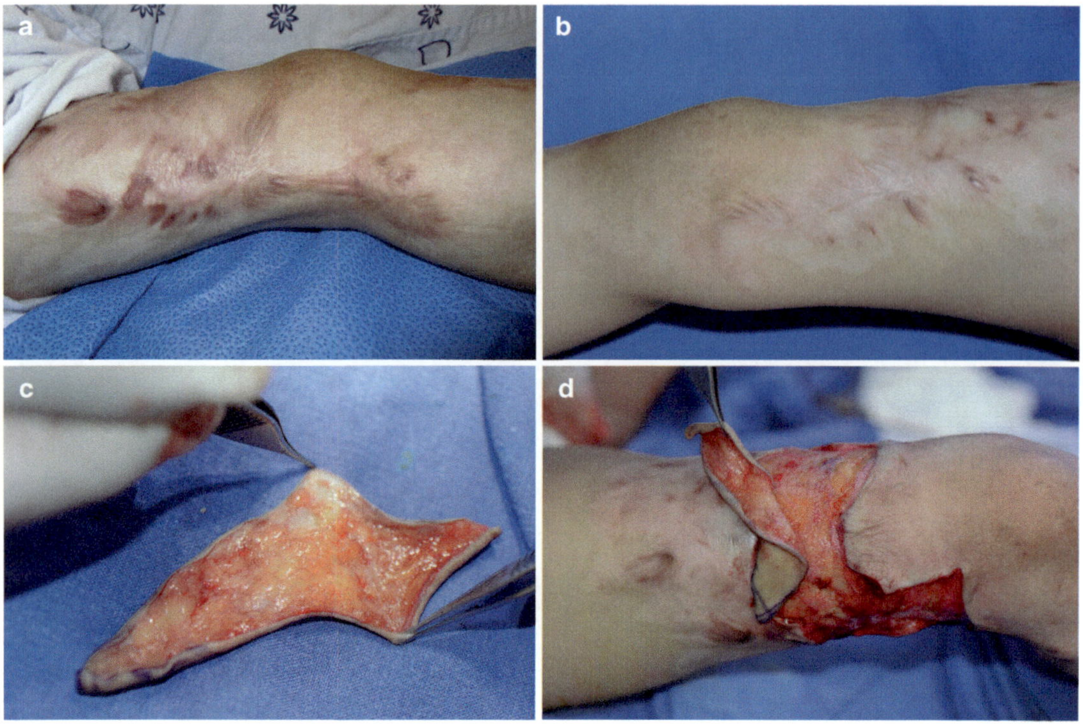

Fig. 2.68 (**a**, **b**) Preoperative view. (**c**) Collected donor skin size 5 × 18 cm attached to the fat layer. (**d**) Intraoperative view

1. The reduction of surgery duration by eliminating the time required for dermal shaving.
2. The cushion effect as soft fat tissue facilitates bleed control, which reduces the incidence of hematoma.
3. Although there is a partial loss of the engrafted skin, it can be restored to the original state while avoiding scarring (Figs. 2.71 and 2.78).
4. The graft survival rate is increased, showing a high take rate of >95% (in recent years, from my experience).
5. The engrafted FTSG skin rapidly softens within 1–3 months, and the maturation period is decreased remarkably (Fig. 2.73).

Further evaluation for scientific evidence is warranted to verify the (mentioned above) clinical findings obtained through my observations for several years.

A 26-year-old male patient suffered an open fracture in the left wrist area, including the radius and ulnar. His main complaint was restriction of motion on his wrist, palm, and thumb because of a fixed titanium plate. Excisional full release and titanium plate removal were performed on the wrist, thumb, and palm areas. The MCP joint on the thumb did not fully recover with full range of motion because of the malunion of the fracture site. FTSG with a fat composite graft was performed along with the removal of the titanium plate. Five days after the operation, the tie-over dressing was removed, and a small hematoma was noted on the palm area, which was evacuated through a slit incision with a compressive saline-soaked gauze dressing (Fig. 2.71). Seven days after the operation, unstable skin colors were noted, and soaking dressing was changed twice a day (white arrow). Two weeks after the operation, almost all of the skin was taken except for the skin in the palm area. Twenty days after the operation, partial upper dermis loss was noted (black arrow). Twenty-four days after the opera-

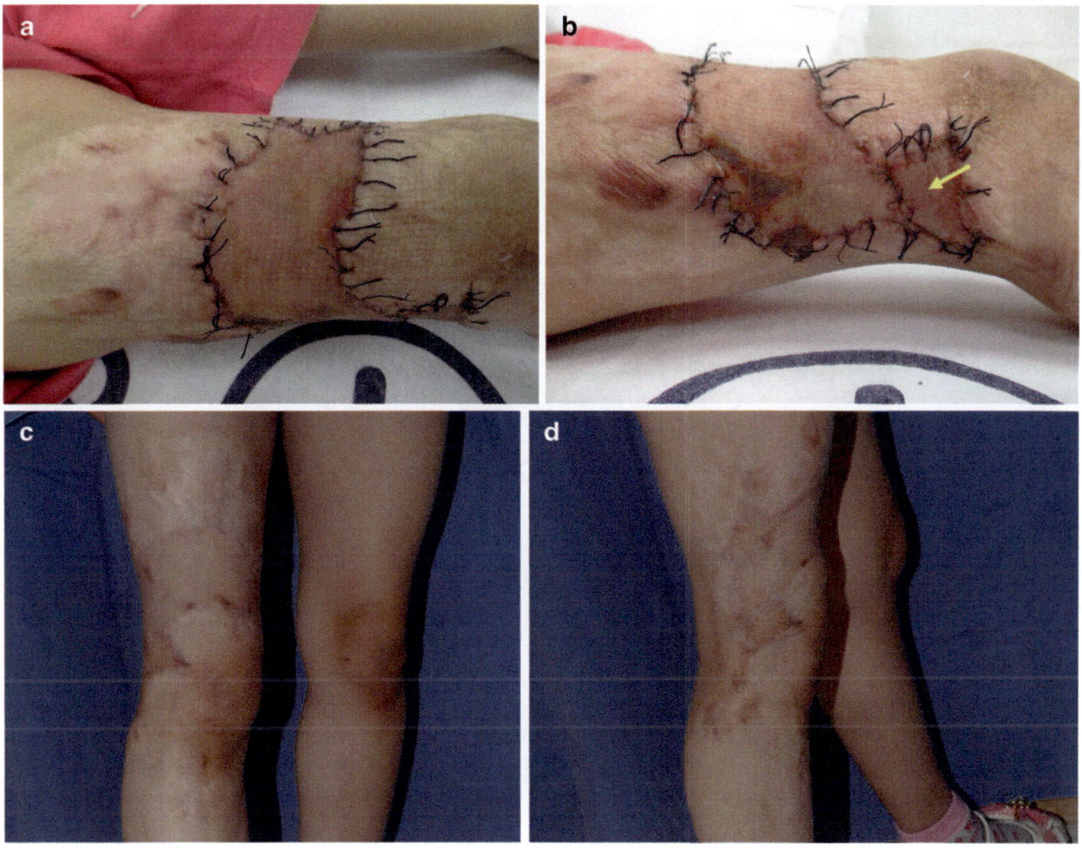

Fig. 2.69 (**a**, **b**) Postoperative 10 days after view, note small engrafted skin region (yellow arrow). (**c**, **d**) Postoperative 1year after view, well-adapted engrafted skin with surrounded wide scar

tion, the skin lesion has completely healed (Fig. 2.72). Two months after the operation, hyperpigmentation was presented in the palm area but no contracture. Three months after the operation, interestingly the pigmentation lesion had disappeared, and the engraftment site had already softened. Ten months after the operation, the palm area was completely recovered, and its original color and texture had been restored, indicating a very fast remodeling process. The previous hematoma with a partial skin loss area (white arrow) recovered completely without scarring, indicating that a composite fat graft is very effective on the wound healing process, with a strong restitutive force and a short remodeling period (Fig. 2.73).

2.4.6 Dermabrasion and Dermal Overgrafting with FTSG

Recently, I obtained successful functional and esthetic outcomes using dermabrasion and dermal overgrafting [57, 58], which have been introduced in Chap. 5, in addition to the approach (mentioned above) of performing FTSG with composite fat graft and an additionally attempted method for obtaining the advantages of volume replacement. This indicates an expansion range of clinical applications of the dermal overgrafting through my years of clinical experience and long-term follow-up observations. It has been sufficiently demonstrated that basic dermabrasion and dermal overgraft-

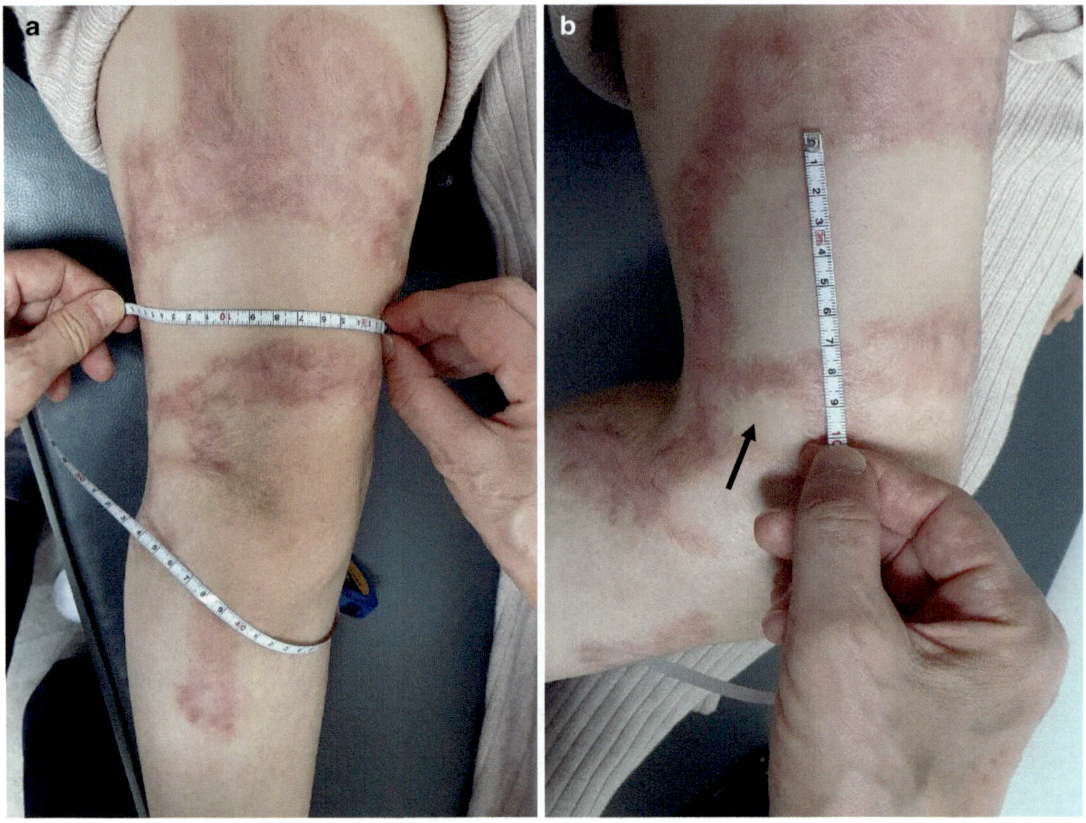

Fig. 2.70 (a) Postoperative 7 years after, marked increasing size length of 20 cm and width of 7.5 cm. (b) Note the seam line and small engrafted skin of the popliteal area (black arrow)

ing with very thin graft as well as FTSG with varying graft thicknesses and composite fat graft can be also performed without any complications, even in cases of inadequate blood supply due to only capillary or pinpoint bleeding in the dermabraded sites. This further elucidates that skin grafting is possible in all forms using FTSG, which has been generally avoided as a technique despite its multiple advantages and, in addition, FTSG with composite fat graft also possible. Another notable point, all types of skin graft can be performed on any type of bed condition regardless of whether the original nature of the recipient skin is the existing old scar tissue, artificial dermal scar bed, so far as bone exposure site, etc., if there are capillary or pinpoint bleeding after dermabrasion, this indicates that the utility range of skin graft has maximally expanded significantly.

Exactly if the capillary bleeding bed is simply generated with a dermabrader, skin graft is possible in all cases, with a much broader range of skin graft area, particularly in terms of esthetic effects as well as functional improvements.

This technique and concepts are closely related to Chap. 5 and interrelated with all the other chapters, please ensure to read them thoroughly and refer to them as and when necessary. I elaborated on the dermal overgrafting on the basis of clinical cases where I could overcome complications by using the previously mentioned techniques.

This female patient developed an irregular, depressed scar on her right cheek as a result of an unknown infectious disease as a child. The depressed site was noted to be noticeably depressed along with a soft tissue defect and an irregular skin surface. I had planned dermabra-

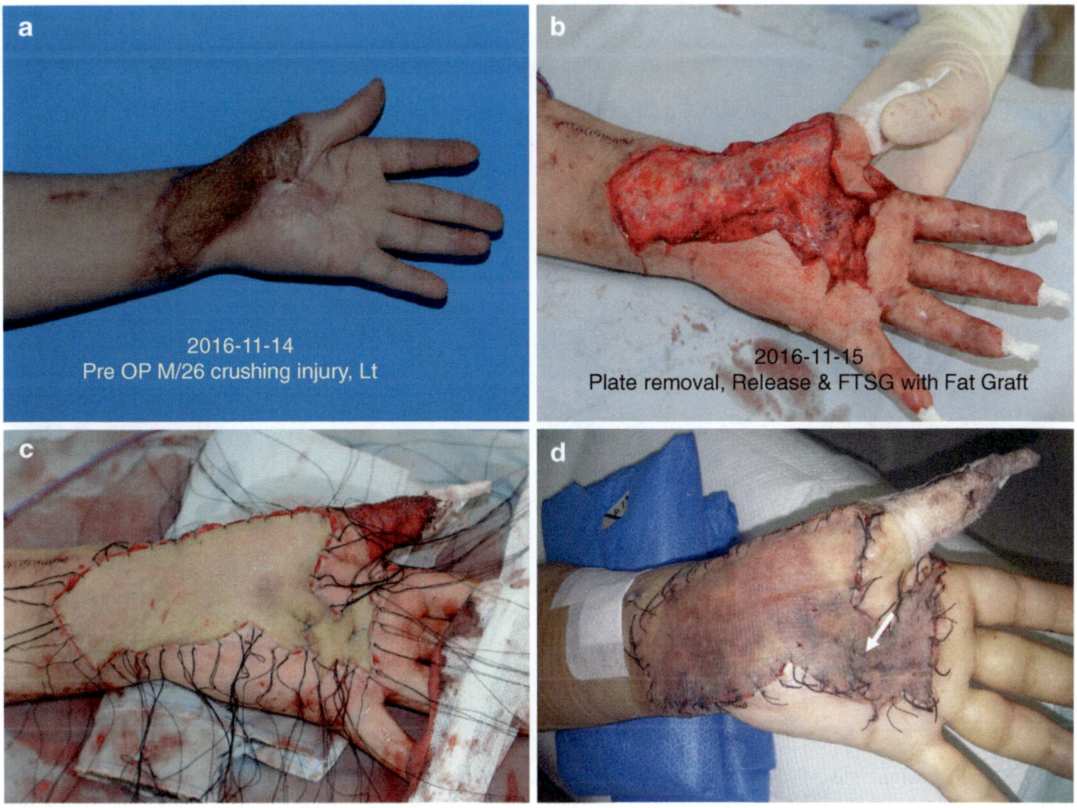

Fig. 2.71 In (**a**) preoperative view. (**b**) Excisional full release and titanium plate removal was performed. (**c**) Full-thickness skin graft with fat composite graft. (**d**) Postoperative 5 days after, small hematoma was noted on the palm area (yellow arrow)

sion and dermal overgrafting with a composite fat graft for the maximum supplement effect of the soft tissue (Fig. 2.74). Initial dermabrasion was performed, and for less conspicuous marginal deformities, scalpel incisional marginal release was performed to achieve accurate edge approximation. A full-thickness skin of 4.5 × 13 cm with fat composite graft was applied. To reduce the stitch mark on the face, 6.0 nylon fine suture and a wide distance tie-over suture were used (Fig. 2.75). Seven days after the operation, there was a small diffuse hematoma which was resolved by diligently applying soaked dressing. Two weeks after the operation, the skin was almost completely taken without any partial loss, but some areas had unstable epidermis and upper dermal layer. One month after the operation, a partially pigmented lesion was noted (Fig. 2.76). Four months after the operation, the pigmented region had gradually regained its original color and texture. The volume replacement of the right cheek was noticeably augmented compared with the left normal side of the cheek (Fig. 2.77). One year after the operation, the pigmented region was markedly improved, and the volume replacement effect was also well maintained compared to the left normal cheek. Excellent color matching and texture were noted on the inconspicuous engraft margin. This case was shown to have a highly effective correction of volume replacement with skin color and texture improvement in a wide depressed scar on the face for esthetic surgery (Fig. 2.78).

In the final case, I would like to introduce full series from acute management to final reconstruction process. This process includes a finger

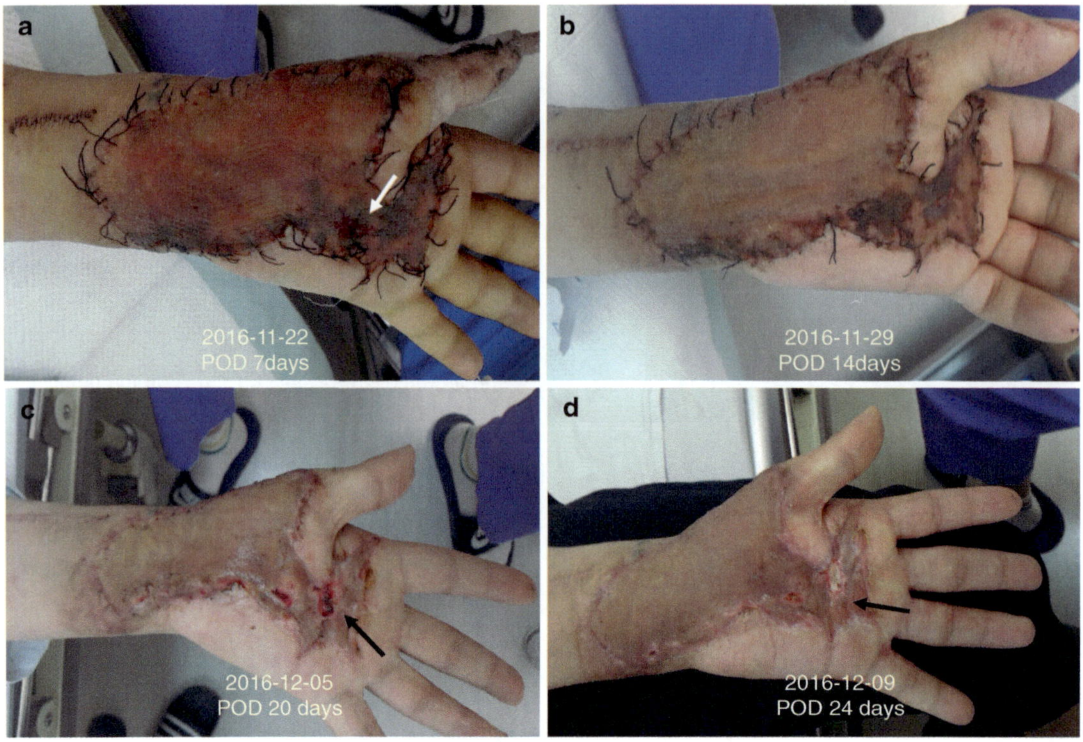

Fig. 2.72 (**a**) Postoperative 7 days, unstable skin color was noted (white arrow). (**b**) Postoperative 2 weeks, almost all skin was taken except the palm area. (**c**) Postoperative 20 days, partial upper dermis loss was noted (black arrow). (**d**) Postoperative 24 days, the skin lesion was completely healed (black arrow)

salvage technique using human dermal matrix, reconstructive surgery for functional recovery of the hand, and finally reinforcement and esthetic graft procedure.

A 51-year-old female patient suffered a gas flame burn in a kitchen, causing an epileptic seizure. We noted full-thickness burns on several fingers and on the dorsum of the hand. We performed a salvage procedure as the patient was adamant about not having her fingers amputated. To preserve the fingers, human allograft was initially applied after necrotic tissue debridement. To maintain functional hand position, allograft removal and electrical drill K-wire interphalangeal bony fixation were performed on post-burn day 12. Human dermal matrix with thin autograft was applied, while keeping the hand in 'funtional hand position' (Fig. 2.79). One year after the procedure, the extensor tendon and 2, 3, 4, and 5 phalangeal bones were almost exposed. Noting sequential wound healing process, postoperative 2, 2.5, and 3 months later view, the exposed tendon and digital bone were covered with granulation tissue and slow epithelialization process of the previously engrafted dermal matrix. In this photo, human dermal matrix is a strong material that can resist infected necrotic tissues of bone and tendon exposure (Fig. 2.80). Eleven months after applying the human dermal matrix graft, FTSG with composite fat graft was performed for MCP joints to restore hand function. The MCP joints were manually reduced after full release on the dorsum of the hand and proximal phalanx area. Six days after tie-over dressing removal, a small hematoma was noted, which was treated with a daily compressive soaking dressing (Fig. 2.81). After 1.5 and 4 months since the operation, the FTSG site had recovered and matured rapidly. Six months after the procedure, the MCP joint function was recovered with reasonable function, although the joints of the digital finger were stiff; she can grip and catch large

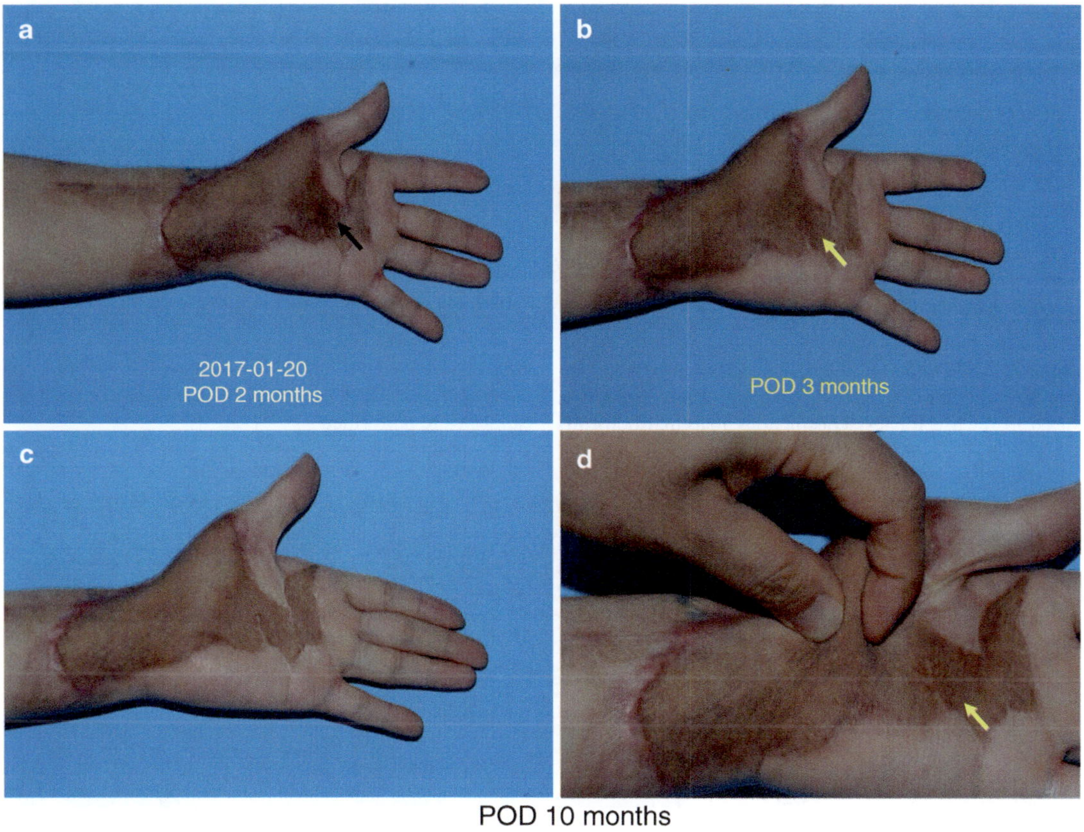

Fig. 2.73 (**a**) Postoperative 2months, the palm area was noted to have hyperpigmentation (black arrow). (**b**) Postoperative 3 months, the pigmentation lesion disappears and engraft site has early softening (yellow arrow). (**c**, **d**) Postoperative 10 months after, the palm area has completely recovered with original color and texture (yellow arrow) with very fast remodeling process

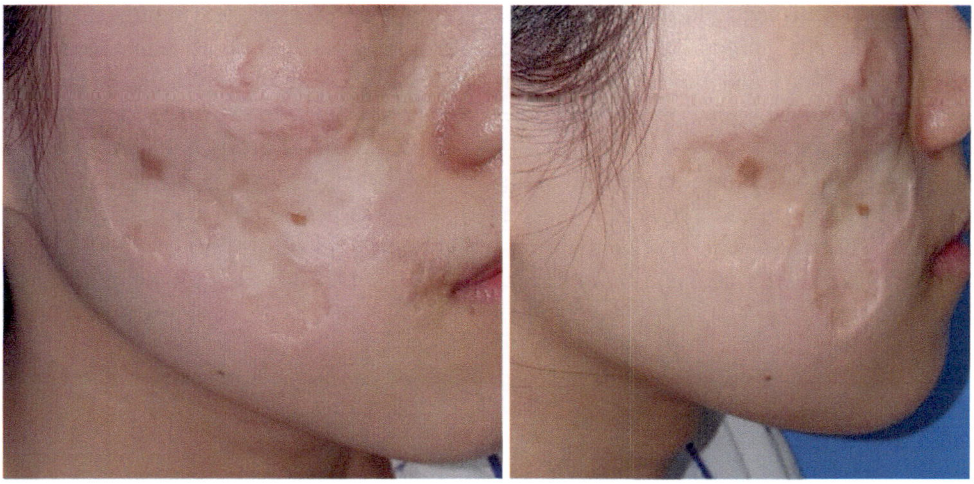

Fig. 2.74 Preoperative view, depressed and irregular skin surface was noted on the right cheek

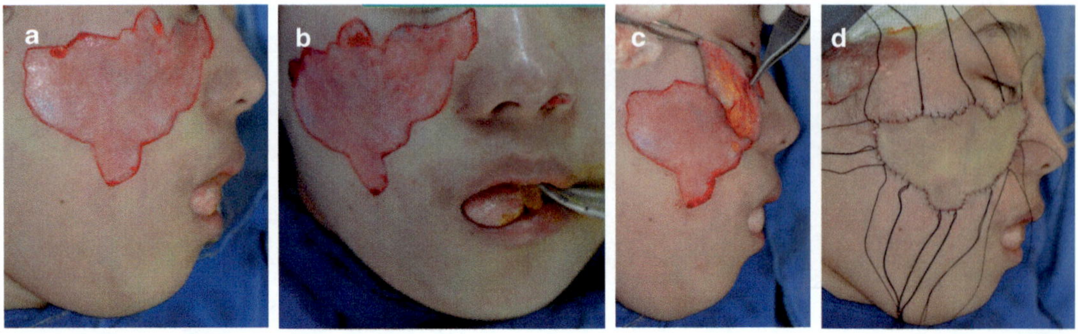

Fig. 2.75 (**a**) Dermabrasion. (**b**) Shallow scalpel incision with accurate edge thickness along the scar margin was sliced to release for less conspicuous marginal deformities. (**c**) 4.5 × 13 cm full-thickness skin and fat composite graft was performed. (**d**) 6.0 nylon fine suture and tie-over suture were performed

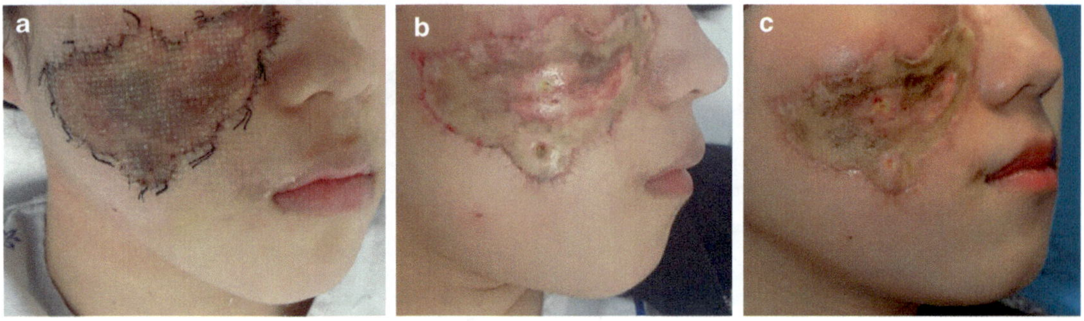

Fig. 2.76 (**a**) Postoperative 7 days, small diffuse hematoma was noted. (**b**) Postoperative 2 weeks after, the skin was almost taken, but in some areas, edematous epidermis and upper dermal layer were noted. (**c**) Postoperative 1monthe later view, partially pigmented lesion was noted

objects. She was satisfied that all of her digits were saved despite functional disturbance (Fig. 2.82). Two years and three months later applying FTSG, we had a final plan to reinforce the dorsal part of the third, fourth, and fifth fingers, this region consists of thin and delicate skin; therefore, it is prone to easy bone and tendon exposure. After dermabrasion, FTSG with a composite fat graft was performed, and 6 days later, the tie-over dressing was removed. One month after the procedure, more stable skin thickness and texture were observed. This case is a very good example to prove that graft can be taken completely on the capillary bled area after dermabrasion (Fig. 2.83).

On completion of Chap. 2 FTSG, I believe that almost all surgeons regard FTSG as a complicated and restricted graft technique, it plays a

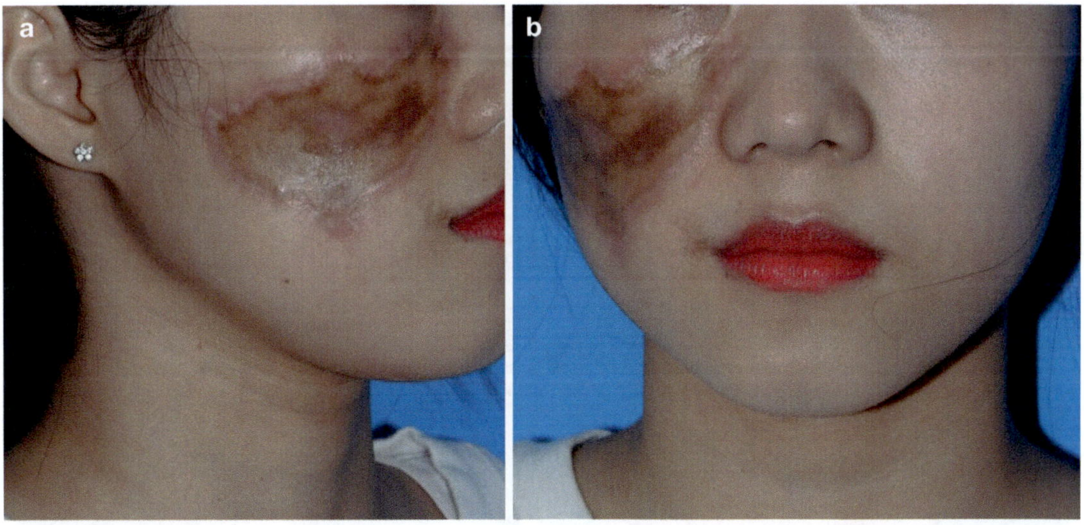

Fig. 2.77 (**a**) Postoperative 4 months later view, the pigmented region has slowly recovered to original color and texture. (**b**) The volume replacement effect was noted compared with the normal side

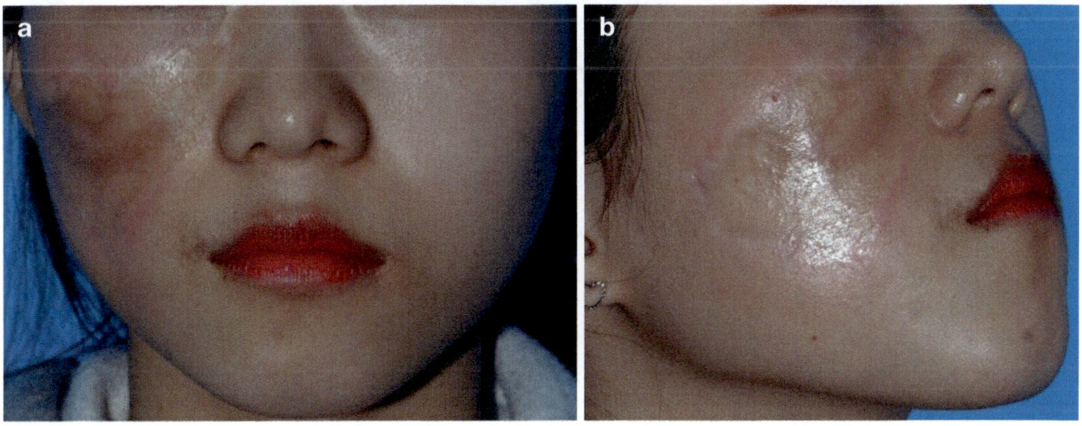

Fig. 2.78 (**a**) Postoperative 1 year after, signs of remarkable improvement of the pigmented region and volume replacement effect. (**b**) The excellent matching of color and texture was noted with inconspicuous engraft margin

critical role in reconstructive surgery among the various skin graft methods. The techniques that have been described here may appear unfamiliar and undetermined, they have been acquired and practiced through long-standing experiences. In particular, if young surgeons who may be hesitant to make attempts at such techniques were encouraged to repeatedly try them to gain confidence and refer to the techniques mentioned in this guide. I believe that they will be able to comprehend my intention.

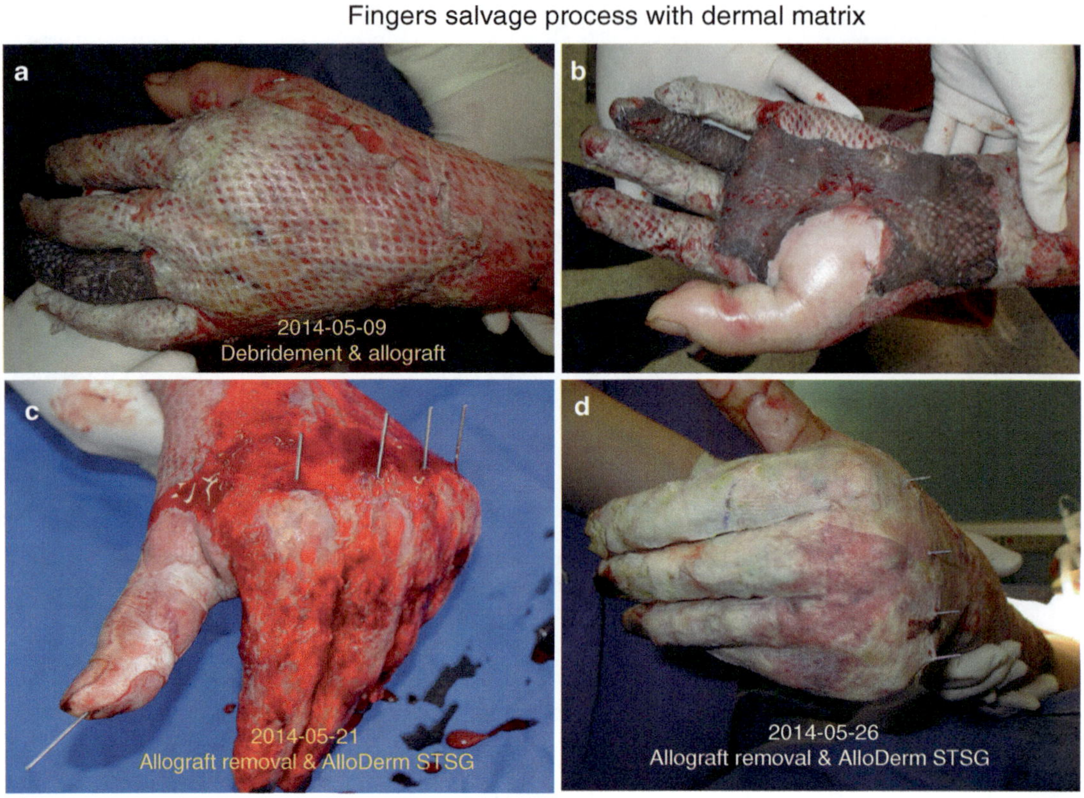

Fig. 2.79 (**a**, **b**) Initially human allograft was applied after necrotic tissue debridement to preserve the fingers. (**c**) Post-burn day 12 after, K-wire interphalangeal bony fixation is done to keep a functional hand position. (**d**) Human dermal matrix with thin autograft

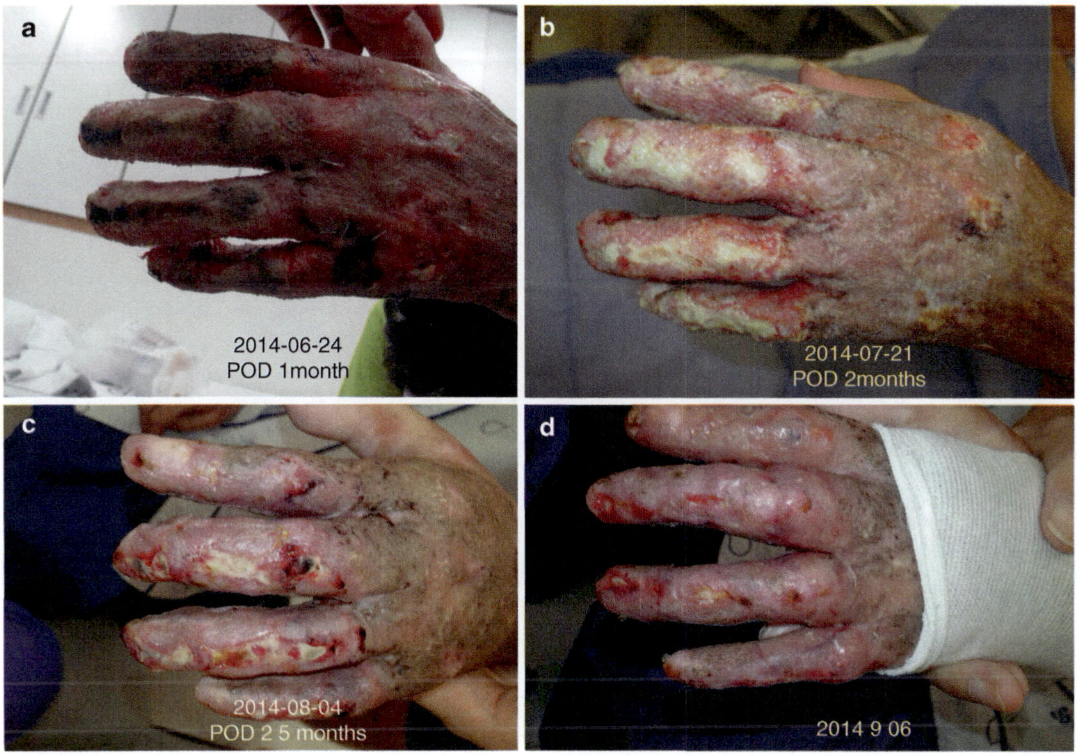

Fig. 2.80 (**a**) 1 month after view, the extensor tendon and second, third, fourth, and fifth phalangeal bones were exposed. (**b–d**) Please note the (**b**) (**c**) (**d**) change of sequential wound healing process, postoperative 2, 2.5, 3 months view, the exposed tendon and digital bone covered granulation tissue and epithelialization process

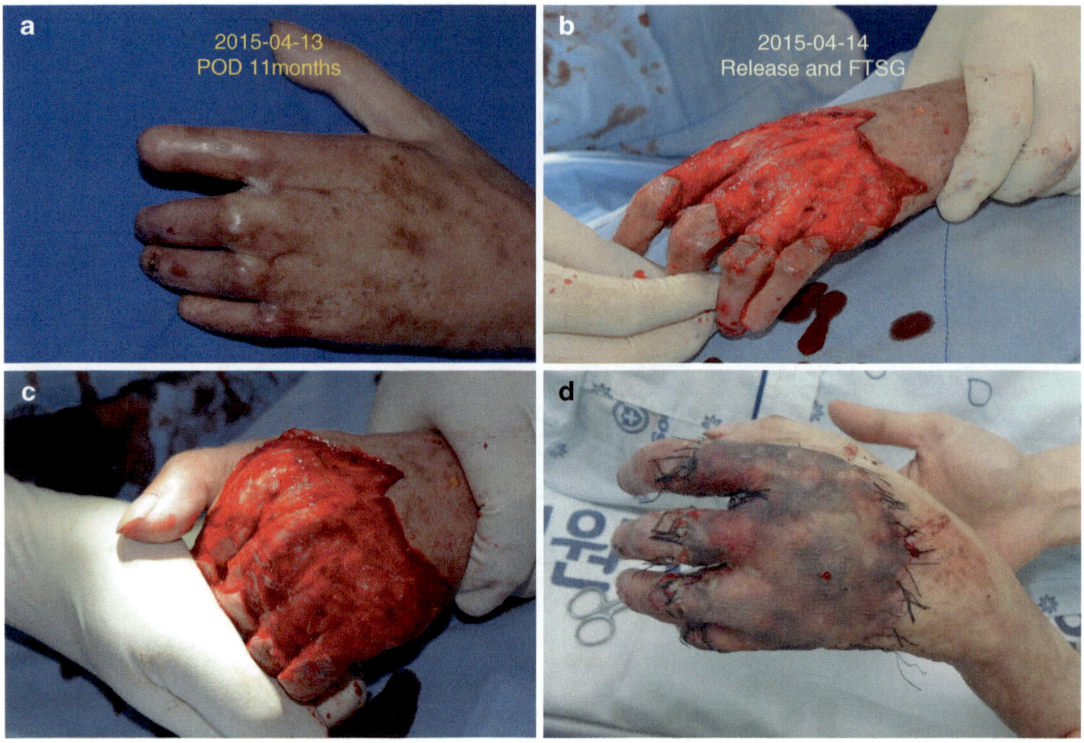

Fig. 2.81 (**a**) Human dermal matrix graft 11 months after view, FTSG with composite fat graft was performed. (**b**, **c**) The MCP joints were manually reduced. (**d**) Postoperative 6 days after tie-over dressing is removed

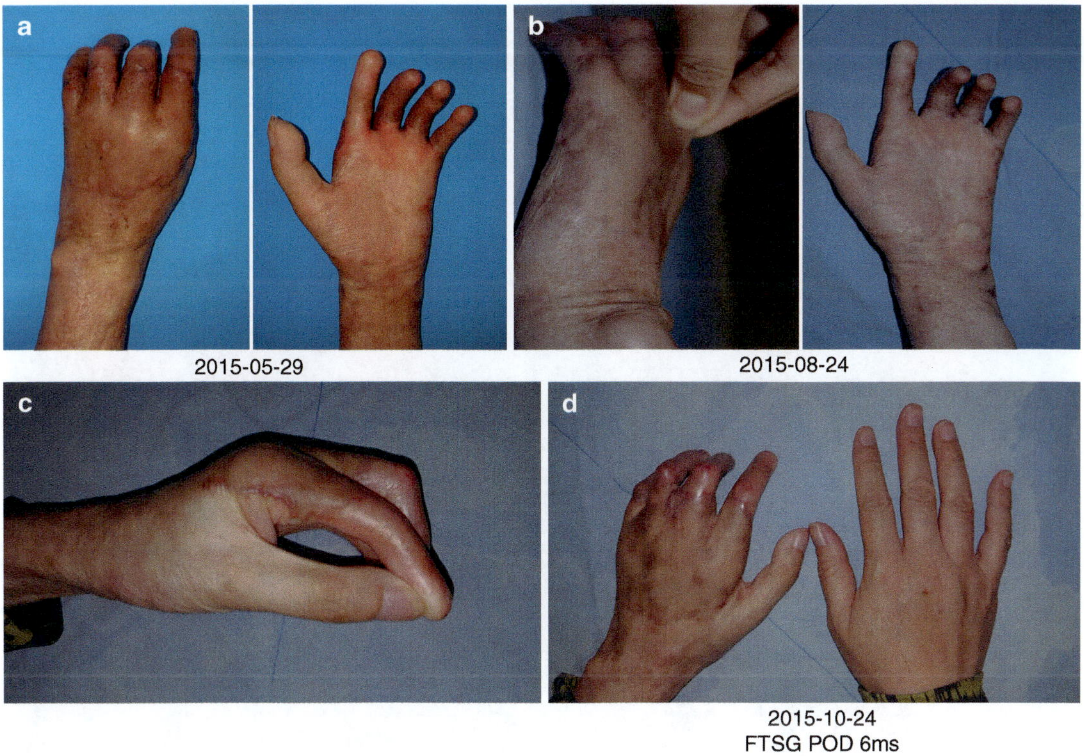

Fig. 2.82 (**a**, **b**) Postoperative 1.5 and 4 months view, FTSG site was noted to have very fast recovery and maturation. (**c**, **d**) Postoperative 6 months view, MCP joint function recovered reasonably even though there was digital finger joint stiffness

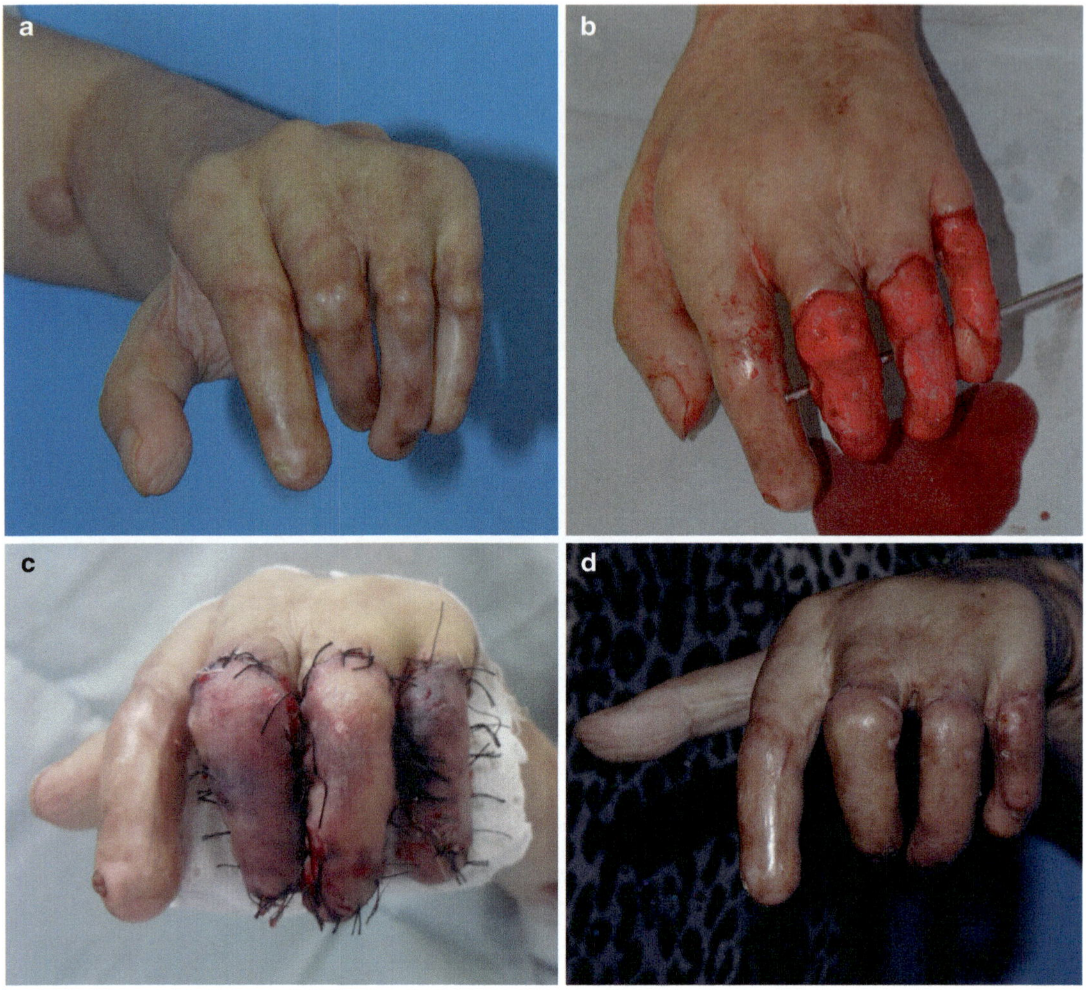

Fig. 2.83 (**a**) Postoperative FTSG 2 years and 3 months after preoperative view. (**b**) After dermabrasion, (**c**) FTSG with composite fat graft. (**d**) Postoperative 1 month after view, more stable skin thickness and texture were noted

2.5 Conclusion

If we expand our horizons regarding a simple skin graft technique, we would be able to overcome complicated challenges that were previously deemed difficult to resolve. I hope that the readers can realize the complications raised in this book can be resolved with ease. I would like to highlight the part where the skin graft area could be considerably expanded by combining dermabrasion and dermal overgrafting with FTSG with composite fat graft. Although this method seems to be a little unfamiliar and unclear approach, if we take a consistence and diligent approach, acquiring these skills and techniques through constant efforts and experiences, I firmly believe that we can continue to improve the outcome results by challenging and really pushing forward all the possibilities.

References

1. Jang YC, Burm JS, Cho JY. Skin-fat composite grafts for reconstructive large full-thickness skin defects. Plast Reconstr Surg. 2023;151(3):635–44.
2. Khan AA, Khan IM, Nguyen PP, Lo E, Chahadeh H, Cerniglia M, Noriega JA. Skin graft techniques. Clin Podiatr Med Surg. 2020;37(4):821–35.
3. Müller W. Split skin and full-thickness skin grafts. Mund Kiefer Gesichtschir. 2000;4(1):314–21.
4. Swaim SF. Skin grafts. Vet Clin North Am Small Anim Pract. 1990;20(1):147–75.
5. Prohaska J, Cook C. Skin grafting. In: StatPearls. Treasure Island: StatPearls Publishing; 2022.
6. Oda T, Kato H, Nakamura M, Morita A. Analysis of biomonitoring data after full-thickness skin grafting. J Dermatol. 2021;48(7):1035–43.
7. Steele L, Brown A, Xie F. Full-thickness skin graft fixation techniques: a review of the literature. J Cutan Aesthet Surg. 2020;13(3):191–6.
8. Pulvermacker B, Chaouat M, Seroussi D, Mimoun M. Tie-over dressings in full-thickness skin grafts. Dermatologic Surg. 2008;34(1):40–3.
9. Cauley RP, Helliwell LA, Donelan MB, Eberlin KR. Reconstruction of the adult and pediatric burned hand. Hand Clin. 2017;33(2):333–45.
10. McCauley RL. Reconstruction of the pediatric burned hand. Hand Clin. 2009;25(4):543–50.
11. Fisher M. Pediatric burn reconstruction: focus on evidence. Clin Plast Surg. 2017;44(4):865–73.
12. Park YS, Lee JW, Huh GY, Koh JH, Seo DK, Choi JK, Jang YC. Algorithm for primary full-thickness skin grafting in pediatric hand burns. Arch Plast Surg. 2012;39(5):483–8.
13. Prasetyono TO, Sadikin PM, Saputra DK. The use of split-thickness versus full-thickness skin graft to resurface volar aspect of pediatric burned hands: a systematic review. Burns. 2015;41(5):890–906.
14. Liodaki E, Kisch T, Mauss KL, Senyaman O, Kraemer R, Mailänder P, Wünsch L, Stang F. Management of pediatric hand burns. Pediatr Surg Int. 2015;31(4):397–401.
15. Palmieri TL. Initial management of acute pediatric hand burns. Hand Clin. 2009;25(4):461–7.
16. Feldmann ME, Evans J. Early management of the burned pediatric hand. J Craniofac Surg. 2008;19(4):942–50.
17. Kuo Y-R, Wang C-T, Cheng J-T, Kao G-S, Chiang Y-C, Wang C-J. Adipose-derived stem cells accelerate diabetic wound healing through the induction of autocrine and paracrine effects. Cell Transplant. 2016;25(1):71–81.
18. Rautiainen S, Laaksonen T, Koivuniemi R. Angiogenic effects and crosstalk of adipose-derived mesenchymal stem/stromal cells and their extracellular vesicles with endothelial cells. Int J Mol Sci. 2021;22(19):10890.
19. Khan S, Villalobos MA, Choron RL, Chang S, Brown SA, Carpenter JP, Tulenko TN, Zhang P. Fibroblast growth factor and vascular endothelial growth factor play a critical role in endotheliogenesis from human adipose-derived stem cells. J Vasc Surg. 2017;65(5):1483–92.
20. Son D, Jeong H, Choi T, Kim J, Han K. A new mechanism associated with compositae graft success. J Plast Reconstr Aesth Surg. 2010;63:1900–9.
21. Kanitakis J. Anatomy, histology and immunohistochemistry of normal human skin. Eur J Dermatol. 2002;12(4):390–9; quiz 400–1.
22. Zilinsky I, Farber N, Weissman O, Israeli H, Haik J, Domniz N, Winkler E. Defying consensus: correct sizing of full-thickness skin grafts. J Drugs Dermatol. 2012;11(4):520–3.
23. Shin J, Jang U, Baek SO, Lee JY. Full-thickness skin graft according to surrounding relaxed skin tension line improves scar quality in facial defect coverage: a retrospective comparative study. Biomed Res Int. 2021;2021:7398090.
24. Smith RO, Dickinson JT, Cipcic JA. Compositae graft in facial reconstructive surgery. Arch Otolaryngol. 1972;95:252–64.
25. Davenport G, Bernard FD. Improving the take of compositae grafts. Plast Reconstr Surg. 1959;24:175–82.
26. Rees TD. The transfer of free compositae grafts of skin and fat: clinical study. Plast Reconstr Surg. 1960;25:556–64.
27. Brown JB, Cannon B. Compositae free grafts of skin and cartilage from the ear. Surg Gynec Ost. 1946;82:253–5.
28. Fazio MJ, Zitelli JA. Full-thickness skin grafts. Clinical observations on the impact of using epinephrine in local anesthesia of the donor site. Arch Dermatol. 1995;131(6):691–4.
29. Lalonde D, Martin A. Epinephrine in local anesthesia in finger and hand surgery: the case for wide-awake anesthesia. J Am Acad Orthop Surg. 2013;21(8):443–7.
30. Denkler KA. Comprehensive review of epinephrine in the finger: to do or not to do. Plast Reconstr Surg. 2001;108(1):114–24.
31. O'Malley TP, Postma GN, Holtel M, Girod DA. Effect of local epinephrine on cutaneous bloodflow in the human neck. Laryngoscope. 1995;105(2):140–3.
32. Ilicki J. Safety of epinephrine in digital nerve blocks: a literature review. J Emerg Med. 2015;49(5):799–809.
33. Larrabee WF Jr, Lanier BJ, Miekle D. Effect of epinephrine on local cutaneous blood flow. Head Neck Surg. 1987;9(5):287–9.
34. Khudr J, Hughes L, Younis F. The what, why and when of wide awake local anaesthesia no tourniquet surgery. Br J Hosp Med. 2022;83(1):1–10.
35. Nielsen LJ, Lumholt P, Hölmich LR. Local anaesthesia with vasoconstrictor is safe to use in areas with end-arteries in fingers, toes, noses and ears. Ugeskr Laeger. 2014;176(44):V04140238.
36. Rutter N. The dermis. Semin Neonatol. 2000;5(4):297–302.

37. Braverman IM. The cutaneous microcirculation. J Investig Dermatol Symp Proc. 2000;5(1):3–9.
38. Timmons MJ. Landmarks in the anatomical study of the blood supply of the skin. Br J Plast Surg. 1985;38(2):197–207.
39. Marsidi N, Boteva K, Vermeulen SAM, van Kester MS, Genders RE. To tie or not to tie-over full-thickness skin grafts in dermatologic surgery: a systematic review of the literature. Dermatologic Surg. 2021;47(1):18–22.
40. Bern R, Serror K, Alvo R, Chaouat M, Mimoun M, Schmidt M, Boccara D. Original and modified technique of tie-over dressing: method and application in burn patients. Burns. 2018;44(5):1357–60.
41. Davis M, Baird D, Hill D, Layher H, Akin R. Management of full-thickness skin grafts. Bayl Univ Med Cent. 2021;34(6):683–6.
42. Yuki A, Takenouchi T, Takatsuka S, Fujikawa H, Abe R. Investigating the use of tie-over dressing after skin grafting. J Dermatol. 2017;44(11):1317–9.
43. Jang YC, Kwon OK, Lee JW, Oh SJ. The optimal management of pediatric steam burn from electric rice-cooker: STSG or FTSG? J Burn Care Rehabil. 2001;22(1):15–20.
44. Pham TN, Hanley C, Palmieri T, Greenhalgh DG. Results of early excision and full-thickness grafting of deep palm burns in children. J Burn Care Rehabil. 2001;22(1):54–7.
45. Brown M, Chung KC. Postburn contractures of the hand. Hand Clin. 2017;33(2):317–31.
46. Kumar S, Khan FAA, Ali H, Kiran S. Surgical management of post burn hand deformities. Pak J Med Sci. 2020;36(6):1387–91.
47. Voulliaume D, Mojallal A, Comparin JP, Foyatier JL. Severe hand burns and flaps: indications. Ann Chir Plast Esthet. 2005;50(4):314–9.
48. Woo SH, Seul JH. Optimizing the correction of severe postburn hand deformities by using aggressive contracture releases and fasciocutaneous free-tissue transfers. Plast Reconstr Surg. 2001;107(1):1–8.
49. Yongwei P, Jianing W, Junhui Z, Guanglei T, Wen T, Chun L. The abdominal flap using scarred skin in the treatment of postburn hand deformities of severe burn patients. J Hand Surg Am. 2004;29(2):209–15.
50. Askari M, Cohen MJ, Grossman PH, Kulber DA. The use of acellular dermal matrix in release of burn contracture scars in the hand. Plast Reconstr Surg. 2011;127(4):1593–9.
51. Choughri H, Weigert R, Heron A, Dahmam A, Abi-Chahla ML, Delgove A. Indications and functional outcome of the use of integra® dermal regeneration template for the management of traumatic soft tissue defects on dorsal hand, fingers and thumb. Arch Orthop Trauma Surg. 2020;140(12):2115–27.
52. Ellis CV, Kulber DA. Acellular dermal matrices in hand reconstruction. Plast Reconstr Surg. 2012;130(5):256S–69S.
53. Kamolz LP, Kitzinger HB, Karle B, Frey M. The treatment of hand burns. Burns. 2009;35(3):327–37.
54. Sando IC, Chung KC. The use of dermal skin substitutes for the treatment of the burned hand. Hand Clin. 2017;33(2):269–76.
55. Shin SH, Kim C, Lee YS, Kang JW, Chung YG. Feasibility and advantages of full thickness skin graft from the anterolateral thigh. J Hand Surg Asian Pac. 2017;22(4):497–502.
56. Rao K, Tillo O, Dalal M. Full thickness skin graft cover for lower limb defects following excision of cutaneous lesions. Dermatol Online J. 2008;14(2):4.
57. Onur Erol O, Atabay K. The treatment of burn scar hypopigmentation and surface irregularity by dermabrasion and thin skin grafting. Plast Reconstr Surg. 1990;85(5):754–8.
58. Maranda EL, Wang MX, Shareef S, Tompkins BA, Emerson C, Badiavas EV. Surgical management of leukoderma after burn: a review. Burns. 2018;44(2):256–62.

3 Dermal Substitutes

3.1 Introduction

Several representative dermal substitutes are Integra®, which is synthesized from pure bovine collagen, and AlloDerm®, which is processed by freeze-drying the dermal layer of cadaver skin after removing all cellular components. In addition, multiple products such as Terudermis® (synthesized from calf skin collagen), Pelnac® (synthesized from porcine atelocollagen), and Matriderm® (synthesized by adding elastin to bovine collagen) are being launched. I have experience in working with all of the products mentioned above. However, in this book, I would like to focus on comparing the clinical practical experience of representative synthetic collagen products which are the first synthetic material, Integra® and AlloDerm®, which are manufactured using acellular human dermis. I have selected these two products because the compositions of their materials are very different and each has unique advantages and effectiveness. Currently, many books and publications have introduced various products mainly for acute wound coverage, with limited examples of operative results and evaluation studies. In this chapter, I aim to describe the differences between the two products in terms of clinical findings from surgeries: aspect of author's experienced graft techniques, new and more variable extended applications, and long-term follow-up results. In particular, I want to draw attention to the use of dermal substitutes Integra® and AlloDerm®, the interpretation of surgical techniques, the expansion of the indications for human dermal matrix AlloDerm® for limb salvage, and the osteomyelitis wound management technique the author developed using AlloDerm® and its utility.

3.2 Dermal Substitutes

3.2.1 General Concept of Dermal Substitute

Integra® (Integra Life Science Corporation, Plainsboro, NJ, USA) is a synthesized pure dermal substitute that was first manufactured by Yanas and Burke [1, 2] in 1981 and popularized in 1996 with the completion of a multicenter clinical trial of Integra® [3]. In contrast, AlloDerm® (Life Cell Corporation, Woodlands, TX, USA) is manufactured by removing all cellular components of the dermis layer of the cadaver skin to prevent any immune reaction and subsequent freeze-drying [4]. It has been used for burn management since 1992 [5, 6]. These two products are very different in terms of their starting materials and clinical applicability. From my experience, if the use of each product is well differentiated, and the appropriate dermal product is selected according to the application, better outcomes can be achieved by maximizing the strong points and characteristics of each product. For example, Integra is very useful and confers a lifesaving benefit in major burns owing to its

Y.-C. Jang, *The Art of Skin Graft*, https://doi.org/10.1007/978-981-97-0017-2_3

early excision and graft characteristics. However, it is susceptible to infection and requires a two-step operation and multiple applications to prevent infection, thereby prolonging the hospitalization period. Human dermal matrix products are very durable against infection and require only a single-step procedure. Despite the relatively low risk of infection and the capacity to overcome infection at the time of occurrence, these products also have disadvantages owing to their different irregular sizes and lengths and prolonged wound coverage time in case of wide wound. In addition, human dermal matrix products, which are quite expensive, cost more than Integra®. In this chapter, I will point out the advantages and disadvantages of each dermal substitute product, their outcomes, and clinical application cases from my clinical experience.

First, the overall concept of artificial dermis needs to be introduced.

3.2.2 Classification

Classification is important since it is related to the uses, advantages, and disadvantages of a product. Generally, products can be classified based on the materials used. Some products are manufactured using the dermis obtained from fresh cadaver skin or are synthetically manufactured by cross-linking animal collagen, such as bovine and porcine materials. Classification is based on the surgical method which can be divided into two: (1) two-step operation, waiting for the artificial dermis to form a neodermis to remove the secondary protective layer, a thin silastic sheet, and then performing a thin split-thickness autograft, and (2) single-step operation, applying a human dermal matrix and performing a split-thickness skin graft (STSG) simultaneously as an immediate single step [7, 8]. When chosen based on the patients' and wounds' conditions, both of these products can be excellent graft materials, which can offset their disadvantage of being more expensive alternatives.

Presently released dermal substitute products on the market and used in clinics include AlloDerm®, a human dermal matrix obtained from the dermis layer of cadaver skin, and purely 100% synthetic products include Integra®, the world's first product manufactured using bovine tissue; Terudermis® (Olympus Terumo Biomaterials, Japan) and Pelnac® (Gunze limited, Japan) are developed in Japan. Another product, Matriderm® (Skin and Health Care AG, Billerbeck, Germany), was recently developed in Germany and is a pure synthetic product bovine collagen that contains elastin and can be used in single-step procedures [9, 10].

3.2.3 General Advantages of Dermal Substitutes

1. Can cover a wide wound area at once, enabling early excision and grafting, thereby improving the survival rate of patients with extensive severe burns [7, 11].
2. Strengthens the dermal component of the STSG, thereby shortening the wound-healing process and reducing scar formation. Minimizes functional disorders and contracture by alleviating the scar contracture that appears on the engrafted site and helps reduce tension in the joint or other areas with high physical activity.
3. Only uses 5–8/1000 in. of a thin STSG and reduces donor site morbidity (Fig. 3.1). Furthermore, a subsequent harvest at the same site is possible.
4. Eschars from burn sites are removed early, and raw surface can be immediately covered. As a result, early mobilization can be performed, thereby reducing the hospitalization period and initiating early rehabilitation. These benefits partially offset artificial dermal products' biggest drawback, which is their exorbitant price [12].
5. Unlike general dressing materials, which are temporary, a dermal substitute is a permanent implantation and does not require a secondary wound coverage operation [13].
6. No clinical cases of rejection have been reported thus far, and the material composition is a safe substance.

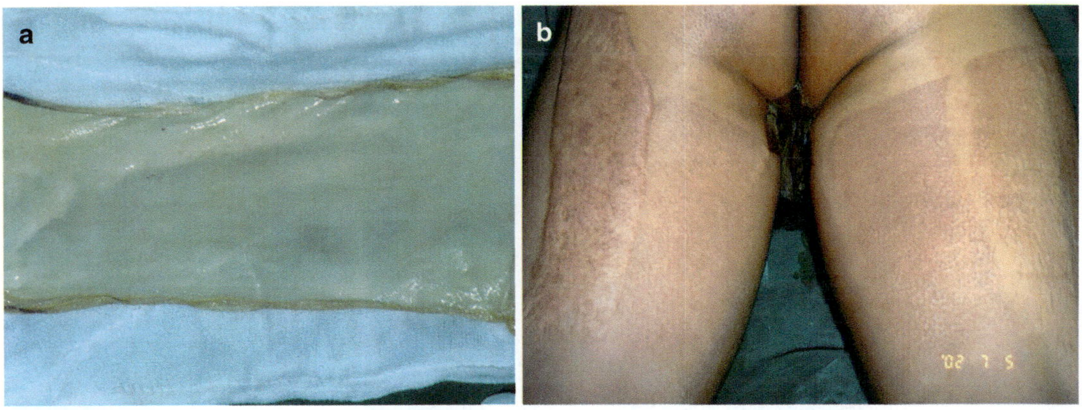

Fig. 3.1 (**a**) Appearance of a 0.15-mm (6/1000 inches) thick harvested skin. (**b**) Compare with donor site scarring on left and right thigh

(a) Appearance of a 0.15-mm-thick harvested skin.
(b) In comparison, the donor site scar on the left is 0.35-mm thick (14/1000 inches), while the right dermal substitute donor site is 0.15-mm thick (6/1000 inches). The left thigh donor area had more hypertrophic scars than the right thigh donor area (Fig. 3.1).

3.2.4 Surgical Indications (Fig. 3.2)

Since dermal substitutes are pricey products, they should only be used when necessary and only after careful consideration, as costs can be reduced by raising the success rate.

1. Deep second- and third-degree burns of joints or lower and upper extremities with a high level of physical activity [14, 15].
2. As effective scar release and grafts for functional recovery in the reconstruction of burns or traumatic scar contractures [16, 17].
3. When total excision and grafting are required owing to severe itchiness or pain from large and severe hypertrophic scarring [18].
4. In chronic ulcerative lesions [19].
5. In skin cancer that requires wide excision and grafting [20].
6. When a wide skin excision needs to be made, such as in the treatment of giant hairy nevi [21, 22].

3.2.5 Considerations of Clinical Indications [2]

1. When performing wound coverage after escharectomy for early excision and grafting in patients with major burns in critical condition.
2. Elderly people aged ≥60 years or young adolescents and infants with thin skin and at risk of prolonged scarring at the donor site.
3. When wishing to improve the outcome of scar contracture correction by adding more dermal layers and obtaining a thick STSG effect.
4. High risk of hypertrophic scarring with severe itchiness and pain and potential donor site morbidity.
5. Populations with deeply pigmented skin, which have a higher risk of hypertrophic scar occurrence, or patients who have experienced hypertrophic scarring from a recent surgery and are expecting severe scarring at the donor site. Before use, it is crucial to carefully examine the patients' circumstances and medical status.

3.2.6 Functions and Uses of Dermal Substitutes for Complex Wound Management

Since the late 1990s, when the first dermal substitute came into active clinical use, to date, various

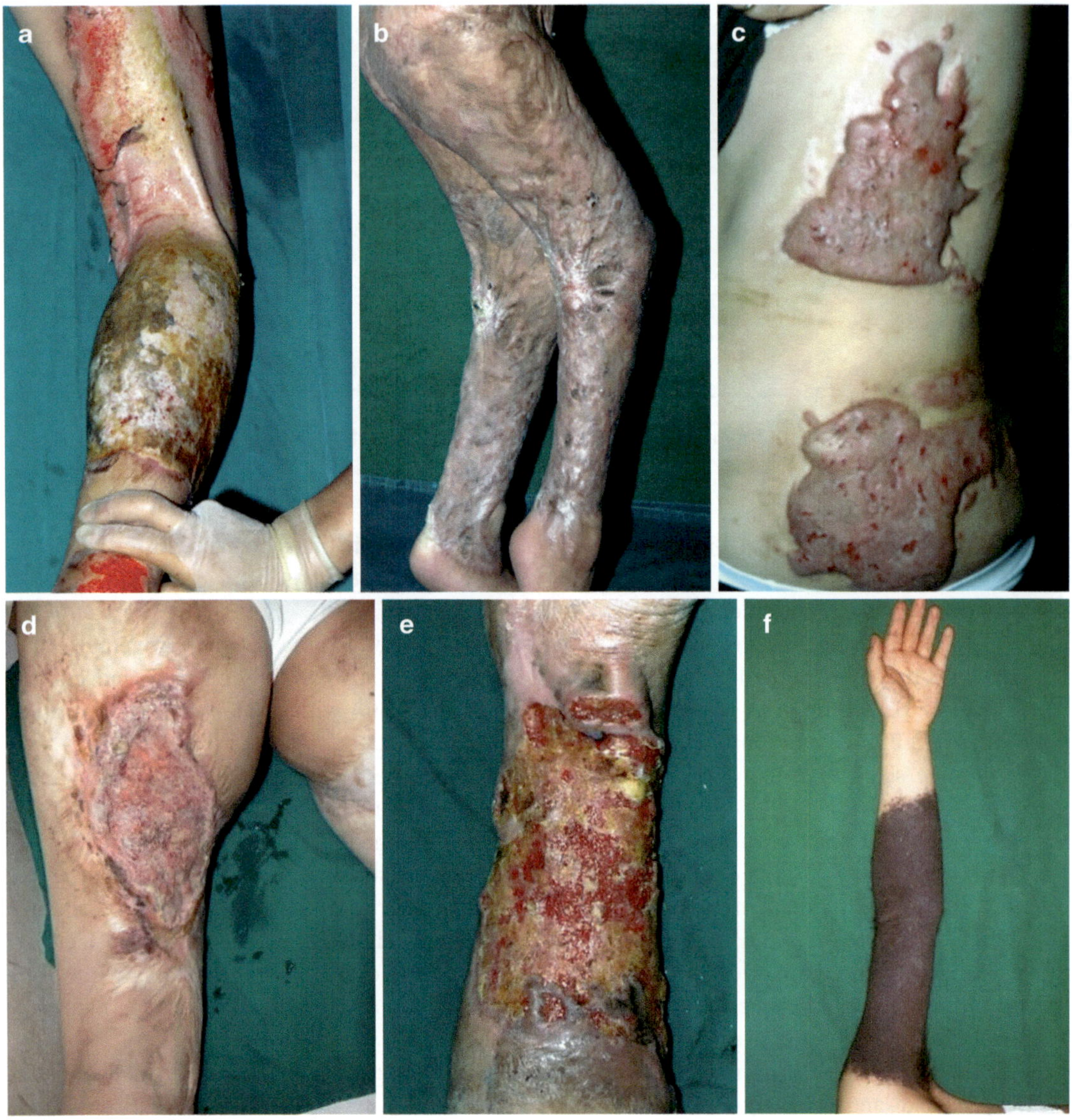

Fig. 3.2 Surgical indications: (**a**) deep second- and third-degree burn, (**b**) severe burn scar contracture, (**c**) severe hypertrophic scar with itching and pain, (**d**) chronic ulcerative lesion, (**e**) skin cancer, (**f**) giant hairy nevus, etc.

artificial dermal products have been developed, and their uses are expanding [23]. These products have been developed primarily for the treatment of burns, but the indications have now expanded to treatments of difficult-to-treat areas, such as the bone, tendons, soft tissues, and chronic wounds, such as diabetic foot, decubitus ulcer, and bed sores [24]. Understanding these properties and selecting the appropriate dermal substitutes are fundamental aspects of the surgery and outcomes of the various surgery methods that will be introduced. This is because the biggest weakness of 100% purely synthetic dermal substitutes is the susceptibility to infections, which has a significant influence on the subsequent usage of products and their outcomes [25]. The biggest advantage of dermal matrices manufactured from the human dermis is their wider usage due to durability against infection. This also means a wider range of usage and a higher treatment efficacy. Hence, they can serve as a turning point or solution for patients with intractable chronic wounds, such as those sustained in extremities with a risk of amputation, bed sores, and chronic osteomyelitis. These products have drawbacks, such as their high cost, low output caused by a scarcity of human tissue, and the time and expense needed for large wounds due to inconsistent sizing. However, by broadening the scope of treatment and addressing stubborn wounds, these drawbacks can be minimized. Thus, I would like to focus more heavily on the indications and usefulness of the human dermal matrix system.

3.3 Allogenic Human Dermal Matrix AlloDerm®

3.3.1 Acute Stage of Wound Coverage with Human Dermal Matrix System

3.3.1.1 Thickness and Types of AlloDerm®

The first human dermal matrix marketed was AlloDerm®, developed by Life Cell. It has been the most widely used human dermal matrix product in burn wound management since 1992 [26]. The most distinct feature of AlloDerm® is that it is manufactured from the epidermis of cadaver skin by removing all components except the basement membrane and splicing the upper layer of dermal components to a thickness of 0.4–0.5 mm (0.015–0.02 in.). All cellular components are removed from the tissue to prevent immune reactions before freeze-drying. The treated dermal layer is then transplanted on the wound bed to form a neodermis, with fibroblast and endothelial cell invasion from the wound bed acting as scaffolds. Human dermal matrix is composed of a dermal structure of collagen, elastin, blood vessel channels, and bioactive proteins. Compared with dermal substitutes synthesized from general animal collagen, human dermal matrix is very compatible with the recipient tissue and suitable for a single-step operation [27]. Moreover, the strong framework of the dermal layer is resistant to infections; even if infection does occur, it can remain functional for 2–3 weeks or more. Thus, the wound can remain protected from the external environment and be able to induce the synthesis of various growth factors required in wound healing, thereby facilitating the wound-healing process. However, products made from pure collagen are extremely prone to infections, and once infected, it is very challenging to stop the entire artificial dermis from dissolving, increasing the risk of total loss. As a result, wound dressing needs to be performed every day, and any infected sections should be immediately removed. Hence, synthetic dermal matrices are not appropriate for use in chronic wounds, infected wounds, or regions exposing bone or ligaments.

Human dermal matrix can be classified based on their thickness and whether they have a mesh or not. In early period, main products are in mesh form to serve the primary development purpose, which is to treat burns. The mesh enables dermal transplantation in parallel with the thin split-thickness autograft for large wounds in order to reduce graft failure and increase the graft intake rate for the single-step operation procedure.

The thickness also plays an essential role in the success rate, and, generally, 0.4–0.5 mm (0.015–0.02 inches) is suitable. From my experience, to make mesh patterns less visible for esthetic purposes, products with a thickness of approximately 0.7 mm or above and non-mesh-type products in the early stages of development can be successful; however, a longer learning curve and more practice with wound dressings are required. Hence, these products are not recommended until the surgeon has gained sufficient experience. Furthermore, no significant differences in contracture rate were observed with different thicknesses, depending on whether the engraftment thickness exceeded 0.5 mm, and the mesh pattern became less visible after graft maturation. Therefore, any steps that jeopardize the take rate or the use of the non-mesh type are not recommended (Fig. 3.3).

Initially, non-meshed AlloDerm® was developed for esthetic skin graft purposes to prevent

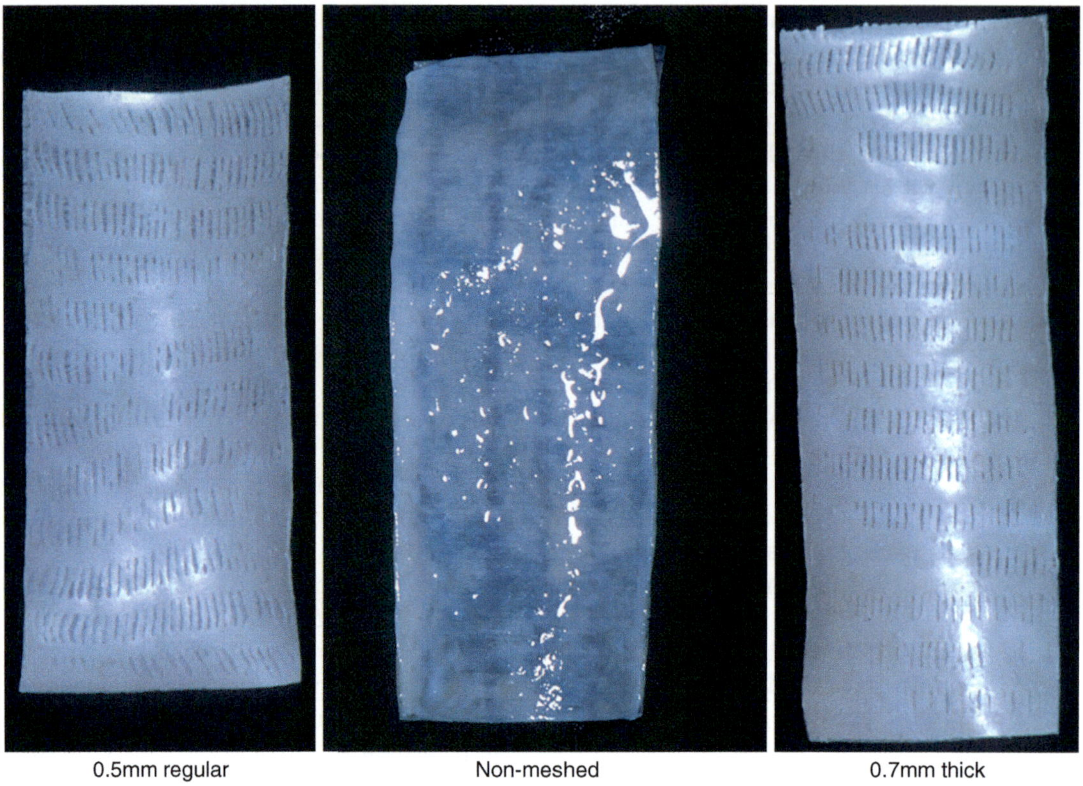

Fig. 3.3 The variable AlloDerm® type and thickness: first is 0.5-mm regular meshed, mid is non-meshed 0.4 mm, and last is 0.7-mm-thick meshed type

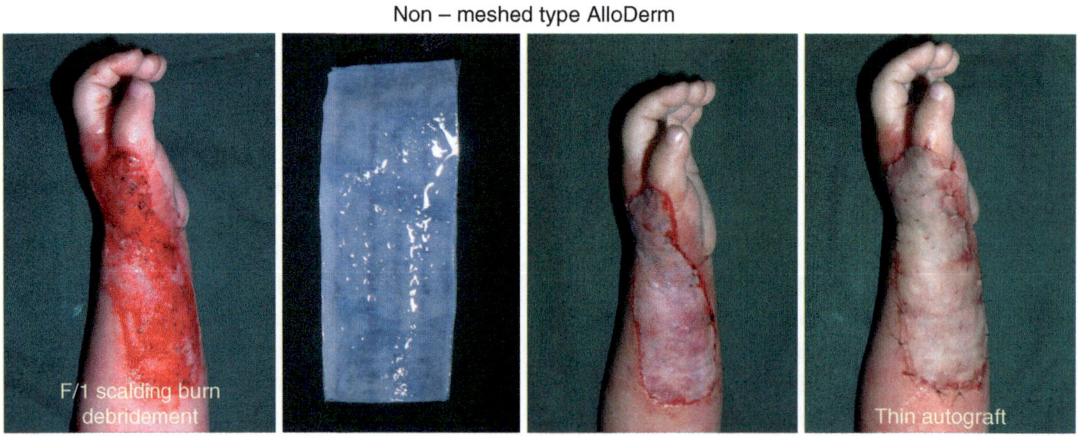

Fig. 3.4 In early period, non-meshed type of AlloDerm® was manufactured but now not in use for graft

visible meshed pattern. But it is no longer used for graft purposes because of lower graft take rate and the minimal difference in the end result between meshed and non-meshed types (Fig. 3.4).

3.3.1.2 Orientation of Engraftment Surface

A further precaution that must be taken before use is determining the orientation of the dermal matrix direction.

These products have been manufactured so that the basement membrane, a biologically important layer between the dermis and epidermis, can help autologous skin grafting and preserve function. The residual basement membrane must face up toward the autologous skin graft. Therefore, correctly determining the orientation of the product, that is, distinguishing the dermal and basement membrane sides, is important in using the products [28]. A few tricks can be used to achieve this. The basement membrane layer appears rough, dull, and buff-colored and repels blood. The dermal layer, which needs to correctly come in contact with the wound bed, appears shiny, smooth, and white and absorbs blood. However, actually differentiating the sides in the operating room is tricky. Hence, a slit marking is placed facing the upper-right or left-bottom corner of the wound bed, or an L-shaped pattern in the mesh is visible with the correct orientation but recently rarely used.

In recent years, printed paper has been attached on top of the basement membrane to maintain the shape of the dermal matrix layer, to help the placement of the basement membrane surface right way up. For thin autografts, the printed paper material is removed, and the autoskin graft is placed on top of the basement membrane (Fig. 3.5).

3.3.2 Acute Stage of Burn Management Using AlloDerm®

3.3.2.1 Basic Technique in Using AlloDerm®

(a) Clean the wound area, and remove any infected or necrotic tissue to ensure a healthy vascularized wound bed, and perform bleeding control to prevent hematoma.

A 42-year-old male suffered deep second-degree flame burns on both hands. Upon examination of the burn after 16 days, eschar

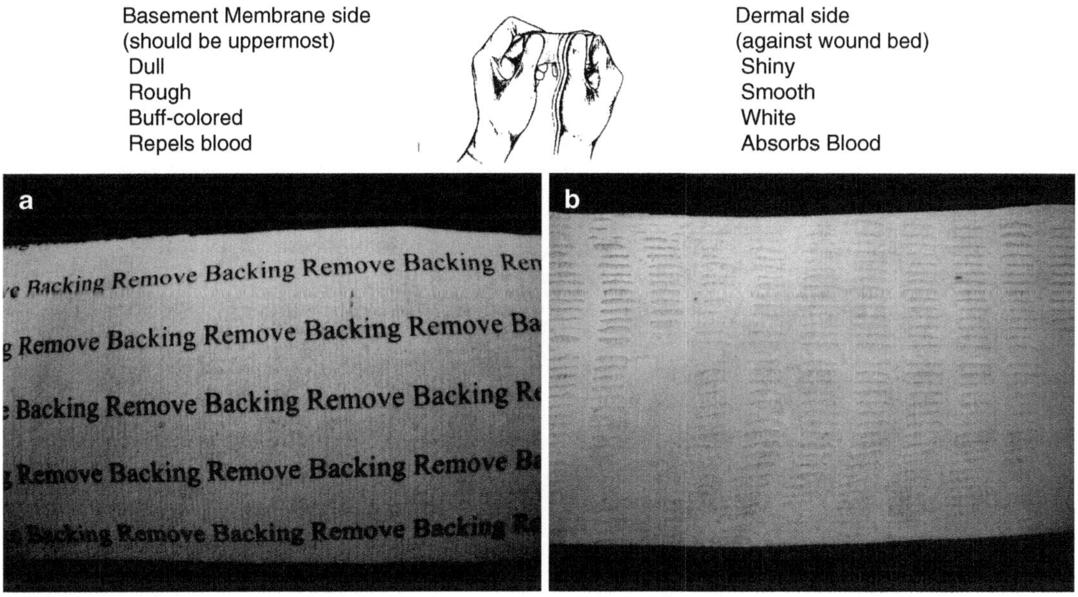

Fig. 3.5 In the past orientation method was distinguished by being dull, rough, and buff-colored, repels blood side is basement membrane side, and shiny, smooth, white, absorbs blood side is dermal side. Recently, orientation of AlloDerm® was more easily checked with (**a**) lettering paper side should be upward and (**b**) dermal side must be against wound bed; for basement membrane constantly keep uppermost position

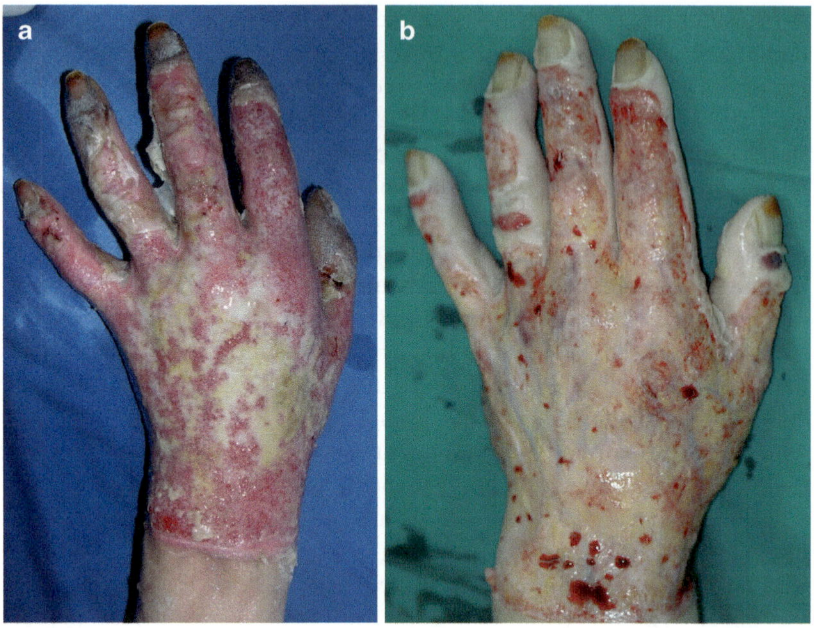

Fig. 3.6 (**a**) Postburn day 16, noted eschar, (**b**) after escharectomy

was noted (left hand; Fig. 3.6). After escharectomy, there was a well-preserved subdermal fat layer and excellent bleeding control using the epinephrine injection technique alone without a tourniquet instrument (Fig. 3.6).

(b) Use a dermal matrix to cover the wound bed as explained above, so that the basement membrane is pointing upward. Take care not to forcefully expand the 1:1 mesh region, but instead allow it to maintain a natural surface to cover the wound with no gap between allografts. This is important for decreasing the wound contracture rate after potential engraftment and for obtaining a good outcome. The reason for mesh incision is made solely to increase the intake rate, not to increase the graft surface. Furthermore, from my experience, the distance between the dermal matrix and wound margin should be precise and approximate as it can be managed and sutured by absorbable suture material to close any gaps between the dermal matrix and matrix. This can decrease the linear contracture rate in the wound margin and encourage a favorable outcome.

AlloDerm® of 0.4-mm thickness was engrafted, and auto-skin of 0.2-mm thickness was harvested. Note the immediate thin autograft thickness in the absence of any slit incision in order to prevent hematoma or fluid collection. There was no expanded meshed dermal matrix, but there were more accurate approximations of each dermal matrix margin for less late linea scar contracture complication. The most ideal hand position is the fist position (Fig. 3.7).

(c) A very thin autologous skin graft can be performed using a sheet or mesh, depending on the variable situation of patients' condition. However, I mostly do not recommend a mesh graft as it causes an increased re-contracture rate and shrinkage of the engrafted surface and reduces the cosmetically surgical outcome. The ultimate goal is to minimize scarring at the donor site by keeping the skin thickness to approximately 0.125–0.2 mm and minimizing scar contracture by supplementing the dermal layer at the wound bed. At the early stage of use, an ultrathin graft is recommended with a thickness of around 0.125 mm. However, my clinical experience has shown

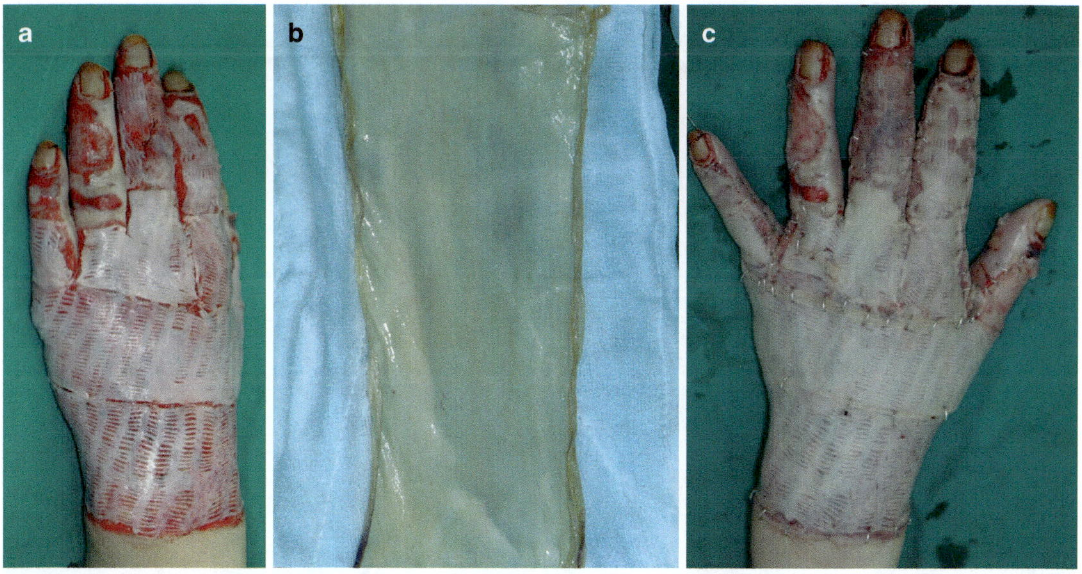

Fig. 3.7 (**a**) 0.4-mm thickness AlloDerm® engraft. (**b**) 8/1000-inches. (0.2-mm) thick harvested skin. (**c**) Immediate thin autograft without any slit incision

that a thin STSG of 0.175–0.2 mm seems to be most appropriate.

The results of the 2-year operation on acutely burned hands managed with human dermal matrix were observed. There was no functional disturbance, and the esthetic results were good, with no scar contracture or deformities. These excellent results emphasize the critical point that the initial proper management of early excision and early graft in the acute stage of hand burn management has a significant impact on functional and esthetic end results (Fig. 3.8).

As a clinical example, I will introduce the dorsum of the hand, which is most exposed to the external environment and has the intensive interphalangeal joints, thus providing essential materials for functional and esthetical recovery. I rarely use dermal substitutes for acute burn management involving the flexor zone of the hand because I believe they have a minimal effect in preventing flexor contracture. The process of wound healing of flexor region is fast combined with scar contracture. A dermal substitute can be considered priority dorsal side rather than flexor side to maximize the use of this expensive material. First, when removing eschar, conduct meticulous debridement of necrotic tissue, so as not to expose any tendon or tendon sheath. In this process, I choose not to use a tourniquet but used only an epinephrine injection to control the bleeding. This is because, when performing debridement, immediate bleeding control is possible under visible active bleeding, and using a tourniquet may lead to rebound bleeding once it is removed. Next, place the AlloDerm® on the graft site without expanding the mesh pattern ensuring no gaps, and between the dermal matrix, use the absorbable 6–0 Vicryl® interrupted sutures side by side where necessary. An even engraftment without gap of a dermal layer can help prevent linear contracture and improve the esthetical appearance of the hand, which is constantly exposed in daily life. On the dorsum of the hands, proper thickness of autograft is 0.2 mm or thicker with better functionally as well as esthetically good texture. Performing the graft while maintaining a fist position is essential to secure a maximal expanded engraft surface and for functional recovery [29].

Next, I would like to discuss a case of how initial treatment played an important role in

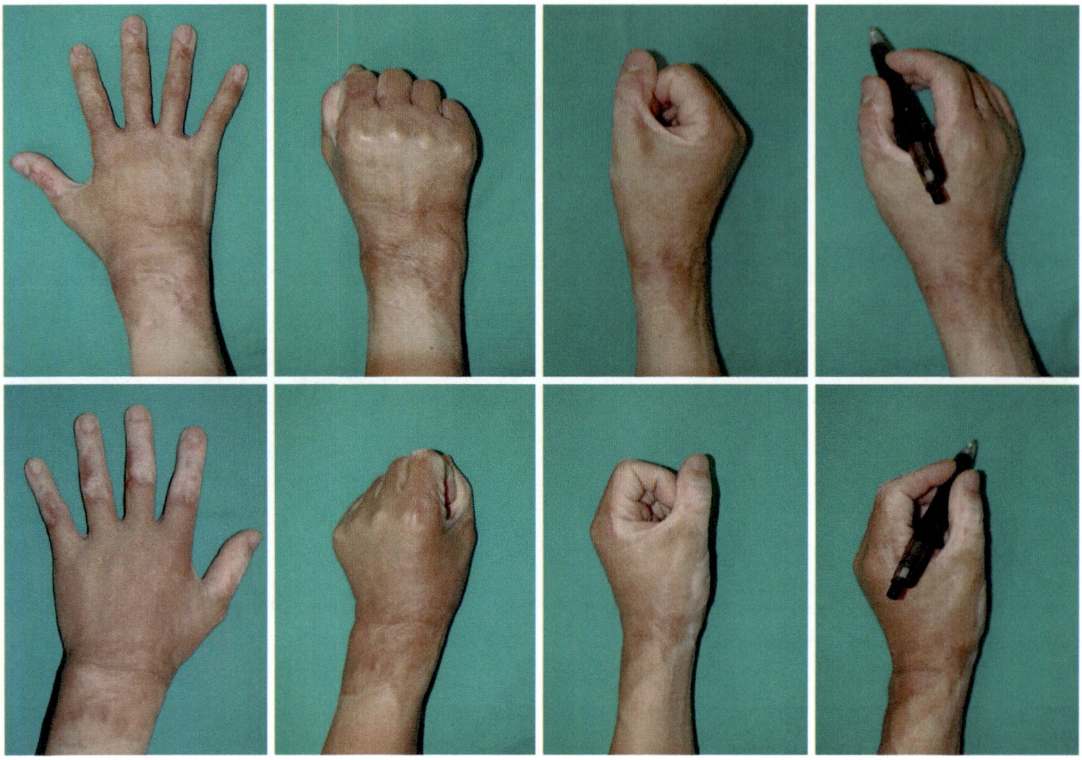

Fig. 3.8 Postoperative 2 year after view. No functional disturbance and also good esthetic results without any scar contracture and deformities

obtaining a good outcome in reconstructive surgery of both hands scarred from strong acetic acid.

Emphasis should be placed on the sequential process of the treatment, as described subsequently. First, during the acute stage, early excision and early grafting were performed using a dermal matrix for rapid wound healing and skin volume supplement [30, 31]. One year after, the postburn scar contracture was corrected with a full-thickness skin graft (FTSG) on the flexor area on both hands. Finally, to promote an esthetic appearance of the dorsum of the hand, dermabrasion and dermal overgrafting were performed to complete the operation. Attention to these sequential procedures may facilitate understanding of the orientation of each chapter to be described.

A 13-year-old female patient was burned by glacial acetic acid, a type of strong acid, on both of her hands. An emergency escharotomy was performed to avoid compartment syndrome and save the fingers. On day 7 after the burn, full-thickness skin necrosis developed on the entire hand, necrotic tissue was removed, and a human dermal matrix graft after wound bed clearance was planned (Fig. 3.9). On day 17 in accordance with the early excision and early graft plan, a single-step human dermal matrix graft was performed on both dorsal and ventral parts of the hands to enhance wound healing and finger preservation. The thickness of the engrafted thin auto-skin graft was 0.15 mm (Fig. 3.10). After performing human dermal matrix system engraftment 1 year later, we observed severe palm contracture and webbing deformities on both hands. Reconstructive surgery using scar contracture release and FTSG was performed on both hands. Reconstructive full-thickness skin grafts on both the palm and fingers resulted in

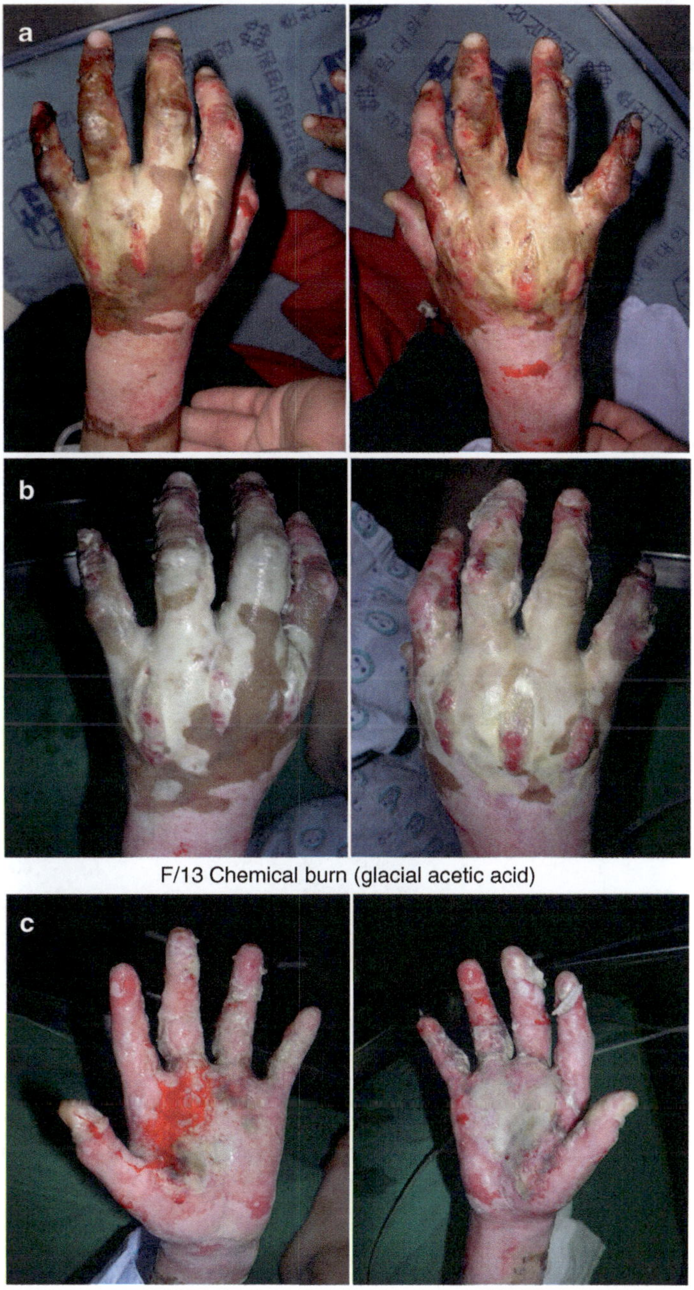

Fig. 3.9 (**a**) Postburn day 7 view. Strong acid chemical burn on both encircled entire hands. Initial emergency escharotomy was performed. (**b**) Postburn day 11 view. (**c**) Postburn day 2 weeks after, both palm side view, preoperative view of human dermal matrix application

good functional recovery. Full functional recovery of the flexor parts on both hands was observed 6 months after surgery (Fig. 3.11). Five years after surgery, both the dorsum of the hands and the flexor parts are functionally and esthetically normal (Fig. 3.12).

Next, I will describe a case of how a dermal matrix system, given its durability against inflammation or infectious state, can be a safe and convenient option in an old infected inflammatory wound with partial bone exposure due to a third-degree deep thermal burn.

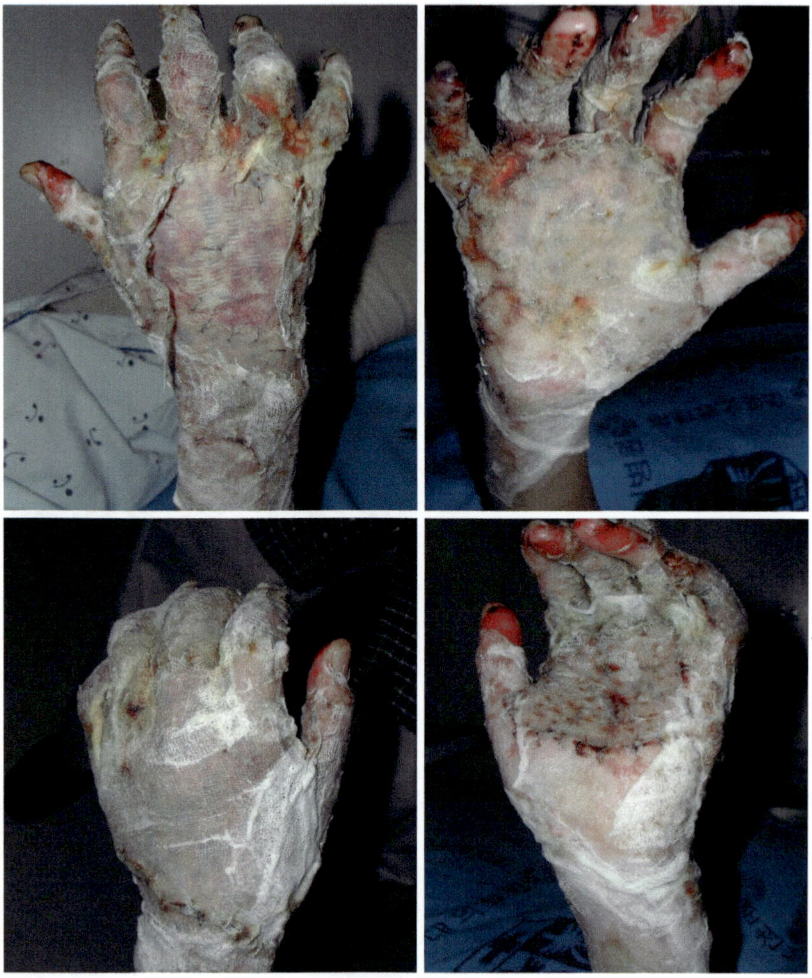

Artificial Dermis AlloDerm Graft

Fig. 3.10 Postburn day 17 view; single-step human dermal matrix graft was performed with 6/1000-inches-thin auto-skin graft

A 21-year-old male was injured 2 months ago and was transferred to our department with burns caused by molten metal on the entire upper back area as well as left partial scapula bone exposure and infected necrotic tissue. Human dermal matrix engraftment was performed after old, infected, necrotic tissue on the back and bony exposure in the right scapular area were debrided. Advantages of human dermal matrix include high resistance to infection and effective protection of the bony exposure area. However, the disadvantage is that irregularly small-sized products necessitate a lengthy engraftment process (Fig. 3.13). A thin auto-skin graft with a 1:1 mesh (0.15-mm thickness) was performed. Three months, 1 year, and 2 months after surgery, the patient had full range of motion in both shoulders and good skin texture with fully covered bone exposure in the scapular area (Fig. 3.14).

3.3.2.2 Treatment of Burn Wounds Accompanied by Exposure of Bone and Ligament, Soft Tissue Defects, and Infected Wound Using AlloDerm®

Generally, surgeons consider flap surgery as first-line treatment when bone or ligaments are exposed. However, I first maximized the wound-healing process and then performed grafting as the ultimate treatment process. This method is one of the most important and interesting points introduced in this book.

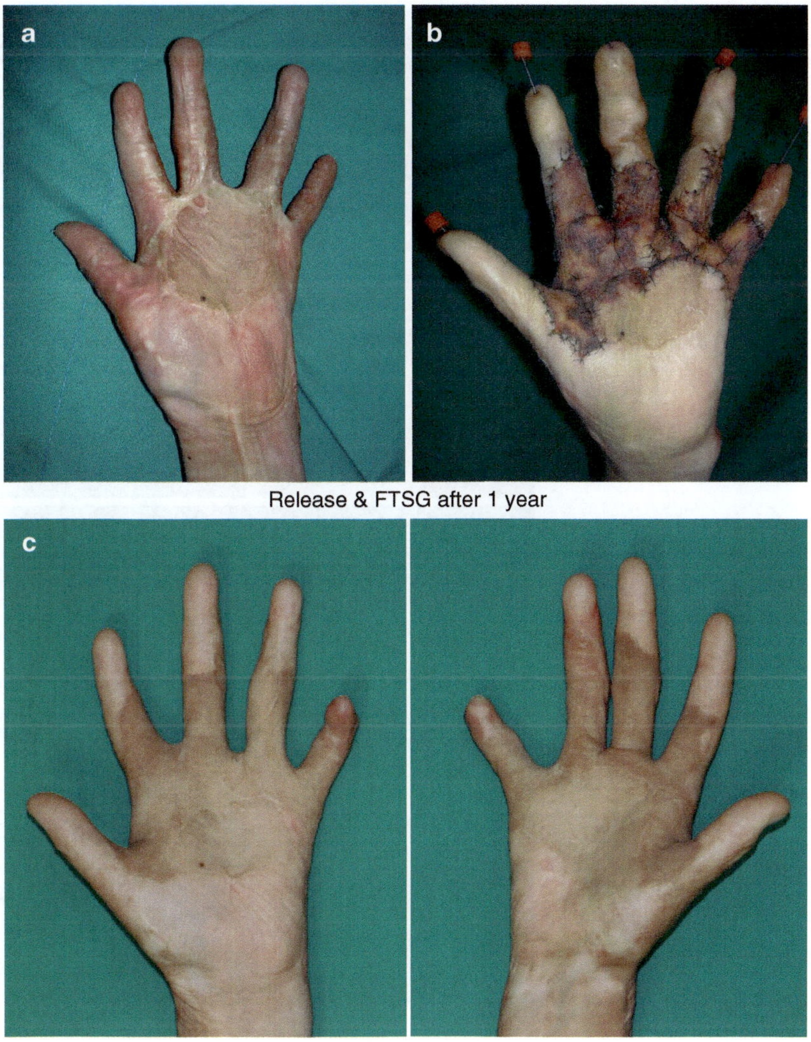

Fig. 3.11 (**a**) Human dermal matrix system engraft 1 year after view; note severe palm contracture and webbing deformities on both hands (in this photo, left hand revealed). (**b**) Release and full-thickness skin graft was performed on both hands. (**c**) Reconstructive full-thickness skin graft on both the palm and fingers was noted with good functional recovery. Postoperative 6-month-later view, full function recovery of flexor part on both hands was noted

The treatment process is as follows:

(a) For an unhygienic necrotic wound, first perform wound debridement several times over to remove all necrotic and nonviable tissue. Then, use saline-soaked gauze to perform wet to dry dressing two to three times a day. The wound condition usually improves in 2–3 days or within a maximum of 1 week. Afterward the use of a human dermal matrix system should be considered.
(b) When the wound contamination is serious, remove all nonviable tissue. However, when the viability of tissues is uncertain, do not actively remove any tissues. Especially for muscle, refraining from any active removal is recommended. From my experience, even pale-colored muscle with no fresh bleeding can recover better than initially expected. Hence, adequate experience in debridement is required for wise decision-making.
(c) When the bone is exposed, remove the cortex with an electrical burr, and confirm pinpoint bleeding of the cancellous bone. Then, perform direct grafting of the dermal matrix, taking precaution that a hematoma does not form. The engraftment outcome is also good when using a thin STSG immediately. The

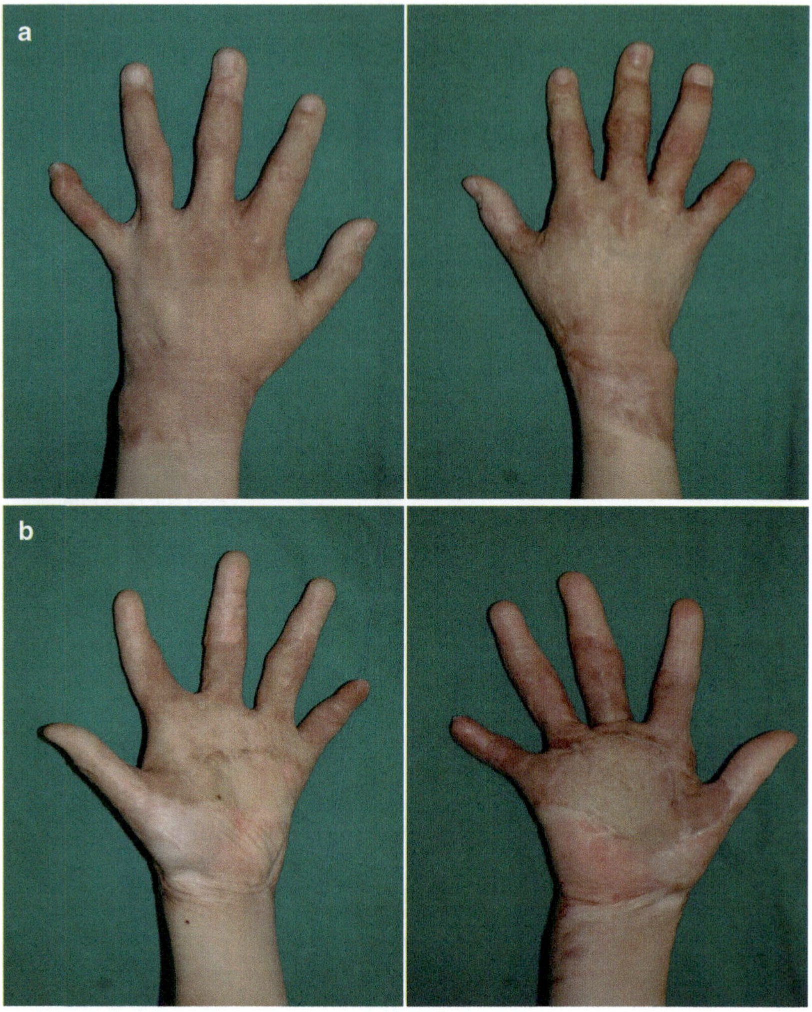

Fig. 3.12 (**a**, **b**) Five years after surgery view: marked improved functional and esthetic outcome on both hands

anterior tibia area, in particular, is a region with most solid bones in the body and is composed of bones and skin with almost no soft tissue. Any soft tissue defects accompanying a fracture with bone exposure must be treated using a muscle flap from the surrounding muscle or a free flap [32, 33]. However, if a third-degree burn involves general soft tissue and full-thickness skin loss in the lower leg, harvesting a muscle flap from the surrounding muscle is unfeasible, and amputation should be considered. I would like to describe a case of an older patient with severe soft tissue loss and full layer of skin loss with bone exposure area with whom a good treatment outcome was achieved using a dermal matrix for wound coverage [34]. This method may serve as a useful option for the treatment of bone exposure in the lower limb on the anterior tibia area.

A 77-year-old female patient suffered a scalding burn with a full-layer, deep thermal burn on her anterior tibia. Three days after the burn, full-layer necrotic tissue death was found on the anterior tibia along with infection. Nineteen days after the burn, an anterior tibia bone exposure with necrotic tissue was observed with lacking of the surrounding skin, and there was no means to cover the bone exposure wound with muscle or a local flap (Fig. 3.15). Necrotic tissue was removed, and the exposed bony part of the anterior tibia

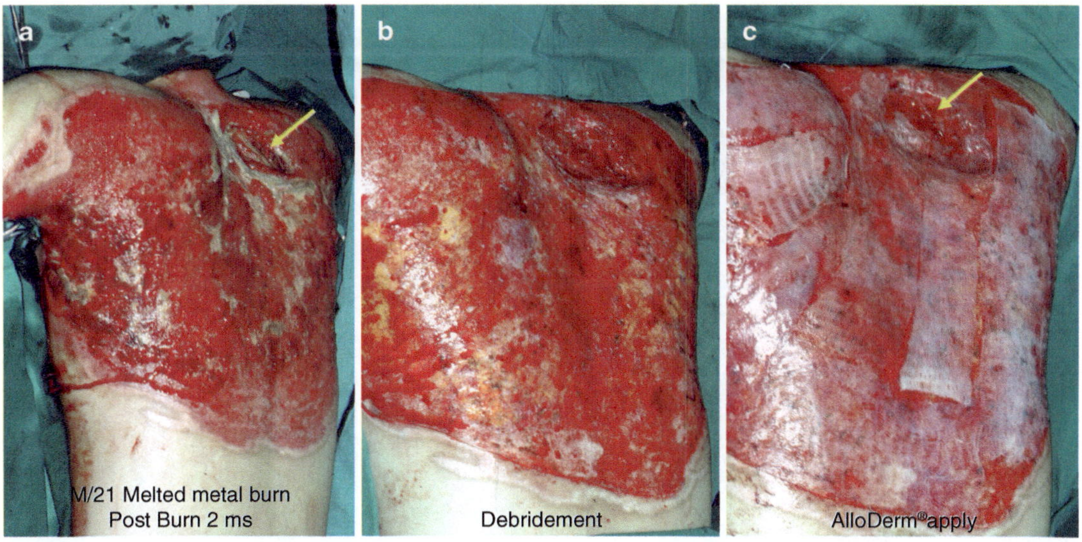

Fig. 3.13 (**a**) Molten metal burn on the entire back area with left partial scapula bone exposure (yellow arrow). (**b**) After total debridement on the back, (**c**) human dermal matrix was engrafted

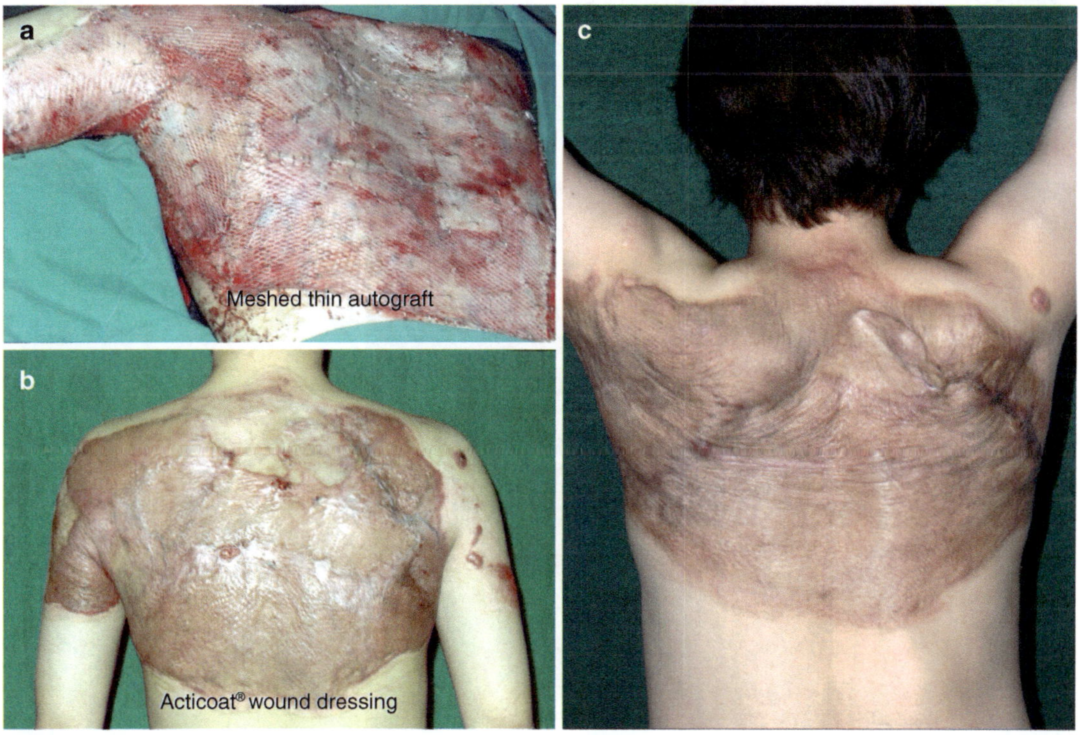

Fig. 3.14 (**a**) 6/1000-inches-thin 1:1 meshed split-thickness autograft, intraoperative view; (**b**) postoperative 3-month-later view; (**c**) postoperative 1.2 years view. The back and both shoulder movement was noted with full range of motion

was ground using an electric burr until cancellous bone exposure and pinpoint bleeding were observed. Immediate wound coverage was achieved using human dermal matrix and thin 1:1.5-meshed auto-skin graft (Fig. 3.16). To improve wound healing, experimentally

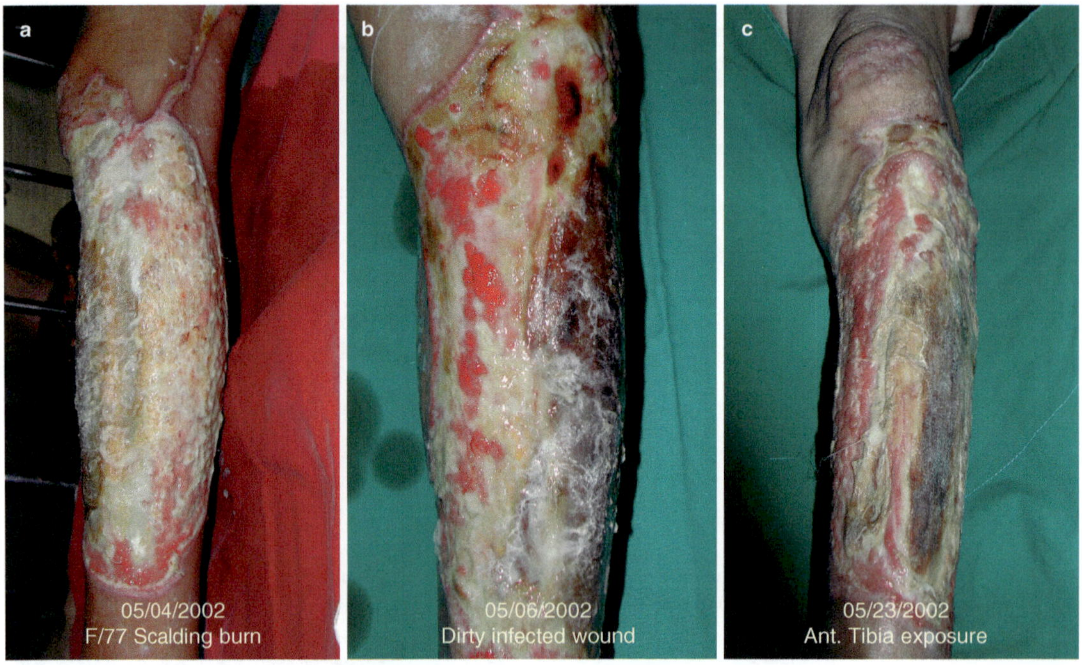

Fig. 3.15 (**a**) Full-layer deep thermal burn on anterior tibia area. (**b**) Postburn day 3, full-layer necrotic death tissue noted on anterior tibia area with infection. (**c**) Postburn day 3 weeks, anterior tibia bone exposure with dirty necrotic tissue was noted

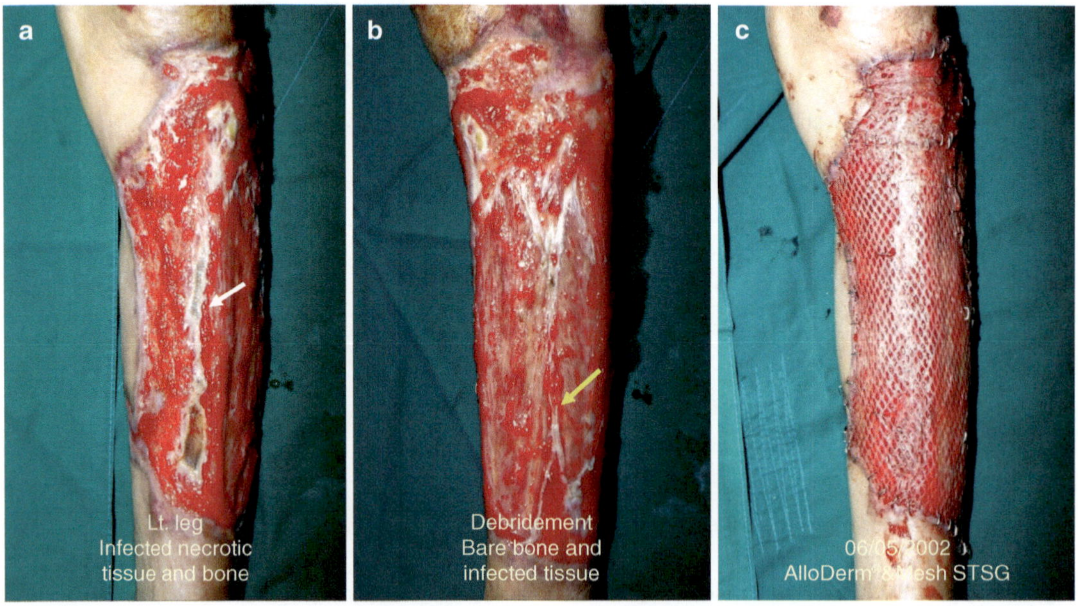

Fig. 3.16 (**a**) Escharectomy after view (white arrow) and (**b**) exposure part of the anterior tibia was ground using electric burr until cancellous bone exposure (yellow arrow). (**c**) Immediate wound coverage with human dermal matrix with thin 1:1.5 mesh auto-skin graft performed

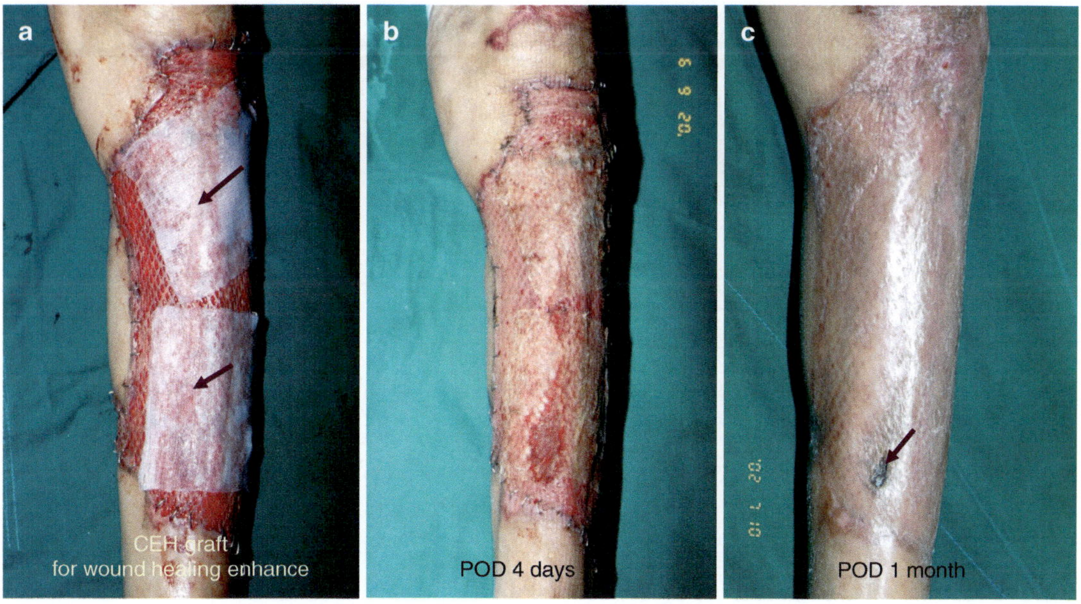

Fig. 3.17 (**a**) Cultured epithelial homograft (CEH) covered on two sites of bony exposure area (black arrow). (**b**) Four days after view, the engrafted mesh skin was almost taken and stabilized operation wound. (**c**) Postoperative 1 month after view, the wound healed without any problems; healed wound (black arrow) in a dimple form left and no need additional flap surgery

cultured epithelial homograft was applied to two sites of the bone exposure area. Four days after the surgery, the engrafted mesh skin was taken almost completely, and the operation wound was stabilized. One month after the surgery, the wound healed without any complications. In this case, the human dermal matrix proved to be a very versatile material for treating difficult wounds (Fig. 3.17).

A 71-year-old male patient suffered flame burns and had a mesh skin graft performed, which encircled the entire left lower leg. However, anterior tibia bone exposure was observed. After removing the cortex of the anterior tibia until pinpoint bleeding was observed, human dermal matrix was engrafted, and a 0.15-mm sheet autograft was applied immediately to cover the bone exposure area (Fig. 3.18). Even though it was a non-meshed sheet graft, the dermal matrix and thin autograft were almost completely removed 7 and 9 days after surgery. Two weeks after the engraftment procedure, the patient was taken completely. This means that this cancellous bone exposure area is ready for good take rate even with non-meshed graft sheet (Fig. 3.19).

These figures show long-term following results with anterior tibia area covered with dermal matrix system. Three and 5 years after surgery, the patient did not face any problems such as recurring bone exposure or an unstable skin lesion during the last 5 years (Fig. 3.20).

(d) When tendons are exposed, a successful engrafting is harder to achieve compared with bone exposure. This is because tendons do not have abundant blood supply, and a granulation tissue bed does not form well. Hence, the intake rate between the tendon and engrafted skin is low. Since directly confirming the viability of the tendon is difficult, the tendon sheath or the surrounding tissue should be preserved if possible in order to implant a dermal matrix graft. In regions where the engraftment is partial in graft loss

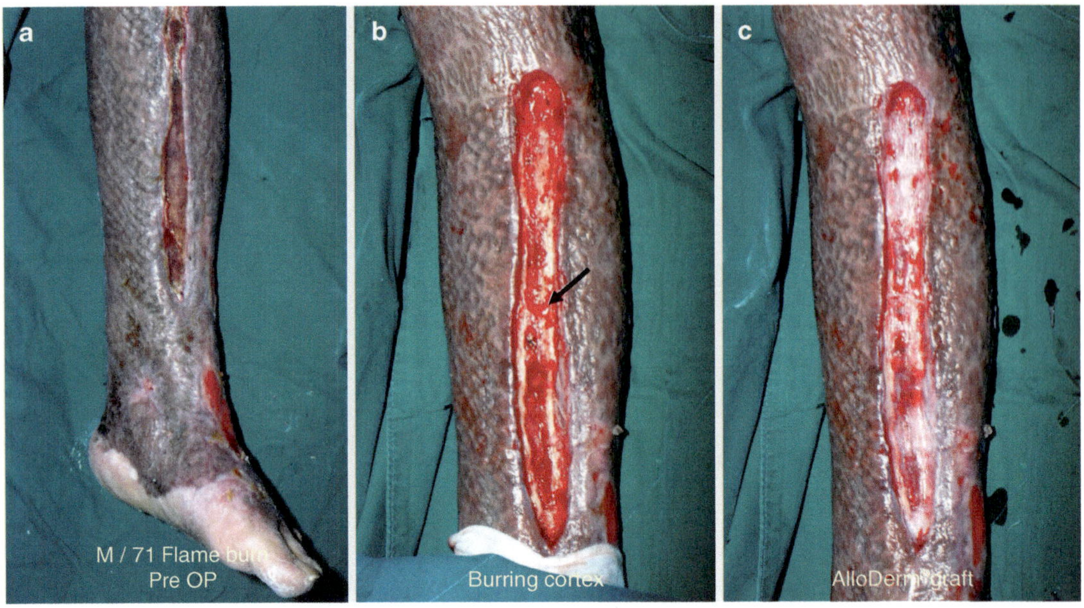

Fig. 3.18 (**a**) Bone exposure with dry necrotic tissue was noted on previous mesh skin graft area. (**b**) After removal of the cortex of anterior tibia with confirmed pinpoint bleeding (black arrow), (**c**) human dermal matrix with 0.15-mm sheet autograft covered immediately

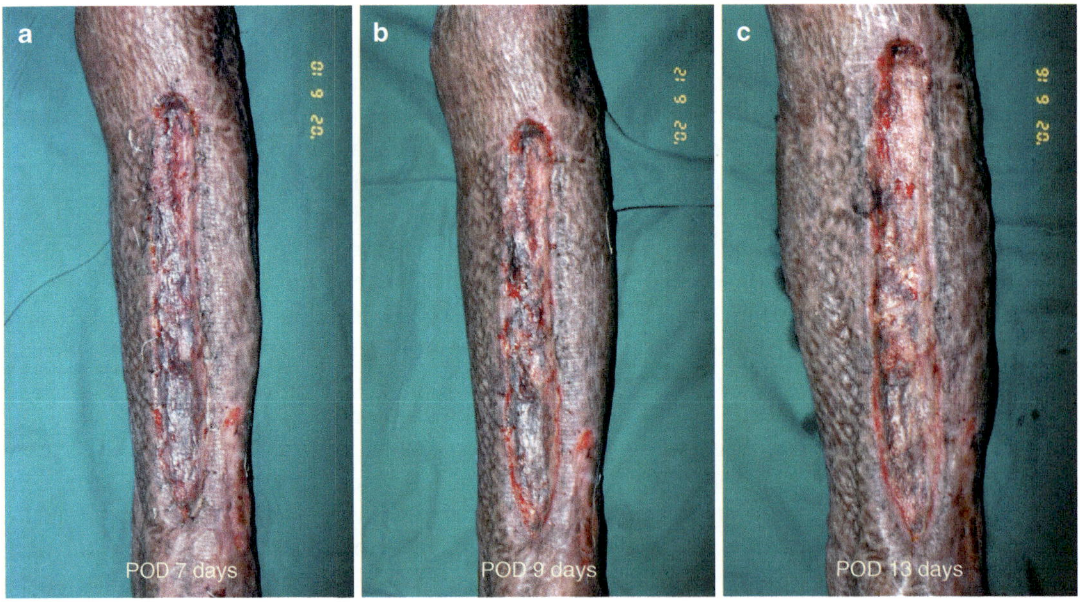

Fig. 3.19 (**a**, **b**) Postoperative 7 days, 9 days were noted dermal matrix and thin autograft is almost taken (**c**) 2 weeks after the engraft was taken completely

area, apply a saline-soaked dressing at least twice a day to clean the wound bed, and make an appropriate environment for granulation tissue to grow. In some cases, two to three more surgeries should be performed to gradually reduce the size of the scar. The sec-

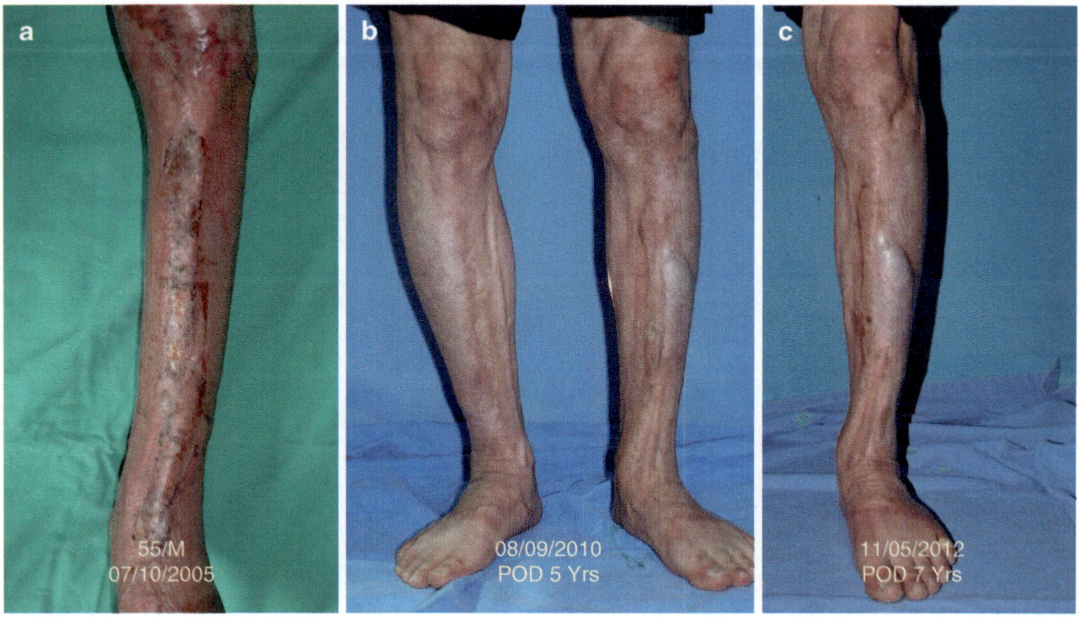

Fig. 3.20 (**a**) Another long-term follow-up case on the left anterior tibia area (**b**, **c**) postoperative 3 years, 5 years after view; there were no problems such as repeat bony exposure or unstable skin lesion during 5 years of everyday life

ond additional engraft is not firm using dermal matrix graft; it can vary case by case according to wound bed condition. Because the primary engrafted dermal matrix will remain even if in small amount, it will be important wound-healing trigger and aid final graft take.

A 31-year-old male patient suffered a deep thermal contact burn on the left wrist. After necrotic tissue debridement on postburn day 13, the healthy granulation tissue and partially exposed flexor tendon were examined. First, a dermal matrix engraft with a thin auto-skin graft was performed to reduce the size of the surrounding wound and protect the exposed tendon and sheath (Fig. 3.21). After 2 weeks, the original wound size was markedly reduced, and 1 week after engraftment, a healthy granulation tissue bed was placed for the second dermal matrix graft. Case 1 underwent dermal matrix engraftment again, but it was not a routine procedure. On day 5 after the second operation, the engrafted skin was safely taken and the tendon exposure area was completely covered (Fig. 3.22).

A 42-year-old male patient had flame burns on his left lower leg and foot as well as a full-thickness skin defect with necrotic tendon exposure on the inner ankle. Dermal matrix and thin autograft were performed 2 days after the operation; however, the center area showed partial skin loss, necessitating a second regraft with auto-skin graft alone. Two weeks after the second surgery, skin graft was taken and no graft loss was observed (Fig. 3.23).

A 2-year-old boy suffered from contact thermal burns on his right palm and wrist. Two days later, a full-thickness thermal burn was observed on the wrist. Twelve days later, the eschar was completely removed, and the partial exposure tendon sheath was covered with dermal matrix and a thin single-sheet auto-skin graft (Fig. 3.24). Four days after the procedure, we observed partial skin loss as well as a well-preserved dermal matrix component in the previously exposed tendon area. Four days later, healthy granulation tissue was covered after daily soaking dressings (one to three times), and there was still dermal matrix on the skin-loss site. Six days later, a simple patch skin graft was successfully performed (Fig. 3.25). Advantages

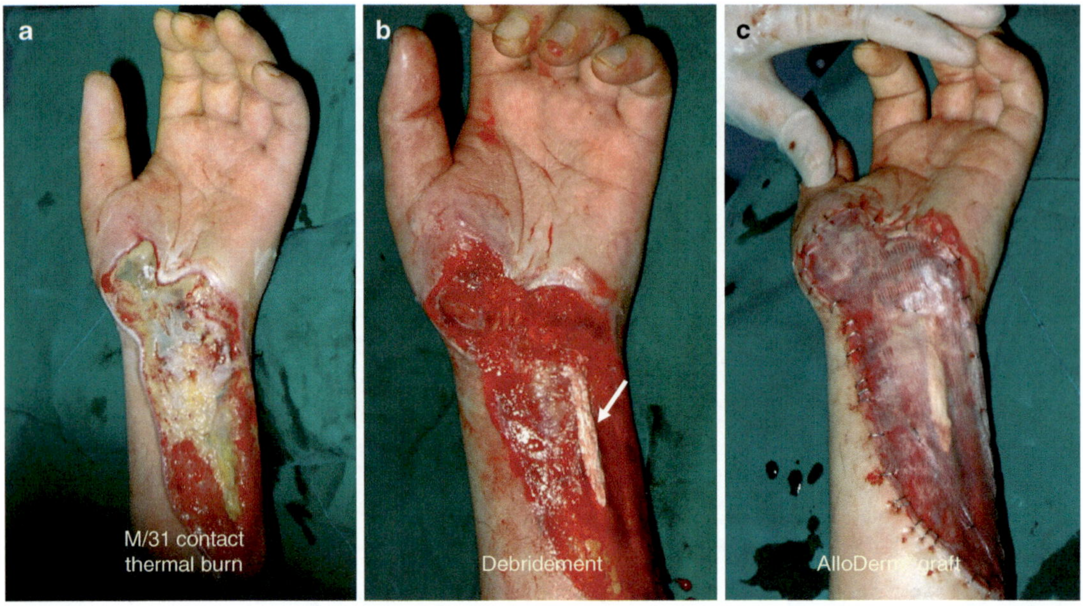

Fig. 3.21 (**a**) Contact deep thermal burn on the left wrist area. (**b**) Postburn day 13, the healthy granulation tissue and partially exposure flexor tendon (white arrow) were noted. (**c**) Priority, dermal matrix engraft with thin auto-skin graft was performed to reduce wound size and for protection of exposure tendon

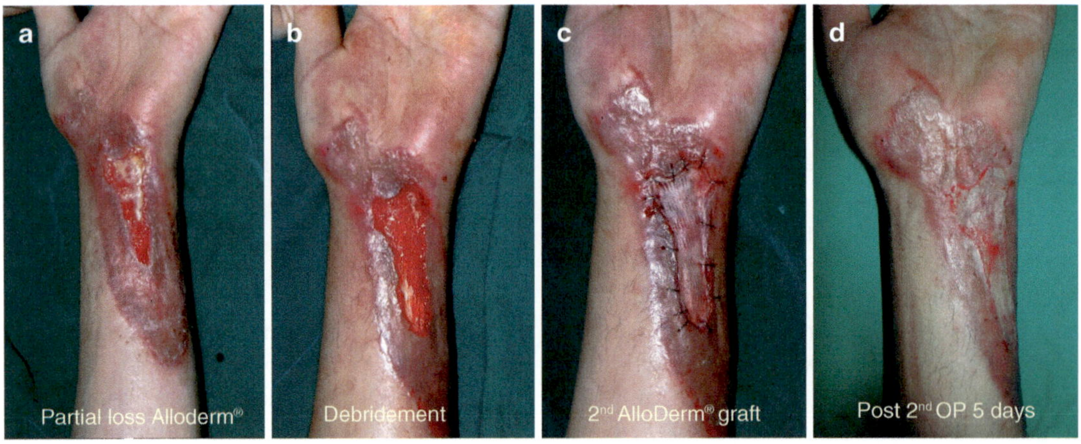

Fig. 3.22 (**a**) After 2 weeks, the original wound size was markedly reduced, and (**b, c**) 1 week after, small part of tendon exposure area was covered with second dermal matrix graft. (**d**) On day 5 after the second operation view

of human dermal matrix are long-standing, strong tissue material and resistance of infection with enhanced granulation tissue growth for possible skin graft.

Two years after the surgery, there was no functional disturbance with tendon adhesion. Four years after the surgery, although children's growth rates are rapid, the engrafted FTSG skin is also well adapted despite the rapid body growth (Fig. 3.26).

Human dermal matrix role is well represented in the case shown above. It is long-standing, strong tissue material that is resistant to infections with the ability to enhance granulation tissue growth for possible skin graft.

Typically in tendon exposure area it is harder for graft to be taken, compared to bone exposed areas or other sites; the author recommends to be more cautious and being aware that tendon exposed areas have higher chances of graft loss.

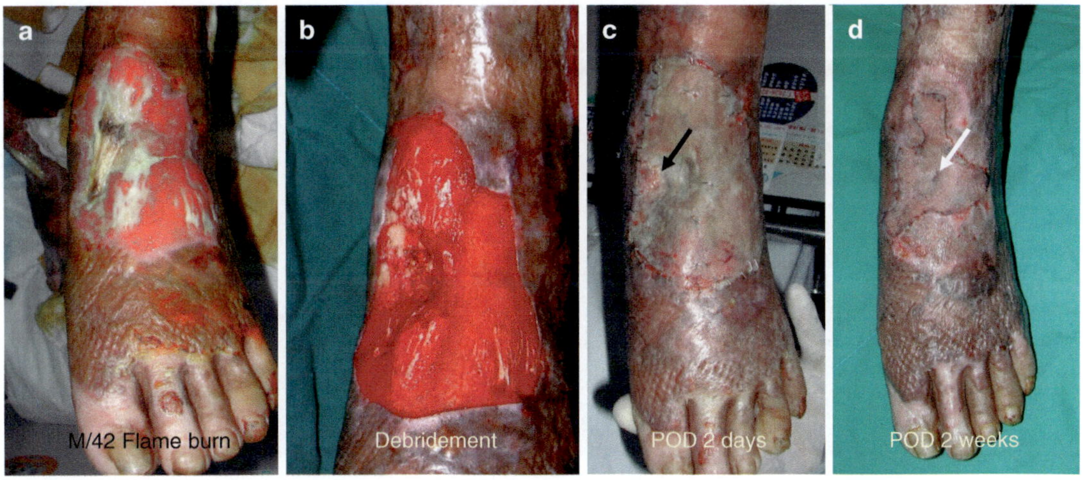

Fig. 3.23 (**a**) Full-thickness skin defect with necrotic tendon exposure was noted on the medial ankle area. (**b**) Human dermal matrix with 0.2-mm sheet auto STSG was performed (**c**) 2 days after operation; center area (black arrow) was partial skin loss (**d**) 2 weeks after the second operation; engrafted skin was taken

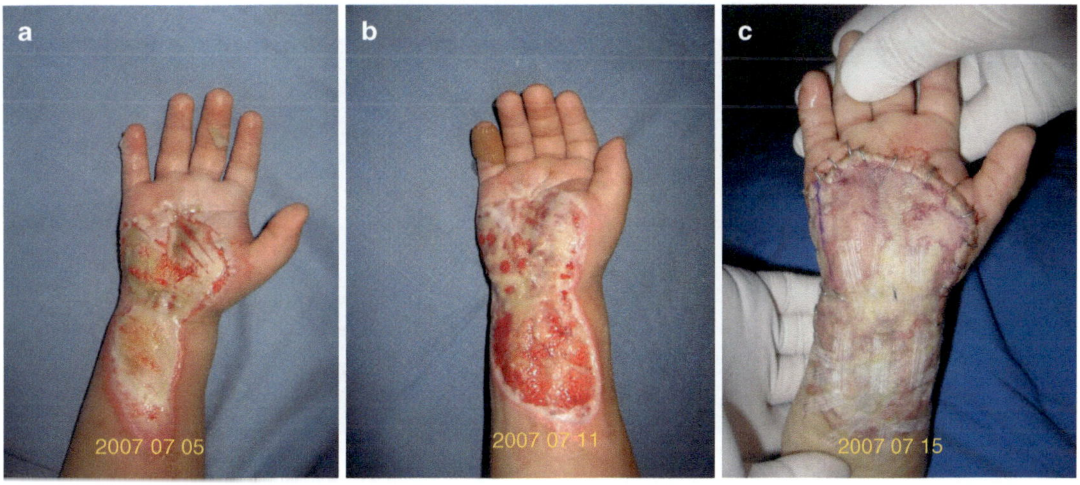

Fig.3.24 (**a**) Postburn 2 days later, full-thickness thermal burn noted on wrist area. (**b**) Postburn day 8 still remainder of thick eschar noted. (**c**) Postburn day 12, total removed eschar with exposure tendon sheath was covered with dermal matrix and single-sheet auto-skin graft

3.3.2.3 The Basic Principle of Difficult Wound Management

The basic principle of difficult wound management can be summarized as follows: once debridement is completed, check the wound bed capillary or pinpoint bleeding in the bone exposure area. Afterward lay out the human dermal matrix and implant a thin auto STSG of approximately 0.2 mm thick. Personally, I prefer a sheet graft when the wound is not too wide because a mesh-type skin graft can affect the esthetic appearance of the dorsum of the hand, forearm, face, neck, lower leg, and parts that are more visible. In general I perform mesh-type graft when the donor site is insufficient unstable infected site, or the size of the wound is immense. I try to avoid using mesh graft, in order to avoid mesh pattern on the healthy skin, which later would need dermabrasion and dermal resurfacing pro-

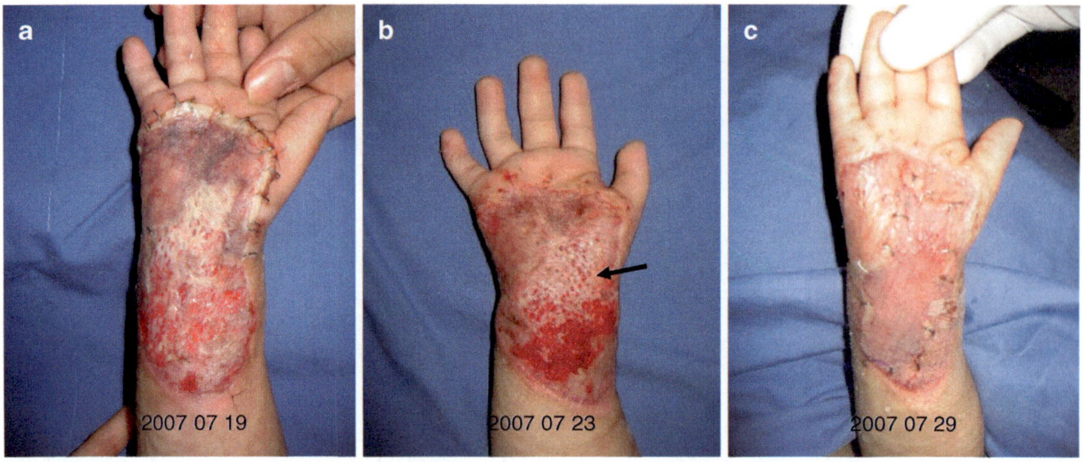

Fig. 3.25 (**a**) Graft 4 days after, partial skin loss was noted with remainder of dermal matrix component on wrist area. (**b**) 4 days after healthy granulation tissue was covered after daily soaking dressing and notice still remaining dermal matrix on skin-loss site (black arrow). (**c**) Six days later, patch skin graft was performed and graft was taken well

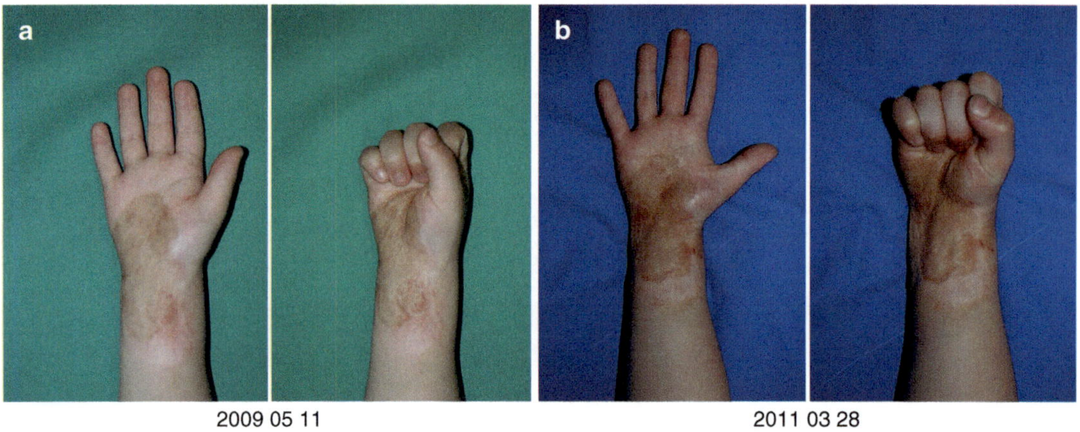

Fig. 3.26 (**a**) Postoperative 2-years-later view, there was no functional disturbance with tendon adhesion. (**b**) Postoperative 4 years later, excellent outcome was noted

cedure. In children or in the axilla, inguinal, or other curved regions of the body where engraftment may be difficult, a vacuum-assisted closure system may be used [35–37].

All surgeons aim for the main goal which is to achieve maximum intake of 100%. However, when the wound situation is very problematic, the first target is to efficiently reduce the wound size. Hence, conducting the procedure several times is recommended to gradually reduce the size of the wound. As the wound size decreases, wound management becomes more efficient, promoting optimal conditions for wound healing in the treated tissues. This technique may prove particularly useful for the coverage of tendon exposure sites.

To summarize, the primary strategy for treating difficult wounds is to first reduce the wound size for more efficient wound management, during which a human dermal matrix system may prove very useful. A strong human dermal matrix facilitates subsequent engraftment by strengthening the tissue, which ultimately leads to the goal of effective wound closure. I would like to emphasize once more time the importance of continuous improvement of the wound bed environment and reduction of the wound size.

In acute major burn management, when insufficient donor skin sites or difficulty in skin graft harvesting is encountered, a wide mesh graft with a dermal matrix graft used at a 1:4 ratio or higher or a combination with a CEA(cultured epithelial autograft) may also be used. This procedure will be covered in greater depth in Chap. 4. Compared with general release and simple STSG method, adding an extra dermal layer for engraftment can decrease the contracture rate and act as a reinforcement at the regions, especially the bone and skin with lack of soft tissue areas like the anterior tibia area, where human dermal matrix can contribute to functional recovery in various ways. This greatly aids the long-term follow-up results and can be especially helpful for hand reconstruction as well as chest and breast reconstruction with a broad corrective margin.

3.3.2.4 Limb Salvage Using Human Dermal Matrix System

The next case introduced is very significant in demonstrating a new potential of the human dermal matrix, its superior contributions to wound management, and its favorable outcomes in limb salvage. I would like to describe a case of severe soft tissue defect in the upper limb with total bone and joint exposure of the right elbow joint, with near impossible survival rate with high possibility of amputation. After persistent efforts and continuous attempts the limb was salvaged. Other orthopedic surgeons may have strongly recommended amputation to prevent unnecessary effort and promote fast recovery in cases of functional disturbance of the arm and hand. My case involved a 32-year-old woman with two rounds of first below-elbow and second above-elbow amputation surgery in the left arm already before her transfer to our department. Limb salvage was planned despite the fact that the right arm had very high chance of no function. The efforts to salvage the limb are to alleviate the psychic trauma and to preserve the hope for functional recovery in the future. To achieve a wider wound coverage by repeating multiple skin grafting to reduce the wound size for easy handling. I believe this case is relevant, demonstrating that the persistent attempts and efforts for limb salvage can discover new potential of nonrecognized application for skin grafts.

This female patient suffered third- and fourth-degree flame burns on her right chest, back, and upper arm and a third-degree deep thermal burn on her entire left arm and chest. Her estimated total body surface area (TBSA) was 25%, and she was admitted to a major burn unit for immediate lifesaving treatment. Escharectomy was performed. One month after the incident, the bones of the right elbow joint and right lateral chest were exposed. The day after the burn accident, escharotomy was performed on the left forearm to prevent compartment syndrome. Thereafter, she underwent below-elbow-joint amputation to prevent wound sepsis development; she underwent orthopedic surgery 1 week after the burn incident (Fig. 3.27). Post-burn day 1month later, serial escharectomy was performed and the wound was covered with a mesh skin graft to reduce the wound size as quickly as possible. A below-elbow amputation on the left arm was performed at the orthopedic department prior to consultation with our department. The right elbow joint and multiple rib bones were exposed with dry necrotic tissue 1 month and 2 weeks after the burn (Fig. 3.28). On postburn month 3, the elbow joint was discovered to have total bone exposure, and the joint capsule was exposed. We removed the dead bone using electrical burrs and an immediate dermal matrix with a thin mesh autograft. On postoperative day 3, the wound bed was significantly improved and stable, with the dermal matrix and mesh pattern auto-skin graft remaining. One month later, a second dermal matrix graft was performed. The human dermal matrix graft was performed three times (2007-05-17, 2007-06-21, and 2007-08-10). In these images, the human dermal matrix is very strong and resistant to unclean wounds and infections, and it promotes granulation tissue growth for proper skin grafting (Fig. 3.29).

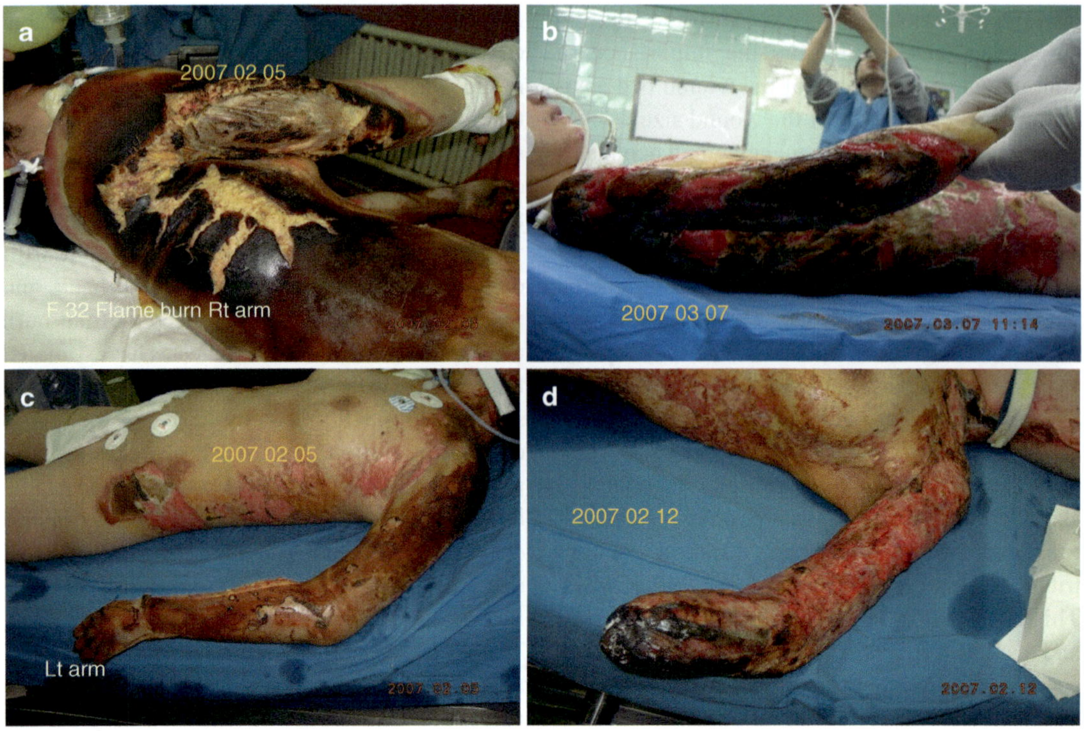

Fig. 3.27 (**a**) Fourth-degree flame burn on the right chest, back, and upper arm. (**b**) Postburn day 1 month later, right elbow and chest area escharectomy underwent partial bone exposure. (**b**) Postburn day 1 month later view. Escharectomy underwent and elbow joint and ribs bone were exposed. (**c**) Escharotomy performed on the left forearm to prevent compartment syndrome on postburn next day. (**d**) After all, she received below-elbow-joint amputation to prevent wound sepsis development at the orthopedic surgery on postburn day 1 week

Multiple rib bone exposures were managed using a mesh graft, and the bare bone area received intense wound care with saline-soaked gauze dressings for growing granulation tissue beds without using the dermal matrix system. Difficulties managing the exposed rib area can be managed with a staged repetition of wound cleansing and soaking dressing, followed by a small-size wound being covered with a simple STSG (Fig. 3.30). On postoperative day 3, a third dermal matrix engraft with an auto-sheet graft was performed. On postoperative month 7, there was no bone exposure, and the wound was successfully closed. During the healing process, a small patch of STSG was applied to aid in the healing process. After 1 year and 2 months from the operation, the final result showed a comparison of the left and right arms. Although her right arm was not fully functional, the quality of her life with both arms amputated may not be comparable to the quality of her life with one arm (Fig. 3.31).

Based on the case mentioned previously, the indication for a human dermal matrix may be expanded to reduce the likelihood of finger and upper and lower extremity amputation [38–41]. Furthermore, above result may provide evidence as an important technique for limb salvage with fingers and toes (Chap. 2, Figs. 2.76, 2.77, 2.78, 2.79).

3.3.2.5 Reconstructive Surgery with Scar Contracture Lesions

While a dermal matrix system is less effective in correcting scar contractures compared with an FTSG, it is resilient against infection and can be very helpful in reducing contracture rate on the usual burn treatment and reconstructive surgery

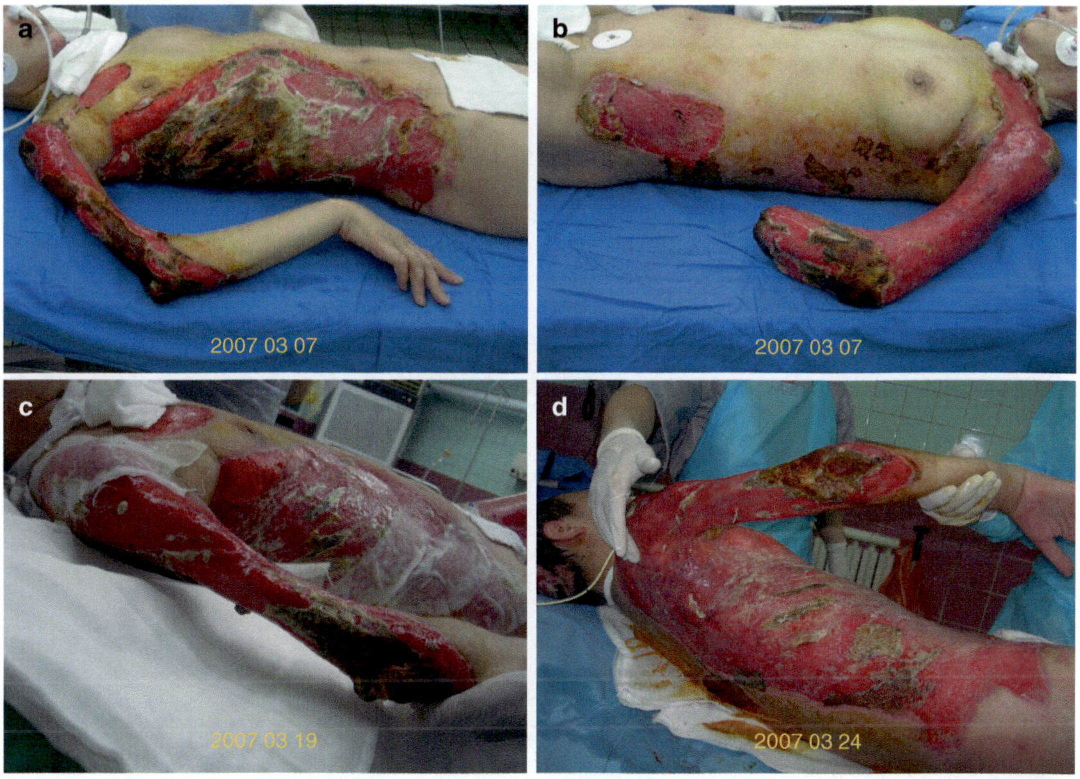

Fig. 3.28 (**a**) Postburn 1 month after, serial escharectomy was performed and covered with mesh skin graft three times (2007-03-08, 2007-03-26, 2007-04-12). (**b**) Below-elbow amputation noted on left arm. (**c**, **d**) Postburn day 1 month 2 weeks after view, right elbow joint and multiple rib bone were exposed with dry necrotic tissue

[42, 43]. Some reconstructive cases that demonstrate the various uses of the human dermal matrix will be discussed.

This female patient suffered flame burns as a child 42 years ago. A chronic ulcerated wound (black arrow) on the midback area was noted as a painless lesion. We planned to completely remove the ulcerated lesion in order to rule out any possible Marjolin's ulcer and reconstruct the back and left axilla area using a dermal matrix system (Fig. 3.32). The ulcerative lesion was completely removed, and a tissue biopsy was performed. After incisional full release, human dermal matrix was engrafted, and an immediate 0.2-mm auto-skin graft was performed (Fig. 3.33). As seen in this image, I did not use an electrocauterization instrument; instead, I used a simple 1:300,000 epinephrine injection and a 1:400,000 epinephrine-soaked gauze, as described in my own bleeding control technique (Chap. 2, Fig. 2.5). On postoperative day 5, there was no skin-loss lesion despite performing a thin-sheet autograft with no multiple slit incisions. One year after the operation, there was no recurrence of contracture, and restricted shoulder and axillary movements improved gradually over time. Because the interdermal matrix gab healed well with no seam line contracture, the author suggests that the meticulous approximate of each dermal matrix with no gap is an important point to prevention of contracture rate of engraftment (Fig. 3.34).

This male patient suffered from flame burns as a child 25 years ago, with recurring, unstable skin lesions and multiple osteomyelitis. Following the removal of the osteomyelitis lesion for biopsy, a thin, unstable skin lesion was observed in multiple areas. Following dermabrasion of the entire skin lesions containing osteomyelitis, a human dermal matrix was engrafted, and an immediate

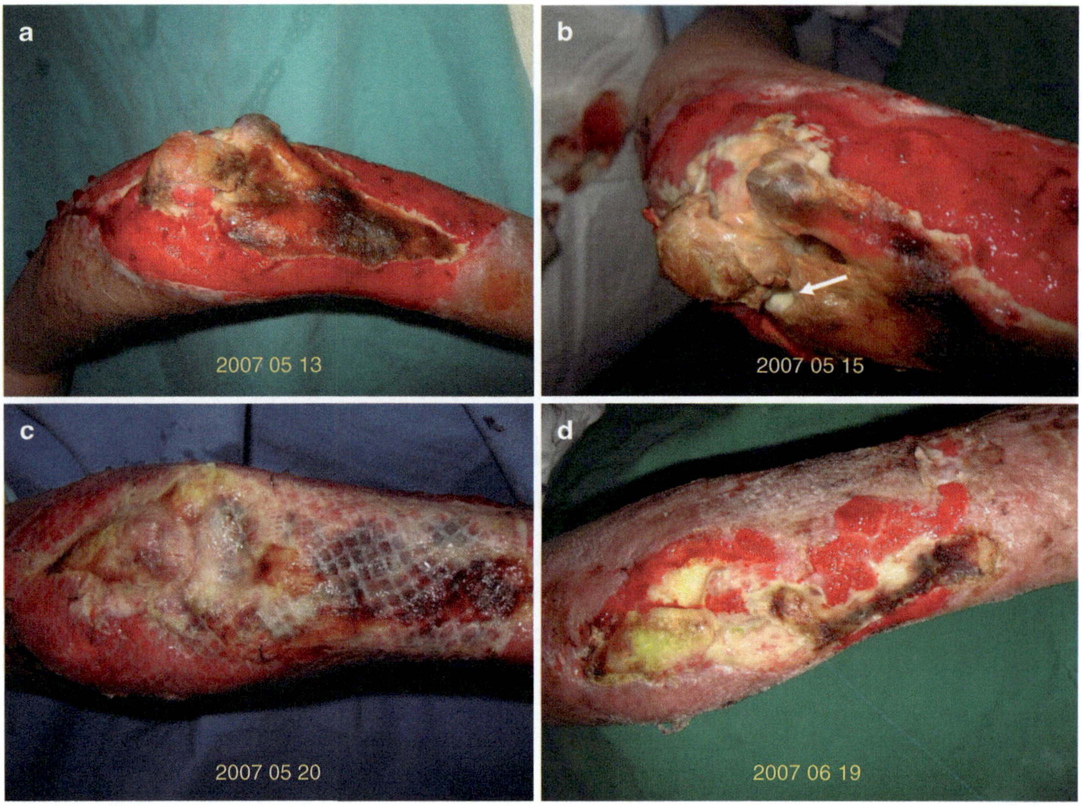

Fig. 3.29 (**a**) Postburn day 3 months after, the elbow joint was noted totally (**b**) with joint capsule opened (white arrow). We performed removal of dead bone using electrical burr and immediate dermal matrix with thin mesh autograft. (**c**) Postoperative day 3, the wound bed was noted markedly improved. (**d**) After 1 month later, second dermal matrix graft was performed, preoperative view

0.2-mm-thin autograft was performed (Fig. 3.35). Three and 8 days after the operation, a small hematoma was noted on day 3; the hematoma was easily removed with a small-slit incision and daily saline-soaked dressing till hematoma resolved. One year after the operation, there were no skin problems, and the texture was stable (Fig. 3.36).

3.3.2.6 Long-Term Follow-Up Results of Human Dermal Matrix

Next, I will describe favorable results from a long-term follow-up for breast and foot reconstruction in childhood. These cases are well-explained on how dermal matrix is useful and the effectiveness with plenty of potency in fast-growing children. The long-term follow-up results of a dermal substitute graft were described in these cases which indicate the usefulness of dermal substitutes may gain more research attention in the future.

A 4-year-old female patient received a mesh skin graft in the acute phase after suffering flame burns. Two years after the operation, a noticeable hypertrophic scar and contracture developed on the right anterolateral chest area (Fig. 3.37). Three years after mesh skin grafting, the contracture developed further due to rapid growth. Excisional release and reconstructive surgery using the dermal matrix system were performed 2 weeks after the procedure. The patient was completely released as there was no skin defect observed with the sheet auto-skin graft (Fig. 3.38). Furthermore, 1.5 years postoperatively, a well-preserved engrafted dermal matrix system and a softened engrafted anterior chest

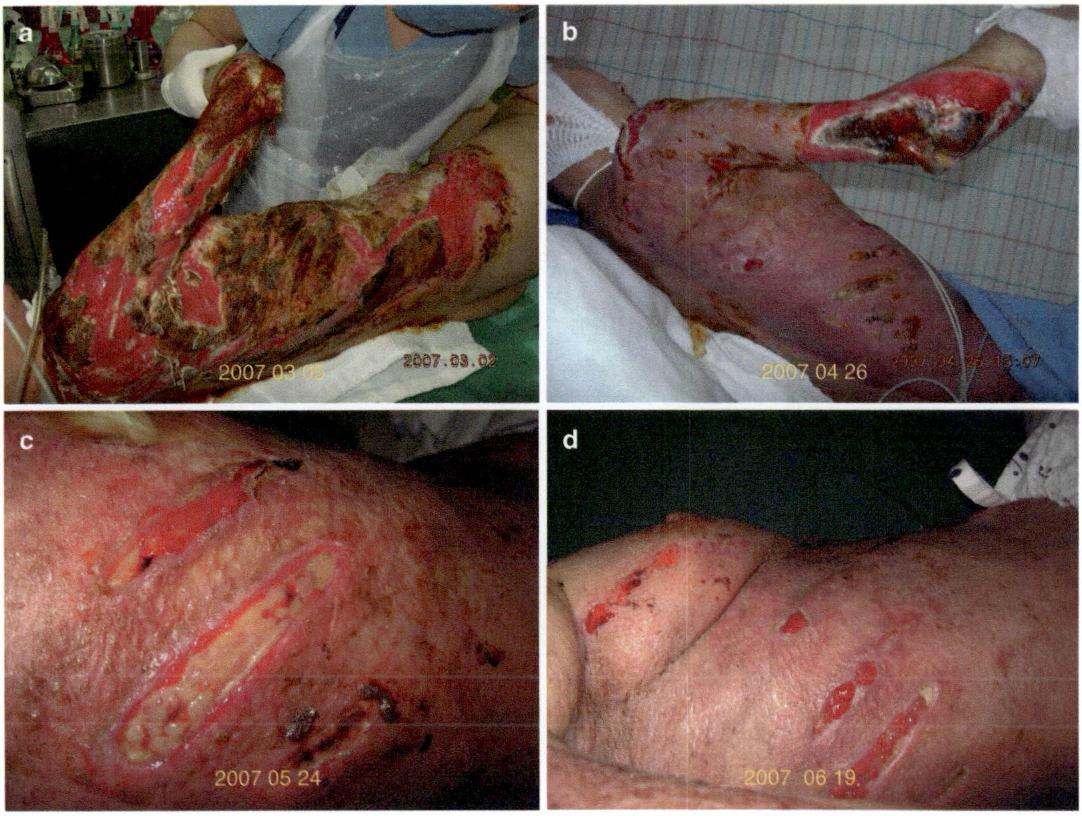

Fig. 3.30 (**a**, **b**) Multiple rib bone exposure can be managed with mesh graft and intense soaking dressing with simple STSG. (**c**, **d**) Continuous periodic debridement was performed on wound bed and soaking dressing was combined and then the remaining small size defect was covered eventually with simple STSG

area were observed, but graft contracture developed during rapid growth. Both breast tissues were slowly developing 5 years after surgery. This indicates that even though the breast tissue is very soft, it can grow with less elasticity due to the dermal substitute skin condition (Fig. 3.39). Seven years after surgery, the breast tissue was developed further and had a better contour, accompanied with good influence on the surrounding scar tissues being more flexible, soft, and smooth. This indicated that dermal substitute materials can effectively help growing children (Fig. 3.40).

A 12-year-old female suffered flame burns. Immediate human dermal matrix engraftment and a 6/1000-in.-thin 1:2 mesh autograft were performed while she was in the acute stage. Three and 7 days after the operation, the engrafted skin was taken and almost in stable condition (Fig. 3.41). On postoperative month 4, the engrafted area shrank significantly relative to the original surface. However, after a postoperative, long-term follow-up 8 years later, the right breast had grown to almost the same size as the opposite left breast, and the surrounding engrafted region has softened without hypertrophic scarring. In such cases, the human dermal matrix system can effectively contribute and is beneficial to breast reconstructive surgery for the fast-growing children, and, even if the breast tissue is very soft and a mesh graft has been performed, it can also develop contour and grow without contracture deformities (Fig. 3.42).

At the time of his first visit to our clinic, a 1-year-old male patient had scalding burns on both legs and a severe scar contracture on the

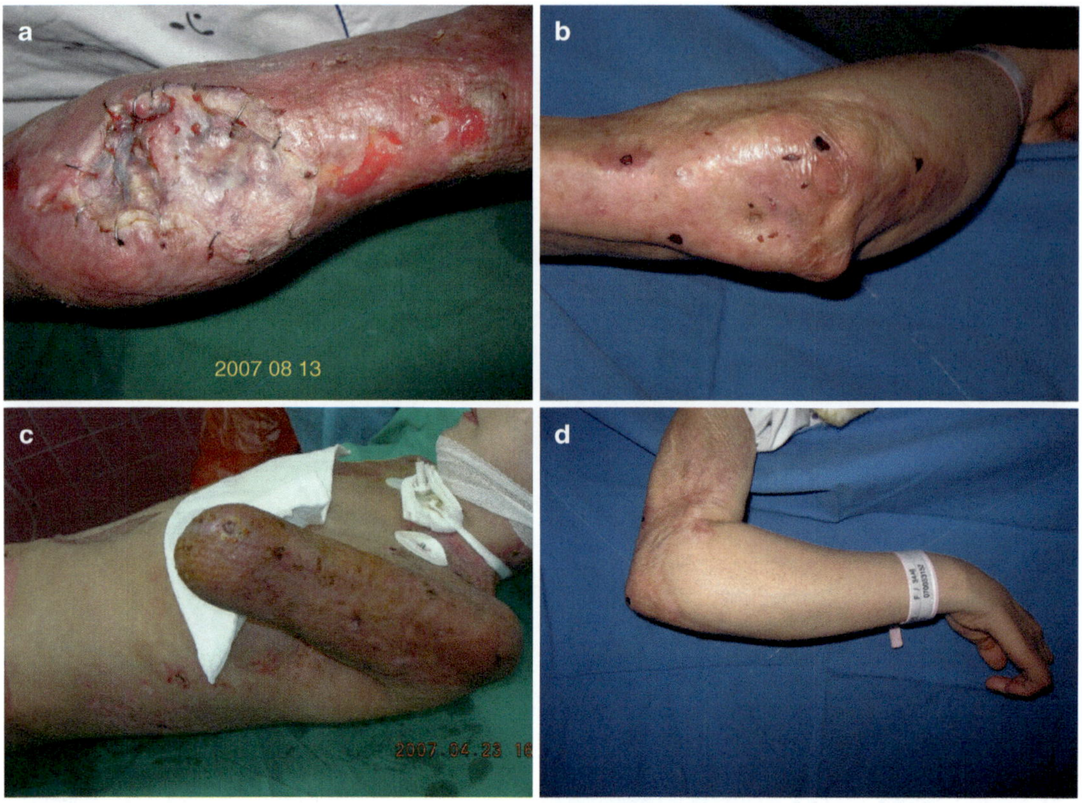

Fig. 3.31 (**a**) Postoperative 3 days after view, third dermal matrix engraft was performed; (**b**) postoperative 7-month-later view, there were no bone exposure and eventually successful closure. (**c**, **d**) Postburn day 1 year and 2 months later, final result was shown compared with left and right arm

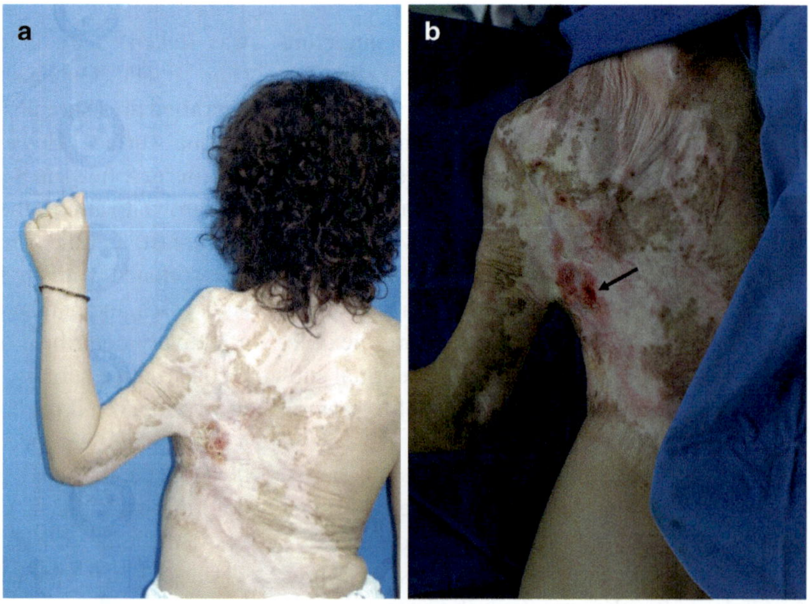

Fig. 3.32 (**a**) Flame burn as a child 42 years ago. (**b**) The chronic ulcerated wound was noted (black arrow) on the mid back area with painless lesion. Rule out any possible Marjolin's ulcer, and full release using dermal matrix system was planned

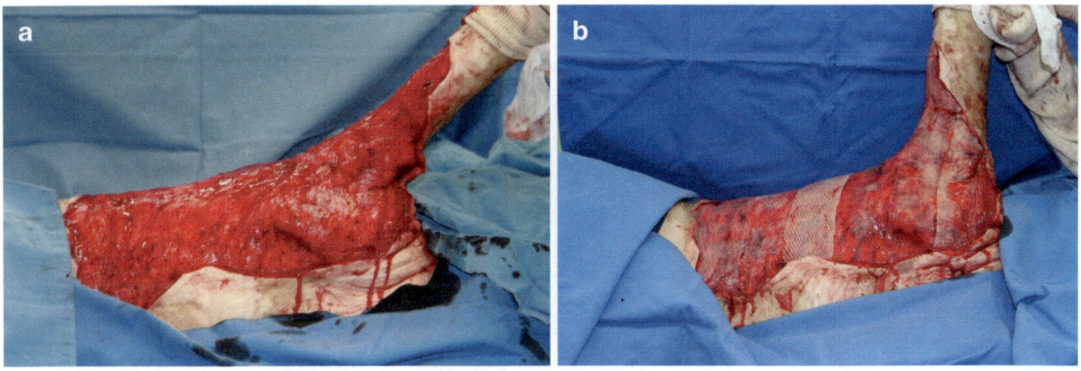

Fig. 3.33 (**a**) The ulcerative lesion was totally removed and tissue biopsy was performed. Note effective bleeding control with epinephrine injection only without electrocauterization (**b**) Human dermal matrix was engrafted, and immediate 8/1000-inches auto-skin graft was performed

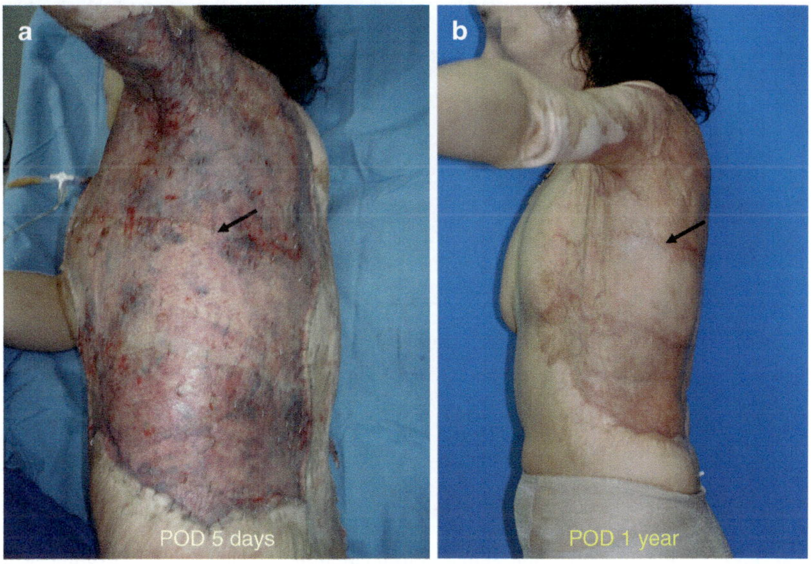

Fig. 3.34 (**a**) Postoperative 5 days after view, there was no skin-loss lesion even though sheet thin autograft without multiple slit incisions. (**b**) Postoperative 1 year after view, note the interdermal matrix gab healed well without seam line contracture (black arrow)

entire foot, lower leg, and knee joint, with multiple macerated raw surfaces (Fig. 3.43). Postburn 1 year and 2 months of waiting for the maturation period, reconstructive surgery was performed using AlloDerm® on both the leg and knee joint areas. There were no skin loss and full scar contracture 9 days and 2 weeks after the procedure (Fig. 3.44). One year later, we planned reconstructive surgery with AlloDerm® on both the foot and ankle. Full release and excisional release were performed on the left ankle and dorsum of the foot. A three-step release of a contracted thick scar and a marginal release (ankle and foot with each individual toes) were performed. Preoperative view, marked contracted deformities were noted on both foots and ankles (Fig. 3.45). Note that subcutaneous k-wire insertion was used to allow for maximal expansion of all five toes to secure the engrafted surface and prevent relapse of the contracted toes (Fig. 3.46). Two weeks and 3 years after the operation, improvements were observed in both contracted toes and the shape and function of both the dorsum of the foot and the ankle (Fig. 3.47). Six years after the operation, dermal matrix-engrafted skin was well adapted to itself, resulting in rapid skin regrowth on the feet and toes. The human dermal matrix is a critical component in reconstructive surgery, especially for

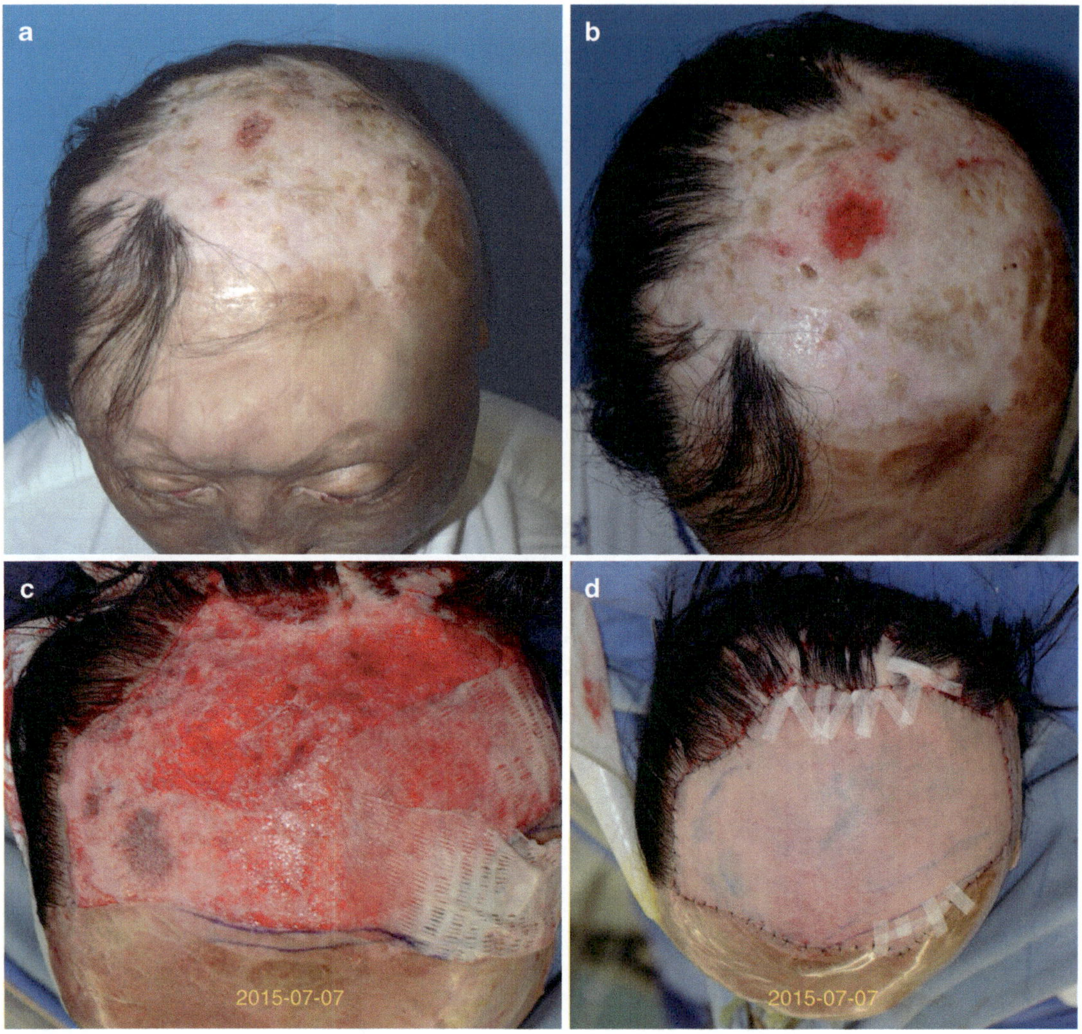

Fig. 3.35 (**a**) Recurring unstable skin lesion and multiple osteomyelitis were noted. (**b**) Biopsy was taken from the osteomyelitis lesion, also thin unstable skin lesion was noted on multiple areas. (**c**) The whole hairless area containing osteomyelitis lesions were dermabraded and human dermal matrix was covered with thin autograft ed. (**d**) Immediate operative view with 0.2-mm thin autograft

the functional recovery and multiple joints of fast-growing children. The next operation will be performed to reconstruct individual toes and the heel area with FTSG, which was preserved for toe reconstruction (Fig. 3.48).

To summarize the long-term follow-up results, early examination period of the dermal substitute showed that wound contracture develops relatively fast. However, in pediatric cases, the effects occurred gradually each year, and after 5 years or more, the contracture region recovered to the original position and size of the engraftment. However, differences may occur, depending on the individual, graft location, and type of dermal substitute. Thus, further evaluation is required to ensure a good successful rate.

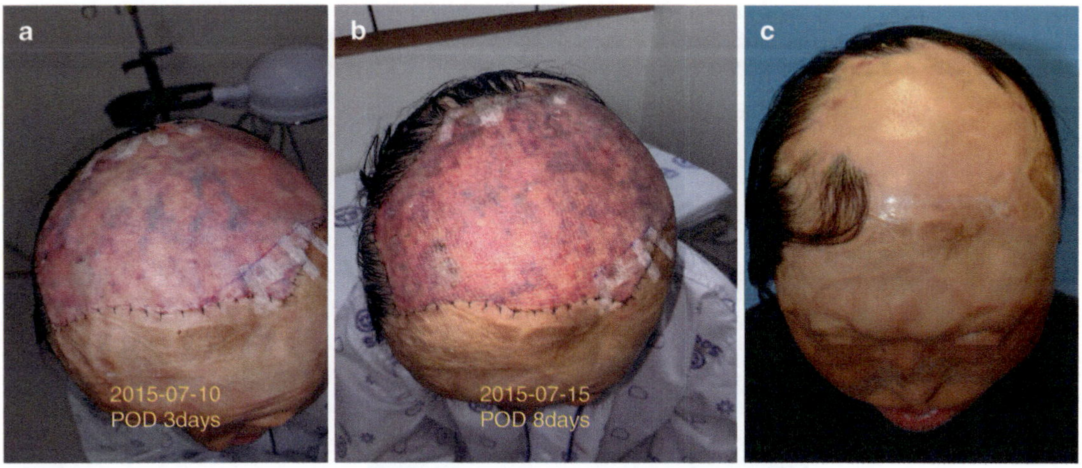

Fig. 3.36 (**a**, **b**) Postoperative 3, 8 days' view, small hematoma lesions were noted, but the hematoma was easily evacuated with small-slit incision and daily saline-soaked dressing. (**c**) Postoperative 1 year after view

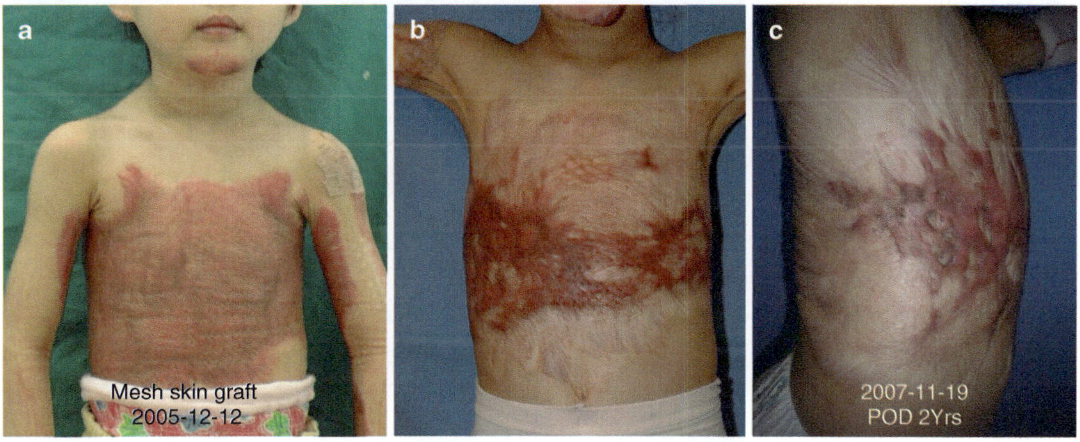

Fig. 3.37 (**a**) Received mesh skin graft at the acute phase. (**b**, **c**) Postoperative 2 years after, marked hypertrophic scar and contracture were developed

3.3.2.7 Diabetic Foot Management with Human Dermal Matrix

This section will introduce a case of diabetic foot ulcer where the wound was covered with using a dermal matrix. Diabetic foot ulcer is a well-known difficult-to-treat wound [43–46]. In most cases, when accompanied by bone exposure, amputation is the first choice of treatment. But my first choice is performing salvage procedure using human dermal matrix and have experienced favorable results. I would like to recommend this technique by studying and selecting the relevant surgical techniques using a human dermal matrix for limb salvage and wound closure, depending on the patients' conditions.

A 62-year-old female patient with a diabetic right foot and necrotic bone exposure was admitted. Serial debridement and soaking dressings were applied to the human dermal matrix system in order to close wounds and prevent above-ankle-joint amputation. Admission 7 days after, healthy granulation tissue was observed on the sole area with metatarsal bony exposured area (Fig. 3.49).

A fourth metatarsal bone exposure with necrotic tissue was observed. Following the

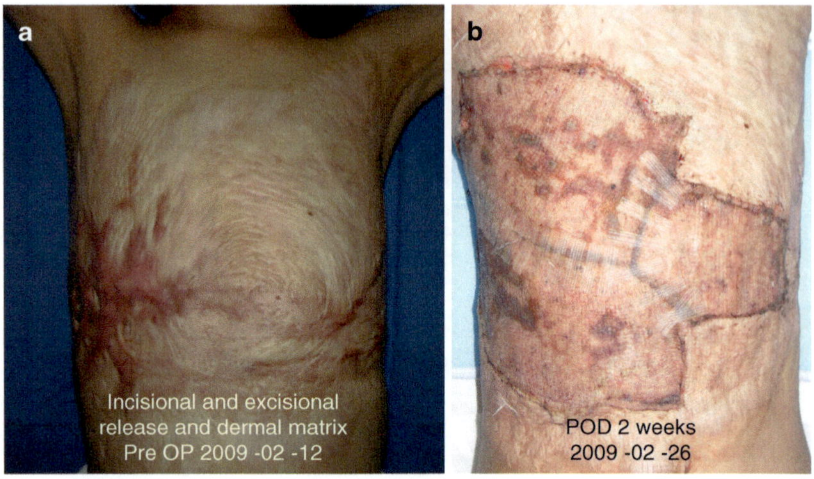

Fig. 3.38 (**a**) Preoperative view, the contracture was developed more according to rapid growing. (**b**) The excisional release and reconstructive surgery using human dermal matrix system and postoperative 2 weeks after view

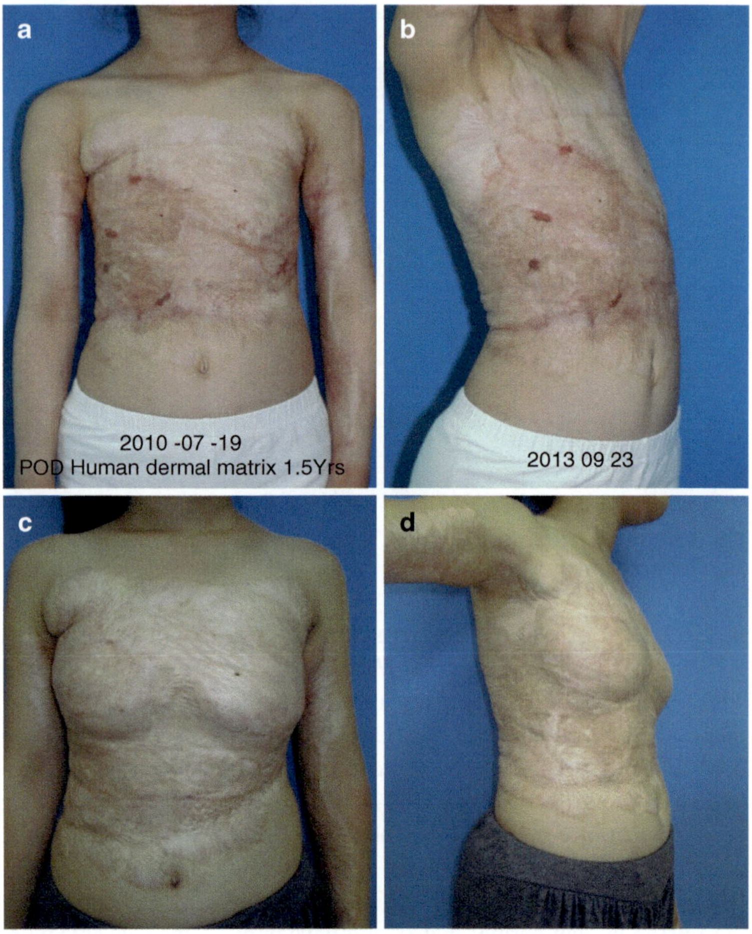

Fig. 3.39 (**a**, **b**) Postoperative1.5 year after view, well-preserved engrafted dermal matrix system and softened engrafted anterior chest area but noted little bit graft contracture developing during rapid growth. (**c**, **d**) Postoperative 5 years after, both breast tissues slowly well developing

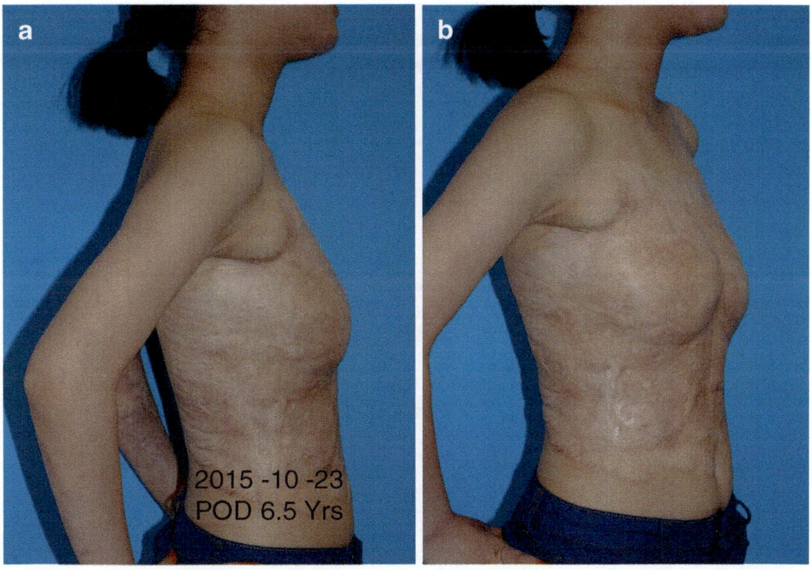

Fig. 3.40 (**a, b**) Postoperative 7 years after view, increased development of the breast tissue and good contour appearance. This shows dermal substitute materials can help effectively growing children as a good dermal replacement material

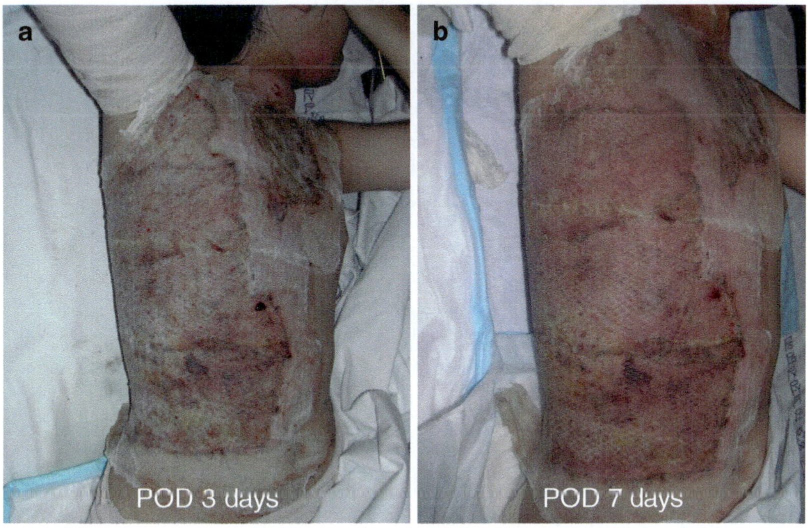

Fig. 3.41 (**a**) Immediate human dermal matrix engraft and 0.15-mm-thin 1:2 mesh autograft were performed, 3 days after operation view. (**b**) Seven days after operation, the engrafted skin was almost taken and stabilized

removal of the fourth metatarsal bone, a dermal matrix and a 0.2-mm single-sheet autograft were applied. One month after the procedure, necrotic skin-loss lesions were noted in the heel, foot, and little toe areas. These lesions were completely covered with a simple patch graft without any wound-healing disturbance. The dermal matrix advantage is extremely effective against infections and enhances wound healing, even in cases of unclean chronic wounds (Fig. 3.50). Three years after the procedure, the engrafted site had improved, with no ulcerative skin lesion. A simple weight-bearing point with hardened skin is indicated by the white arrow. If the patient wants to reinforce the hardened area, we can perform additional surgeries such as dermabrasion and dermal resurfacing using the fat composite graft to reinforce the weight-bearing site (white arrows) (Fig. 3.51).

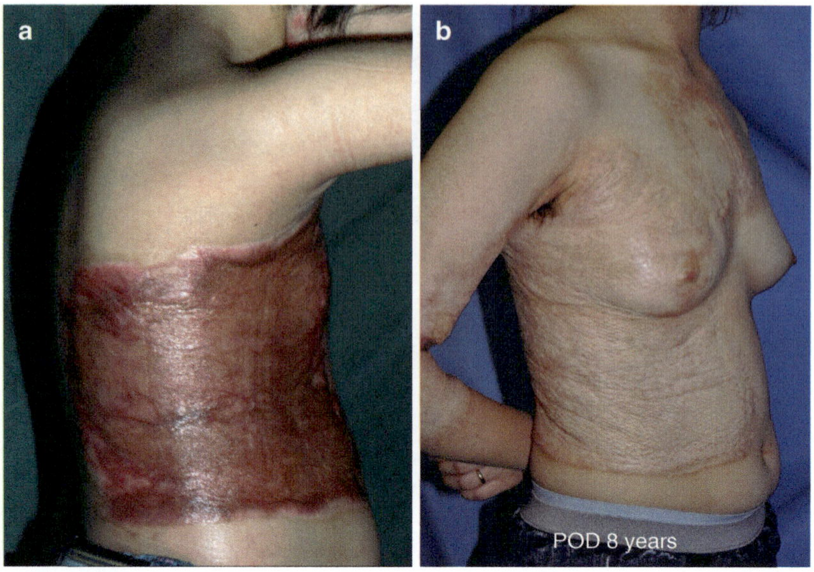

Fig. 3.42 (**a**) On postoperative month 4, engrafted area shrunk in size compared to its original engrafted size. (**b**) But postoperative long-term follow-up 8 years later, the right breast had grown to almost the same size as the left breast

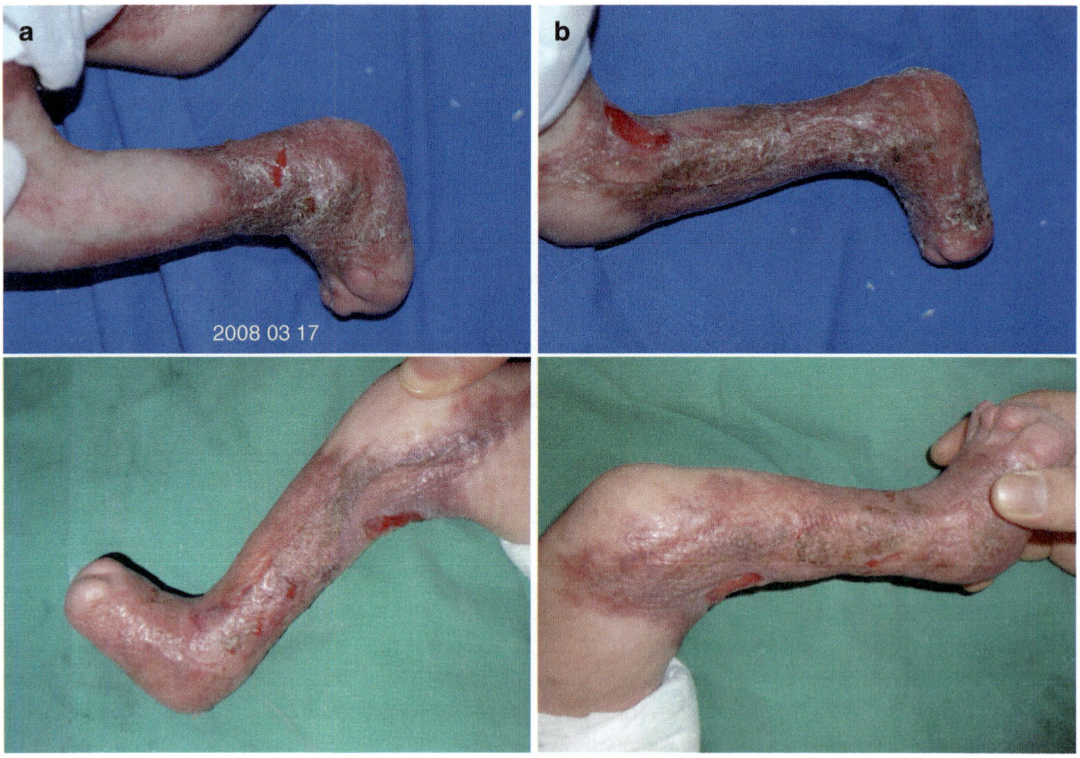

Fig. 3.43 (**a**) Severe scar contracture noted on both the entire foot and lower leg with multiple macerated raw surface. (**a**) Right inner and outer view of the leg and foot; (**b**) left outer and inner view of leg and foot

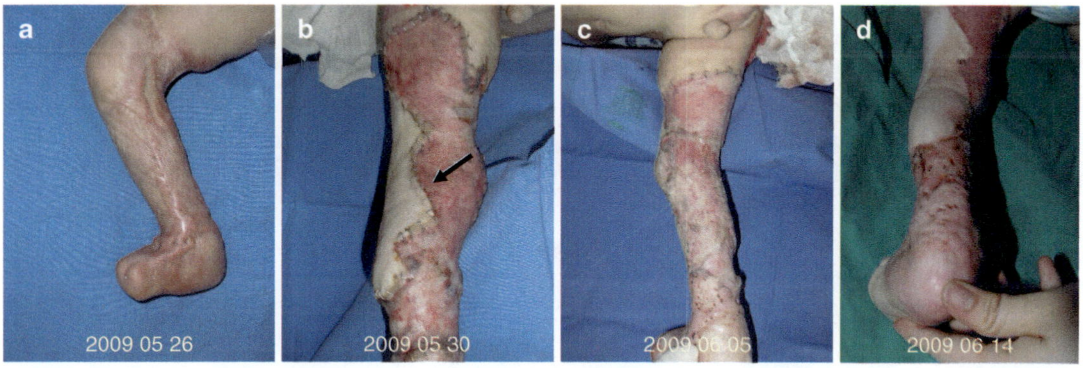

Fig. 3.44 (**a**) Preoperative view right side; (**b**) postoperative 4 days after, 6/1000-in.-thin auto-sheet graft was applied on the thigh and leg and ankle area. Note the zig-zag triangular flap to prevent linea scar contracture (black arrow); (**c**, **d**) postoperative 9 days and 2 weeks after view

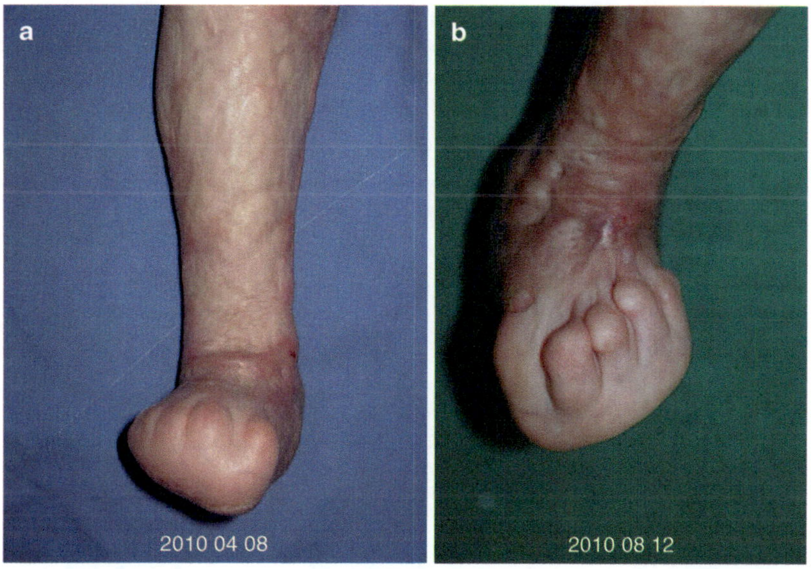

Fig. 3.45 One year after, reconstructive surgery with AlloDerm® on both foot and ankle area. (**a**) Preoperative right foot view (**b**) and left foot view

3.3.2.8 Management of Chronic Osteomyelitis Using AlloDerm

Finally, I would like to describe a patient who had been suffering for over 40 years from severe burn scar contracture and chronic osteomyelitis of the elbow joint since childhood. The indication for the human dermal matrix was expanded to the treatment of chronic osteomyelitis, as several good outcomes have already been observed in old burn scar contracture reconstruction and chronic osteomyelitis treatment. Furthermore, the effectiveness of the human dermal matrix in diabetic foot treatment has already been proven many times. Adding to this, dermabrasion and dermal resurfacing FTSG with a fat composite graft were performed for final durable tissue supplementation which was introduced in Chap. 5. In this case I have applied many of my skin graft techniques and methods that I have developed and refined throughout my career.

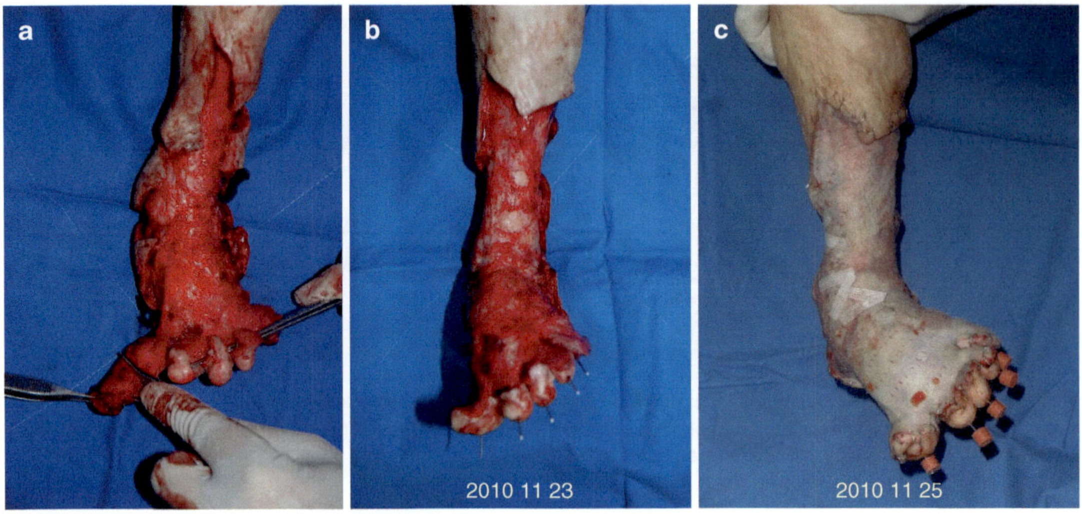

Fig. 3.46 Full release and excisional release on the left ankle and dorsum of foot. (**a**) Note three-step release on contracted thick scar and marginal release on the ankle and foot with each individual toes. (**b**) Note subcutaneous k-wire insertion to keep position of maximal expansion of each toes. (**c**) 0.15-mm-thick auto-sheet skin graft, postoperative 3 days after view

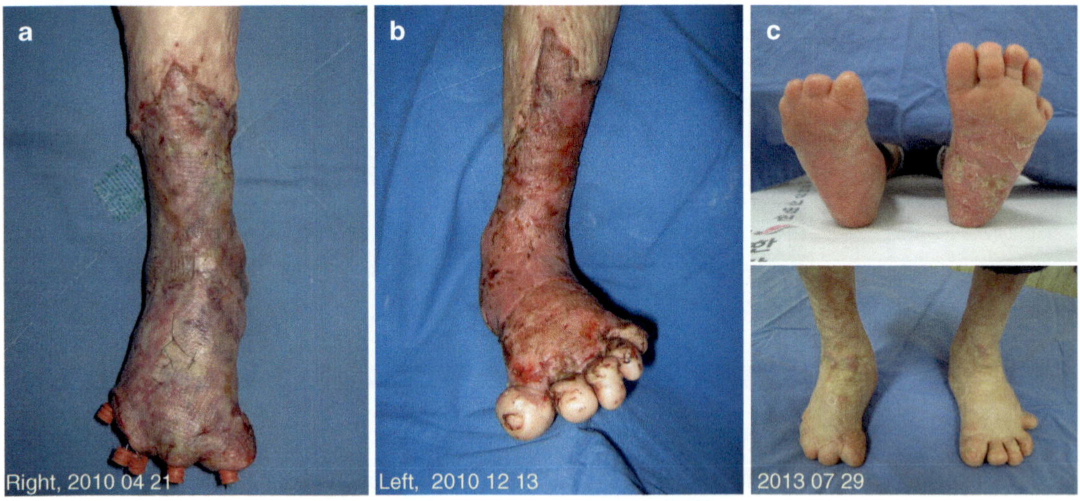

Fig. 3.47 (**a**, **b**) Postoperative 2 weeks view and (**c**) postoperative 3 years later, well grown up both contracted toes and marked improved shape and function on both the dorsum of the foot and ankle area

A 52-year-old female patient suffered scalding burns at the age of 4. Severe disfigurement was observed on the right upper arm and axilla area, which was markedly underdeveloped, as well as chronic osteomyelitis on the elbow joint (black arrow) that took a long time to heal and recur (Fig. 3.52).

First, the right upper arm, axilla, and trunk areas were treated with burn scar contracture release and human dermal matrix with a thin auto-skin graft. Note the chronic osteomyelitis lesion on the elbow joint to reinforce the skin lesion with the human dermal matrix system (Fig. 3.53). One year and 3 months later, we per-

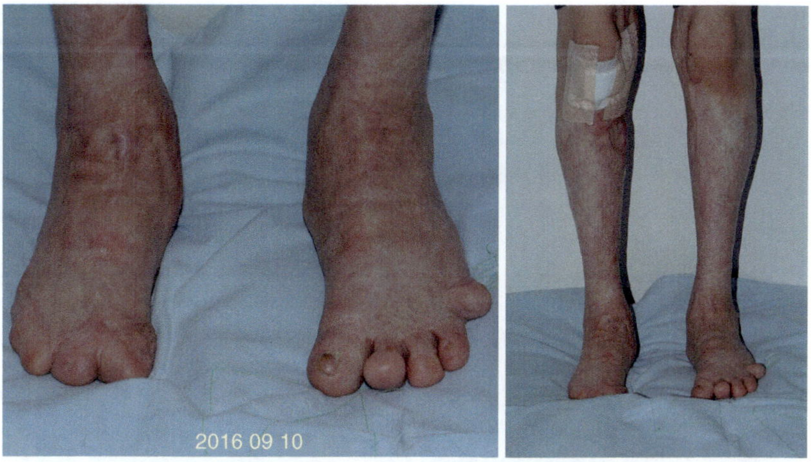

Fig. 3.48 Postoperative 6 years later, well-adapted and grown dermal matrix-engrafted skin

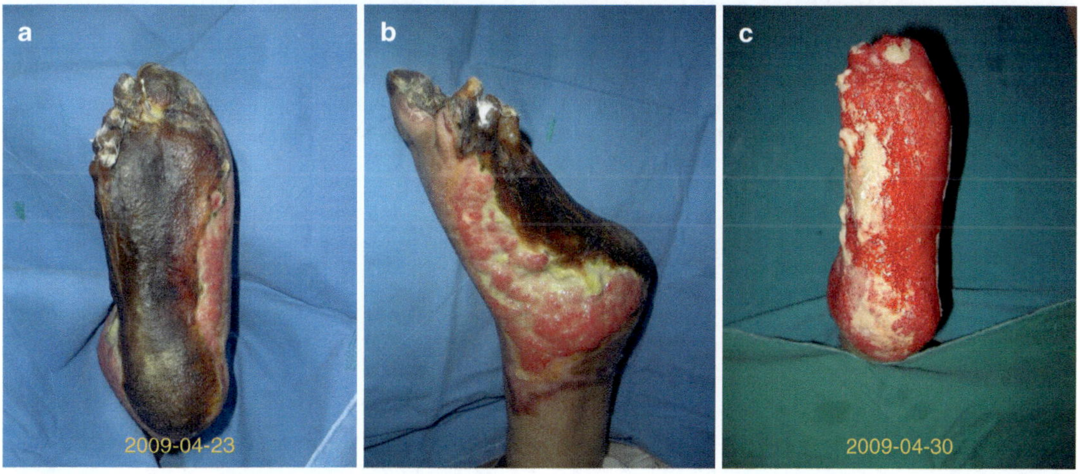

Fig. 3.49 (**a**) Diabetic foot on the right foot with necrotic bone exposure. (**b**) Serial debridement and soaking dressing were performed. (**c**) Admitted 7 days after, the healthy granulation tissue was noted

formed FTSG to release the axilla and upper inner arm area for more moveable functional recovery; we used dermabrasion and dermal overgraft with human dermal matrix system engraft to reinforce an unstable skin lesion on the elbow-joint area. It is possible to repeat the same technique on the previously engrafted skin area to increase skin thickness (Fig. 3.54). We planned to completely correct the osteomyelitis lesion 1 year later. The skin around the elbow-joint area was dermabraded and dermalized over full-thickness skin with a fat composite graft for reinforcement of skin thickness in order to correct the bone and skin lesion. For the treatment of chronic osteomyelitis after necrotic bone curettage on the inner humeral malleolus, the dead space was sufficiently packed with AlloDerm® sheet (5 × 5, 5 × 6 cm two sheets, two sites). After completing this procedure, dermal over FTSG with a fat composite graft reinforced and cushioned the elbow-joint area (Fig. 3.55). Sixteen days after the procedure, the FTSG with a composite fat graft was taken completely. Six months after the procedure, the osteomyelitis open wound was closed completely without a discharge entrance (Fig. 3.56). Three and half years after the procedure, functional and posture recovery was observed on the

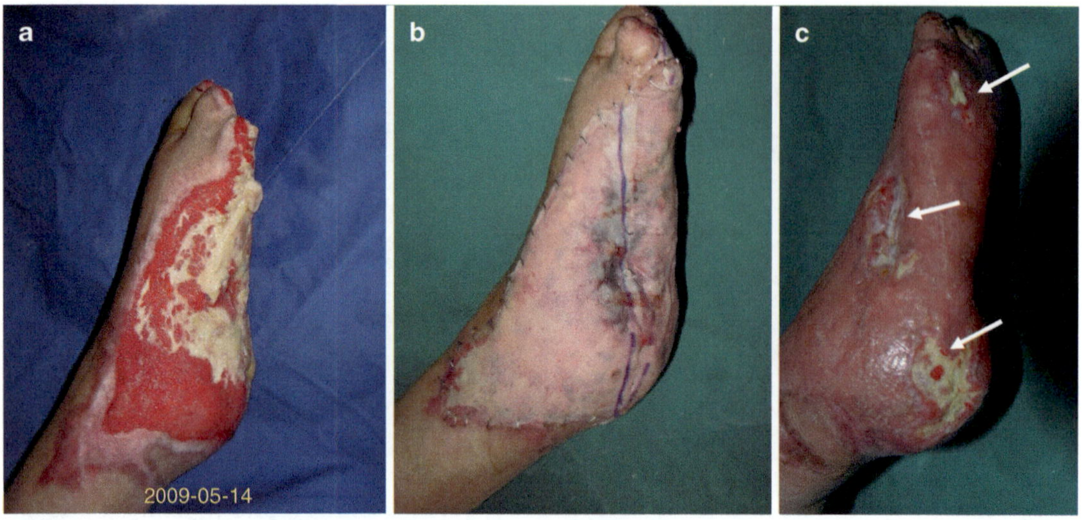

Fig. 3.50 (**a**) Preoperative operation finding. Note fourth metatarsal bone exposure with necrotic tissue. (**b**) After removal of fourth metatarsal bone, dermal matrix and 0.2-mm auto single-sheet skin graft was applied; postoperative 3 days later view. (**c**) Postoperative 1 month later, the necrotic skin-loss lesions were noted in the heel, foot, and little toe area (white arrows). These lesions were covered completely with simple patch graft without any wound-healing disturbance

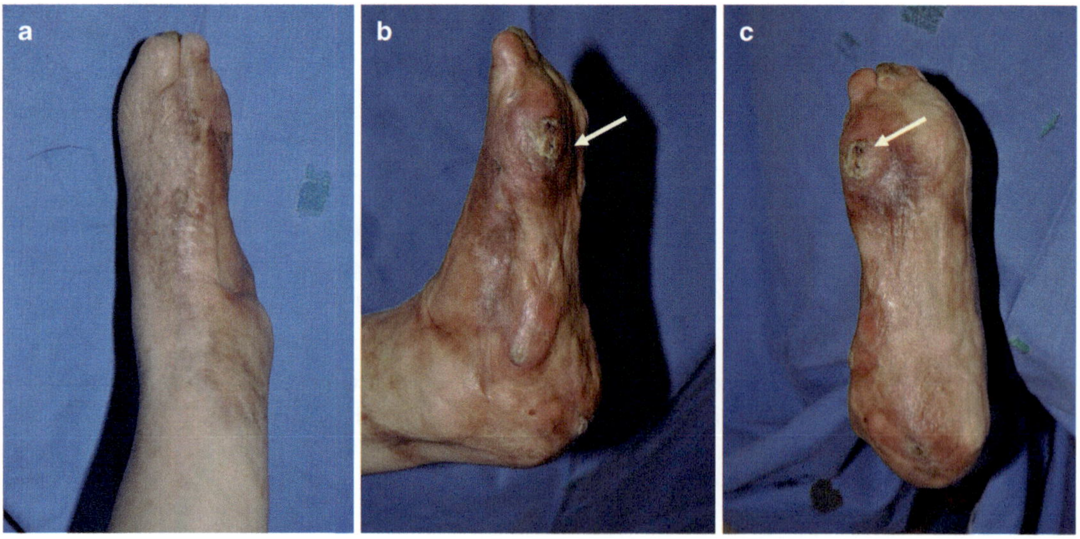

Fig. 3.51 Postoperative 3 years later, (**a**) dorsal, (**b**) lateral, and (**c**) ventral view, the engrafted operation site was well adapted without ulcerative skin lesion

right upper arm and axilla area. The elbow-joint area was found to have stable and normal full-thickness skin texture, with no recurrence of chronic osteomyelitis (Fig. 3.57).

This case is a good example showing all processes of skin graft techniques I have introduced in this book such as dermal substitute graft and FTSG for reconstructive case and finally highlighting dermabrasion and dermal overgraft fat composite graft technique for reinforcement coverage and in chronic osteomyelitis problem-solving method.

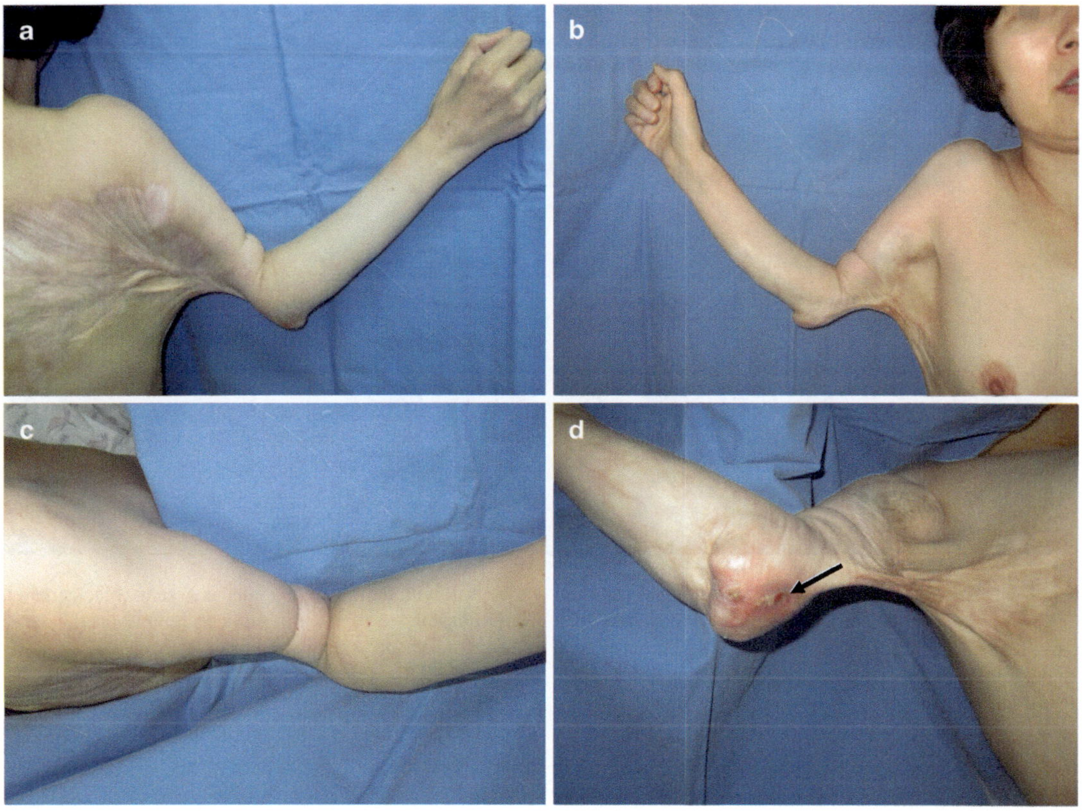

Fig. 3.52 (**a**–**c**) Severe disfigurement noted on the right upper arm and axilla area which was markedly underdeveloped and (**d**) chronic osteomyelitis on the elbow joint (black arrow)

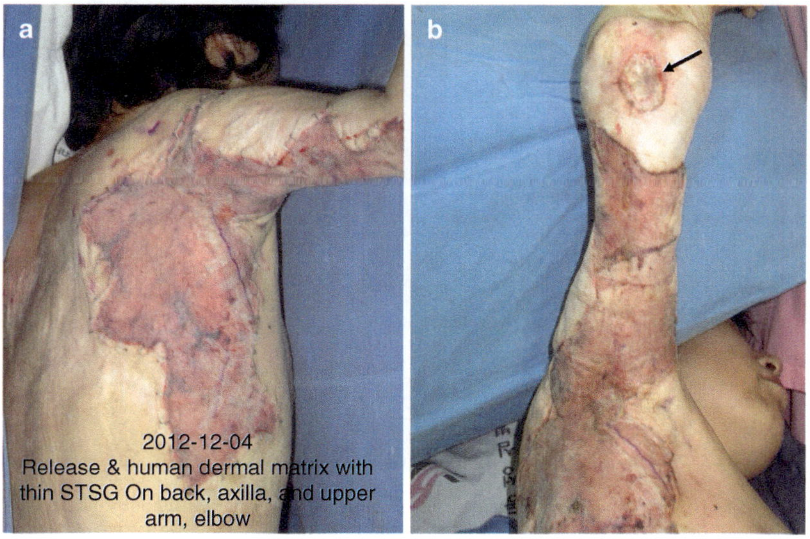

Fig. 3.53 (**a**) Release and human dermal matrix with thin auto-skin graft were performed on the right upper arm, axilla, and trunk area. Postoperative 10 days after, the engrafted skin was taken mostly, (**b**) postoperative 1 month later. Note the chronic osteomyelitis lesion on the elbow joint to reinforce with human dermal matrix system (black arrow)

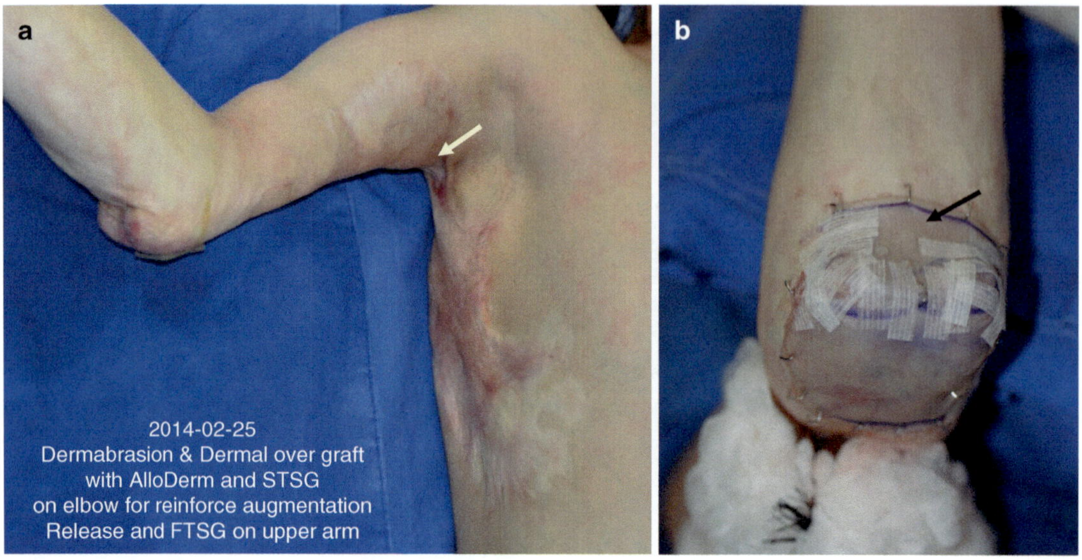

Fig. 3.54 (**a**) One year and 3 months after, FTSG for release on the axilla and upper inner arm area (white arrow), and (**b**) reinforce unstable skin lesion on the elbow-joint area with repeats of dermabrasion and dermal overgraft with human dermal matrix system (black arrow). It is possible to repeat the same technique on the same place for reinforcement adding skin thickness

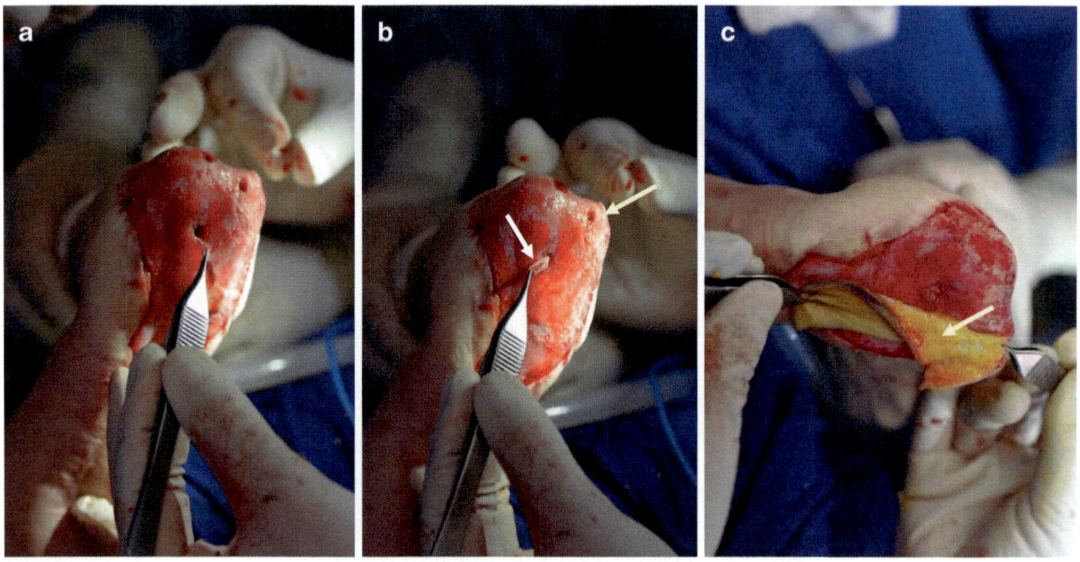

Fig. 3.55 (**a**) One year later, we had a plan to correct the osteomyelitis lesion completely. The surrounded elbow-joint area skin was dermabraded for dermal over FTSG for reinforcement of skin thickness. (**b**) After the necrotic bone curettage on inner humeral malleolus, the dead space was sufficiently packed with AlloDerm® sheet (5 × 5, 5 × 6 cm two sheets, two sites white arrow)). (**c**) Dermal over FTSG with fat composite graft for reinforcement strong and cushion effect (white arrow)

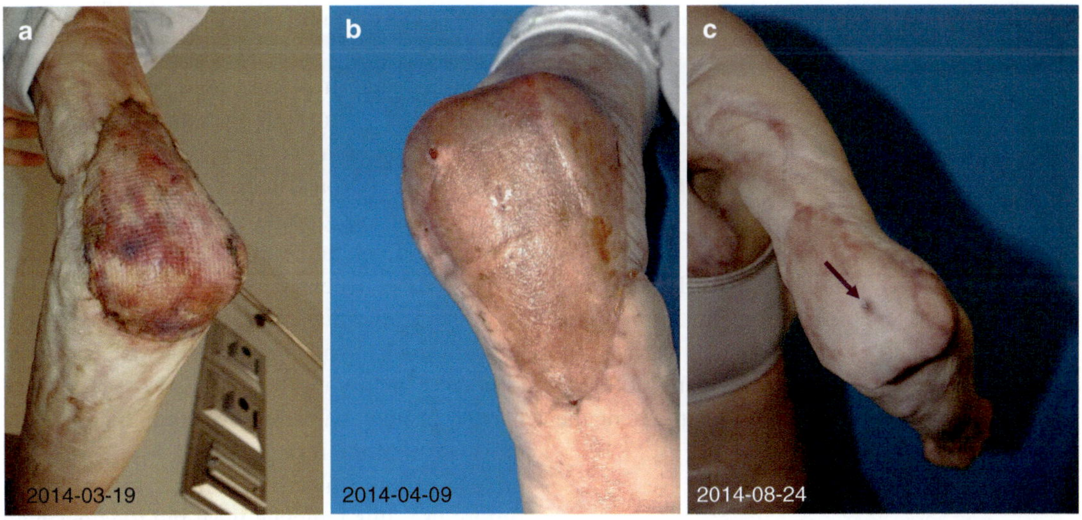

Fig. 3.56 (**a**) Postoperative 16 days after, the FTSG with composite fat graft was taken completely; (**b**) postoperative 1 month and (**c**) postoperative 6 months later view, the osteomyelitis open wound was closed (black arrow)

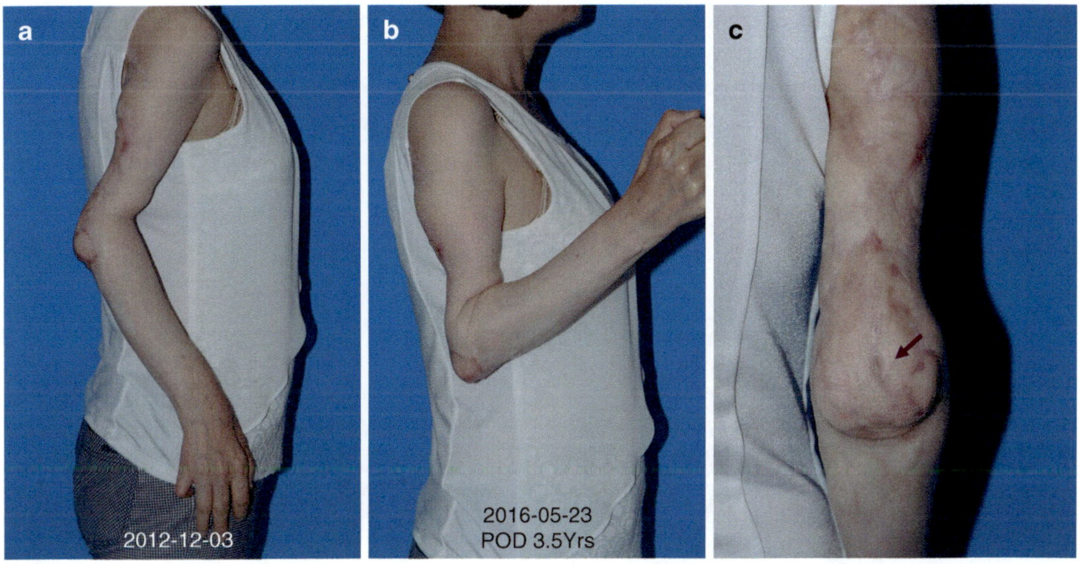

Fig. 3.57 (**a**, **b**) Postoperative 3 years 6 months later, the functional and posture recovery was noted on the right upper arm and axilla area. (**c**) Elbow-joint area was noted stable with normal full-thickness skin texture

Next, I will introduce Integra®, which is synthesized purely from bovine collagen and is very distinct from the human dermal matrix system. Significant differences in terms of surgical and dressing methods due to the characteristics of this material will be introduced. The overall dermal substitute system can be applied more selectively and efficiently once the different features of each product are understood.

3.4 Integra® (Life Sciences Corporation, Plainsboro, NJ, USA)

Integra® was developed in the early 1980s at the Massachusetts General Hospital by John Burke and Ioannis Yannas as a dermal substitute for permanently covering burn wounds using collagen extracted from bovine tissue to supplement the dermal layer of the skin [7, 13, 47].

3.4.1 Structure and Mechanism

Integra® is a bilayer product, with the main layer being a dermal regeneration template approximately 2-mm thick and presenting a white, spongelike appearance, which faces the wound bed side. It is composed of bovine collagen and glycosaminoglycan (chondroitin 6-sulfate). Integra is composed of a three-dimensional porous matrix 70–200 μm size, which is an appropriate porous size for fibroblasts, endothelial cells, and macrophages, among others, to enter from the wound bed and form the neodermis [26, 48]. The outer layer is a 0.1-mm-thick synthetic polysiloxane polymer (silicone) membrane that acts as a mechanical barrier against bacterial invasion, helps retain moisture until the formation of a neodermis, and protects from physical damage or infection. Before use, this template is stored together with alcohol in an aluminum foil and rehydrated in normal saline (Fig. 3.58). The formation of the neodermis takes approximately 2–3 weeks or more. When the color of the engrafted Integra®

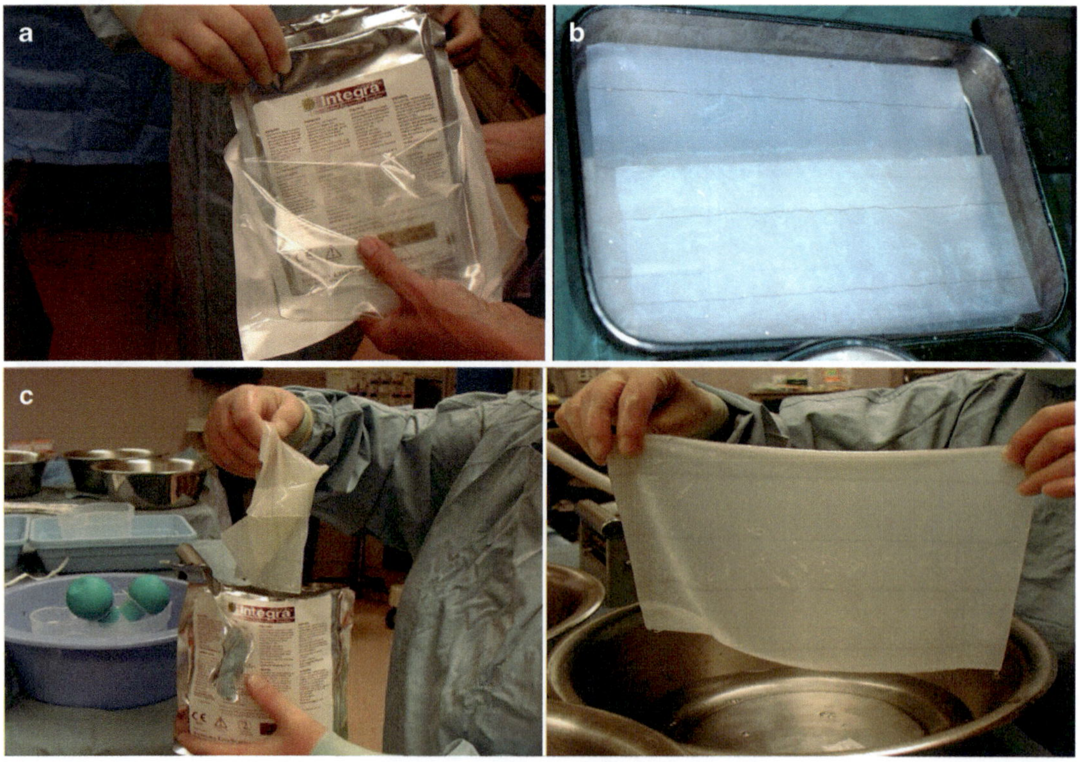

Fig. 3.58 (**a**) Integra® is preserved in aluminum foil and (**b**) composed of two-layer template which is white spongelike glycosaminoglycan, and out layer is 0.1-mm-thin silicone sheet for role of protection. (**c**) Before using this product, rehydrate in normal saline

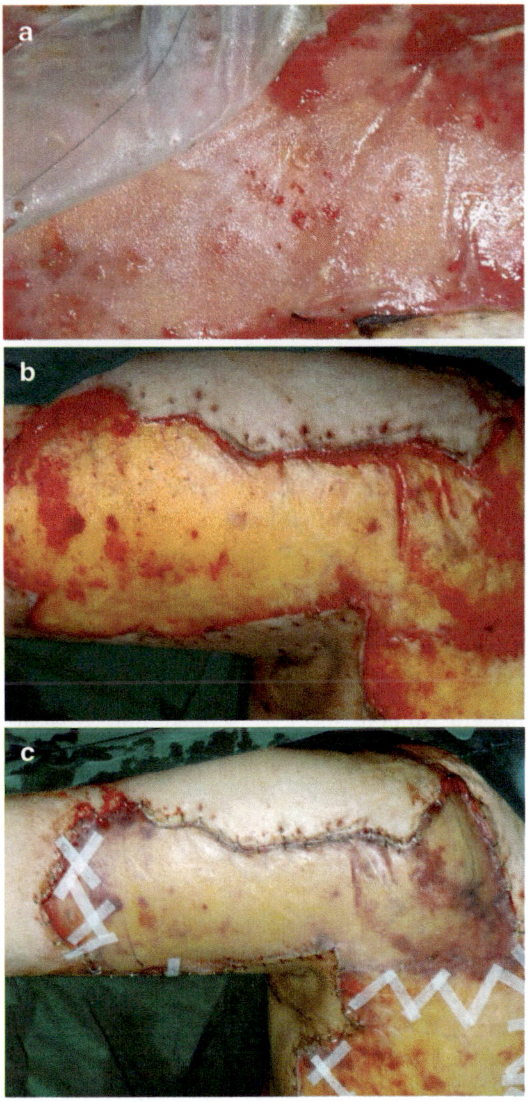

Fig. 3.59 (**a**) When neodermis is formed completely during 2–3 weeks, the outer silicone sheet is easily peeled off; (**b**) light orange color change indicates proper state of engraftment with auto-thin graft. (**c**) Usual second stage of auto-skin graft thickness is 5–8 inches/1000

gradually turns yellowish-orange and the silicone membrane acting as an epidermis can be easily peeled, a thin skin autograft of about 0.125–0.2 mm is performed, thereby completing the skin graft and strengthening the newly formed dermal layer (Fig. 3.59). I prefer thin-sheet auto-skin graft rather than mesh auto-skin graft because mesh graft is more fragile when engrafted on the Integra® compared to AlloDerm®.

3.4.2 The Author's Surgical Technique from the Perspective of Plastic Surgery

I began my clinical experience with Integra® when I participated in a multicenter clinical trial at Washington University Harborview Medical Center in 1996 [49]. Since 1998, I have been accumulating experiences in both acute burn management and reconstructive surgery at the Burn Plastic Surgery Center (Hallym University, Hangang Sacred Heart Hospital, Burn Center, Seoul, Korea) to which I belonged. The reason I am revealing this is to describe the differences in the management strategies that I implemented and experienced in the surgical approach and applications in using Integra®, which has now been established as a general procedure the protocol for the use of Integra® in the early days after its development. Since the initial clinical trials of Integra® mainly focused on major burn management, I would like to discuss some differences between the burn wound management and Integra® grafting techniques used at the general burn center and viewpoint of the plastic surgery department (Hallym University, Hangang Sacred Heart Hospital, Burn Plastic Surgery, Plastic and Reconstructive Surgery, Seoul, Korea). The two key differences were a) whether to preserve the fat layer or remove it completely in deep thermal acute burns to prevent infection and to facilitate bleeding control, thereby preventatively setting the extent of escharectomy to a fascial level that removes all the fat layer and b) breaking the silicone barrier, which is very durable against bacterial invasion, into mesh forms to prevent hematoma or fluid discharge accumulation. Generally, many surgeons consider fat tissue too soft and easily damaged in major burn management, which not only provides a good culture medium for bacteria but can also interrupt graft intake. Hence, removing fat tissues as a preventative measure is a prevailing idea [50, 51]. However, from my experience in the plastic surgery department, fat tissue does not interrupt the skin graft intake rate at all but aids it. This is proven through several cases described in Chap. 2

using FTSG with a fat composite graft. In the acute state, checking the viability of fat tissues is difficult; however, instinctively removing a large amount of soft tissue will adversely affect the functional and esthetic results of reconstructive surgery in the long term. Therefore, I judge the extent of escharectomy by judging the level of glossy grease in the fat layer and recommend it to be preserved if possible. In fact, in the early application of Integra® during the management of a case with a major life-threatening injury, the most important points are saving the patient's life and preventing infection if at all. However, in burns affecting less than 20% of the TBSA, intensive wound management is possible, and high incidence of infection is relatively low. The preservation of soft tissue is also very important for the surgical outcome from the perspective of the plastic surgery department [52, 53]. From a plastic surgeon's perspective, I would like to recommend selecting the surgical method only after thoroughly assessing the situation of burn patients, I chose Integra® for wound management out of all the choices.

As my grafting experience increased, the impact of soft tissue preservation on the results became very clear, especially in the extremities; hence, I hope to further expand the scope of preservation of soft tissue in acute wound management by continuing to accumulate my experiences. In recent years, my accumulated experiences in the management methods of major burns have varied widely; thus, the technique may be different for each burn center. However, the process of setting Integra® in early days involved a series of difficulties and required a considerable learning curve in burn management. For example, during the early days of Integra® usage at our burn center, escharectomy was performed on day 1, and bleeding was controlled within 1 or 2 full days after; when the patient became stable, a non-mesh Integra grafting method would be adopted, and, in some cases, it has been established as a standard protocol in our burn center. Another different approach is whether we have to make mesh or not on the entire Integra® surface. The thin silicone membranous barrier is an important guard for infection, but in the opposite point of view, for prevention of hematoma and fluid collection control, making mesh is more advanced in this situation. Many of the the global burn centers are making mesh on the Integra® routinely [54] and operation wound dressing soaked with strong antibacterial solution of 0.1% mafenide acetate (Sulfamylon™) for infection control [55] and prevention of hematoma and Integra® dry up, etc. But the author does not make mesh on the Integra for prevention of hematoma; on the contrary, the author preserves silicone sheets with no mesh and no gap on the engraft seam line. For this reason, the author has many experiences with bleed control and effective dressing technique without meshed Integra.

In addition, in the management of minor burns (20% or less of the total body surface), infection control is possible with wound dressing; thus, destroying the strong silicone barrier is unnecessary. In case of signs of hematoma, the Integra silicon sheet is scoped out. Soaking dressing is applied on the cutout region. The point of this is to partially remove the silicone immediately after a sign of infection is detected and to apply a saline-soaked gauge dressing twice a day until infection is controlled. If these measures are delayed, the infection will rapidly spread underneath the silicone membrane, resulting in a total loss of engrafted Integra® in one or two days.

Since the main purpose of Integra® dermal replacement is to save the life of patients with major burns, acute burn management should be mainly considered first. However, if the surgeon knows how to use Integra for localized acute deep thermal burns and for reconstruction of burn scar contracture, very useful results can be obtained; thus, I will describe the procedure.

3.4.3 Integra® Usage in Acute Burn Management

The most important procedure in acute burns is the efficient removal of dead tissues. This is because Integra® itself is very susceptible to infection, and when infection progresses, not only are expensive materials squandered, but the surgical outcomes also become poor. When handled by inexperienced surgeons, it can cause stress and wasted expensive materials. Thus, thorough knowledge and devotion to wound management are required. This resolute manner is an important progression in the learning curve such as mastering the usage of Integra to obtain the product's maximum benefits. The bleeding control tip is to use intradermal epinephrine injection at a dilution of 1:200,000–400,000 in which I had introduced subdermal epinephrine injection technique. The above technique has a higher bleeding risk than the scar tissue wound bed in reconstructive surgery, but it is sufficiently possible to carry out a rapid escharectomy using an electric dermatome or a Blair or Humby knives followed by elastic bandage compression. Even in a wide wound area from deep second- or third-degree burns, if the necrotic burned tissues are selectively removed, the viable tissue can be preserved at the usual escharectomy level or at least superficial subcutaneous fat layer level. In my experience, in most cases of deep second- or third-degree burns, the subcutaneous fat layer is less severely injured, so I would like to recommend escharectomy to be precisely performed with gaining experience. The usual escharectomy level is not too much deep; hence, escharectomy involving the subcutaneous fat layer beyond the reticular dermis is not usual. Once bleeding is controlled, fasten the Integra® to the wound margin with staples as soon as possible rapidly. Performing wound coverage quickly and shortening the operating time using a very large-sized template are possible, which is one of Integra®'s advantages. For fixation, it is best to slightly elevate Integra® margin and the wound margin to each other as if it were completely sealed to prevent the wound surface from being exposed. I usually would undermine the wound margin approximately to 1 cm or more inside and create an elevation eversion with Integra® to fix it with a tightening staple suture. This kind of manipulation provides room for freeing the wound margin later, which is helpful in preventing contracture progression on the engrafted wound margin. This is a very important technique because it prevents infection or margin of wounds from drying out until a new dermis is formed.

If the wound area is larger than the size of Integra sheet, the sheets must be joined together as soon as possible to reduce the number of the staples, which damages the silicone barrier and prevent infection by making sure the seam does not open or overlap. Entire surgical wound fixation after engrafting Integra® is very important in preventing hematoma; hence, the use of Surgifix® (Colorline, Italy) is recommended. Surgifix® has an elastic net structure suitable for the process.

In case of localized deep thermal burns, (a) if possible, the subcutaneous fat tissue and reticular dermis preserve differently in wide major burn cases. (b) Use Integra® in engraft immediately as soon as possible with tightened staples with no intergrafted gap space. Integra® engraftment requires a limited number of staples to avoid breaking the silicone barrier and exposing the source of infection. (c) I prefer using Surgifix® for hematoma prevention, surgical wound protection, and fixation (Fig. 3.60).

I do not use the very expensive Sulfamylon™ solution and have previously used Acticot™ (Smith & Nephew, England), which is a nanocrystalline silver dressing material for covering the wound margin to prevent infection. However, I have not used Acticot™ in recent years, except in acute cases. Since infection is the most important factor in the success of the grafting surgery, if possible, keep the Surgifix® fixation on for 3–7 days after surgery; if hematoma forms, make a slit incision for evacuation, and check for infection daily through the transparent silicone film. If infection occurs, remove the silicone film from the infected area immediately, and make a wound window to remove the infected area. Controlling the infection before it spreads is very important; hence, in some cases, daily dressing with Sulfamylon™ solution is recommended, or a silver dressing material that is effective in infection control is used. However, my preferred method is a daily saline-soaked gauze dressing. Depending on the degree of infection, applying the dressing two or three times a day is sufficient to control the infection. The success of the operation is

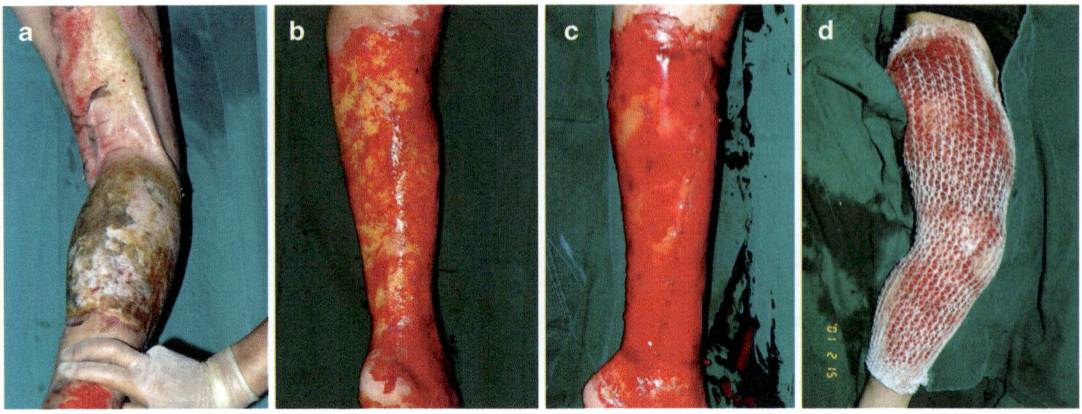

Fig. 3.60 (**a**) Acute case of deep thermal burn; (**b**) in case of localized deep thermal burns, if possible preserve the subcutaneous fat tissue and reticular dermis. (**c**) Integra® engraftment is tightened and without intergrafted gap space. (**d**) Using Surgifix® is very effective to prevent hematoma and surgical wound protection and fixation

determined by the successful removal of necrotic tissue, thorough effective hemostasis, and the complete removal of the cause of infection source. If signs of infection are observed, refrain from using Integra® until the infection is under control. The formation of a new dermis takes 2–3 weeks, depending on the environment. However, using the recently developed VAC device [37, 56, 57], the duration of secondary surgery can be shortened, and the need for everyday continuous wound management can be eliminated, increasing the engraftment success rate. Thus, VAC has become a frequently used method. But the disadvantage of VAC is its cost, and the need to consistently check for keeping negative pressure state, infection, and hematoma during the first week or longer would stabilize the engrafted Integra condition. Shortened hospitalization period and increased successful take rate make VAC popular and used widely [58]. When a neodermis is formed, the graft turns into a pale-orange color instead of red, and the thin silicone film can be easily separated. For the second step operation, a thin split-thickness skin autograft is performed at a thickness of about 0.125 mm and has become more common in recent years, at 0.2 mm. I do not prefer a mesh skin graft to preserve the advantages of dermal substitutes and esthetic results but will recommend a mesh graft with a low ratio if possible.

In a localized deep thermal burn case I handled, debridement and infection control that minimized bleeding determined the success of the grafting. Within 2 weeks, when the dead tissues are well demarcated and the granulation tissue grows healthily with frequent debridement and burn wound dressing, consider using Integra®. To remove granulation tissue, prepare an epinephrine injection and gauze soaked in epinephrine, remove the tissue bluntly using the back of a knife, and, if possible, quickly cover with Integra® to seal the cut blood vessels. In partial tendon exposure was noted, but no special measures were taken in anticipation of granulation tissue growing within the 2-week period of neodermis formation.

(a) A 57-year-old male patient suffered hot metal burns on his left foot; 2 weeks after surgery, granulation and partial tendon exposure (white allow) were observed. (b) Granulation tissue was removed via blunt escharectomy. (c) Directly applied Integra® with non-meshed manipulation. In this figure, the wound has a bloody appearance after the operation but indicates that there is no active bleeding or hematoma. The image depicts bloody findings, but no hematoma was found except for capillary bleeding from the wound bed (Fig. 3.61). Seventeen days after the procedure, a neodermis with a slightly orange color was observed with a cov-

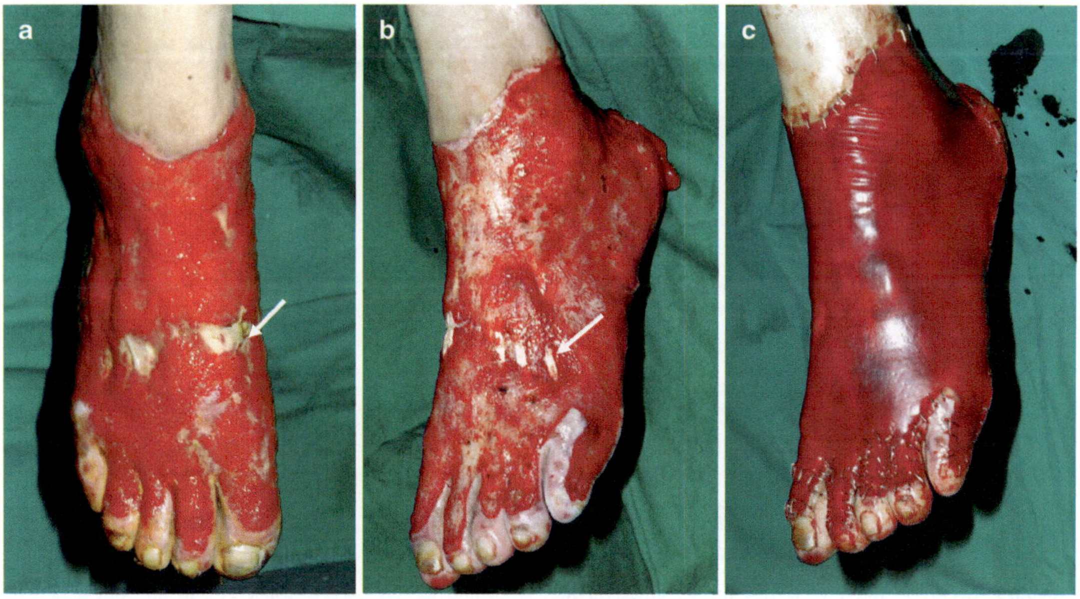

Fig. 3.61 (**a**) Hot metal burn on the left foot, postburn 2 weeks after view, partial tendon exposure (white allow). (**b**) Blunt escharectomy. (**c**) Integra® applied, postoperative immediate view

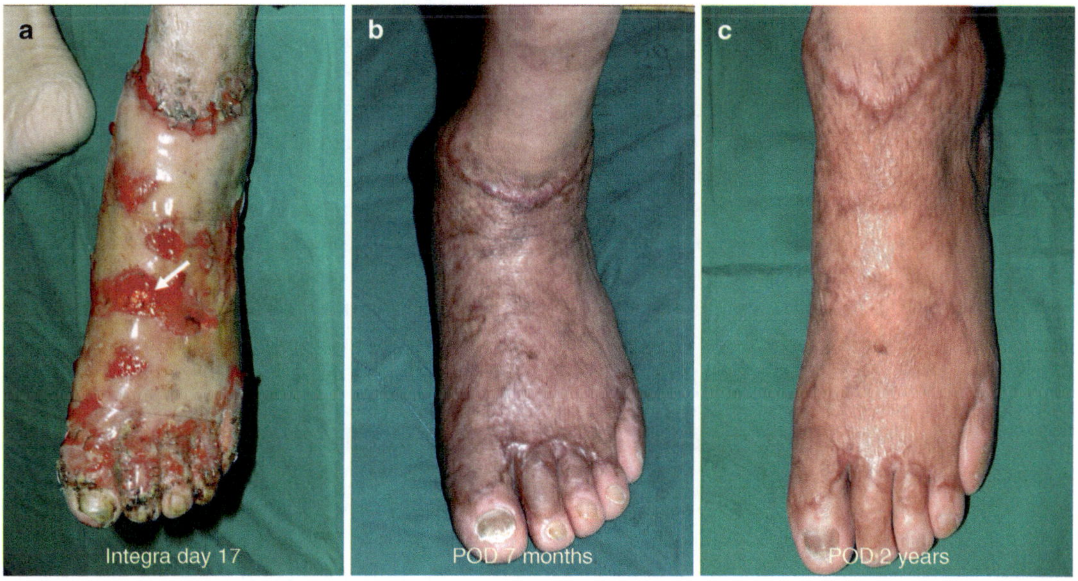

Fig. 3.62 (**a**) Whitish-orange-colored neodermis, small window of partial loss area (white arrow) on day 17; (**b**) 7 months after operation and (**c**) 2 year after view, there were no significant complication and well-covered partial tendon exposure area

ered tendon exposure area, and infection control was partially performed through small open windows. In cases such as the one discussed, my standard method does not change even if the wound area is large. Even 2 years postoperatively, no signs of scar contracture could be observed in such cases, which indicates that the dermal substitute was effective (Fig. 3.62).

The next case has shown a long-term follow-up of 8 years from acute burn management with

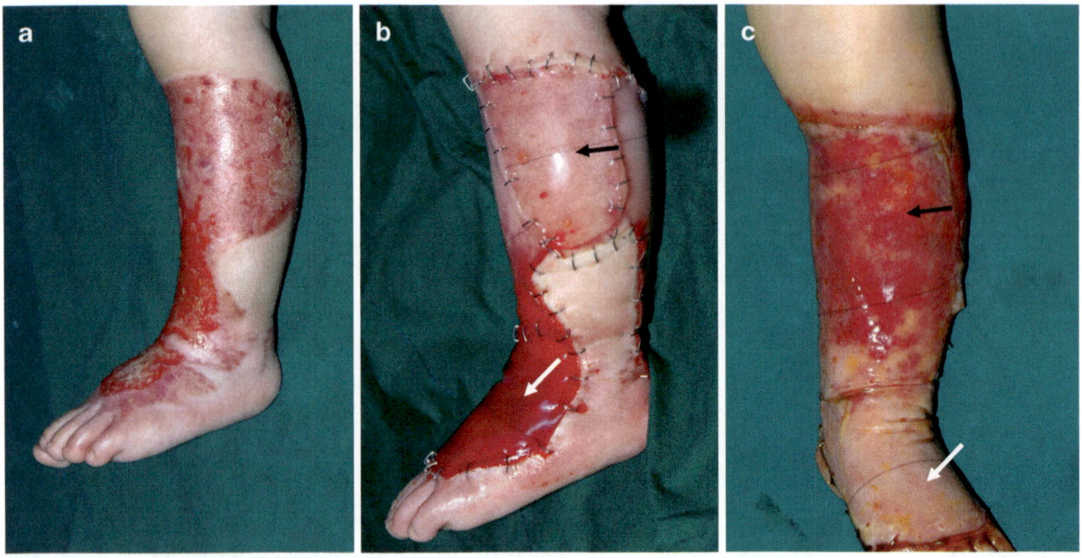

Fig. 3.63 (**a**) Preoperative view, raw surface noted on the dorsum of the foot and epithelialized leg area. (**b**) Integra® applied immediate postoperative view. (**c**) Sixteen days after surgery, well-formed neodermis is observed in the foot and leg area. Note especially in the foot area with well-formed neodermis (white arrows) with whitish-orange color than red color on leg area (black arrows)

Integra® to final reconstruction with FTSG on the ankle area.

(a) A 1-year-old female suffered a scalding burn on her left lower leg. Preoperative view, thin unstable epithelialized and a raw surface were observed on the leg and dorsum foot. (b) After the removal of the eschar on the wound bed and Integra® applied, intra-operative view. As seen in this image, more extensive debridement was performed to prevent contracture deformity in fast-growing children. (c) Sixteen days after surgery, a well-formed neodermis was observed on the foot and leg. The foot area, in particular, had a well-formed neodermis (white arrows) with a whitish-orange color rather than the red color on the leg area (black arrows) (Fig. 3.63).

Postoperative 1-month, 2-month, and 8-month findings revealed a slightly contacted hypertrophic scar in the ankle and dorsum of the foot. However, 1 year and 10 months later, the skin was well matured and smooth, indicating that as time passes, the engrafted Integra adapts even in the case of growing children (Fig. 3.64). During the 5-year, long-term follow-up, there was no severe scar contracture or growth disturbance (Fig. 3.65). However, 8 years after the procedure, there were contracture deformities on the ankle joint and on the fourth and fifth toes. These deformities were corrected with FTSG. In this Integra® case, 8 years after the procedure, the fourth and fifth toes of the left foot and the ankle area had mild retracted contractures (white arrows). We have a plan for reconstructive surgery with release and FTSG at the ankle and dorsum of the foot (black arrows). Note the triangular flap to prevent re-contracture (yellow arrow). Two weeks after the procedure, we observed well-engrafted FTSG and fully released toes (white arrow). Long-term follow-up demonstrated the success of reconstructive surgery following the observation of significant co-growth in growing children (Fig. 3.66).

3.4.4 Integra® Usage in Reconstructive Burn Surgery

In my experience, Integra® is practical for reconstruction surgery [2, 59–61], I will describe a

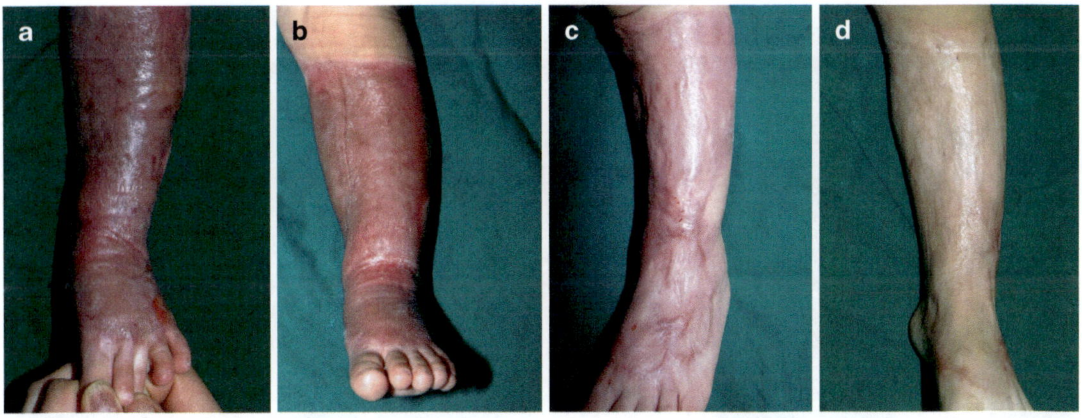

Fig. 3.64 Postoperative (**a**) 1-month, (**b**) 2-month, and (**c**) 8-month finding, slightly contacted with hypertrophic scar was noted in the ankle and dorsum of foot area. (**d**) But 1 year 10 months after view, well-matured and smooth skin texture were noted

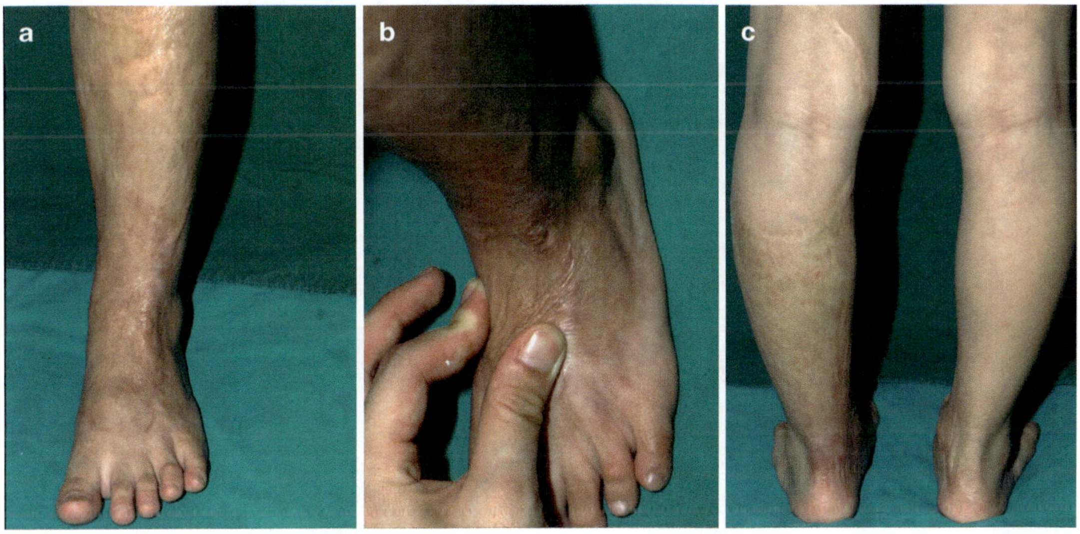

Fig. 3.65 (**a**) Postoperative 5 years later view, (**b**) note softened and good texture and (**c**) well-adapted growth

case and its findings from long-term follow-up observations. Integra® has many advantages of lower risks of infection than acute burns and is more convenient dermal replacement with variable larger sizes. However, as a human dermal matrix, it requires many small pieces to be applied and is more costly, which are its disadvantages. In my long-term follow-up experience, the contracture rate and end results are similar and cheaper to that of AlloDerm®, and I will personally recommend Integra® in reconstructive surgery involving large area even long hospitalization caused by two-step operation.

The reconstruction case used basically the same method described previously, but the success or failure of the surgery is greatly affected by the dissection technique. Thus, refer to the dissection technique described in Chap. 2.

The author has had interest about the breast reconstruction on burn scar contracture deformi-

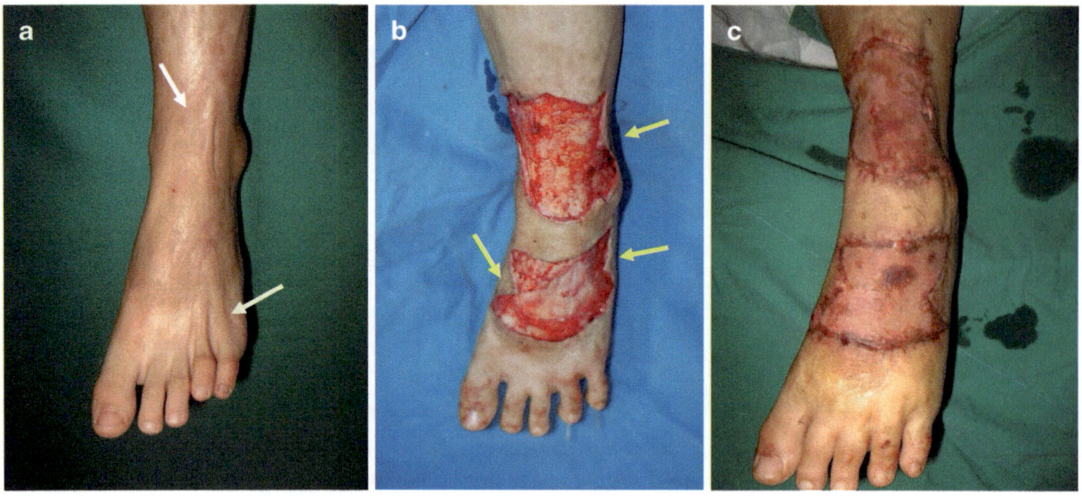

Fig. 3.66 (**a**) Postoperative 8 years later view, the fourth and fifth toes and ankle area were noted with mild retracted contracture (white arrows). (**b**) Note triangular flap to prevent re-contracture (yellow arrows). (**c**) Postoperative 2 weeks later, the ankle and toes were noted returning to original positions

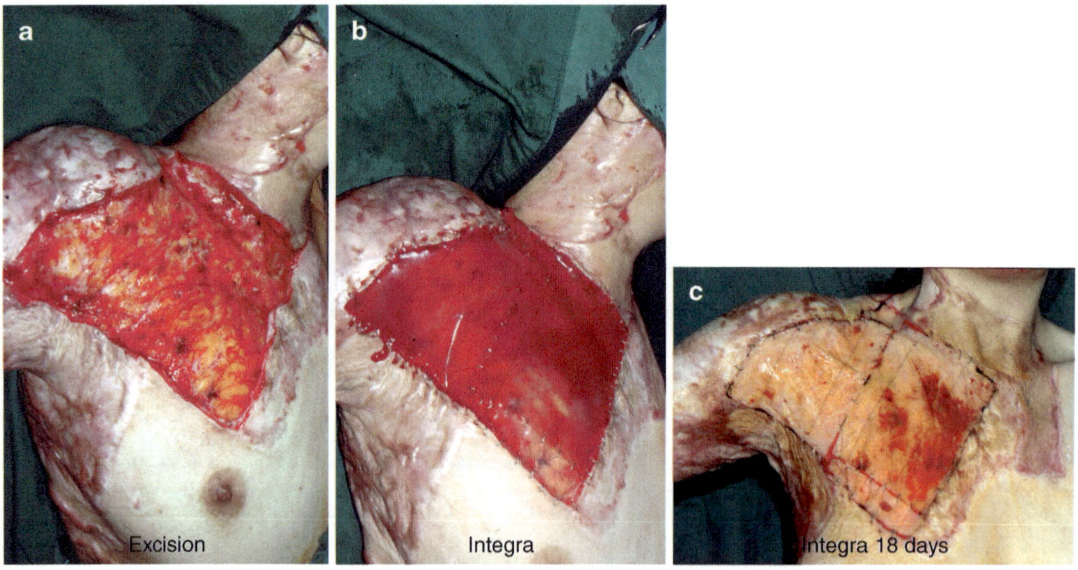

Fig. 3.67 (**a**, **b**) Right upper anterior chest and axilla area were fully released and Integra® applied (**c**) postoperative 18 days after, well-formed orange-colored neodermis was noted. In this case, the Integra was engrafted with two sheets, very fast and convenient

ties because of reasonable advantages [62, 63]. The next is the introduction of clinical cases of the breast and chest area reconstruction with connected shoulder and axilla.

A 31-year-old female patient suffered flame burns several years ago. An incisional full release was performed on the right upper anterior chest and involved the axilla area. Integra® was applied. Eighteen days after the procedure, a well-formed, orange-colored neodermis was noted. In this case, Integra® was engrafted using only two sheets; this procedure was quick and convenient (Fig. 3.67). After 17 months and 22 months of the procedure, the operation site was noted with

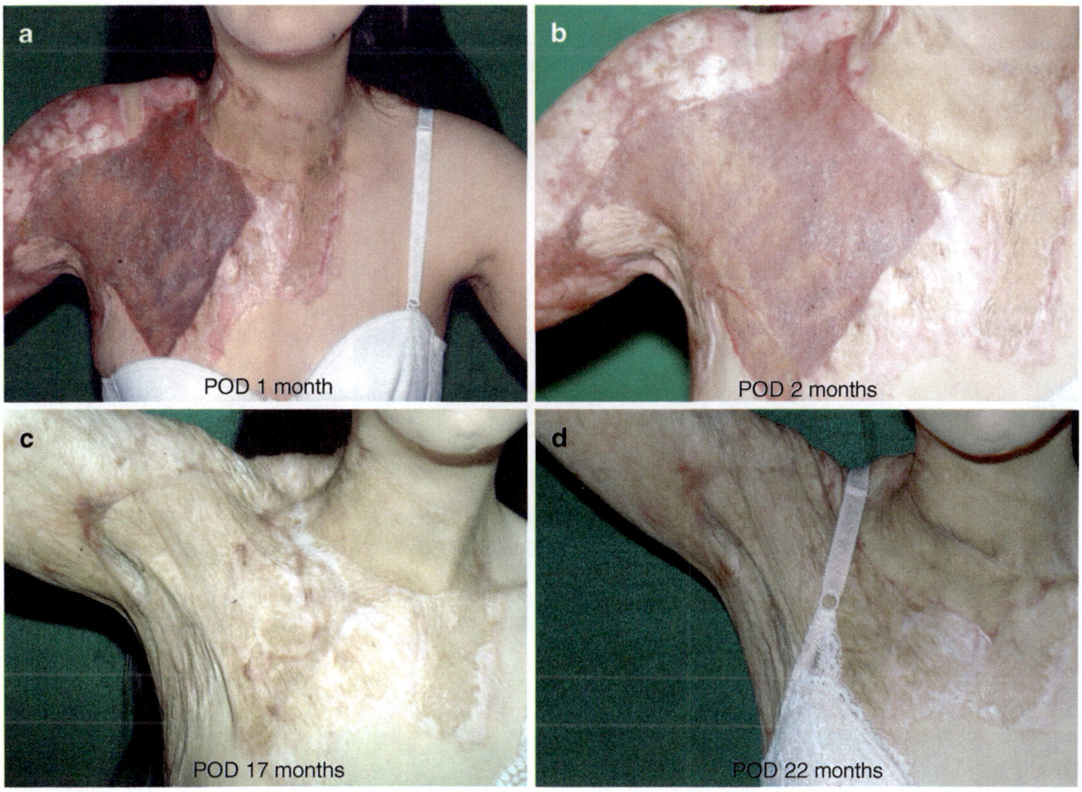

Fig. 3.68 (**a**, **b**) Postoperative 1 month, 2 months view, (**c**, **d**) postoperative 17 months and 22 months view

good functional result and has recovered with full range of motion in the upper chest and axilla areas (Fig. 3.68). In this case, the author recommends Integra as a highly effective and effective material for extensive reconstructive surgery.

A 32-year-old female patient suffered scalding burns on her right breast and axillary area 20 years ago. After full release of the upper chest and axillary areas, a clean wound with preserved fat layer that had minimum bleeding was left. Only diffuse epinephrine injection was used to control bleeding without any electric cauterization in this area. The benefit of maximum size of Integra® (500 cm^2) is that it can cover larger operation wound with only one site of seam line, which is convenient and effective. I performed my own release technique with almost incisional release and only a small amount of scar tissue excision. Furthermore, I did not use an electric surgical knife or cauterization (Fig. 3.69). The Integra®-engrafted site was secured with Surgifix®, which is a very practical protective and compressive dressing material. Eighteen days after the procedure, a well-formed neodermis was noted on the entire Integra®-engrafted site. Six months after the procedure, the right breast had reshaped and was almost back to its normal size compared to the left breast (Fig. 3.70).

A 29-year-old female patient suffered scalding burns on the right breast and shoulders as a child. Severe retractions of the breast and nipple areolar complex were observed. When releasing the contracted nipple areolar complex, the release points must be taken with great consideration (Fig. 3.71). After performing Integra engraftment 18 days later, a well-formed neodermis and an immediate thin, non-meshed autoskin graft were observed. Three months after the procedure, the right breast size recovered by almost 80% compared to the opposite breast. There was a three-quarter view full release and

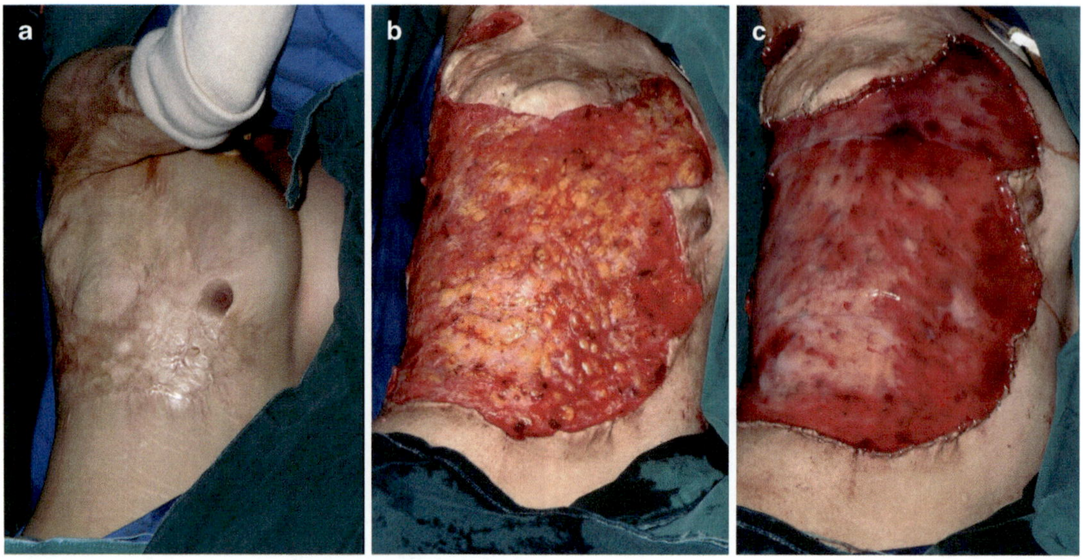

Fig. 3.69 (**a**) Preoperative view. (**b**) After full release upper chest and axillar area, there was noted clean wound with less bleeding and preserved fat layer. (**c**) Integra® applied was noted just one site seam line because of maximal size of Integra® product (500 cm^2)

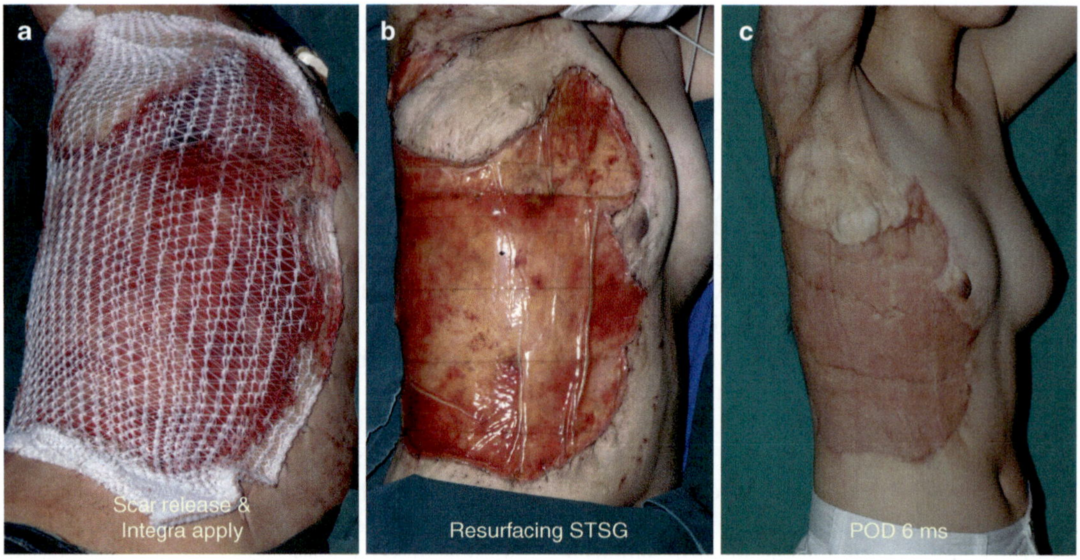

Fig. 3.70 (**a**) The Integra®-engrafted site was secured with Surgifix® which is a very useful protective compressive dressing material. (**b**) Postoperative 18 days, well-formed neodermis was noted in the entire Integra®-engrafted site. (**c**) Postoperative 6 months after, the right breast had reshaped and almost back to its normal size compared to the left breast

anatomical functional recovery of the left shoulder area. In this case, I recommend that when releasing the three-dimensional breast tissues, each relationship between the anatomical position of the nipple areolar complex and breast tissue be considered (Fig. 3.72).

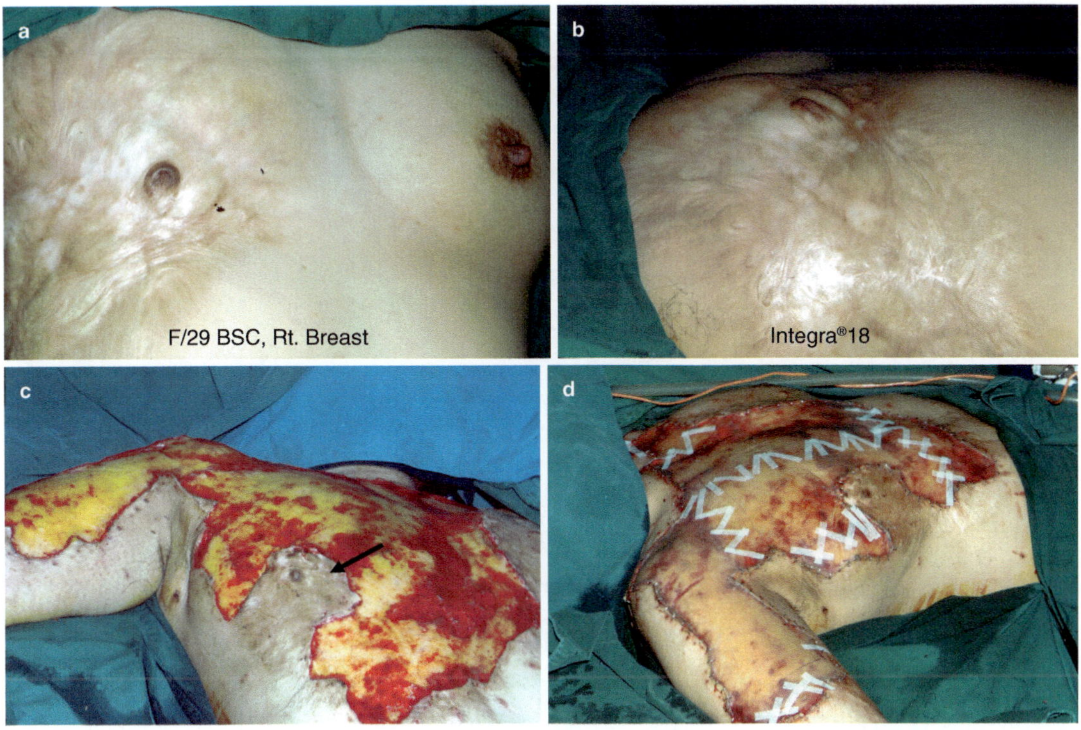

Fig. 3.71 (**a**) Preoperative view. (**b**) Note severe retracted breast and nipple areolar tissue. (**c**) Note the repositioned nipple areolar complex with designed flap (black arrow). Eighteen days after Integra® engraft, well-formed neodermis was noted and (**d**) immediate thin non-meshed auto-skin graft

The next case will introduce severe scar contracture in the lower extremities where it is difficult to obtain good results with general release and STSG.

A 7-year-old male patient was observed to have severe burn scar contracture on his right lower leg and ankle. Scar contracture was released, and the total excision of scar tissue was performed. With a well-preserved subcutaneous fat layer, no tourniquet or electrodessication is used: only usage of epinephrine injection technique. After release, Integra was engrafted immediately. The site had a bloody appearance, but there was no active bleeding or hematoma. Twenty days after the procedure, an orange-colored, well-formed neodermis was observed (Fig. 3.73). Three weeks later, a 0.15-mm-thick, thin auto-skin graft was performed. Two and three years after the procedure, there was good adaptation with no functional disturbance, despite the fact that the patient was a growing child (Fig. 3.74).

3.4.5 Reconstruction of the Neck Area

A 21-year-old male patient suffered flame burns on 35% TBSA, and severe scar contracture was noted on the anterior neck, chest, axilla, and upper arm areas. On the three-quarter view, cervico-mental angle was blunted due to a contracted upper chest and anterior neck (Fig. 3.75). Excisional and incisional release were performed with a well-preserved subcutaneous fat layer, and Integra® was applied immediately. Eighteen days after the procedure, an orange-colored neodermis was noted on the entire operated area. Postoperative two months later view, contour of

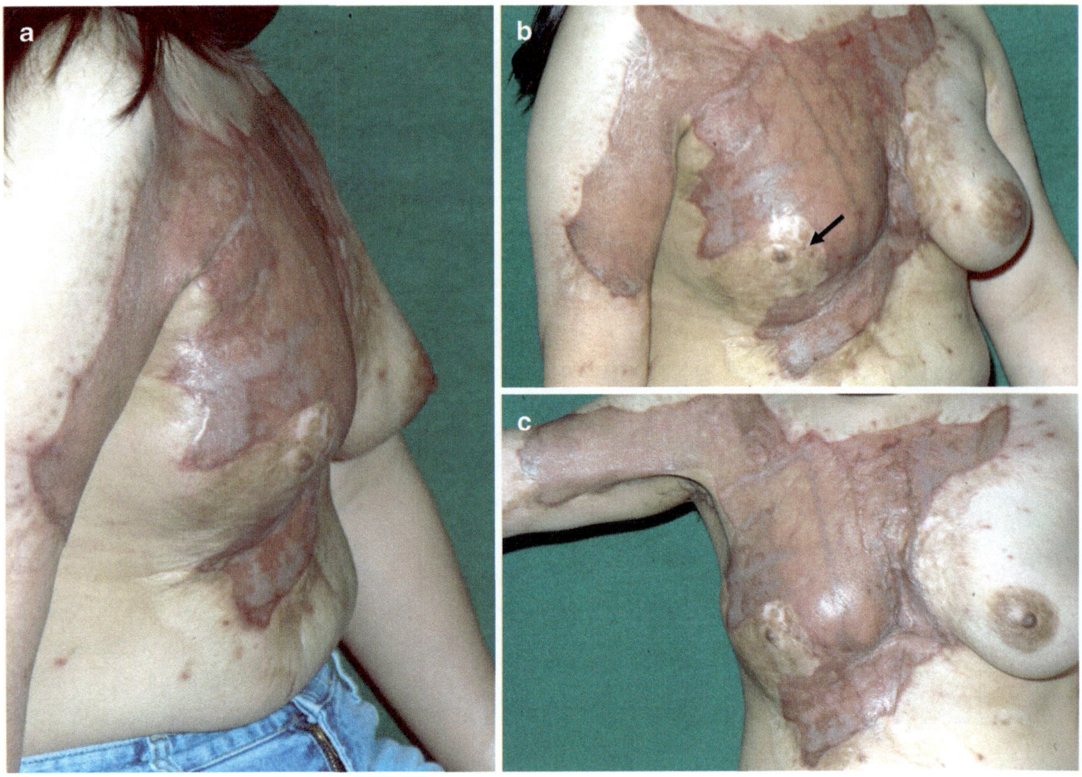

Fig. 3.72 (**a**) Postoperative 3 months after, the right breast size recovers almost 80% compared with opposite breast. (**b**) Three-quarter view; note the nipple areolar complex position (black arrow). (**c**) Full release and functional recovery noted on the right shoulder area

the anterior neck and upper chest area were observed to have noticeable improvement but additional FTSG is required for reconstruction to achieve more natural appearance and functional mento-cervical angle recovery of the anterior neck and submental areas (Fig. 3.76).

Next, mento-cervical angle reconstructive procedure will be introduced by many plastic surgeons considering a high probability of failure that is difficult to obtain natural appearance of mento-cervical angle with one-stage reconstruction.

A 34-year-old female patient presented to our clinic with the complaint of anterior neck contracture, which was treated with platysma muscle Z-plasty (the authors' own developed technique that manipulated platysma muscle vertical lengthening with Z-plasty) and Integra engraft. Seventeen days after the procedure, a well-formed yellowish-orange neodermis was observed after silicone sheet removal. Three days later, a 0.2-mm-thin auto-skin graft was performed (Fig. 3.77). After 6 weeks and 3 months of the procedure, there were no re-contracture deformities, and a well-formed mento-cervical angle was observed (Fig. 3.78). Thirteen months after the procedure, the mento-cervical angle was well preserved which is a difficult area, especially in the case of a one-stage operation. The engrafted, new dermal substitute skin was soft and pliable in the hyperextension position. However, readers should keep in mind that the excellent result in this case is a very important factor in scar release using my technique of platysma muscle manipulation (Fig. 3.79).

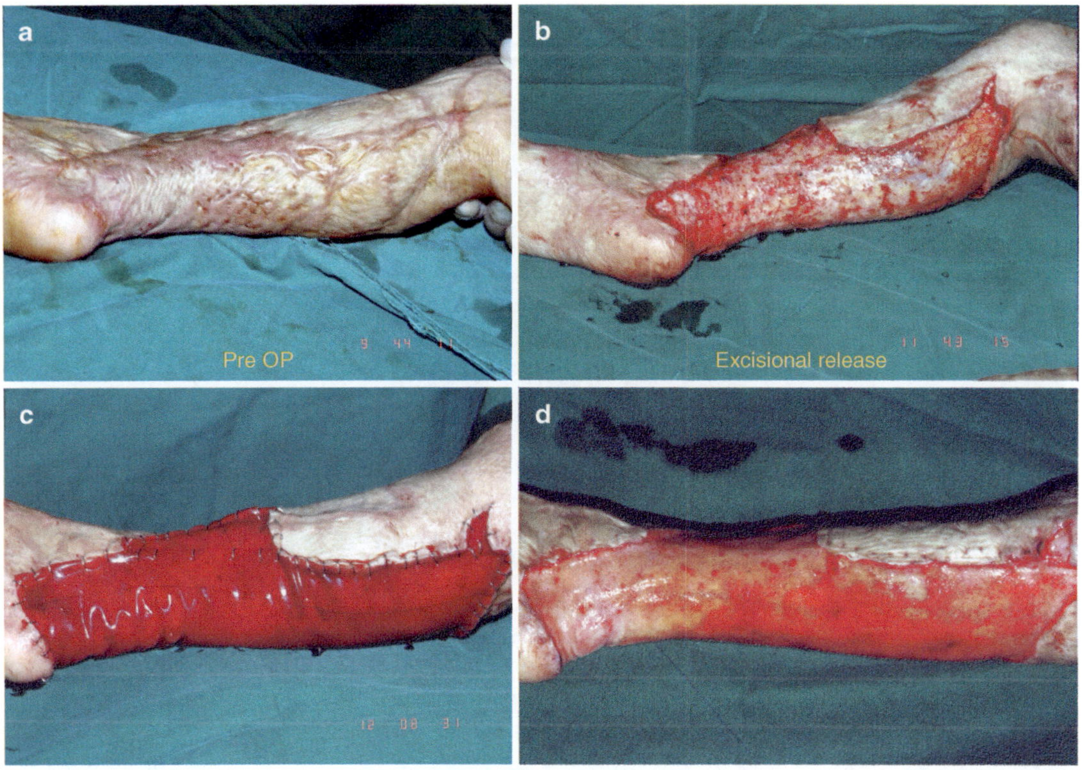

Fig. 3.73 (**a**) Severe burn scar contracture on the right lower leg and ankle area. (**b**) Release and total excision of scar tissue. (**c**) Integra was engrafted. (**d**) Postoperative 20 days after, the neodermis well-formed with orange color change

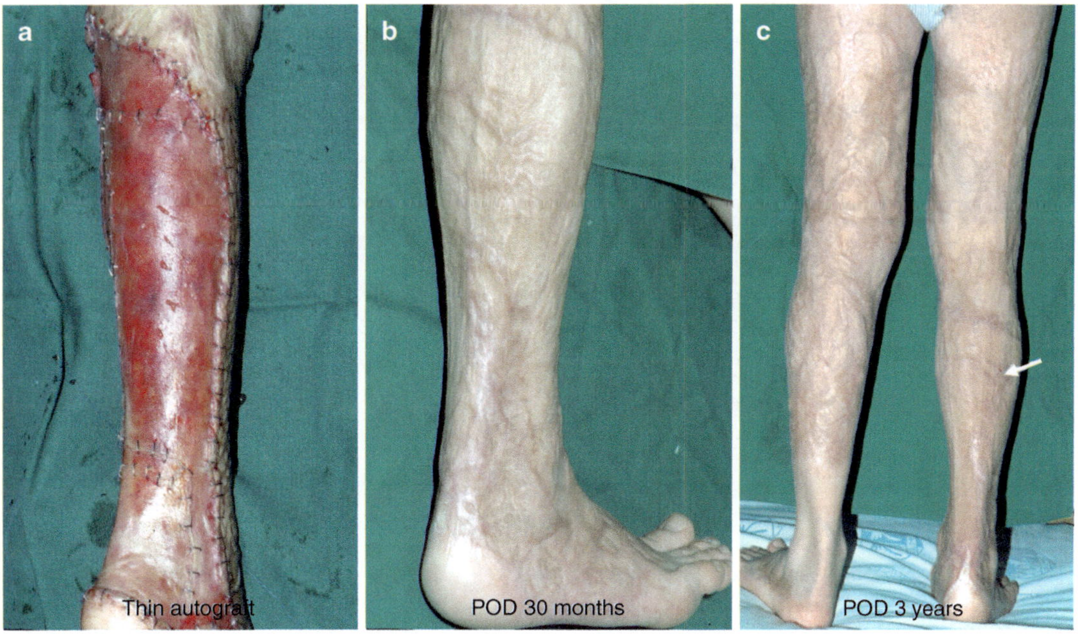

Fig. 3.74 (**a**) Three weeks after surgery, thin auto-skin graft was performed with 6/1000-in. thickness; (**b**) postoperative 2 years after view and (**c**) postoperative 3 years after view, good adaptation without functional disturbance even though repaid growing children (white arrow)

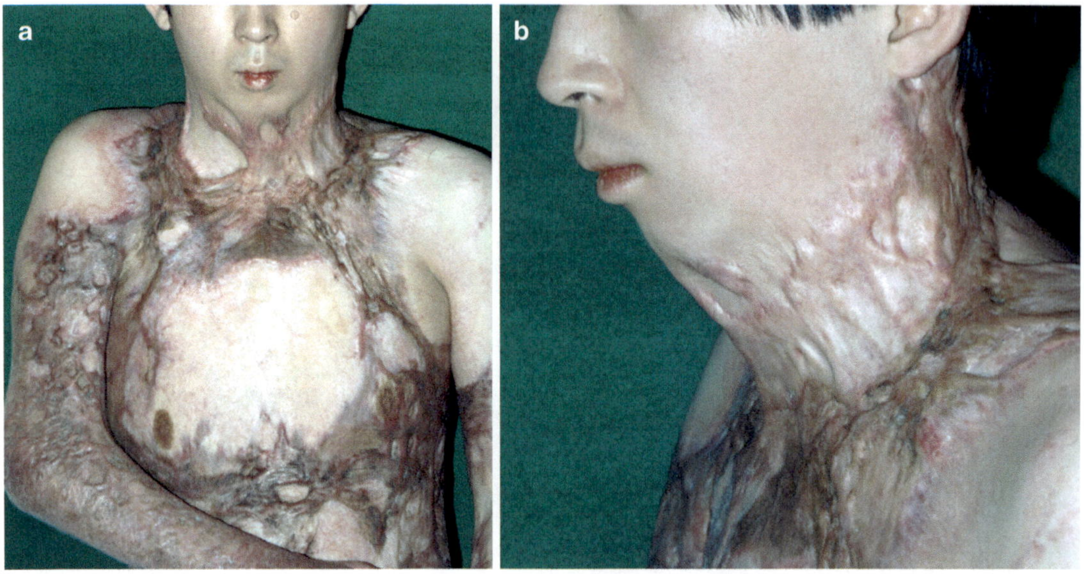

Fig. 3.75 (**a**) Severe scar contracture noted on the anterior neck, chest, axilla, and upper arm area. (**b**) Cervico-mental angle was blunted due to contracted upper chest and anterior neck

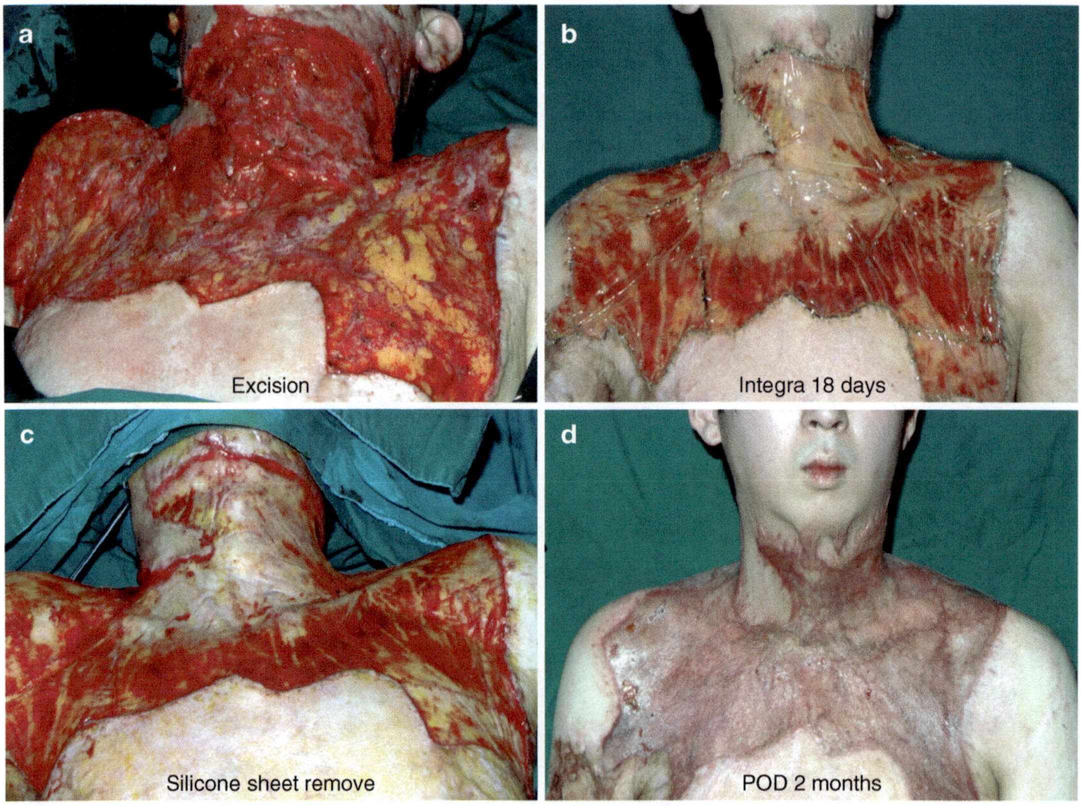

Fig. 3.76 (**a**) Excisional and incisional release was performed with well-preserved subcutaneous fat layer. (**b**) Postoperative 18 days later, orange-colored neodermis was noted. (**c**) 0.15-mm non-meshed thin autograft was performed. (**d**) Postoperative 2 months later, marked improved contour of anterior neck and upper chest area

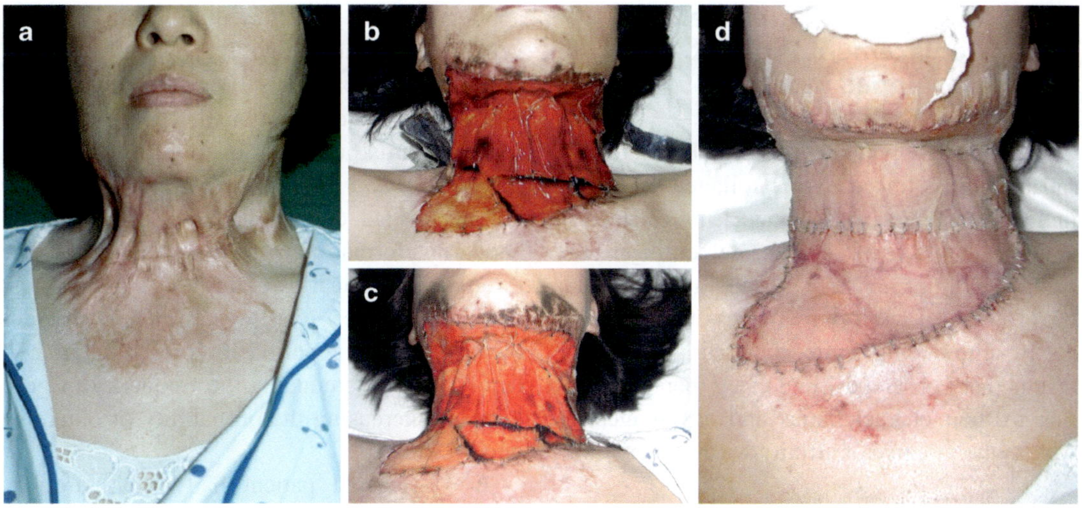

Fig. 3.77 (**a**) Preoperative view, anterior neck scar contracture. (**b**) Release and platysma muscle Z-plasty and Integra® engraft 17 days after view and (**c**) well-formed yellowish-orange-colored neodermis was noted. (**d**) 0.2-mm-thin auto-skin graft was performed, 3 days after surgery view

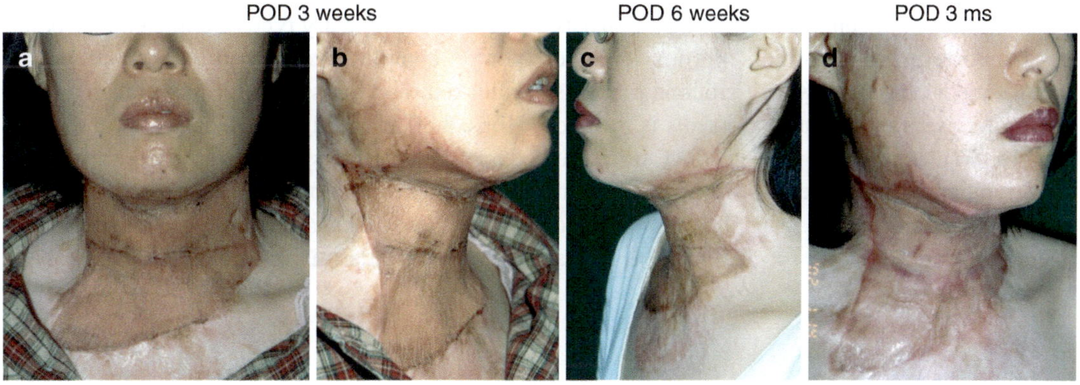

Fig. 3.78 (**a**, **b**) Postoperative 3 weeks after view of anterior and three-quarter view. (**c**, **d**) Postoperative 6 weeks, 3 months after view

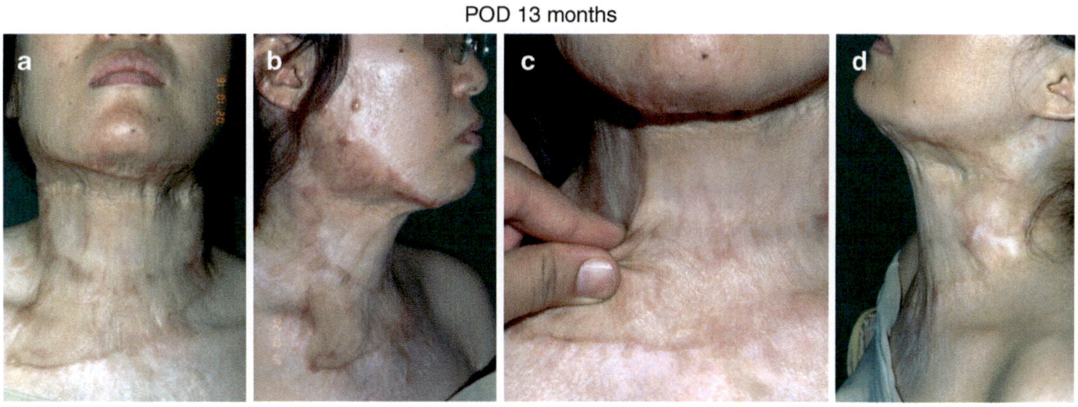

Fig. 3.79 (**a**, **b**) Postoperative 13 months after view, the mento-cervical angle was well preserved. (**c**, **d**) Note soft and pliable engrafted skin and hyperextension position

3.5 Dry-Type Collagen Dermal Replacement Product Developed in Japan

Terudermis® (Olympus Terumo Biomaterials, Japan), a cross-linked bovine collagen developed in Japan, and Pelnac® (Gunze Limited Japan), which is made from porcine atelocollagen, are being used in some clinical trials in Asian countries [64–66]. I will briefly discuss these materials by introducing some characteristics of the results that I observed while using them, in addition to their characteristics and advantages, as well as their degree of affinity with tissues.

3.6 Terudermis®

Terudermis® (Terumo Co. Ltd., Tokyo, Japan) is made of low-antigenic atelocollagen obtained from calf hide collagen. Like Integra®, it consists of a two-layer, 3-mm-thick porous collage sponge and a very thin layer of silicone that acts as a protective film until a new dermis is formed [46, 49, 67]. It is a dry-type product stored at room temperature and used by simply soaking it in regular saline before transplantation in the operating room [68]. The surgical method for its application does not differ significantly from the general dermal substitute. It can simply be rehydrated for approximately 10 seconds and applied directly to the surgical wound. The formation of the neodermis takes less or more than 3 weeks (Fig. 3.83), and the resulting granulation tissue is well-formed on the wound bed. Shortening neodermis formation by up to 14 days is possible through the application of the VAC system (VAC, Instill: KCI, Inc.) [52], which in turn shortens the hospitalization period and prevents fluid collection, thereby reducing the frequency of graft loss and increasing the probability of obtaining good results.

A 42-year-old patient had a hypertrophic, depigmented scar on the entire back, with contracture and motion limitation in both the frank and axilla. Immediately after surgery, Terudermis was applied to the left flank and right upper chest. The whitish material was noted on both operation sites because the dry type of collagen matrix had not yet completely absorbed tissue fluid, but the color returned to tissue color in less than an hour (Figs. 3.80 and 3.81). Three days after the procedure, the VAC™ system was used to improve neodermis formation and hematoma prevention. Twenty-two days after the procedure, a well-preserved neodermis was noted in the postopera-

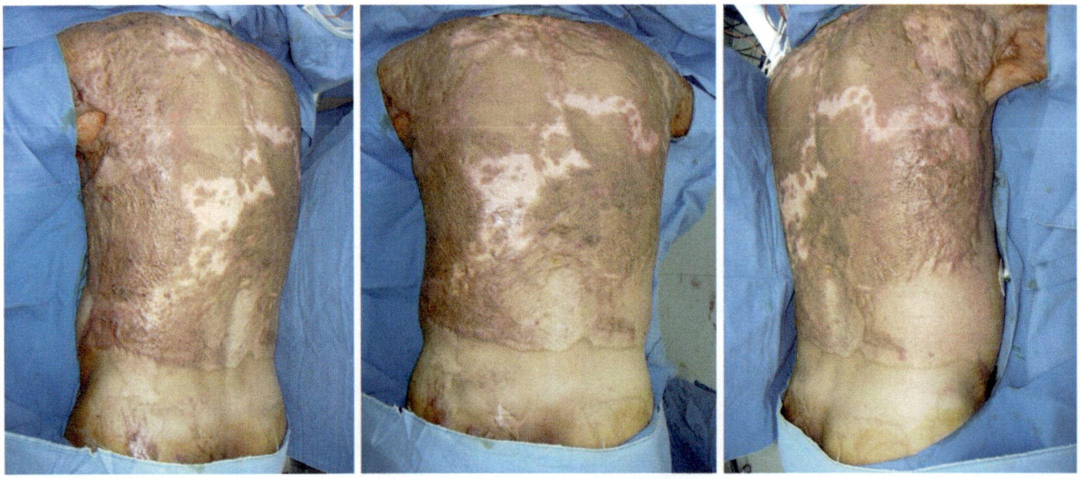

Fig. 3.80 Hypertrophic, depigmented scar was noted on the entire back with contracture and motion limitation in frank and axilla

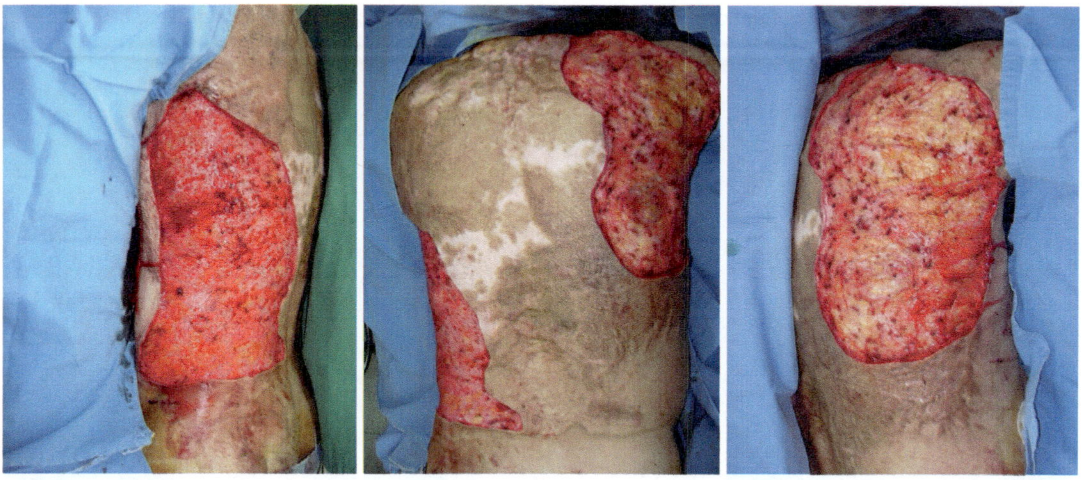

Fig. 3.81 Excisional release underwent on the left flank and right upper back for relaxation of both shoulder movements

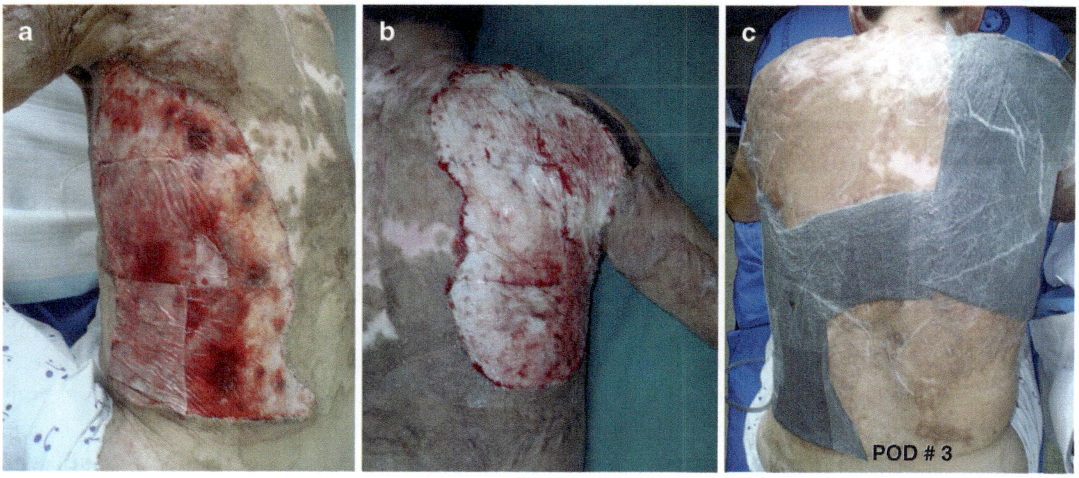

Fig. 3.82 (**a**) Terudermis® was applied on the left flank, (**b**) right upper chest area. (**c**) Postoperative 3 days after VAC™ system applied to enhance the neodermis formation and hematoma prevention

tive immediate 0.2-mm auto-skin engraft view (Figs. 3.82 and 3.83).

Clinically, the results from the use of Terudermis® show little differences to those of Integra®. However, in terms of long-term post-operative follow-up, the surgical site is slightly more contracted and more susceptible to infection during neodermis formation, and the granulation tissue tends to form faster. Nevertheless, differences occur depending on the individual and the condition of the surgical site. So it may be hard to conclude its end results and contracture rate and need for further evaluation study.

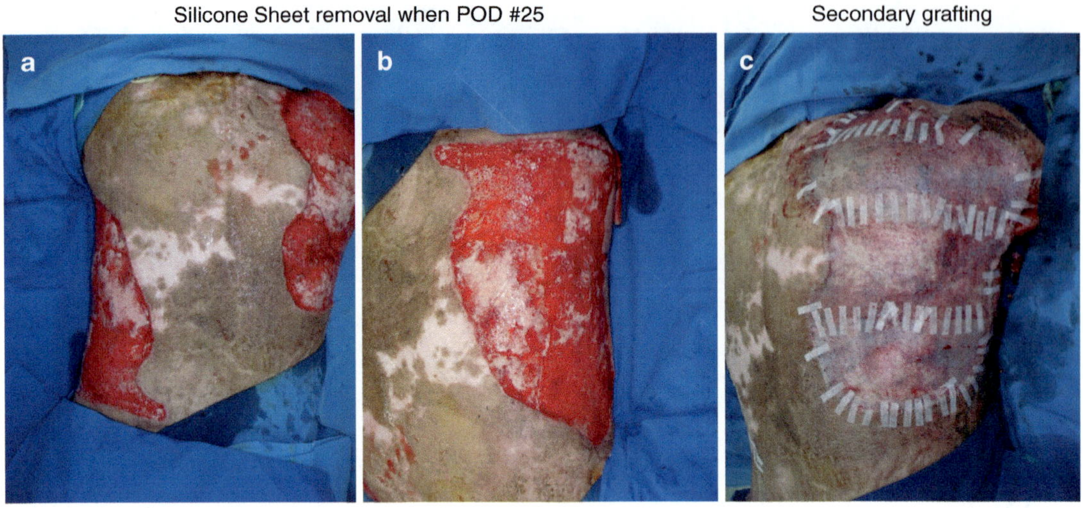

Fig. 3.83 (**a**, **b**) Postoperative 22 days after well-preserved neodermis was noted. (**c**) 0.15-mm auto-skin graft was performed

3.7 Pelnac®

Pelnac® (Gunze Ltd., Japan) is also applied using a very similar method to Terudermis®. Both products were developed in Japan, but for those who are reluctant to use Terudermis due to concerns of bovine spongiform encephalopathy, Pelnac can be used instead like in Islamic culture, where the use of porcine collagen is prohibited for religious reasons. Pelnac is also introduced as a dry-type porcine atelocollagen with a single silicone layer, and it is compatible to human tissue [56, 69–71]. The method of application and its strengths and weaknesses are similar to Terudermis®, but it tends to form granulation tissue faster because of its fast absorption and biocompatibility with human tissue [56]. As I presented at my 2006 clinical presentation of 44 cases, the duration of a secondary thin autograft was 14 ± 1.8 days, which was 3–4 days earlier than those of Integra® and Terudermis® (Fig. 3.84). Therefore, Pelnac promotes better wound management, with good neodermis formation and tissue affinity. Pelnac can also be used frequently with VAC since it enables a more stable neodermis formation over a large area while shortening the formation period and reducing complications.

A 23-year-old female was admitted for breast scar contracture correction. After full release of both contracted breasts, nipple areolar tissue was preserved. Pelnac was engrafted (Fig. 3.85), and the VAC system was immediately applied to reduce the formation of short neodermis (Fig. 3.86). Sixteen days after the procedure, a well-formed, clear, orange-colored neodermis was noted without partial loss. After 3, 6, and 12 days of operation, there were no issues with the healing process. These images indicate that the VAC system has many advantages, including a shorter neodermis formation period, stability, less fluid collection, simple operation, and wound management without daily wound checks (Fig. 3.87).

However, Terudermis® and Pelnac® tend to have a slightly higher contracture rate in the early postoperative stages in my experienced opinion.

(a) A 6-year-old male patient suffered scalding burns, and severe scar contracture was noted on the abdomen, anterior chest, and right

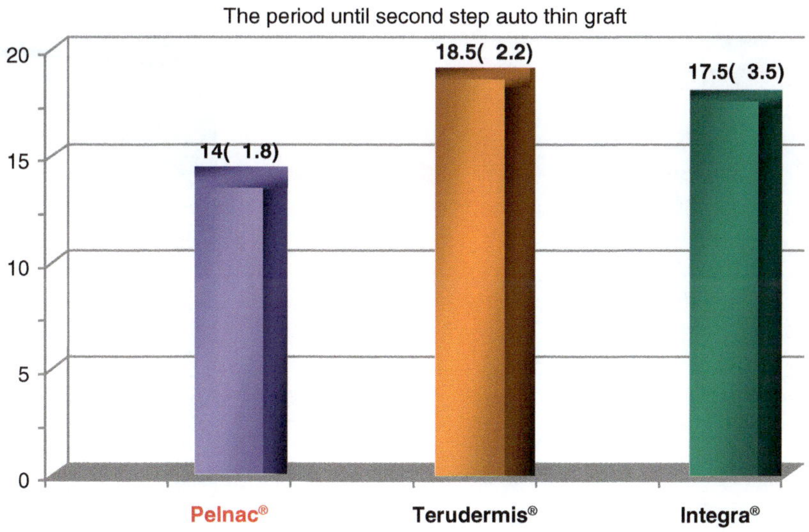

Fig. 3.84 My 2006 clinical presentation of 44 cases in small and medium-sized materials—Total patients No; Male: Female (38:17)—Area: 620 cm^2 (35-1000 cm^2)—Infection; 12 cases (total:2, partial:10) was evaluated—the duration of a secondary thin auto graft was 14 ± 1.8 days in Pelnac® cases, which was 3–4 days earlier than those of Integra® and Terudermis®

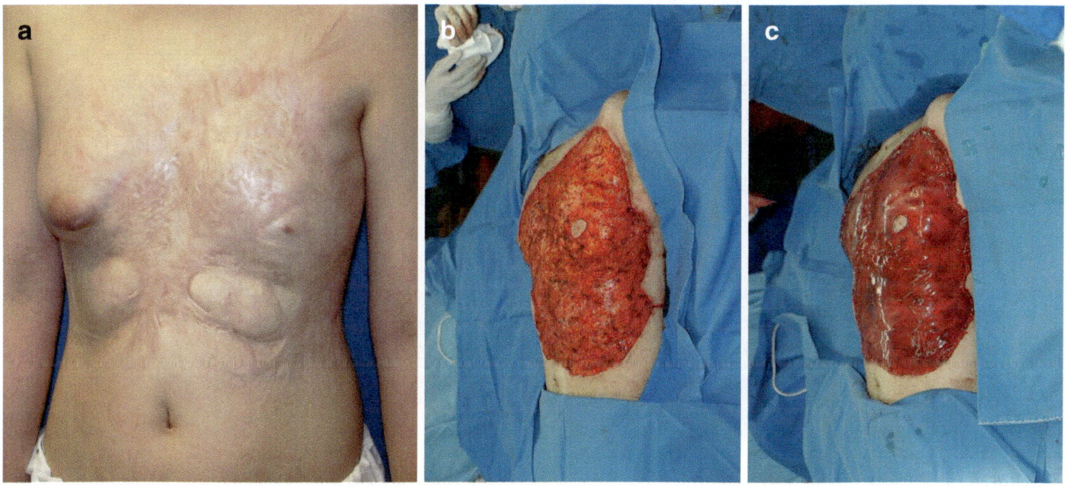

Fig. 3.85 (**a**) Preoperative view, severe scar contractures were noted both breast and anterior chest. (**b**, **c**) After full release, Pelnac® application

axilla. (b) Excisional full release was performed, and Pelnac® was immediately applied. (c) The whitish color (black arrow) of Pelnac quickly faded when body fluid was absorbed from the wound bed. Two and three months after the procedure, the engrafted size was noticeably reduced, and a shrinking contracture band was noted on the left frank and axillary area. The author routinely strongly recommends wearing the pressure garment continuously for at least 1 year or more especially for growing children cases (Figs. 3.88, 3.89, 3.90).

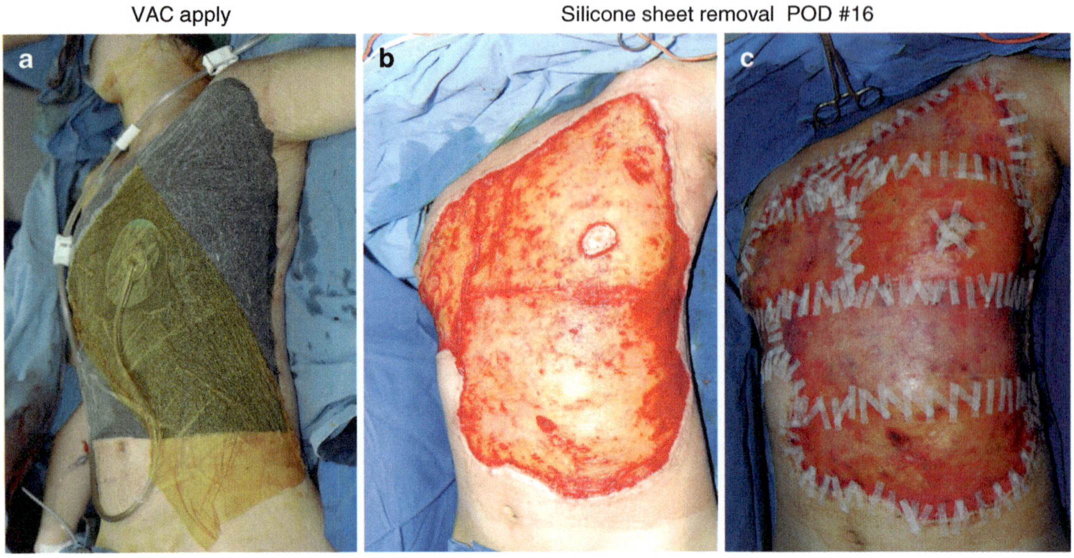

Fig. 3.86 (**a**) VAC system was applied and (**b**) postoperative day 16, well-formed clear orange-colored neodermis was noted; (**c**) thin non-meshed autograft was performed

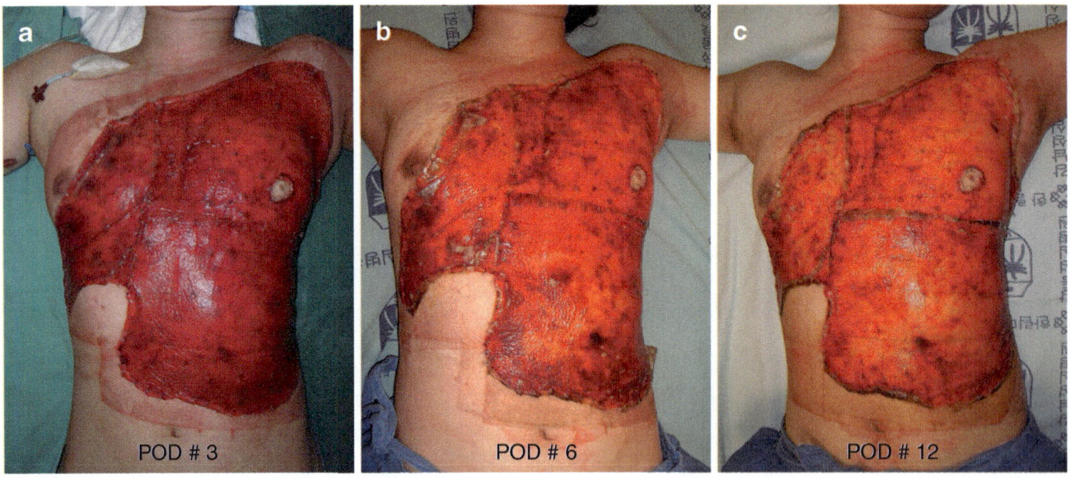

Fig. 3.87 (**a**) Postoperative 3, (**b**) 6 days and 12 days, (**c**) good healing process was noted without complication

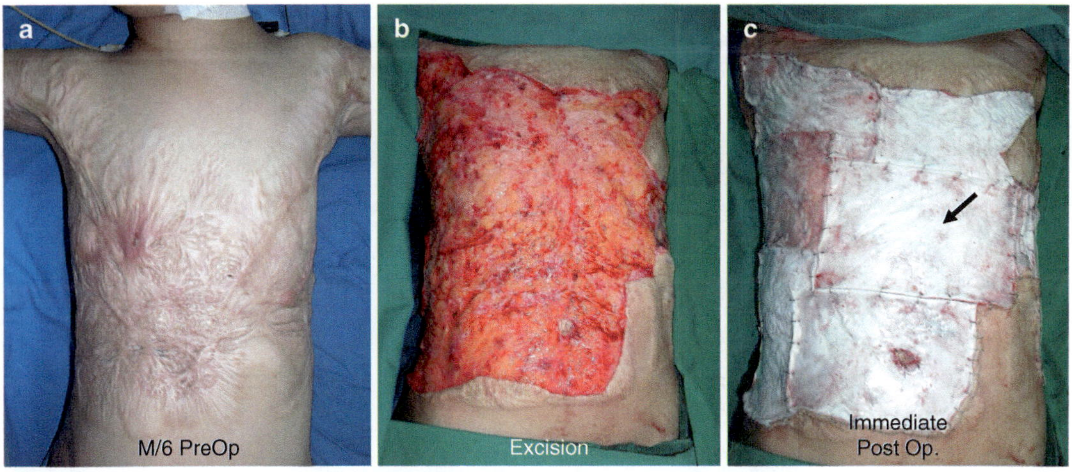

Fig. 3.88 (**a**) Severe scar contracture was noted on the abdomen, anterior chest, and right axilla. (**b**) Excisional full release and (**c**) Pelnac applied was noted

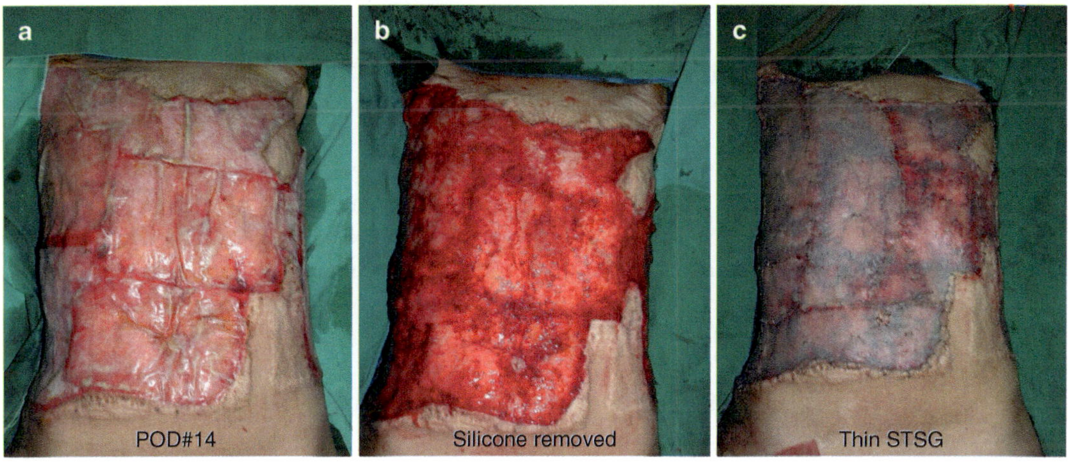

Fig. 3.89 (**a**) Postoperative day 14, neodermis was well-formed for preparation of auto-thin skin graft. (**b**) After removal of silicone sheet, (**c**) 0.15-mm auto-skin sheet graft was applied

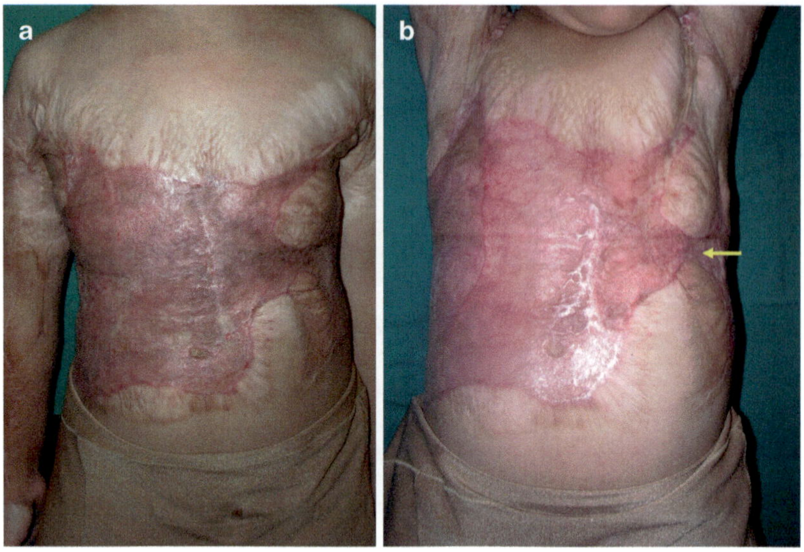

Fig. 3.90 (**a**) Postoperative 2 months, (**b**) 3 months after view, the engrafted size was noticeably reduced, and shrink contracture band was noted on left frank and axilla area (yellow arrow). Note the pressure garment to prevent postoperative contracture and enhance graft remodeling

3.8 Collagen Synthetic Dermal Substitute Matriderm® Is Suitable for Single-Step Surgery

3.8.1 Matriderm®

Matriderm® is a material that is gaining attention in recent years for its noteworthy properties. It is used to support dermal regeneration by impregnating bovine collagen types 1, 2, and 3, as well as elastin components [72]. Matriderm® was manufactured so that a single-step operation like the human dermal matrix was possible, circumventing a two-stage operation, which has been the biggest drawback of animal collagen products [73, 74]. In particular, while using this product, I focused on the two different thicknesses, 1 and 2 mm, and the differences in the results attributable to the different thicknesses. I found that intake of a thin autograft was sufficient, even with the 2-mm version, without any major problems. When comparing the results between the two thicknesses, the contracture rate was not significantly affected, but as data on long-term follow-up comparisons are limited, I personally expect further evaluation studies of the two implant thicknesses in the future. The product is manufactured in a wet condition to aid its adaptation to the wound bed and also has absorptive power; this slightly helps with bleeding control. The immediate skin autograft is 0.125–0.2-mm thickness and employs the same application method as the general dermal substitute. In acute burn wound management, Matriderm® is well adapted to bleed control and simple to use. With a single-step autograft, it shortens the hospital stay and promotes a higher intake rate. As I was already aware of the operability and convenience of Matriderm®, I described some observations from clinical trials evaluating the contracture rate and results of the two types of thicknesses. The benefit of an immediate auto-skin graft with a single-step procedure is that no notable findings were found in the care of acute burns with Matriderm®, other than the simplicity of the procedure and reduction in operation time. As a result, analysis was done with a focus on the variations in autograft take rate between the 2-mm and the 1-mm options. However, it was found that there was no big difference in the graft take according to the thickness.

More clinical evaluations with long-term follow-up on the scope of application according to anatomical region and reconstruction rate of the surgical site are needed. Although the evaluation of the differences in contracture rate between the two thicknesses is important, unfortunately, the

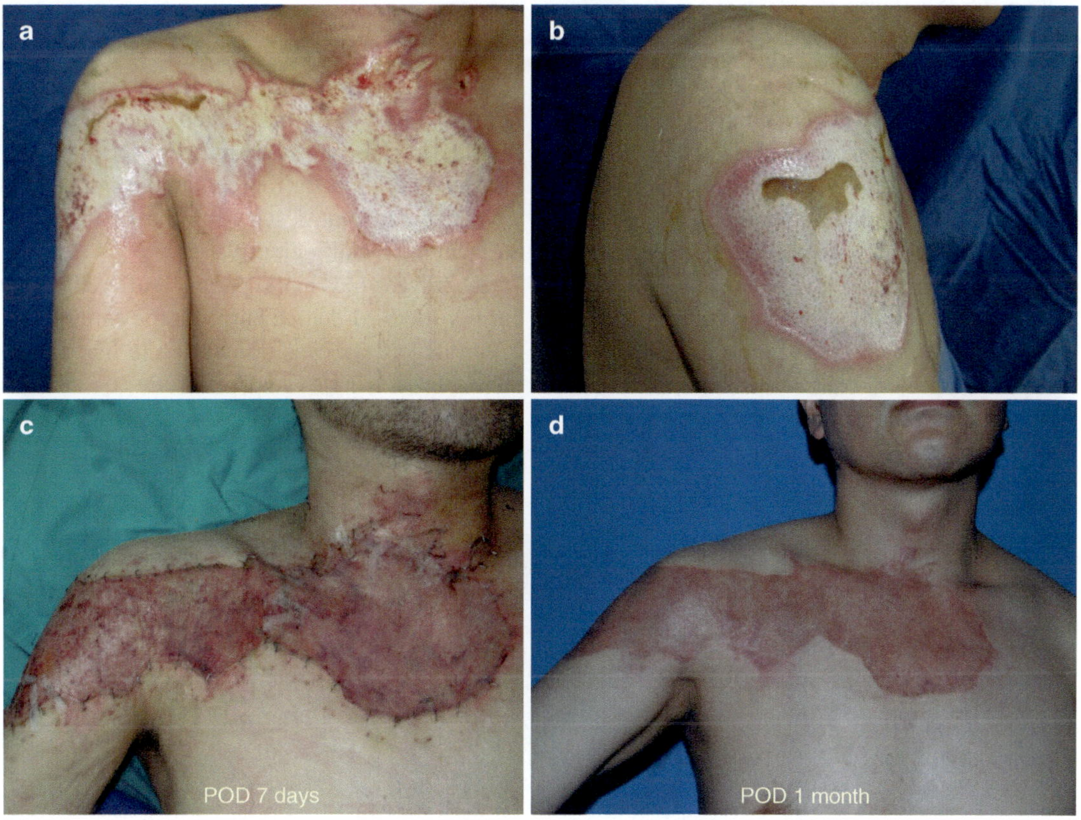

Fig. 3.91 (**a**, **b**) Flame burn on the right upper chest and shoulder area. (**c**) 1-mm thickness of Matriderm® and single-step 0.125-mm autograft were applied. (**c**) Postoperative 7 days after view, the auto-skin graft was taken completely; (**d**) 1 month after the operation, the engrafted space was preserved compared with original wound size

clinical evidence cannot be clearly presented. Although an accurate comparison between the postoperative contracture rates I obtained with those of other dermal substitutes is difficult, the contracture rate was slightly higher in a case of localized deep thermal burns in the shoulder region, but confirmation is difficult to obtain with only a few cases. Given the impression that an engraftment with 2-mm thickness will not significantly affect the contracture rate, I believe that doubling the thickness will not affect the contracture less.

A 41-year-old male patient suffered flame burns on the right upper chest and shoulder area. A dermal substitute was applied with a 1-mm-thick Matriderm, and a single-step 0.125-mm-thick autograft was applied. Seven days after the procedure, the auto-skin graft was taken completely. One month after the procedure, the engrafted space was nearly preserved in comparison with the original wound size. The author's impression was that the healing process with other types of dermal substitutes was almost identical (Fig. 3.91).

A 19-year-old male patient suffered scalding burns on the anterior chest and upper abdominal area during childhood. Incisional rather than excisional release was performed, with multiple triangular advance rotational flaps created to reduce scar re-contracture. A 2-mm-thick Matriderm was applied, followed by an immediate single-step 0.125-mm-thick auto-skin graft. Seven days after the procedure, there was a good appearance without any problems, even though Matriderm® was 2-mm thick. Thirteen days after the procedure, an unstable inflammatory lesion was noted on the right middle area, which eventually healed without skin loss. Two months after the procedure, a noticeable re-contracted lesion with hypertrophic scarring was noted, and the entire engrafted area was contracted (Figs. 3.92, 3.93). In this case, precise postoperative wound management without inflammation or partial skin loss is strongly recommended to prevent and to improve scar contracture (Fig. 3.94). In my experience, the thickness of Matriderm of 1 mm or 2 mm made little difference in contracture rate, and there was no difference in the take rate between 1 mm and 2 mm of thickness. We need to further research on long-term follow-ups and tissue scar analysis.

The following is a case of deep thermal burns in the facial region, which indicates that Matriderm® has many advantages especially single-step operation for rapid wound coverage and yielded significant results for the treatment of burns in the facial region [9, 75].

A 26-year-old male patient suffered flame burns with third-degree burns on the entire face.

On day 12, he was transferred to our department. In a single step, necrotic tissue was removed and a 2-mm-thick Matriderm with a 0.125-mm-thick auto-skin graft was placed.

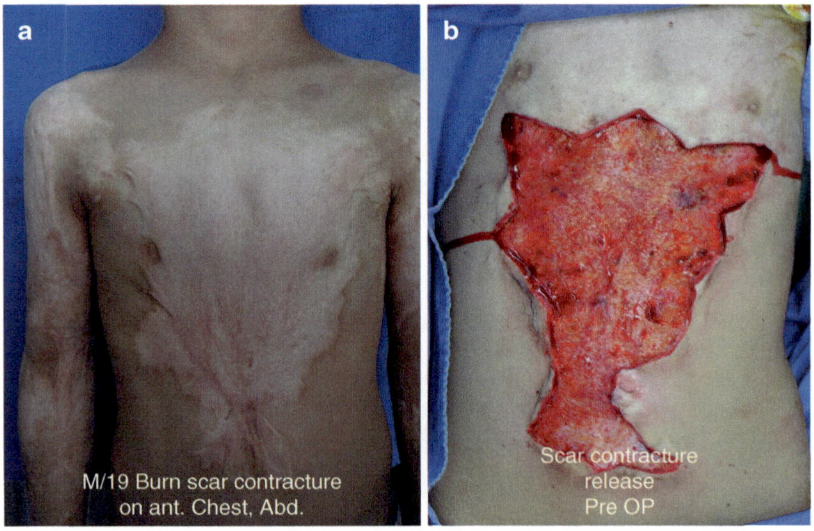

Fig. 3.92 (**a**) Scar contracture was noted on anterior chest and upper center of the abdominal area. (**b**) Incisional rather than excisional release was performed with multiple triangular advance rotational flaps

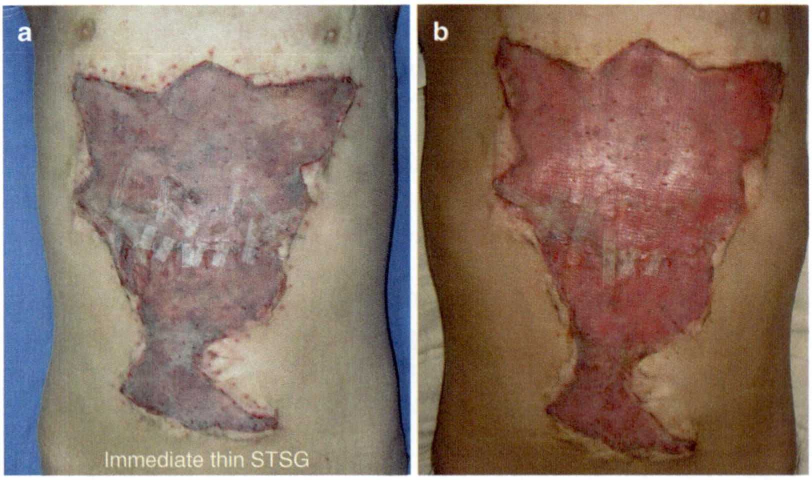

Fig. 3.93 (**a**) 2-mm thick Matriderm® applied and then single-step 0.125-mm-thick auto-skin graft was performed immediately; (**b**) postoperative 7 days after there was noted good taken appearance without any problems

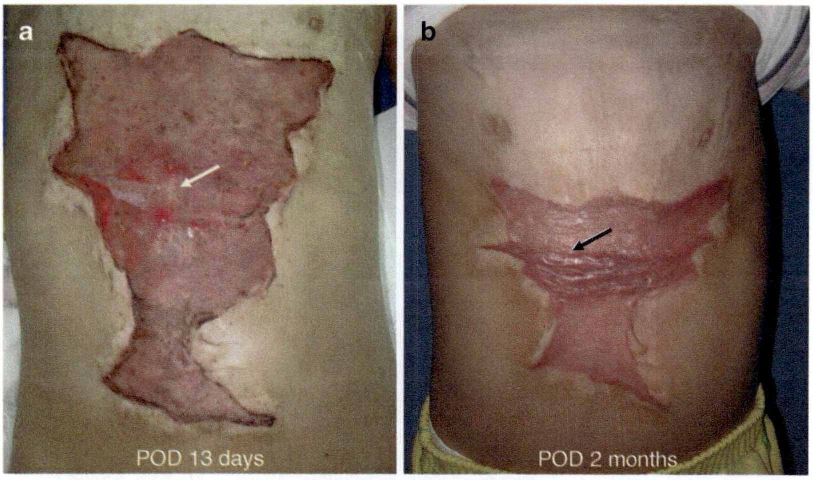

Fig. 3.94 (**a**) Postoperative 13 days later, unstable inflammatory lesion (white arrow) was noted on right middle area but eventually healed without skin loss. (**b**) Postoperative 2 months later, marked re-contracted lesion with hypertrophic scarring (black arrow) was noted, and also whole engrafted area was contracted

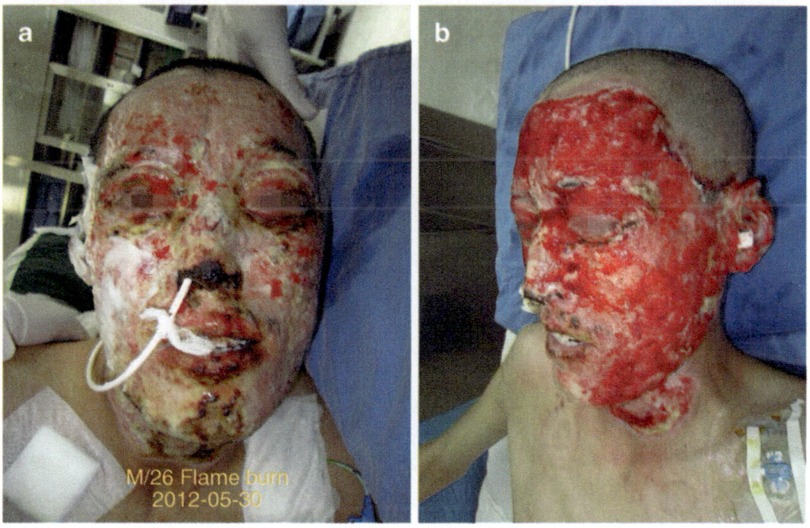

Fig. 3.95 (**a**) Postburn day 12, he was transferred to our department. (**b**) Postburn day 16, all necrotic tissue was debrided, preoperative view, 2-mm Matriderm® with single-step 0.125-mm-thick auto-sheet engraft was performed

Four days after the procedure, the engrafted Matriderm and the thin autograft were completely removed, with no engrafted skin loss. The skin was divided and engrafted according to the esthetic unit on the face. One month after surgery, lower lid ectropion, loss of both ala nasi, and microstomia on the upper and lower lips developed. We planned a reconstructive surgery for correction of these deformities (Figs. 3.95, 3.96, 3.97). After 2.5 years of the procedure, both lower lid ectropion were corrected using thick STSG and corrective FTSG on the anterior neck, and the lower lip area was corrected with thick STSG. Both eyebrow reconstructions were performed with single-hair transplantation techniques under local anesthesia. In the future, we intend to correct the upper lip and reconstruct the philtrum with a triangular fossa from the ear using a composite graft (Fig. 3.98).

A 59-year-old male patient suffered a 22,000-volt electrical burn. The inlet was discovered on the right thumb and mummified in a nonviable state. Immediate escharotomy was performed to prevent the compartment syndrome. Eighteen days after the procedure, a 1-mm-thick Matriderm was applied. One year after the procedure, good skin texture and color match were observed with no functional disruption. Pinching the engrafted

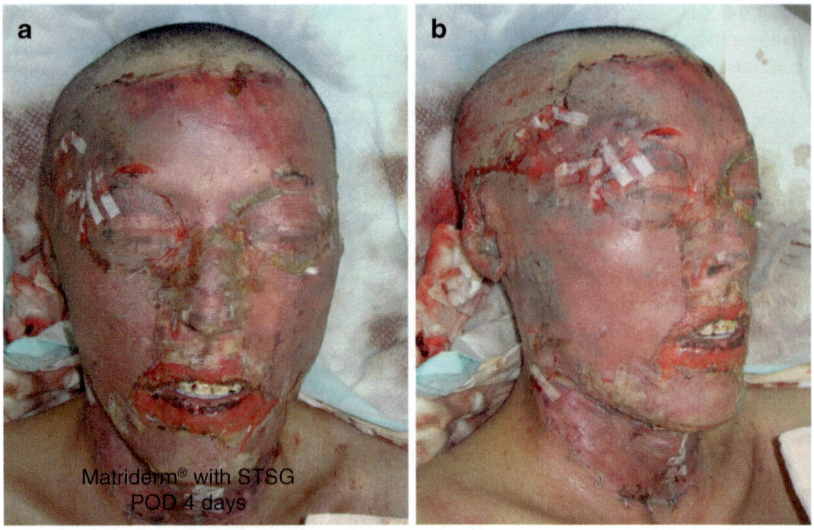

Fig. 3.96 (**a, b**) Four days after procedure, the engrafted Matriderm® and thin autograft were taken with no eventually. The engraftment was divided engraft according to esthetic unit on the face

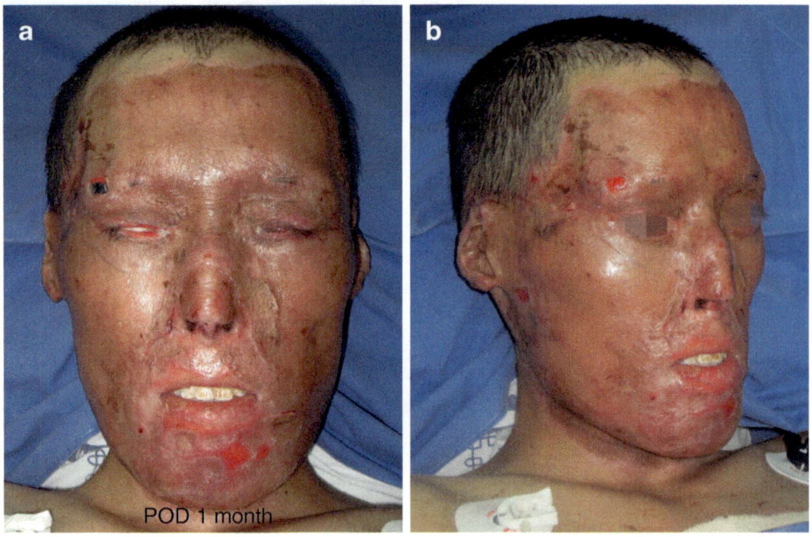

Fig. 3.97 (**a, b**) Postoperative 1 month later, lower lid ectropion, loss of both ala nasi, and developed microstomia on the upper and lower lips were noted

skin revealed good skin texture and elasticity (Figs. 3.99, 3.100, 3.101, 3.102). In this case, the Matriderm was very effective on the massive burn injury, hospitalization time was reduced with a single-step operation, and good skin texture and elasticity were observed.

As introduced above, a wide variety of artificial dermal products are being developed, and the frequency of their application is rapidly increasing. However, these uses require a learning curve and are still expensive treatments. Thus, its advantages and disadvantages should be considered before using them. The various types of artificial dermis I have used have their own unique strengths and weaknesses [76–78]. Rather than recommending one, selection of the most suitable option will have to be made according to the characteristics of the wound and situation. To briefly summarize my experience,

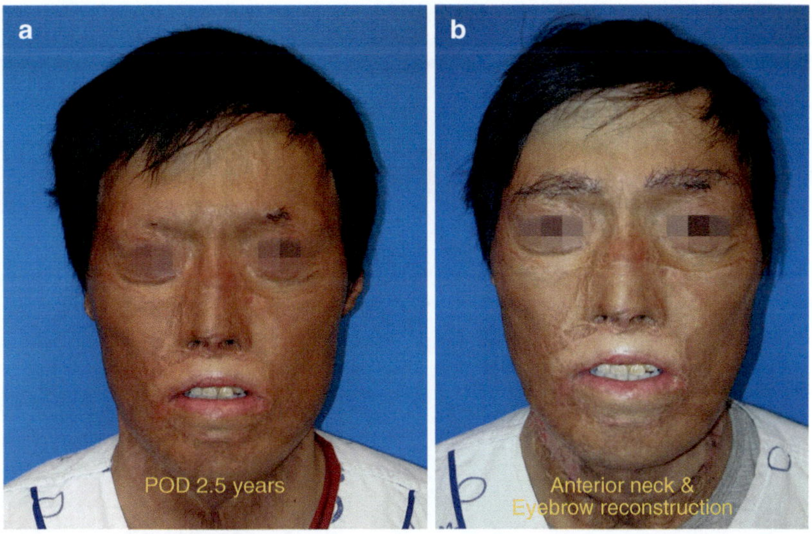

Fig. 3.98 (**a**) Postoperative 2.5 years view, lower lid was corrected with thick STSG; (**b**) anterior neck was corrected with FTSG and eye brow reconstruction with single-hair transplantation. Remark: He received FTSG on the upper lip area in another hospital. Notice and compare with upper and lower lip difference of dimensional contour

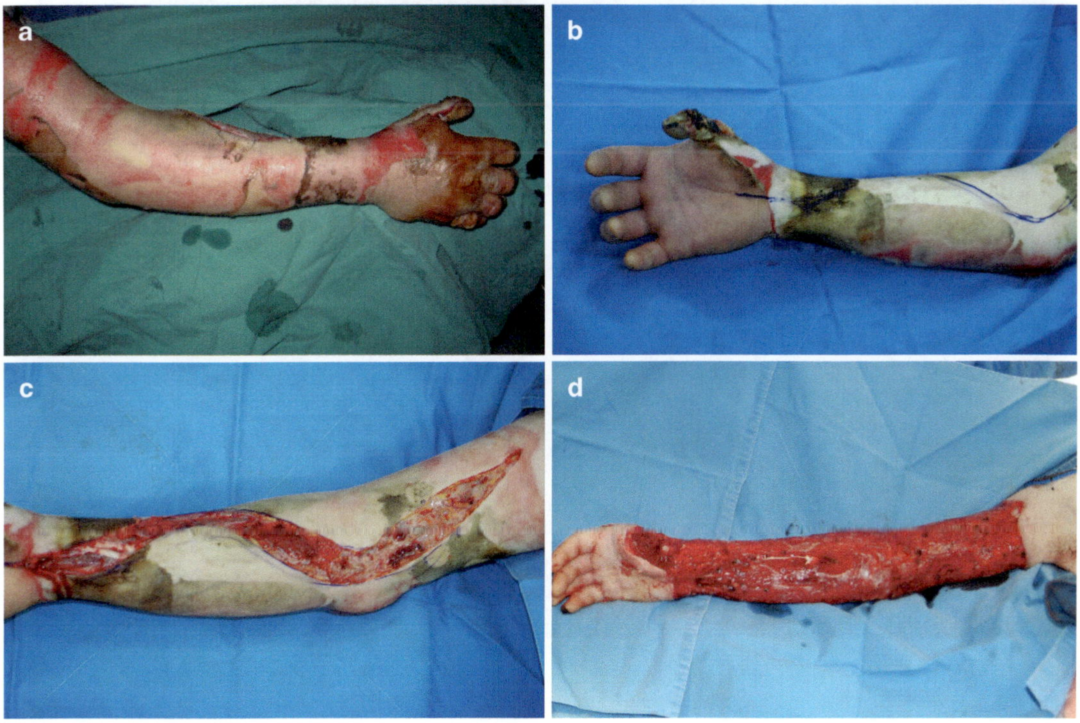

Fig. 3.99 (**a**) 22,000-volt electrical burn was noted full-thickness thermal burn. (**b**) The inlet was noted right thumb and mummified nonviable state. (**c**) Immediate escharotomy to prevent compartment syndrome. (**d**) Postburn day 18, escharectomy was performed to prepare Matriderm application

1. In order to use dermal substitutes, a learning curve required for skill acquisition is essential. In my experience, the most important aspect is to gain professional knowledge on wound management, which is an integral element of infection, bleeding, and dressing control.

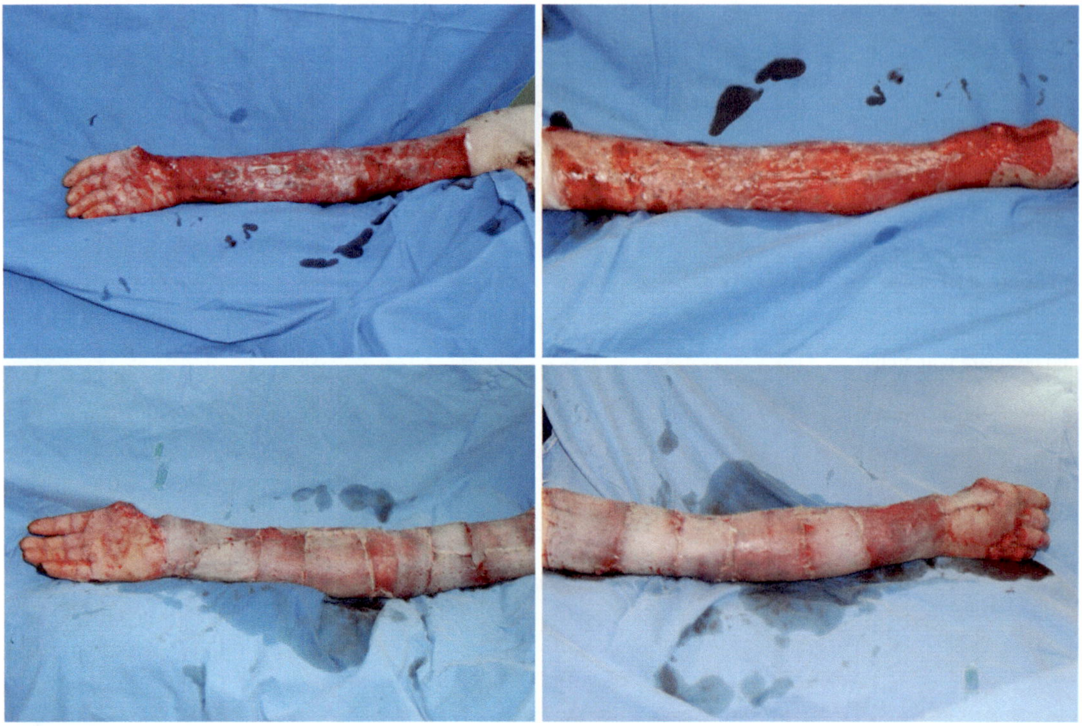

Fig. 3.100 1-mm Matriderm with 0.2-mm-thick sheet autograft was performed

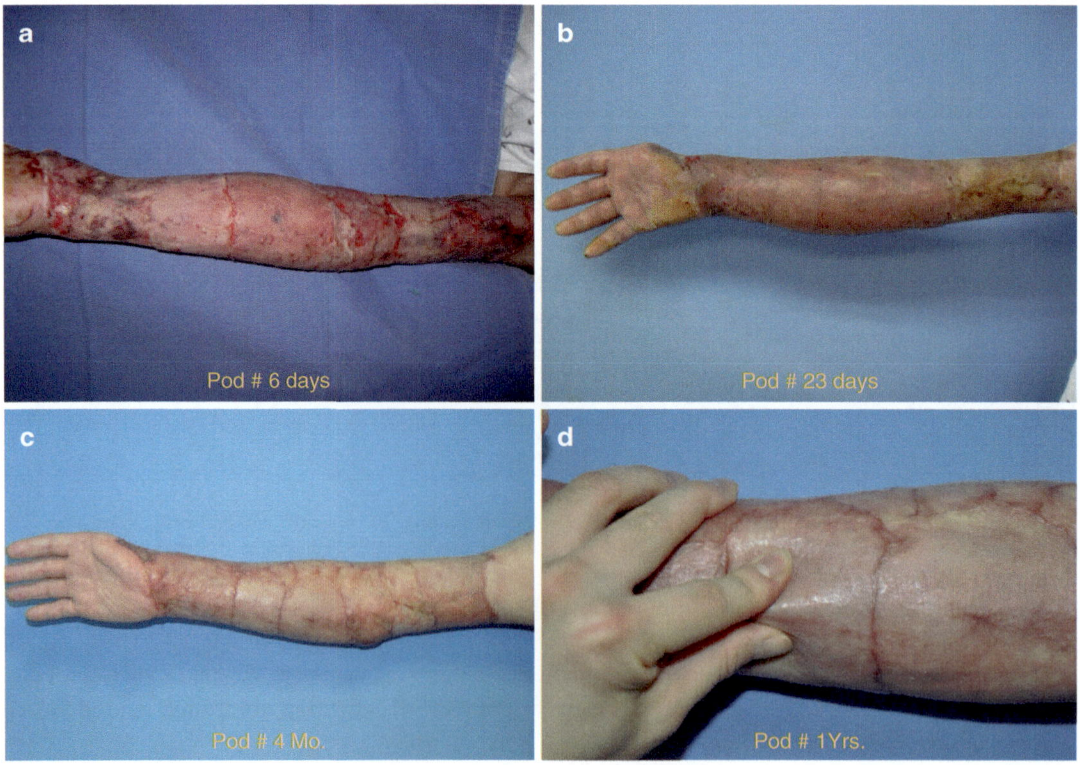

Fig. 3.101 (**a**) Postoperative 6 days, (**b**) 23 days, (**c**) 4 months, and (**d**)1 year after view

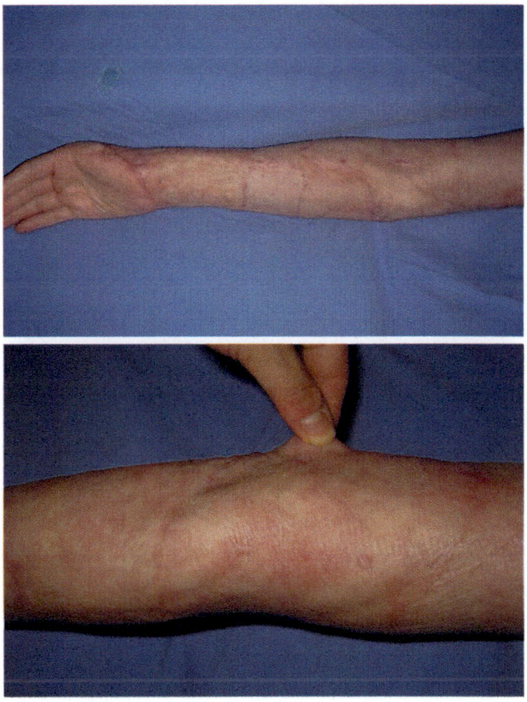

Fig. 3.102 Postoperative 1 year after, good skin texture and color match without functional disturbance. Pinching the engrafted skin revealed good skin texture and elasticity

2. In order to increase the success rate of the dermal substitutes, caution should be taken to not allow it to completely cover the wound surface, if possible, so that the gap of graft to graft does not widen. So, as to cover the artificial dermis, the lower surface of the wound should be staunched thoroughly, and, if possible, a compressive elastic net (Surginet®) should be used to fix the lower surface and maintain it well in order to prevent hematomas and fluid collection from forming. If possible, observe the condition of the wound every day, and if signs of infection or suspicious infections are noted, remove the silicone layer from the infected area immediately, and create an open window through which to apply antibacterial dressing material Sulfamylon® solution, or proceed with simple compressive dressing with saline-soaked gauze twice a day.
3. Use of a human dermal matrix is highly recommended for areas with exposed ligaments and bone where skin engraftment is difficult or with signs of infection [79]. In my experience, it can be especially beneficial for chronic wound management in such cases as limb salvage, diabetic wounds, and osteomyelitis [80, 81].
4. Integra is very useful in complementing the concept of early excision and grafting in the treatment of major burns. However, it is very susceptible to infection; hence, the wound should be checked daily at least for 10 days or longer, and the necessary dressing should be applied until the neodermis is formed. My evaluation of long-term biopsy for Integra® showed that the structure and properties of collagen remained even for several years, and the graft contracture rate was less than those of other pure synthetics, such as Pelnac, Terudermis®, and Matriderm®. It can be very useful in reconstructive surgery, especially for breast reconstruction that needs a wide and three-dimensional moveable area.
5. Matriderm's key feature is the ability to perform a single-step surgery, and recently, other businesses have started to develop and produce products with similar capabilities. However, a detailed analysis of the engrafted contracture rate with long-term follow-up is still needed. Furthermore, the effects of usage on different anatomical regions and in late deformity reconstruction and the comparison of the intake and contracture rates for the 1-mm and 2-mm options still need to be established. In my experience, I found no significant difference in the intake and contracture rates between the two thicknesses.
6. Since the condition of a very thin autograft is much more vulnerable to external stimuli than a general skin graft, meticulous postoperative skin care is essential. When maceration is observed, wound healing should be actively facilitated, or wound covering should be conducted to prevent damage to the newly formed dermis, so that the engrafted contracture rate can be reduced. For adjuvant therapy, pressure garments or silastic gel sheets and laser therapies are essential in reducing the engrafted contracture rate and enhancing the scar maturation.
7. By using the VAC system, which has recently gained research attention for its high efficacy

in promoting wound healing, the engraftment period of the artificial dermis can be shortened significantly, hematomas can be prevented, and the risk of infection can be reduced, resulting in better results.

3.9 Conclusion

In recent years, a wide variety of dermal substitutes have been developed and have been very useful in clinical practice. However, only an insufficient amount of information has been established about their costs and the surgical outcomes after their application, which could help in assessing their overall advantages and disadvantages and in their more effective and appropriate application. I have participated in the early clinical trials of Integra® since 1996 and have described the use, advantages, and disadvantages through long-term follow-up and clinical experiences of most of the products developed so far. However, many controversies remain, and standard guidelines have not been established. Although the introduction to these products through my experience may be controversial depending on the pros and cons, the technique and results of the clinical trials are worth noting. In particular, I have extensively compared Integra and AlloDerm, which have been introduced in the initial development, and described their advantages and disadvantages, as well as the long-term follow-up results, and introduced guidelines for their extended applications to more variable conditions. Viewed specifically from a plastic surgery perspective, Integra obtained remarkable results for especially breast reconstruction and other soft and three-dimensional wide regions. The human dermal matrix, which is composed of completely different materials and suitable for single-step operation, presents the disadvantage of having to attach smaller pieces individually and is expensive compared to relatively synthetic dermal substitutes. However, it is very useful for special cases, such as in the treatment of a diabetic foot or a difficult wound where the bone and tendons are exposed. In addition, it has been introduced as a new treatment due to the remarkable results in several cases of chronic osteomyelitis I had encountered in clinical practice. Matriderm® has been recently manufactured specifically for a single-step operation to overcome the shortcomings of dermal substitutes using animal collagen, and I have described here my clinical experience with the product. Moreover, the uses of Terudermis® and Pelnac®, which were developed in Japan and used in some Asian countries, were also briefly described. This discussion on dermal substitutes in the context of my clinical experience emphasizes the importance of determining their correct usage by determining their material composition and various properties.

Although new dermal replacement systems are being continuously introduced, the development of a purely artificial skin graft is still a distant prospect. Thus, I will finish this chapter with earnest anticipation for groundbreaking research and development in the near future.

The author found through a recent analysis of postburn scars following treatment with dermal substitutes that, when compared with STSG or conservative treatment, treatment with dermal substitutes produced regeneration that was closer to the natural skin in elastin, collagen III, stromal CD31, and α-SMA; CD31 vessel width and stromal α-SMA; vessel quantity and width; and laminin. This chapter thus articulates evidence of the important role of dermal substitutes in the development of future burn treatments.

References

1. Yannas IV, Orgill DP, Burke JF. Template for skin regeneration. Plast Reconstr Surg. 2011;127(Suppl 1):60S–70S.
2. Chang DK, Louis MR, Gimenez A, Reece EM. The basics of integra dermal regeneration template and its expanding clinical applications. Semin Plast Surg. 2019;33(3):185–9.
3. Heimbach D, Luterman A, Burke J, Cram A, Herndon D, Hunt J, Jordan M, McManus W, Solem L, Warden G, et al. Artificial dermis for major burns. A multi-center randomized clinical trial. Ann Surg. 1988;208(3):313–20.
4. Wainwright DJ. Use of an acellular allograft dermal matrix (AlloDerm) in the management of full-thickness burns. Burns. 1995;21(4):243–8.

5. Shin HS, Kim MK, Lee JW, Jang YC, Kim DC. Clinical experience in reconstruction of post burn scar contracture using AlloDerm. J Korean Soc Aesthet Plast Surg. 1999;5(1):147.
6. Tsai CC, Lin SD, Lai CS, Lin TM. The use of composite acellular allodermis-ultrathin autograft on joint area in major burn patients—one year follow-up. Kaohsiung J Med Sci. 1999;15(11):651–8.
7. Winfrey ME, Cochran M, Hegarty MT. A new technology in burn therapy: INTEGRA artificial skin. Dimens Crit Care Nurs. 1999;18(1):14–20.
8. Dantzer E. Role of skin substitutes in surgical repair of the sequelae of burn injuries. Ann Chir Plast Esthet. 2011;56(5):369–81; (We review the technical characteristics of collagen matrixes (Intégra(®)—Matriderm(®)) and their method of use).
9. Jackson SR, Roman S. Matriderm and split skin grafting for full-thickness pediatric facial burns. J Burn Care Res. 2019;40(2):251–4.
10. Demircan M, Cicek T, Yetis MI. Preliminary results in single-step wound closure procedure of full-thickness facial burns in children by using the collagen-elastin matrix and review of pediatric facial burns. Burns. 2015;41(6):1268–74.
11. Shakespeare P. Burn wound healing and skin substitutes. Burns. 2001;27(5):517–22.
12. Ayaz M, Najafi A, Karami MY. Thin split thickness skin grafting on human acellular dermal matrix scaffold for the treatment of deep burn wounds. Int J Organ Transplant Med. 2021;12(1):44–51.
13. Lataillade JJ, Bey E, Thepenier C, Prat M, Leclerc T, Bargues L. Skin engineering for burns treatment bull. Acad Natl Med. 2010;194(7):1339–51.
14. Henning JA, Liette MD, Laklouk M, Fadel M, Masadeh S. The role of dermal regenerative templates in complex lower extremity wounds. Clin Podiatr Med Surg. 2020;37(4):803–20.
15. Liu Y, Panayi AC, Bayer LR, Orgill DP. Current available cellular and tissue-based products for treatment of skin defects. Adv Skin Wound Care. 2019;32(1):19–25.
16. Juhasz I, Kiss B, Lukacs L, Erdei I, Peter Z, Remenyik E. Long-term followup of dermal substitution with acellular dermal implant in burns and postburn scar corrections. Dermatol Res Pract. 2010;2010:210150.
17. Téot L, Otman S, Trial C, Brancati A. The use of non-cellularized artificial dermis in the prevention of scar contracture and hypertrophy. Wound Repair Regen. 2011;19(Suppl 1):s49–58.
18. Moyer HR, Yezhelyev M, Ingram WL. Bilayer dermal matrix for the treatment of painful burn scars. Wounds. 2011;23(8):236–42.
19. Jones JE, Nelson EA, Al-Hity A. Skin grafting for venous leg ulcers. Cochrane Database Syst Rev. 2013;2013(1):CD001737.
20. Chalmers RL, Smock E, Geh JL. Experience of Integra(®) in cancer reconstructive surgery. J Plast Reconstr Aesthet Surg. 2010;63(12):2081–90.
21. Opoku-Agyeman J, Humenansky K, Davis W 3rd, Glat P. Use of integra for reconstruction after nevi resection: a systematic review and pooled analysis of reported cases. Surg Res Pract. 2019;2019:9483627.
22. Schiestl C, Stiefel D, Meuli M. Giant naevus, giant excision, eleg(i)ant closure? Reconstructive surgery with integra artificial skin to treat giant congenital melanocytic naevi in children. J Plast Reconstr Aesthet Surg. 2010;63(4):610–5.
23. Goodarzi P, Falahzadeh K, Nematizadeh M, Farazandeh P, Payab M, Larijani B, Tayanloo Beik A, Arjmand B. Tissue engineered skin substitutes. Adv Exp Med Biol. 2018;1107:143–88.
24. Dai C, Shih S, Khachemoune A. Skin substitutes for acute and chronic wound healing: an updated review. J Dermatolog Treat. 2020;31(6):639–48.
25. Gonzalez SR, Wolter KG, Yuen JC. Infectious complications associated with the use of integra: a systematic review of the literature. Plast Reconstr Surg Glob Open. 2020;8(7):e2869.
26. Boyce ST, Kagan RJ, Meyer NA, Yakuboff KP, Warden GD. The 1999 clinical research award. Cultured skin substitutes combined with integra artificial skin to replace native skin autograft and allograft for the closure of excised full-thickness burns. J Burn Care Rehabil. 1999;20(6):453–61.
27. Sarkozyova N, Dragunova J, Bukovcan P, Ferancikova N, Breza J, Zilinska Z, Koller J. Preparation and processing of human allogenic dermal matrix for utilization in reconstructive surgical procedures. Bratisl Lek Listy. 2020;121(6):386–94.
28. Bello YM, Falabella AF, Eaglstein WH. Tissue-engineered skin. Current status in wound healing. Am J Clin Dermatol. 2001;2(5):305–13; (basement membr).
29. Burm JS, Chung CH, Oh SJ. Fist position for skin grafting on the dorsal hand: I. Analysis of length of the dorsal hand surgery in hand positions. Plast Reconstr Surg. 1999;104(5):1350–5.
30. Robinson EP, Chhabra AB. Hand chemical burns. J Hand Surg Am. 2015;40(3):605–12; quiz 613.
31. Choi M, Armstrong MB, Panthaki ZJ. Pediatric hand burns: thermal, electrical, chemical. J Craniofac Surg. 2009;20(4):1045–8.
32. Barret JP, Dziewulski P, McCauley RL, Herndon DN, Desai MH. Dural reconstruction of a class IV calvarial burn with decellularized human dermis. Burns. 1999;25(5):459–62.
33. Chun MK, Jang YC, Ko JH, Seo DK, Lee JW, Choi JK. Reconstruction of the bone exposed soft tissue defects in lower extremities using artificial dermis (AlloDerm). J Korean Soc Plast Reconstr Surg. 2009;36(5):578–82.
34. Soldatos NK, Stylianou P, Koidou VP, Angelov N, Yukna R, Romanos GE. Limitations and options using resorbable versus nonresorbable membranes for successful guided bone regeneration. Quintessence Int. 2017;48(2):131–47.
35. Kantak NA, Mistry R, Varon DE, Halvorson EG. Negative pressure wound therapy for burns. Clin Plast Surg. 2017;44(3):671–7; (vac).

36. Menn ZK, Lee E, Klebuc MJ. Acellular dermal matrix and negative pressure wound therapy: a tissue-engineered alternative to free tissue transfer in the compromised host. J Reconstr Microsurg. 2012;28(2):139–44.
37. Leffler M, Horch RE, Dragu A, Bach AD. The use of the artificial dermis (integra) in combination with vacuum assisted closure for reconstruction of an extensive burn scar—a case report. J Plast Reconstr Aesthet Surg. 2010;63(1):e32–5.
38. Ribeiro LM, Serras R, Guimarães D, Vilela M, Mouzinho MM. Bilateral third-degree burn of the legs: lower limb salvage with dermal regenerative matrix. Ann Burn Fire Disasters. 2018;31(3):228–32.
39. Aguilera-Saez J, Lopez-Masramon B, Collado JM, Monte-Soldado A, Rivas-Nicolls D, Serracanta J, Barret JP. Severely damaged lower limb salvage in a critically ill burned patient. Lessons learned. Int J Burn Trauma. 2020;10(5):191–200.
40. Dalla Paola L, Cimaglia P, Carone A, Boscarino G, Scavone G. Use of integra dermal regeneration template for limb salvage in diabetic patients with no-option critical limb ischemia. Int J Low Extrem Wounds. 2021;20(2):128–34.
41. Ali B, Wu J, Borah G, Wu E. Temporary use of acellular dermal matrix in upper extremity salvage. Plast Reconstr Surg Glob Open. 2020;8(7):e2965.
42. Walden JL, Garcia H, Hawkins H, Crouchet JR, Traber L, Gore DC. Both dermal matrix and epidermis contribute to an inhibition of wound contraction. Ann Plast Surg. 2000;45(2):162–6.
43. Karakol P, Bozkurt M. Recent strategic approach in postburn extremity scars and contractures. J Plast Surg Hand Surg. 2021;55(3):153–61.
44. Guo X, Mu D, Gao F. Efficacy and safety of acellular dermal matrix in diabetic foot ulcer treatment: a systematic review and meta-analysis. Int J Surg. 2017;40:1–7.
45. Campitiello F, Mancone M, Cammarota M, D'Agostino A, Ricci G, Stellavato A, Della Corte A, Pirozzi AVA, Scialla G, Schiraldi C, Canonico S. Acellular dermal matrix used in diabetic foot ulcers: clinical outcomes supported by biochemical and histological analyses. Int J Mol Sci. 2021;22(13):7085.
46. Winters CL, Brigido SA, Liden BA, Simmons M, Hartman JF, Wright ML. A multicenter study involving the use of a human acellular dermal regenerative tissue matrix for the treatment of diabetic lower extremity wounds. Adv Skin Wound Care. 2008;21(8):375–81.
47. Sefton MV, Woodhouse KA. Tissue engineering. J Cutan Med Surg. 1998;3 Suppl 1:S1-18-23.
48. Bessho K, Murakami K, Iizuka T. The use of a new bilayer artificial dermis for vestibular extension. Br J Oral Maxillofac Surg. 1998;36(6):457–9.
49. Hori K, Osada A, Isago T, Sakurai H. Comparison of contraction among three dermal substitutes: morphological differences in scaffolds. Burns. 2017;43(4):846–51; Multicenter study.
50. Shin HS, Lee JW, Jang YC. Clinical experiences in acute burns using Integra® artificial skin. J Korean Burn Soc. 2000;3(1):1.
51. Cho YH, Lee JW, Oh SJ, Jang YC. Clinical experiences of artificial dermis, Integra® in acute burn on hand and foot. J Korean Soc Reconstr Hand Surg. 2001;6(2):1.
52. Lee JW, Jang YC, Oh SJ. Use of the artificial dermis for free radial forearm flap donor site. Ann Plast Surg. 2005;55(5):500–2.
53. Jang YC, Lee JW, Han KW, Han TH. Burns in epilepsy: seven years of experience from the Hallym burn center in Korea. J Burn Care Res. 2006;27(6):877–81.
54. Khan S, White PM, Street JH 3rd, Light TD, Jordan MH. Seven years' experience with integra as a reconstructive tool. J Burn Care Res. 2007;28(1):120–6.
55. Afshari A, Nguyen L, Kahn SA, Montgomery AC, Shinha T, Stratton C, Summitt B. The effective duration of antimicrobial activity of mafenide acetate after reconstitution. J Burn Care Res. 2018;39(5):736–8.
56. Kashimura T, Nagasaki K, Horigome M, Yoshida K, Soejima K. Selection of artificial dermis for shortening treatment period: integra versus pelnac. Plast Reconstr Surg Glob Open. 2021;9(6):e3599.
57. Eo SR, Kim YS, Cho SH. Vacuum-assisted closure improves the incorporation of artificial dermis in soft tissue defects: Terudermis(®) and Pelnac(®). Int Wound J. 2011;8(3):261.
58. Stiefel D, Schiestl CM, Meuli M. The positive effect of negative pressure: vacuum-assisted fixation of integra artificial skin for reconstructive surgery. J Pediatr Surg. 2009;44(3):575–80.
59. Scalise A, Torresetti M, Di Benedetto G. Reconstruction of full-thickness soft tissue defects with integra: risk factors and treatment algorithm. Plast Reconstr Surg Glob Open. 2020;8(9):e3099.
60. Martínez L, Ros Z, López-Gutiérrez JC, Díaz M, Quezada B, Perdiguero M, Hernández F, Rivas S, Tovar JA. Integra artificial dermis in pediatric reconstructive surgery. Cir Pediatr. 2002;15(3):97–100.
61. Palao R, Gómez P, Huguet P. Burned breast reconstructive surgery with integra dermal regeneration template. Br J Plast Surg. 2003;56(3):252–9.
62. Tsoutsos D, Stratigos A, Gravvanis A, Zapandioti P, Kakagia D. Burned breast reconstruction by expanded artificial dermal substitute. J Burn Care Res. 2007;28(3):530–2.
63. Gronovich Y, Maisel Lotan A, Retchkiman M. Post-burn breast reconstruction using an artificial dermis-a long-term follow-up. Burns Trauma. 2016;4:12.
64. Ko JH, Lee JW, Jang YC, Oh SJ. Reconstruction of the tibial exposure by using terudermis in extensive deep burned patients on lower extremities. J Korean Burn Soc. 2003;6(2):164.
65. Lee JS, Lee JW, Jang YC, Ha JW. Coverage of donor site defect of radial forearm free flap by using Terudermis®. J Korean Soc Plast Reconstr Surg. 2001;28(3):357.
66. Nam YO, Lee JW, Hyu J, Koh DKS, Oh SJ, Jang YC. Burn management and reconstruction using

artificial dermis Pelnac^{R}. J Korean Burn Soc. 2006;9(2):115–7.
67. Frame JD, Still J, Lakhel-LeCoadou A, Carstens MH, Lorenz C, Orlet H, Spence R, Berger AC, Dantzer E, Burd A. Use of dermal regeneration template in contracture release procedures: a multicenter evaluation. Plast Reconstr Surg. 2004;113(5):1330–8.
68. Yurugi S, Hatoko M, Kuwahara M, Tanaka A, Iioka H, Niitsuma K. Usefulness and limitations of artificial dermis implantation for posttraumatic deformity. Aesthetic Plast Surg. 2002;26(5):360–4.
69. Lisa AVE, Galtelli L, Vinci V, Veronesi A, Cozzaglio L, Cananzi FCM, Sicoli F, Klinger M. Adoption of a newly introduced dermal matrix: preliminary experience and future directions. Biomed Res Int. 2020;2020:3261318.
70. Lyu QB, Xiao GX, Bao YM, Hu L. Analysis of clinical effects of artificial dermis in functional reconstruction in the late stage of extremely severe burn. Zhonghua Shao Shang Za Zhi. 2019;35(7):517–24.
71. Agostinis C, Spazzapan M, Vuerich R, Balduit A, Stocco C, Mangogna A, Ricci G, Papa G, Zacchigna S, Bulla R. Differential capability of clinically employed dermal regeneration scaffolds to support vascularization for tissue bioengineering. Biomedicines. 2021;9(10):1458.
72. Kolokythas P, Aust MC, Vogt PM, Paulsen F. Dermal substitute with the collagen-elastin matrix matriderm in burn injuries: a comprehensive review. Handchir Mikrochir Plast Chir. 2008;40(6):367–71.
73. Ryssel H, Germann G, Kloeters O, Gazyakan E, Radu CA. Dermal substitution with Matriderm(®) in burns on the dorsum of the hand. Burns. 2010;36(8):1248–53.
74. Lamy J, Gourari A, Atlan M, Zakine G. Use of Matriderm® 1mm in reconstructive surgery. Series of 31 cases. Ann Chir Plast Esthet. 2013;58(3):235–42.
75. Ryssel H, Gazyakan E, Germann G, Ohlbauer M. The use of MatriDerm in early excision and simultaneous autologous skin grafting in burns—a pilot study. Burns. 2008;34(1):93–7.
76. Lee MY, Kim H, Kwak IS, Jang Y, Choi Y. Immunohistochemical analysis of postburn scars following treatment using dermal substitutes. Anal Cell Pathol (Amst). 2022;2022:3686863.
77. Kwak IS, Choi YH, Jang YC, Lee YK. Immunohistochemical analysis of neuropeptides (protein gene product 9.5, substance P and calcitonin gene-related peptide) in hypertrophic burn scar with pain and itching. Burns. 2014;40(8):1661–7.
78. Choi YH, Kim KM, Kim HO, Jang YC, Kwak IS. Clinical and histological correlation in post-burn hypertrophic scar for pain and itching sensation. Ann Dermatol. 2013;25(4):428–33.
79. Lucich EA, Rendon JL, Valerio IL. Advances in addressing full-thickness skin defects: a review of dermal and epidermal substitutes. Regen Med. 2018;13(4):443–56.
80. Reyzelman AM, Bazarov I. Human acellular dermal wound matrix for treatment of DFU: literature review and analysis. J Wound Care. 2015;24(3):128; 129-34.
81. Rupert P. Human acellular dermal wound matrix for complex diabetic wounds. J Wound Care. 2016;25(4):S17–8; S20-1.

Cultured Epithelial Cell Therapy

4

4.1 Introduction

Cultured epithelial cell therapy was applied to human clinical studies in 1981 after human keratinocytes were first cultured in 1975 and became a stepping stone for lifesaving treatments for patients with massive burns [1, 2]. Since then, the cultured epithelial homograft (CEH) was developed in 1989 and has been recognized for its usefulness as a wound dressing material (the wound treatment effect of CEH) [3]. However, this homograft is not yet popularized in practice owing to the fact that they are considerably expensive for routine clinical applications and require expertise for successful utilization. In cultured epithelial autograft (CEA), the disappointing take rates fewer than 20% at early stages suggest that additional research and development are required, despite the observation of gradually increasing take rates [4]. Culture techinque still needs to be improved and furter developed to make real dermal-epidermal combination to acheive skin that is closer to real skin structure. This is because CEA needs to be well connected to the epidermal and dermal layers to function in a manner similar to the real skin. For the same, several research and development activities are currently underway; however, we still remain a long way off from reaching our goals [5–9]. Since 2003, the author has conducted clinical trials as a principal investigator of Kaloderm® (TEGO Science, Inc., Seoul, Korea) which is a CEH, under the supervision of the KFDA (Korea Food & Drug Administration, MFDS; Ministry of Food and Drug Safety) [10]. Furthermore, the author has successfully conducted a clinical trial on Holoderm® (TEGO Science, Inc., Seoul, Korea), which is a CEA, as a subsequent clinical research assignment. Since then, the author has researched and developed a cellular spray technique conducting a clinical trial to cover wide surface areas with ease. This method has been proven to show great effects on treatment of patients with massive burns. Furthermore, combination trials which will prove useful in the future are being conducted to apply CEA to second-degree burns, esthetic surgery, and laser therapy, among others, by further expanding the range of applications and by compensating for and reducing the disadvantages of its long cell culture time and high cost. Based on these experiences, the author would be describing a variety of clinical experiences and technical problems arising during the process of these clinical trials.

4.2 Cultured Epithelial Cell Therapy

4.2.1 History of Cultured Epithelial Cell

Cultured epithelial cells, which currently play a very important role in the treatment of burns, were first cultured in 1975 by James Rheinwald and Howard Green, who succeeded in culturing human

Y.-C. Jang, *The Art of Skin Graft*, https://doi.org/10.1007/978-981-97-0017-2_4

keratinocytes [11]. Subsequently, in 1979, they successfully developed keratinocyte sheets that are suitable for grafting after separating keratinocytes from skin tissue and culturing them for approximately 2 weeks. In their experiment, a method for separating keratinocyte sheets from culture plates using an enzyme called dispase was developed, which enabled clinicians to culture and transplant these sheets. The clinical trial involved an animal study in 1980, and a graft to a human body was attempted at Brigham and Women's Hospital in Boston, USA, in 1981 [12, 13]. Since its first successful transplant in a pediatric patient with 95% TBSA (total burn surface area) at the Shriner's Hospital, Boston, in 1984, this graft has been applied in clinical practice worldwide [14, 15]. These can now be obtained with an area 10,000 times the size of the initial skin biopsy (1 cm^2) within 14 days (TEGO Science, Inc.). This indicates how culture techniques have improved to such an extent that it is now possible to cover the entire body surface of a patient in 3–4 weeks, thereby allowing these grafts to play an important role in saving the lives of patients with major burns. The development of cultured keratinocytes began in 1975 with Dr. Rheinwald and Dr. Green, which was first successfully cultured as a graft able sheet in 1979 [16]. Since then, the technology has improved considerably. The first animal study was conducted in 1980 and the human clinical trial study during the following year. In 1984, it was first used in a lifesaving case of a 95% TBSA pediatric patient. Currently, this cell culture technology is commonly used in burn treatment and has gradually extended to esthetic fields as well. In 1989, the CEH was introduced as a temporary wound dressing [17, 18]. The CEH is a type of cultured allograft which is derived from neonatal foreskin.

4.3 Cultured Epithelial Homograft (CEH)

The author has conducted a clinical trial on Kaloderm®, which is a CEH under the supervision of the KFDA (present MFDS) since July 2003.

CEH was developed in 1989 for use as a dressing material in clinical practice [19]. It provides constantly proliferating stem cells which are obtained from infant foreskin. This is not a treatment method in which a graft is integrated into the wound area but instead peels off naturally after temporarily promoting the wound healing process. This is a dressing material, through which temporarily grafted keratinocytes provide various growth factors and cytokines required for wound healing. These then stimulate the cells around the wound to trigger the wound healing process, thereby promoting re-epithelialization [20, 21]. Therefore, although they do not permanently become part of the skin, they can be used flexibly to promptly produce the desired treatment effect by compensating for the biggest disadvantage of CEAs. Furthermore, the culture time required by this graft is at least 2–3 weeks, and it is costly. The possible reasons that an immune response does not occur in CEH are that it typically exists in the epithelium, and Langerhans cells providing antigens to T cells are removed without being attached to plates during culturing. Therefore, the resulting cultured cells do not include Langerhans cells when they are cultured for more than 7 days [22, 23]. This indicates that owing to the not existence of Langerhans cells, which normally present major histocompatibility complex (MHC) class II antigens. Class II HLA-DR antigens are not expressed, thereby preventing immunorejection even though they are not histologically suitable. However, CEHs with an identical HLA (human leukocyte antigen) type are eventually rejected in the human body. If blood group antigens are different from the MHC, CEHs are rejected in 14.5 days after they are grafted to third-degree burns and a donor site, which is as safe as it is 4–5 days later, compared to a human allograft skin (human cadaver skin) graft. DNA analyses, among other tests, have verified that keratinocytes in engrafted homograft are completely substituted by grafted patient cells after a period ranging between 2–4 weeks and 6 months. Therefore, it is imperative to focus on the point where CEHs applied to wounds do not remain grafted, unlike CEAs, but still substantially affect the wound healing process [24].

Before initiating the application of CEH, it is necessary to be familiar with certain concepts owing to the fact that treatment using cultured epithelial cells involves the most important part of biological dressings.

4.3.1 Biological Dressing

The recent trend in wound treatment over the last 20 years has involved the use of synthetic polyurethane dressing materials, which maintain a wet wound condition by increasing oxygen permeability and by retaining water molecules. However, recent research approaches to wound treatment have been focused on wound healing through the use of various substances, including infinitesimal amounts of growth factors and cytokines secreted by various cells, such as fibroblasts, endothelial cells, and macrophages, among others, which play important roles in wound healing. Additionally, autocrine effects on the cells themselves, paracrine effects on the surrounding cells, and endocrine effects on the distant cells of the whole body are utilized [25–27]. The cells directly involved in treatment and changes in the surrounding cell environment have also garnered considerable attention, and thus, many studies have been performed to examine these changes, along with identifying the receptors expressed in cellular membranes, which respond to the various types of extracellular matrices, including collagen, fibrin, fibrinogen, laminin, fibronectin, vitronectin, etc. [28–34]. Furthermore, per the recent trend in wound treatment, numerous studies have also focused on treating wounds by inducing changes in the cells of the surrounding environment of the wounds rather than treating them directly. The author will introduce CEH, which is the primary component of biologic dressings that stimulate and are directly involved in the wound healing process described above.

4.4 CEH: Kaloderm®

The wound healing efficacy of Kaloderm® was validated in the official clinical trial approved by the MFDS in 2003 and showed significant reductions in wound healing time and scar formation, thereby obtaining manufacturing product permission from the MFDS in 2005. Subsequently, its safety and effectiveness have been revalidated through post-marketing surveillance (PMS) over 6 years, and it is the only product in the world covered by national insurance restrictively for certain indications.

Next, the results which were obtained from clinical trials as well as the study results which were helpful in verifying such results are introduced. Kaloderm®, which consists of a CEH, is petrolatum gauze with attached cell sheets acquired through in vitro serial cultivation of keratinocytes up to passage 6 which are isolated from neonatal foreskin tissue obtained from a single donor.

The product is a 7.5 × 7.5 cm cell sheet attached to meshed petrolatum gauze for easier handling. This sheet is made up of five to six keratinocyte cell layers (Fig. 4.1).

Kaloderm® is currently covered by government health insurance in Korea and is widely used as a biological burn wound dressing. Their wound healing mechanisms include secretion of growth factors such as TGF-α, TGF-β, and FGF. These were reported by a molecular biological study to be directly and indirectly involved in the wound healing process, as well as the production of cytokines such as IL-1, IL-6, IL-8, and GM-CSF and also the secretion of the matrix protein fibronectin [35]. Accordingly, they play a role in promoting migration or proliferation of keratinocytes remaining in the wound edge or hair follicles and engage in the wound healing process by stimulating pre-existing stem cells.

The wound healing mechanism of CEH is as follows: it secretes various types of growth factors and cytokines, promotes migration and proliferation of keratinocytes, and also stimulates stem cells on recipient wound bed. In an animal study involving rats, the CEH-treated case had well-regenerated epidermis compared to the non-CEH-treated control case (black arrow) (Fig. 4.2).

The results of the in vitro experimental study on the factors secreted by CEH have been mentioned below (Kaloderm®) In in vitro experimental study (ELSA), we confirmed that there are various growth factors and MMP (matrix metal-

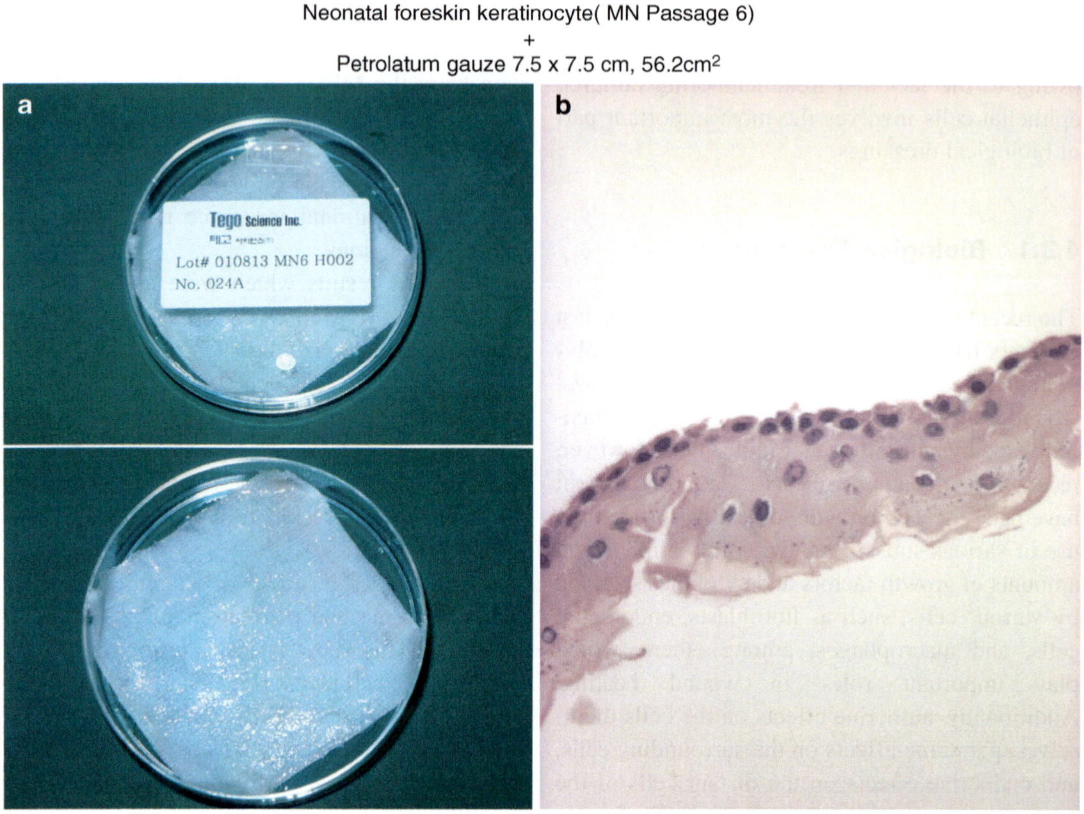

Fig. 4.1 (**a**) This product is 7.5 cm by 7.5 cell sheet attached on the meshed petrolatum gauze for easier handling. (**b**) This sheet is composed of 5 to 6 keratinocyte cell layers

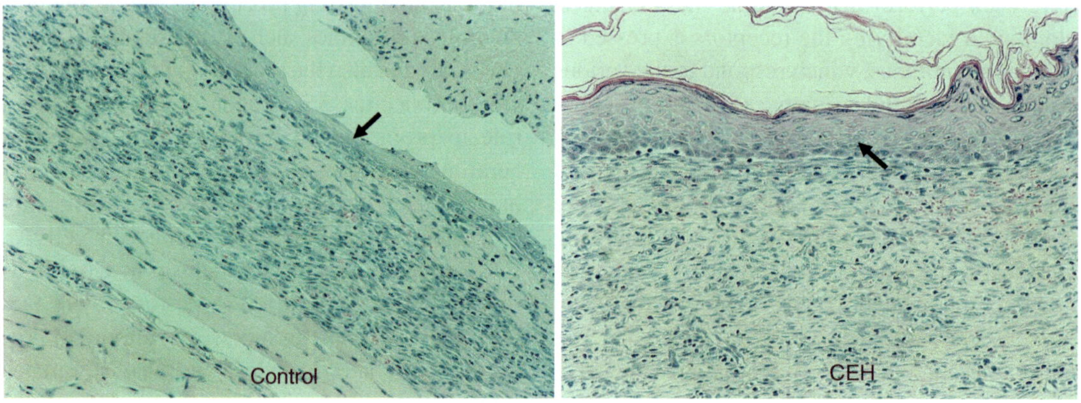

Fig. 4.2 In an animal study involving rats, the CEH-treated case had well-regenerated epidermis compared to the non-CEH-treated control case (black arrow)

loproteinase) and TIMP (tissue inhibitor matrix metalloproteinase) secreted by CEH (Fig. 4.3).

The wound healing mechanism of Kaloderm® acts as a membrane preventing the outflow of moisture in the same manner as other general dressing materials. This property consequently prevents dehydration, protects wounds from infections or physical stimuli, and ensures the timely supply of the appropriate amount of proteins required in the entire wound healing process.

Secreted Factors by CEH (Kaloderm®)

bFGF	3790.9 pg
IL-1α	4496.0 pg
PDGF-BB	89.3 pg
TGF-α	1698.4 pg
TGF-β	359.0 pg
VEGF	4142.0 pg
MMP2	316.0 ng
MMP9	109.3 ng
TIMP1	258.9 ng
TIMP2	913.8 ng

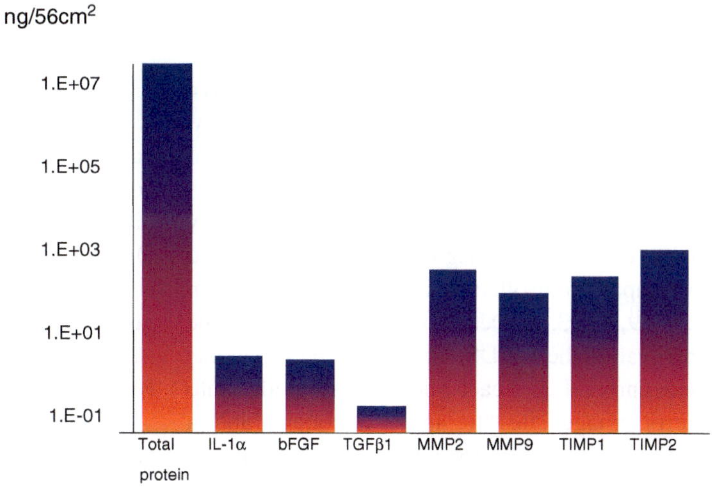

Fig. 4.3 In in vitro experimental study (ELSA), we confirmed that there are various growth factors and MMP (matrix metalloproteinase) and TIMP (tissue inhibitor matrix metalloproteinase) secreted by CEH

Wound healing progresses through the processes of (1) inflammatory reaction, (2) cell proliferation, and (3) cellular and tissue remodeling, where cytokines and extracellular matrixes are secreted in large amounts, which promote the proliferation and migration of undamaged stem cells from the areas surrounding the wound and the sebaceous organs of the skin, such as hair follicles, sebaceous gland, sweat gland, etc., and stimulate fibroblasts, which induce the synthesis of extracellular matrices, such as collagen. Additionally, they secrete matrix metalloproteinase including MMP1, MMP2, and MMP9 and also secrete TIMP (tissue inhibitor matrix metalloproteinase) 1 and 2 to regulate excessive synthesis of collagen, thereby inhibiting the production of hypertrophic scars. However, considering that Kaloderm® is also effective for the treatment of diabetic ulcers, diabetic foot ulcers were added to its indications in 2010, and from 2011, they have been sold in various sizes (9, 16, 25, and 56 cm²). Accordingly, they are currently being used for burns and diabetic foot ulcers in burn centers and in general hospitals across the country, as well as for treatment of skin damage, such as ulcers, abrasion wounds, and laser therapy.

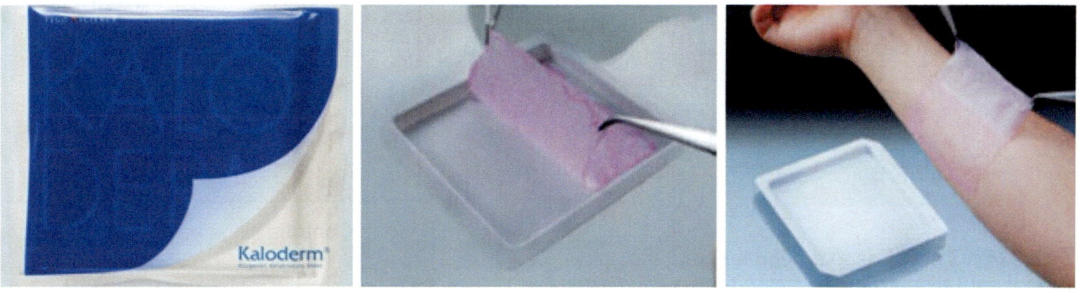

(Photo. 1)

1. The appearance of the package.
2. Kaloderm in the form of sheets.
3. An example of a clinical application.

Epithelial cell therapy, CEH in particular, is available immediately for the treatment of burns or foot ulcers, without the waiting time of >2 weeks for the culture. They can also be used to promote cornea or skin regeneration after laser therapy, as a tool for cosmetic surgery and for gene therapy. Therefore, the demand for the product is expected to further increase progressively.

For CEH, the phase III clinical trial for efficacy and safety on second-degree burns was conducted to compare controlled sites on each patient from July 29, 2003 to December 29, 2003 with the approval of the MFDS. Thirty-five burn patients were enrolled, and each subject was divided into mirror image sites to apply a control and a CEH. Effectiveness was compared in 33 subjects (excluding three dropouts), and the results indicated that the median healing time to 100% re-epithelialization was 11 days for the control and 7.5 days for the CEH, showing a significant improvement in healing time in the CEH group.

Clinical outcomes of trial of Kaloderm® (Figs. 4.4 and 4.5).

A phase III clinical trial of Kaloderm® for efficacy and safety on deep second-degree burns was conducted at the single burn center of Hangang Sacred Heart Hospital from July 29, 2003, to December 29, 2003. The results showed that the control group took 11 days and the Kaloderm® group took 7.5 days to heal, indicating that the healing process was faster (by 3.5 days) in the Kaloderm® group.

This is a summary of the CEH clinical trial study conducted between 2003 and 2004 in order to obtain approval from the MFDS (former Korea Food and Drug Administration).

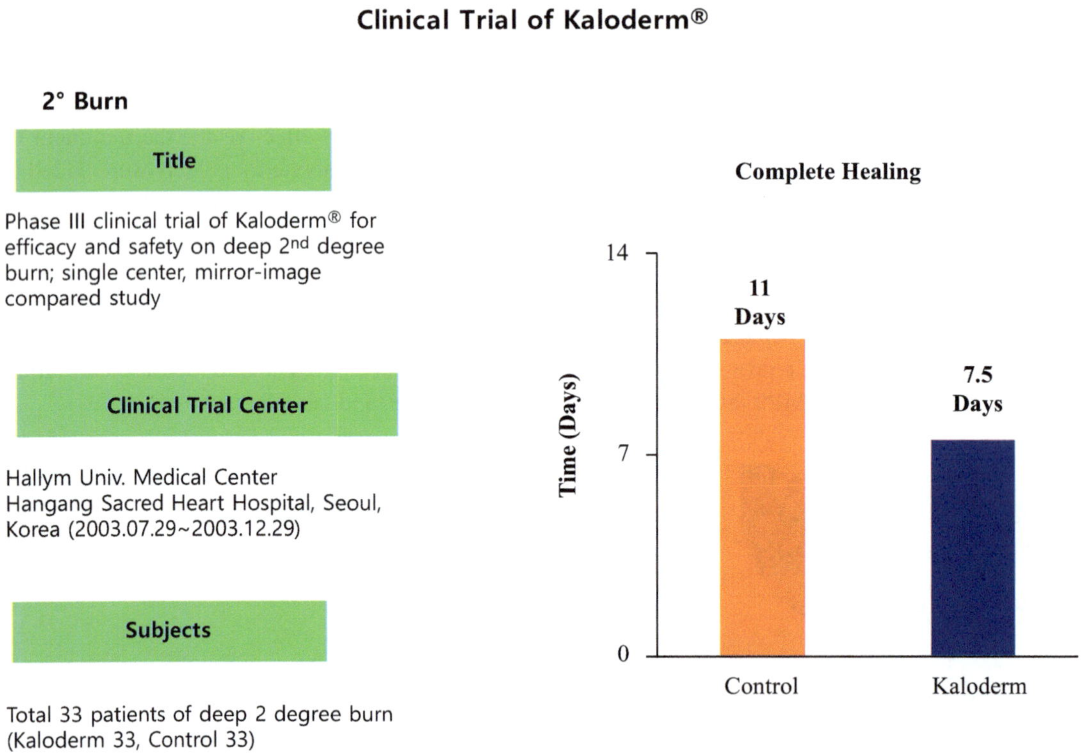

Fig. 4.4 A phase III clinical trial of Kaloderm® for efficacy and safety on deep second-degree burns was conducted at the single burn center of Hangang Sacred Heart Hospital from July 29, 2003, to December 29, 2003. The results showed that the control group took 11 days and the Kaloderm® group took 7.5 days to heal, indicating that the healing process was faster (by 3.5 days) in the Kaloderm® group

Result (Sheet Type of CEH)

(July 2003 – Jan. 2004)

• Number of Patients	35
• Mean Age (yrs)	26.3 (1-80)
• Mean TBSA burned (%)	5.9±3.7
• Mean size of CEHs used (cm²)	58.9±57.3
• Mean healing days(CEH)	8.3±2.8
• Mean healing days(control group)	11.7±3.3

Fig. 4.5 This is a summary of the CEH clinical trial study conducted between 2003 and 2004 in order to obtain approval from the MFDS (former Korea Food and Drug Administration). A total of 35 subjects were included in the study, and the mean healing time was 8.3 days for the CEH group and 11.7 days for the control group. It is approved by the KFDA and covered by the National Health Insurance Reimbursement Program for treating patients with minor second-degree burns and major burns

A total of 35 subjects were included in the study, and the mean healing time was 8.3 days for the CEH group and 11.7 days for the control group. It is approved by the KFDA and covered by the National Health Insurance Reimbursement Program for treating patients with minor second-degree burns and major burns.

In this section, clinical experiences encountered while conducting the clinical trial are introduced.

A 2-year-old female patient suffered a scalding burn on the left dorsum of her foot, which was accompanied by deep second-degree burns. The use of CEH and Acticoat® (Smith & Nephew, England) was planned 3 days post-injury after reduction in exudation and edema, and a comparative clinical trial was conducted as an experimental comparison with Acticoat®, which is a nanocrystal silver dressing material. As a result, CEH treatment of the burn site was completed on post-burn day 13, whereas Acticoat® treatment was completed on post-burn day over 16, indicating that CEH is effective for second-degree burn treatment (Fig. 4.6).

Meanwhile, in a study on split-thickness skin graft (STSG) donor-site healing, the wound healing process with CEH progressed rapidly, even for a 76-year-old patient, showing 70% healing on day 3 of its application (Fig. 4.7) and complete healing on day 8. The control site (Fig. 4.8a (black arrow)) was healed completely 5 days later on day 13 (Fig. 4.8c (black arrow)), demonstrating that CEH's epithelialization ability was excellent (Fig. 4.8).

In another case of donor-site healing, there was a difference of 4–5 days because the complete healing time was 8 and 12 days in the CEH and control groups, respectively. A 66-year-old female patient with a STSG donor site participated in a comparative study. Two days after the exudate controlled on donor, CEH was applied on the left half side (dashed line) of the STSG donor site (black arrow) only. Seven days later, the left CEH site was completely healed compared to the right side with a simple dressing of petrolatum gauze, indicating that the CEH-treated site healed faster than the control site by 5 days (Fig. 4.9).

In terms of the wound healing effect of CEH, recovery was proven to be rapid, even in the thick-split donor site of 0.5 mm 20/1000 in. This suggests that CEH can play an important role in the wound healing process along with epithelialization. A thick, split-thickness donor site (0.5 mm thickness) was noted postoperatively. Two days after the surgery, the discharge noticeably diminished and CEH was applied. After 8 days, the wound healing process and epithelialization of the CEH-treated site were observed to be faster than those of any other thick-split donor sites. Eighteen days after CEH application, the donor site appeared to have a quick and stable wound healing process (Fig. 4.10).

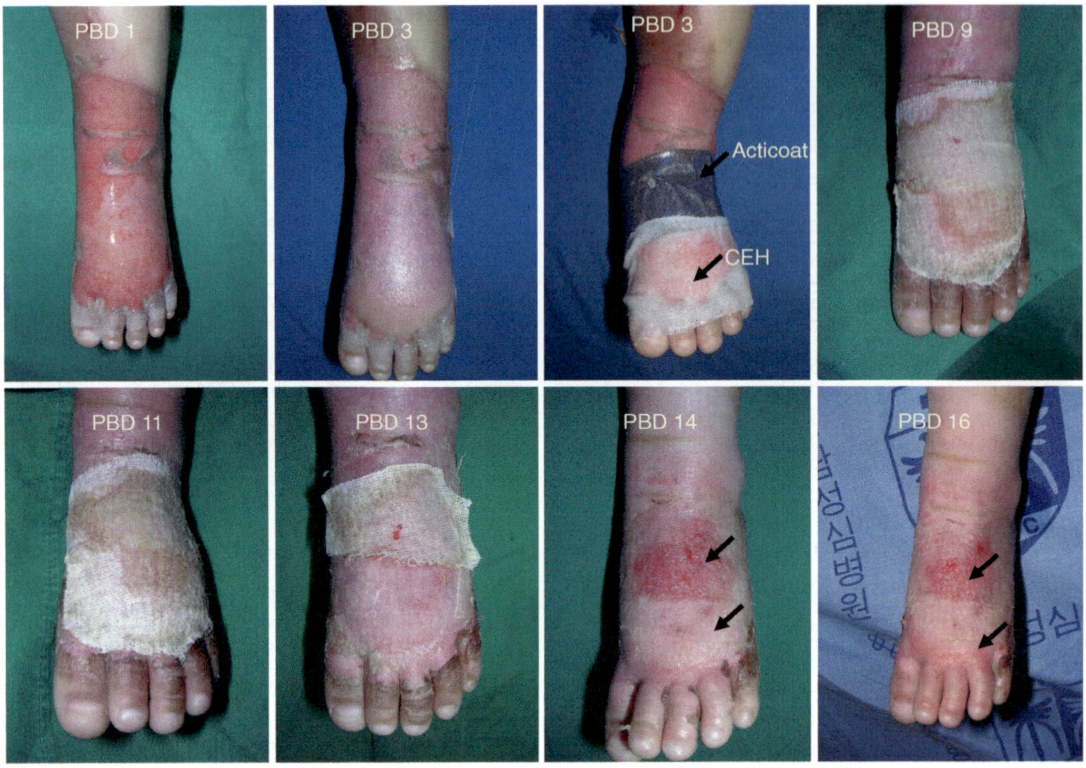

Fig. 4.6 Deep second-degree scalding burn on left dorsum of foot. CEH and Acticoat® were applied on burn wound at post-burn day 3. Post-burn day 9 and 11, the CEH region shows reduced discharge and faster wound healing process. Post-burn day 13, the CEH region is healed completely compared to the control of Acticoat® site (black arrows)

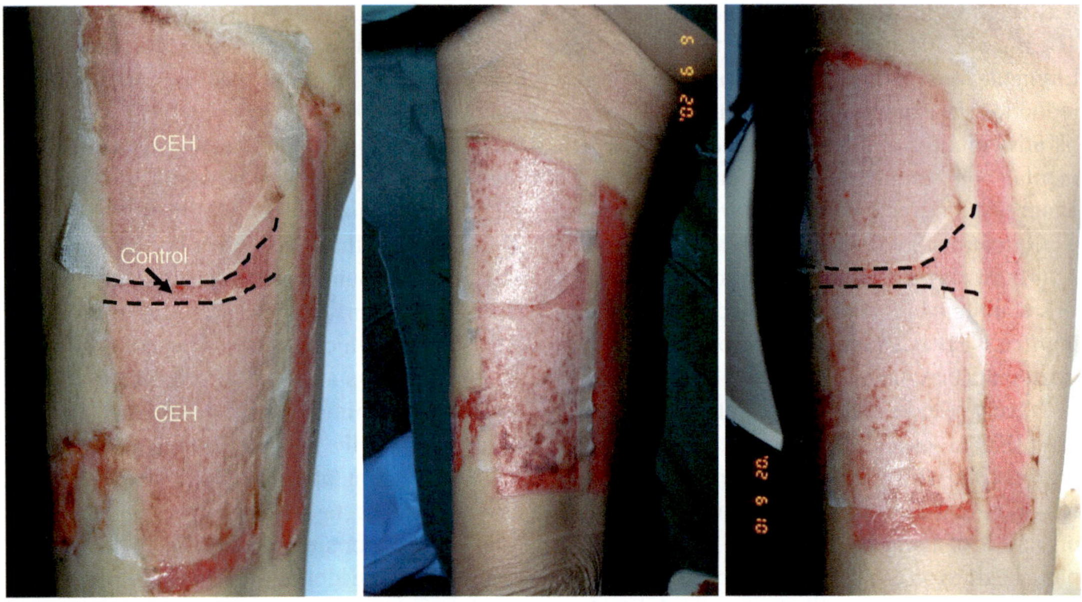

Fig. 4.7 2 sheets of CEH were applied on split-thickness skin donor site and the control site (black arrow) is where CEH is not applied (space between dashed black lines)

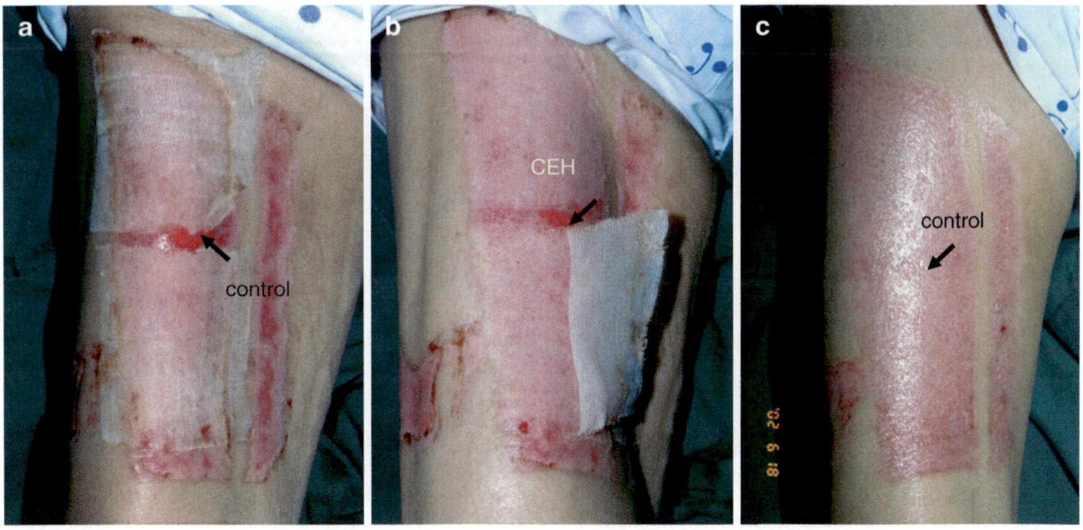

Fig. 4.8 (**a**, **b**) After 8 days, CEH applied site was healed completely but the control site is still in healing process (black arrows). (**c**) On 13th day, the control site is still not healed completely (black arrow)

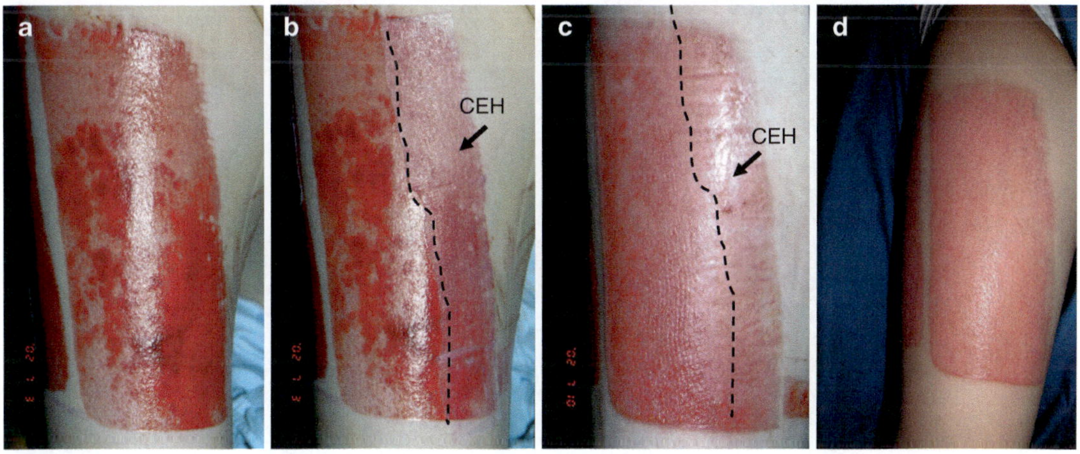

Fig. 4.9 (**a**) Comparison study in split-thickness skin graft donor site, (**b**) postoperative 2 days after the CEH was applied on STSG donor site (black arrow) only. (**c**) post CEH 7 days after view left CEH site was completely healed. (**d**) the CEH applied site is healed 5 days faster than the control site

A 41-year-old male patient received a right-side above-the-knee amputation after a traffic accident. A 0.2-mm-thick 1:3 mesh graft was used for single-step coverage after using human dermal matrix (AlloDerm®) in the wide wound coverage process. To promote the wound healing process, a sandwich technique was used, where two CEH sheets of 7.5 × 7.5 cm were used as a control to cover the upper and lower parts to compare with surrounding mesh only area, but the sheet on the lower part was removed a day later accidentally. The wounds were checked regularly. Seven days after CEH application, the wounds were mostly healed, including the wounds on the control site; however, it is worth noting that slightly different manifestations of epithelialization were found, thereby warranting continued follow-up (Fig. 4.11). The CEH graft site clearly shows different mesh patterns than the control site, indicating that CEH was involved

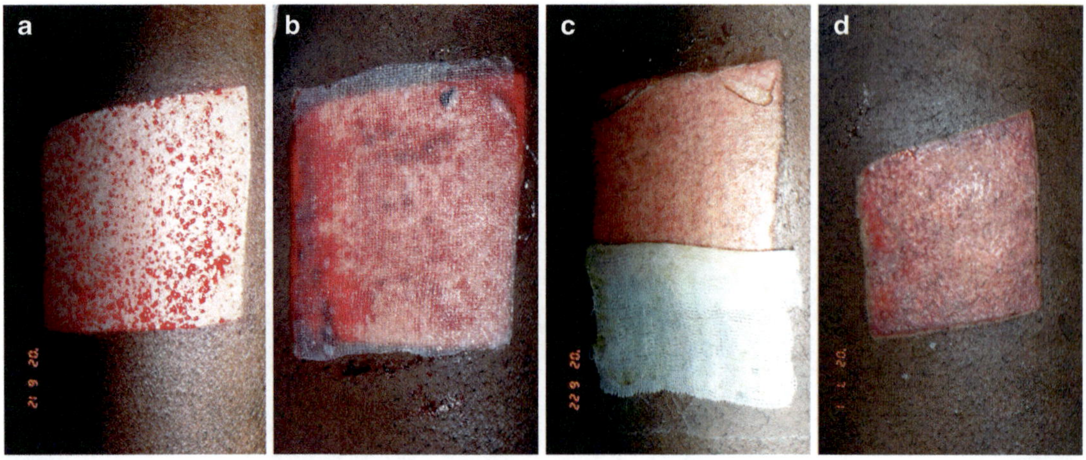

Fig. 4.10 (**a**) Thick split-thickness harvest donor site (0.5 mm thickness) was noted, notice and remember the pin point bleeding pattern (**b**) 2 days after the operation, CEH was applied (**c**) CEH 8 days after view, (**d**) 18 days after CEH procedure, the donor site observed quick and stable wound healing

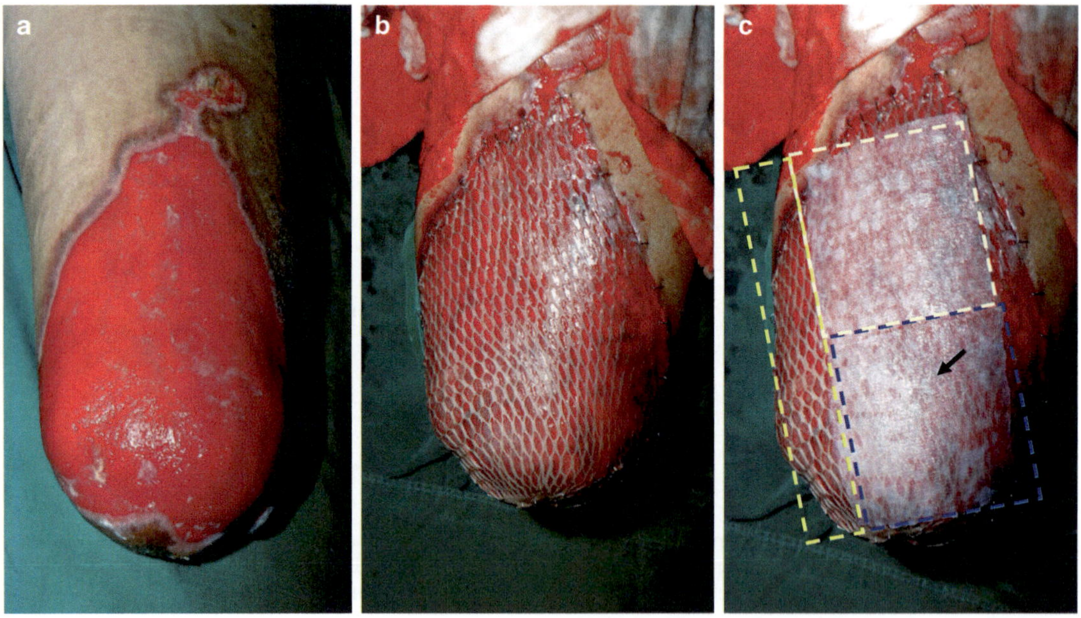

Fig. 4.11 (**a**) Full-thickness skin defect observed on the AK amputee right thigh. (**b**) Human dermal matrix with 0.2 mm thick 1:3 meshed auto graft was covered on the skin defect site. (**c**) 2 sheets of CEH were covered to promote the wound healing. But the sheet on the lower part was removed a day later accidentally (black arrow). The other sheet remained intact for 7 days

in wound healing. Seven days after CEH application, the top region where CEH was applied healed with less visible mesh patterns (upper part of dashed line). Ten days after CEH application, two sites appeared to have a more distinct epithelialization healing process (Fig. 4.12). In the follow-up after 2 weeks, the mesh healing pattern was found to be slightly different, with a flattened healing space and a more visible mesh pattern. After 3.5 months, the CEH-engrafted

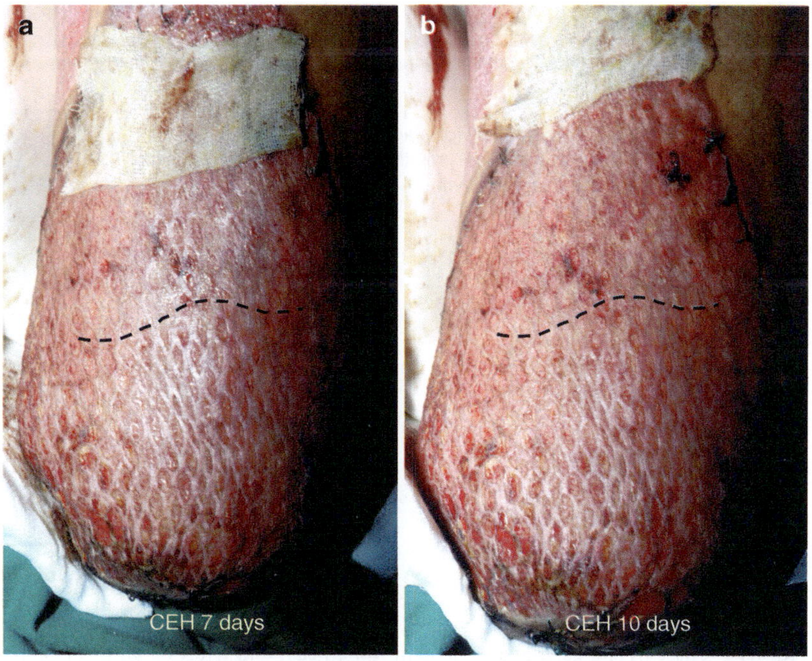

Fig. 4.12 (**a**) 7 days after CEH application, the top region where CEH was applied healed with less visible meshed patterns (upper part of dashed line). (**b**) 10 days after CEH application, two sites showed apparent more distinct epithelialization healing process

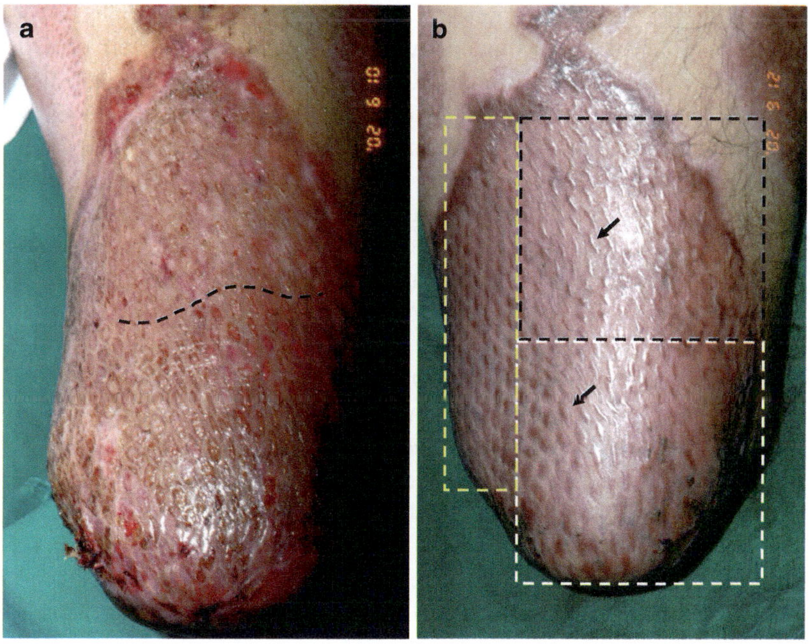

Fig. 4.13 (**a**) Meshed healing pattern was noted little bit different with flattened healing space and more visible mesh pattern day 14. (**b**) The CEH region (black dashed squire) shows the meshed patterns more compact compared to the non-CEH (white and yellow dashed squire) applied region after 3.5 months later view

mesh pattern appeared slightly denser and more compact, indicating that the CEH is directly involved in the wound healing process (Fig. 4.13). This finding provided the basis for a CEH sandwich technique with a 1:4 wide mesh for major burn treatment, which the author developed later.

Summarizing the CEH clinical trials which have been performed so far, it began with a phase III clinical trial conducted between July 2003 and

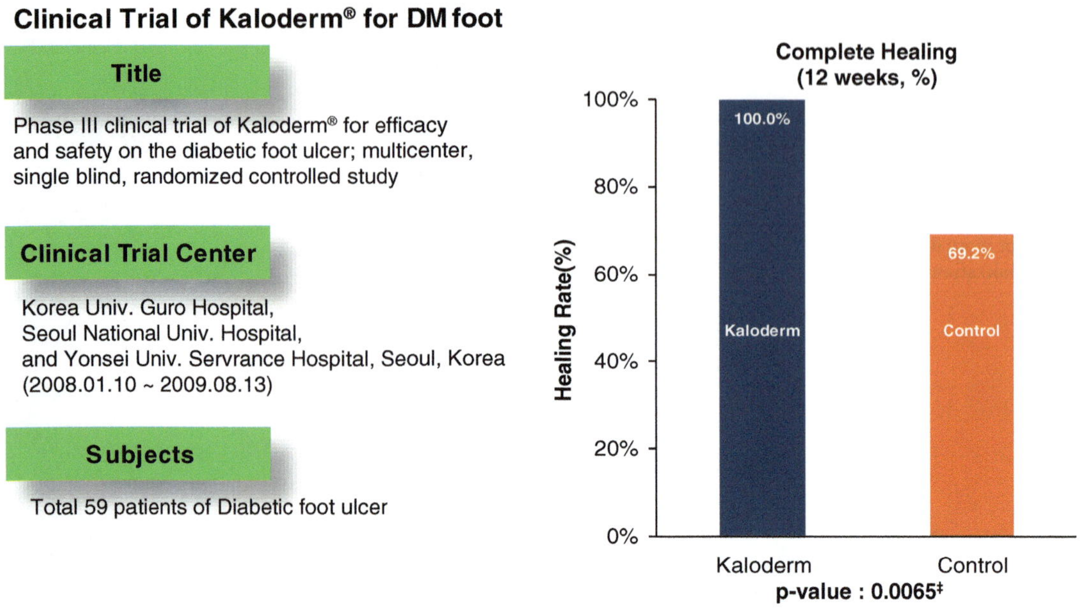

Fig. 4.14 Phase III clinical trial of Kaloderm® for efficacy and safety on the diabetic foot ulcer was performed in 2008. 01. 10 to 2009. 08. 13 by multi-center single blind randomized controlled study

December 2003 and marketing approval for CEH for second-degree burns in March 2005. This was followed by approval for Workers' Compensation Reimbursement in March 2007 and National Health Insurance Reimbursement in April 2007. Since these approvals, CEH has been used in clinical practice. Additionally, for the approval of its use as a treatment for diabetic foot, a phase III clinical trial was conducted for DM (diabetes mellitus) foot between January 2008 and August 2009, and marketing approval for DM foot was granted by the MFDS in June 2010. Additionally, in February 2012, a PMS was conducted, and approval was granted for second-degree burns by the MFDS. The PMS report for DM foot was submitted to the MFDS in September 2014. Since approvals were granted following the clinical trials, CEH is now being used for 20,000 grafts annually in major burn centers and DM foot clinics.

For DM foot, a phase III, multi-center, single-blind, randomized and controlled clinical trial was conducted to examine the efficacy and safety of Kaloderm®. The results have been presented below. In terms of the clinical information for DM foot, 59 patients with leg ulcers of grade 1 or 2 (according to the Wagner classification) were enrolled in the trial from among patients with both types 1 or 2 diabetes, and a control or CEH was applied for 12 weeks. The effectiveness was compared between 21 patients in the control group, and 26 patients in the test group, except for dropouts, and as a result, the cure rate after 12 weeks was 69.23% in the control group and 100% in the CEH test group. This result reflected a significantly higher rate in the CEH group (Fig. 4.14).

The summary of the clinical results for Fig. 4.14 was as follows:

Phase III clinical trial of Kaloderm® for efficacy and safety on the diabetic foot ulcer was performed on January 10, 2008 to August 13, 2009 by multi-center single blind randomized controlled study.

CEH plays an important role as a dressing material, but since it falls off naturally, it is limited in its usability as a permanent graft material. Thus, a clinical trial for CEH as a permanent engraftment material is crucial. The author will describe CEA next.

4.5 CEA-Holoderm® (TEGO Science, Inc., Seoul, Korea)

The cell culture technique called the Green and Rheinwald method (Green culture method) involves the cultivation of keratinocytes in monolayer culture using fibroblasts as feeders, where the cells are held firmly together mutually and cell sheets are formed solely by keratinocytes. Using this technique, cultured skin that is large enough to adequately cover the whole body of an adult can be produced in approximately 2 weeks (TEGO Science, Inc.). Through clinical outcomes and tissue biopsies conducted worldwide over the past 30 years since its application in clinical practice, it has been proven that skin stem cells present in cultured skin were grafted to patients, which then became a stable part of the skin lasting for decades. In early years when CEA was introduced in the past, the take rate was around 20 to 30%, and the results were not satisfactory due to the absence of dermal components. A continuous tissue biopsy study confirmed that the epidermis and basement membrane formed within a month and that the dermis partially regenerated between 2 and 5 years [36].

Currently, cultured skins have been produced using a different method (without the use of fibroblasts), i.e., the Green culture method; however, there are no study results that have verified that the resulting stem cells are stable in the human body. Namely, the Green culture method is the only culture method for skin cells through which skin stem cells can be grafted to the human body. This is a cell therapy developed from a technique that can culture more than 10,000 cm^2 of skin from a 1 cm^2 skin tissue sample within 2–3 weeks. Therefore, in this therapy, a small amount of skin tissue is collected from the patient, and cells are separated, cultured, and later grafted to an affected area.

Partially cultured cell lines are preserved in a cell bank; hence, these cells can be used whenever needed for additional surgery without requiring additional skin biopsy. The confluent keratinocyte sheet has 1 × 10^7 cells.

The size is 7.5 × 7.5 cm of meshed petrolatum gauze with vital clip fix for easy handling.

This sheet can be stored in the range of 4 °C–25 °C for up to 48 h, and the price is reasonable compared with that in other countries. It is approximately $12/cm^2. CEA permanently takes to the wound, enhancing the wound healing process and epithelialization compared with CEH.

CEA can be cultured using a biopsy section of 1–3 cm^2.

Partially cultured cell lines are preserved in a cell bank so that they can be used for additional surgery without requiring an additional skin biopsy. There are one- to four-fold cells in the confluent keratinocyte sheet.

The meshed petrolatum gauze measures 7 × 7.5 cm and has a clip fixation for easy handling.

This sheet can be stored at temperatures ranging from 4 °C to 25 °C for up to 48 h, and the price is reasonable in comparison with other countries. It costs approximately 12 dollars per cm^2 (Fig. 4.15).

This is an order-made product customized for each patient to be grafted directly onto an affected site. It is cultivated to a designated size, and once grafted to the human body, the patient's own skin stem cells are engrafted to become a permanent part of the patient's skin. Additionally, since this is CEA cultivated from a patient's own skin cells, graft rejection never occurs, and the level of engraftment and skin tissue regeneration is excellent. This is mostly used for patients with severe second- or third-degree burns and is the only lifesaving measure for patients in whom autograft is not possible with burn sites >50% TBSA. This is the second product in the world that has been successfully commercialized for use in burn patients and is being marketed with the product name of Holoderm®.

- 1 time of skin biopsy of 1 - 3 cm² ➡ preserved at cell bank
- Culture time: 2-3 weeks
- Confluent keratinocyte sheet: cell numbers 1 - 4 x 10^7
- 7.5 x7.5 cm on meshed petrolatum gauze with vita clip fix
- Storage condition: 4 - 25° C for 48 hours
- Price: ~ $12 / cm²

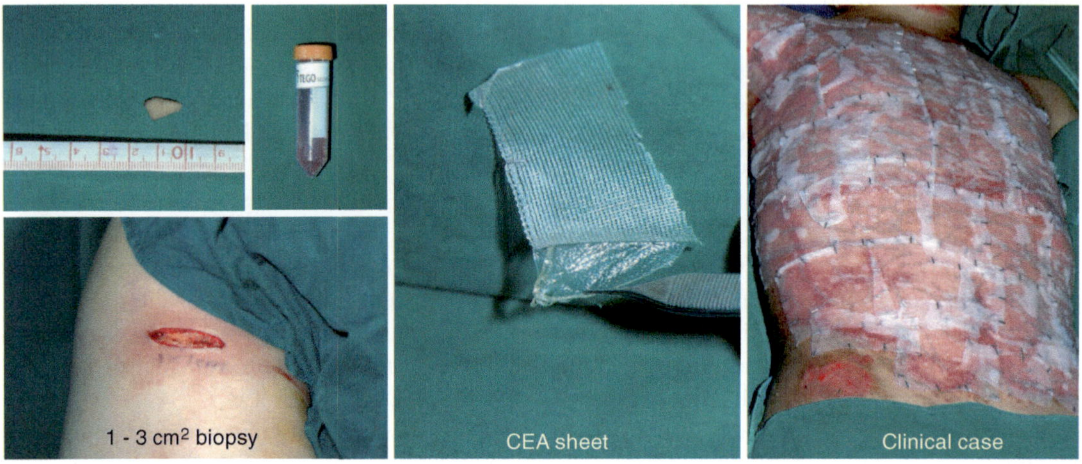

Fig. 4.15 CEA, can be cultured with biopsy of 1 to 3 cm². The confluent keratinocyte sheet has 1 to 4 times ten to the seventh power number of cells. The size is 7.5 cm by 7.5 cm of meshed petrolatum gauze with vital clip fix for easy handling. This sheet can be stored in the range of 4 to 25 Celsius for up to 48 h and the price is reasonable compared to other countries. It is around 12 dollars per square centimeters

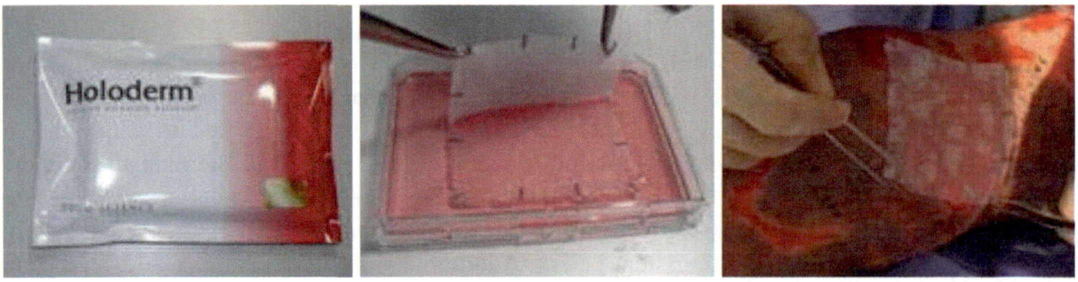

(Photo. 2)

1. The appearance of the package.
2. CEA made in the form of sheets.
3. An example of clinical applications.

4.6 CEA-Holoderm®

The history of Holoderm® is as follows. It obtained marketing approval from the MFDS on the condition of "post-approval clinical trial" in December

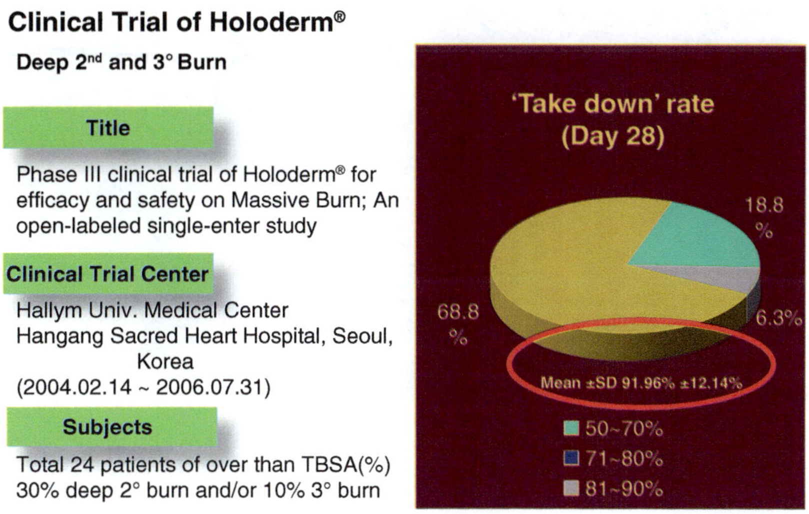

Fig. 4.16 The takedown rate had a mean ± SD of 90.21% ± 13.66% according to analysis of 16 subjects in ITT (intention-to-treat) settings

2002. Later, a phase III clinical trial was conducted in a burn center from April 2003 to December 2007. Worker's Compensation Reimbursement was permitted by the MFDS in March 2007. It was then approved via reexamination by the MFDS in August 2010 following a 6-year period of PMS. As a result, the efficacy of Holoderm® was officially validated, and it has been used in more than 850 burn patients since its approval in 2002, contributing greatly to saving lives.

For Holoderm®, a phase III open-label clinical trial was conducted on massive burn patients with deep second- or third-degree burn injuries under approval of the MFDS between February 12, 2004 and July 31, 2006. Holoderm® was applied to 16 subjects, including eight minors aged ≤19 years. Excluding those who withdrew consent or died before the Holoderm® was grafted, 24 patients with massive burns enrolled in the clinical trial, and its effectiveness was then evaluated. The average burn area among the 16 patients was 5902.9 cm^2 (TBSA 46.13%), and the average of the third-degree burn area was 4165.7 cm^2 (TBSA 33.91%). Holoderm® was applied to burn sites of 1420 cm^2 on average.

The clinical outcomes revealed that after 4 weeks from the first application of Holoderm®, the take rate of CEA was 90.21% on average. The success rate of engraftment was determined based on the assumption that no subsequent surgeries would be necessary and was determined to be 93.75%. The following results are from a phase III clinical trial of Holoderm® on its efficacy and safety of Holoderm® in patients with major burns: according to an analysis of 16 subjects in intention-to-treat (ITT) settings, the takedown rate had a mean ± SD of 90.21% ± 13.66% (Fig. 4.16).

4.6.1 Preparation for CEA

In terms of preparation for CEA, 1–3 cm^2 of skin was collected through a full-thickness skin biopsy from the body and was preserved in a donor cell bank so that the cell lines could be used whenever necessary without requiring an additional biopsy. But recently in the author's experimental study, split-thickness skin biopsy also can be used without any issues compared with full-thickness skin biopsy. The culture took approximately 2–3 weeks, and the cell numbers of confluent keratinocyte sheets were nearly $1–4 \times 10^7$. The cultured cells were transferred to petrolatum gauze sized 7.5 × 7.5 cm, i.e., 56.2 cm^2, and made into a sheet to facilitate grafting.

4.6.2 Clinical Application of CEA

Currently, the take rate of CEA has increased significantly compared to its rate in the past, with a

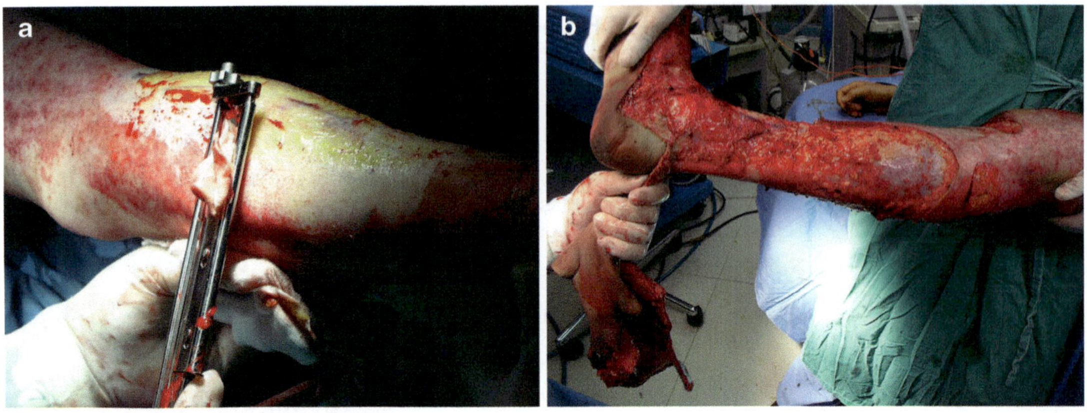

Fig. 4.17 43-year-old male patient suffered flame burn 60% TBSA. First, early selective escharectomy performed on full-thickness burn areas either by tangential (**a**) or fascia level excision on the right lower leg (**b**)

take rate of >90% in most cases. However, since they are composed of a single keratinocyte layer, there are still numerous obstacles to overcome to actually function fully as skin. To that, many studies and clinical trials are required. Currently, since the treatment of massive burn patients should be focused and prioritized on wound coverage, efficient and prompt graft techniques are required so that the rates of wide mesh of >1:6, or even 1:9, according to the percentage of TBSA, can be used. Permanent wound coverage of massive burn patients takes at least 2–3 weeks for a culture of CEA. Thus, focusing on saving the patients' life by combining tangential excision and sequential excision as a concept of early excision and early graft, human allograft is performed using cryopreserved allograft (CPA) which utilizes human cadaver skin, or GPA (glycerol-preserved allograft), which can be preserved for a longer period of time and maintained at average room temperature. This is an important period in both burn wound treatment and patient lifesaving and requires securing time for cell culturing. Human allograft corrects electrolyte imbalance in patients, prevents water vaporization, promotes the formation of granulation tissue in the wound bed, and peels off in 2–3 weeks. Peeling occurs naturally in most cases, but if there is a partial take, it is not necessary to remove it by excision because it does not hinder wound healing even when it is not fully removed by force. This can be explained because allografts may take generalized immunity declines in major burn patients [37]. During this period, CEA can be produced in a large amount of CEA sheets, which can cover the body surface area of patients, thereby making it possible to proceed to permanent wound coverage. For this procedure, the use of human dermal matrix and dermal substitutes, such as Integra®, can be combined to minimize scar contracture [38].

According to the clinical examples introduced previously by the author, a 43-year-old male patient suffered from a flame burn of 60% TBSA. First, early selective escharectomy on full-thickness burn areas is performed by tangential excision (a) or fascia-level excision on the right lower leg (b). It is rare to perform an excision up to the fascia level (Fig. 4.17). After selective escharectomy, CPA or GPA is engrafted immediately (Fig. 4.18), and the culture is prepared by collecting 1–3 cm^2 of skin. Once CEA has been fully cultured, the rate of mesh autograft, which can be obtained from the donor site in patients, is determined, and the mesh size ratio required to cover wounds is determined using a mesher (Brennen Skin Graft Mesher, USA) (Fig. 4.19). The allograft was completely removed 23 days after the CPA allograft, and engraftment with a wide-mesh autograft (mesh size ratio: 1:4 or 1:6) was performed, followed by the application of a CEA-sheet graft. After approximately 3 weeks, 1:6 wide-mesh autograft with sheet-type CEAs was applied on granula-

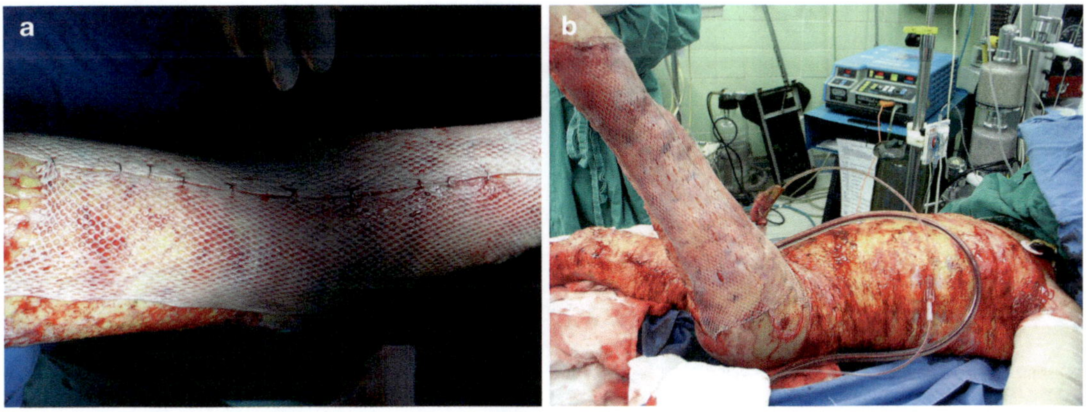

Fig. 4.18 (**a**) After selective escharectomy, cryopreserved allograft was engrafted on excised areas as a temporary biological dressing. (**b**) The allograft will be removed after 2 to 3 weeks while keratinocytes are being cultured

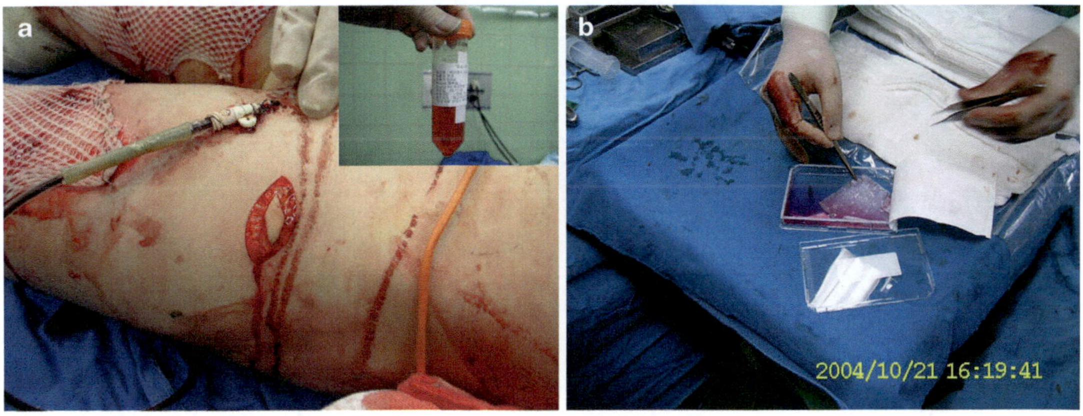

Fig. 4.19 (**a**) Small skin biopsy 1–3 cm^2 was obtained for culturing CEA. After 3 weeks, (**b**) CEA sheets were ready and it is provided on top of mesh petrolatum gauze

tion-forming areas after the allograft skin was removed. Prior to the introduction of CEA, wide-mesh autograft was used, which resulted in poor healing and unsatisfactory results. However, CEA is now a very useful wound dressing material on a wide mesh of engrafted auto-skin, with good results (Fig. 4.20).

The biggest disadvantage of CEA is the absence of the dermal layer, which results in several problems, including unstable wound coverage, severe wound contracture, and an unsightly appearance. As seen in the figure, CEAs were simply applied to a 1:6 wide-mesh autograft [39]. Note the different mesh ratios in the leg and knee joint areas to reduce joint contracture. They can be repaired using small staples (Fig. 4.21). But for areas such as large joints or the neck that has lot of movements and where scar contracture should be minimized, it is encouraged to combine human dermal matrix, which can be achieved in a single-step operation, in order to supplement the dermal layer, thereby minimizing scar contracture and aiding in reinforcement. However, the high cost of this technique is one of its disadvantages that must be overcome (Fig. 4.22). In large joint areas such as the knee joint or axilla, human dermal matrix is partially used to minimize post-burn scar contracture. However, if it is financially feasible, the author encourages dermal matrix to be engrafted in a sufficient amount without any gaps, whenever possible, which delivers better outcomes. The engrafted petrola-

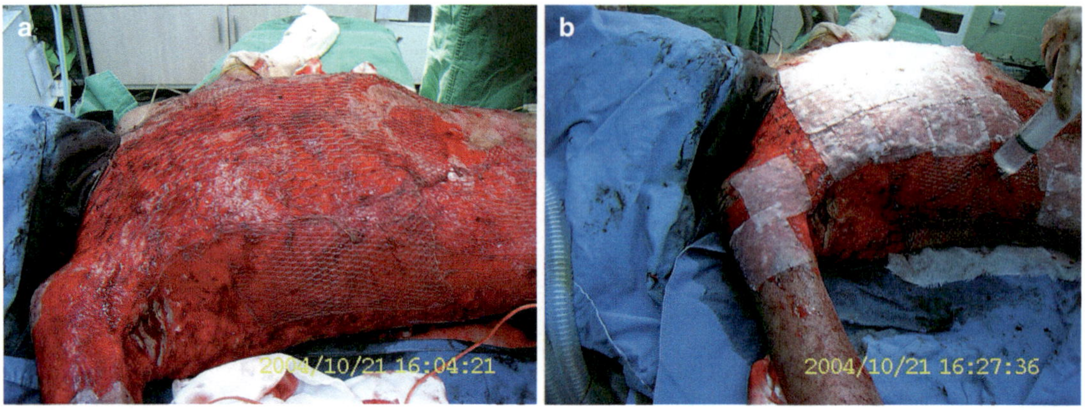

Fig. 4.20 (**a**, **b**) After around 3 weeks, 1:6 wide meshed autograft with sheet type of CEAs was applied on granulation formed areas after the allograft skin was separated

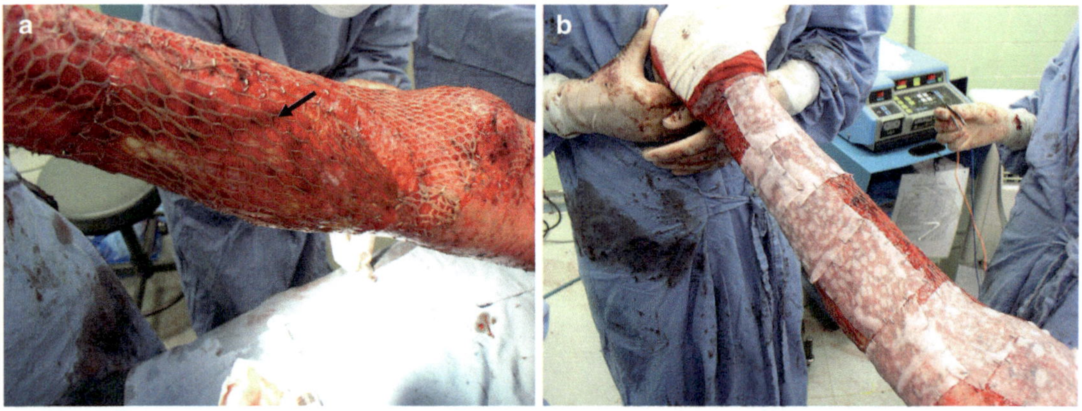

Fig. 4.21 (**a**) CEAs were simply applied on 1:6 wide meshed autograft (black arrow). (**b**) CEA sheets can be fixed using small-sized staples

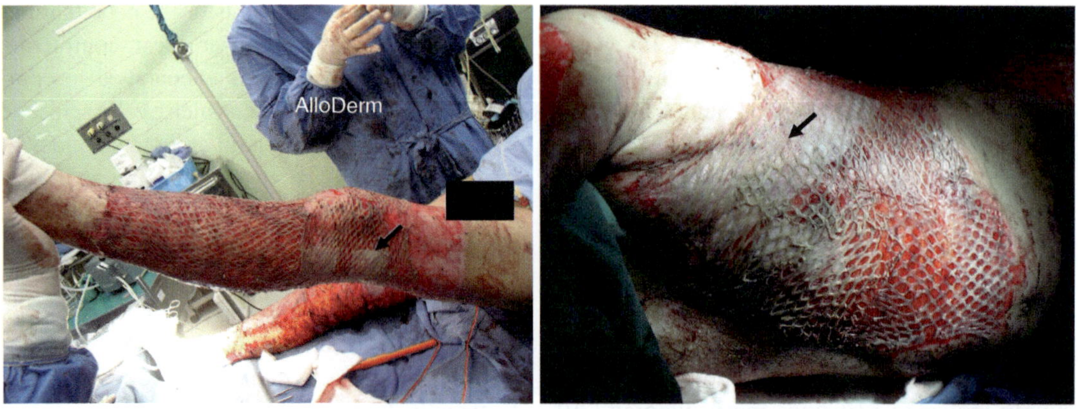

Fig. 4.22 Acellular dermal matrix such as AlloDerm® was concurrently used on joint areas to minimize post-scar contractures and deformity (black arrows)

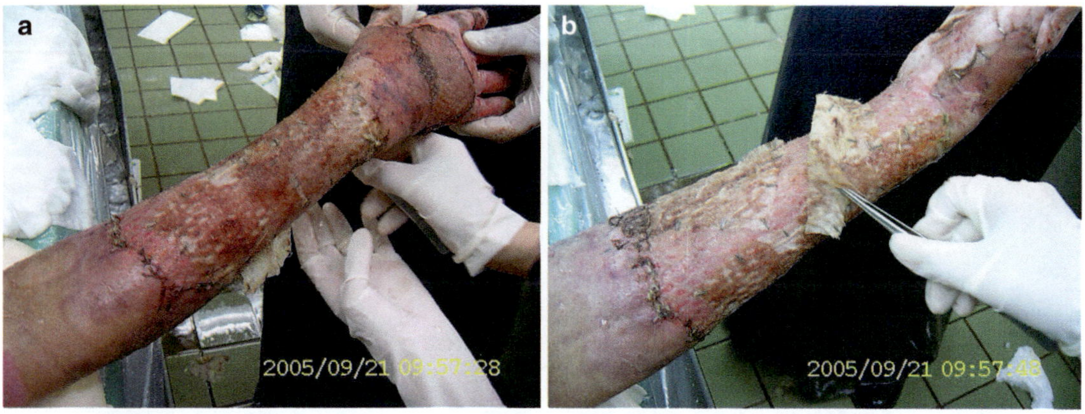

Fig. 4.23 (**a**) 7 days after application of CEA. Petrolatum gauze of CEAs was removed after 4 to 9 days according to wound condition. (**b**) But it is better to leave it intact until wound healing is stabilized

tum gauze of CEAs is typically removed between days 4 and 9, but it is better to leave it intact until wound healing is stabilized, if possible, and then slowly remove it (Fig. 4.23).

To avoid exhaustion, operations on children with major burns should be performed more carefully by dividing the process into stages. A scalding burn on a 1-year-old male patient resulted in 67% TBSA. Post-burn day 2, escharectomy and immediate CPA were performed on the left upper arm and trunk area. After 3 weeks, the engrafted allograft was removed, and a 1:6 wide-mesh skin graft and CEA sheets were applied to the chest and flank areas using the sandwich technique. Furthermore, 9 days after the first mesh skin graft site healed, a 1:6 mesh graft with CEA sheets was performed as a second operation to improve joint function disturbances in the lower and upper extremities using human dermal matrix. On day 8 after applying the CEA-sheet graft, the site appeared to have almost healed, and on day 21 after the second skin graft, the site had completely healed (Figs. 4.24 and 4.25).

The following case involves a 37-year-old male patient with a 51% TBSA flame burn and a mild inhalation injury. On the fifth day after the injury, escharectomy was performed in the anterior neck, chest, and trunk areas, followed by an allograft of glycerol-preserved cadaver skin (GPA) (Fig. 4.26). On day 16 after the burn, a 1:5 wide-mesh autograft with CEA was performed in the well-formed granulation tissue. On day 11 after applying the meshed skin autograft (Fig. 4.27), the findings revealed that it had almost healed. Fourteen days following the first auto-skin graft, the second auto-skin graft was performed using human dermal matrix AlloDerm ® with a 1:1 mesh autograft without a CEA-sheet graft on the remaining anterior neck area in order to minimize neck scar contracture (Fig. 4.28).

The following table is a summary of the results from a phase III clinical trial of Holoderm® conducted between February 12, 2004 and July 31, 2006 (Tables 4.1, 4.2, and 4.3).

For this clinical trial, a total of 24 subjects were enrolled from one clinical trial site, and 16 subjects from an ITT group completed a clinical trial after Holoderm® was grafted. The main analysis of the effectiveness evaluation variables was conducted on 16 subjects from the ITT group (Table 4.1). The first of the effectiveness evaluation variable in this clinical trial was the success rate of engraftment during the fourth week (28 days), and the take rate was defined as the percentage of the engrafted area of the total graft area with CEA (Table 4.2). The success of engraftment was defined as being when researchers decided to follow up since no additional operations were needed because the take rate was >50% and the graft site showed signs of healing (Table 4.3).

In the ITT analysis of 16 subjects, the take rate during the fourth week was 90.21 ± 13.66%. Since the minimum take rate was 60% and the maximum was 100%, engraftment was consid-

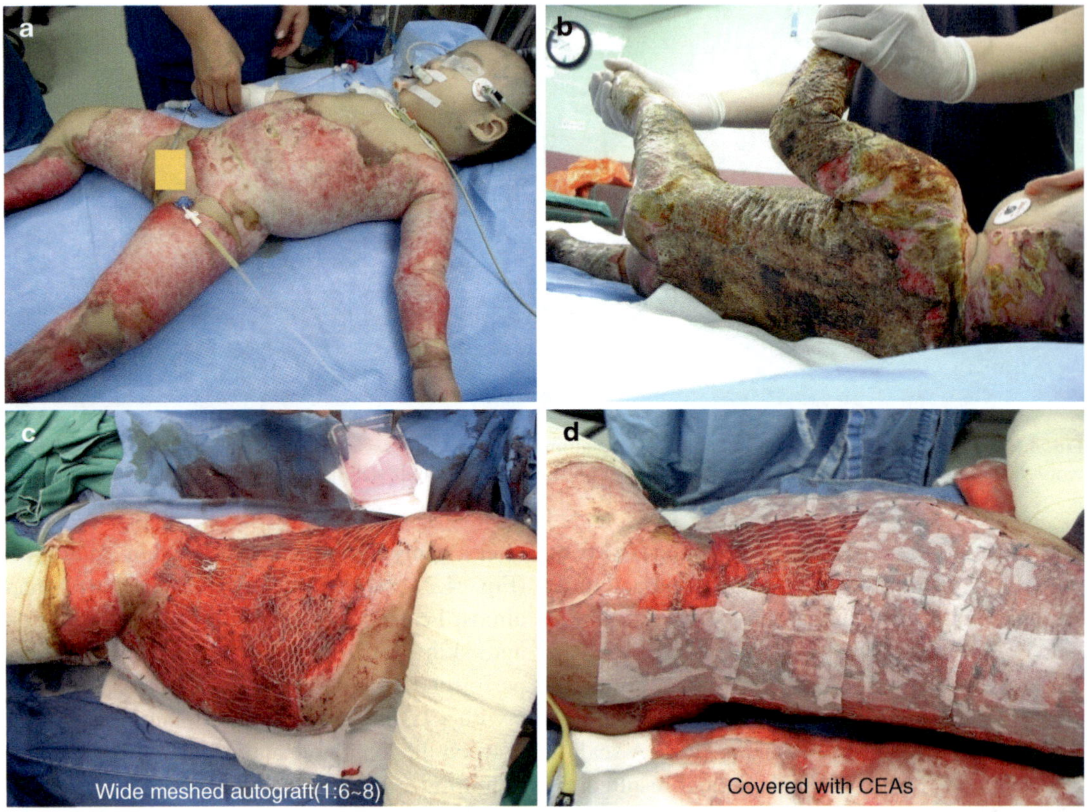

Fig. 4.24 (**a**) 67% TBSA by scalding burn. (**b**) Post-burn day 2, cryopreserved allograft was applied after escharectomy. (**c**) Around 3 weeks after, allograft was removed and 1 to 6 mesh autograft was applied. (**d**) The CEA sheets were covered over wide meshed autograft

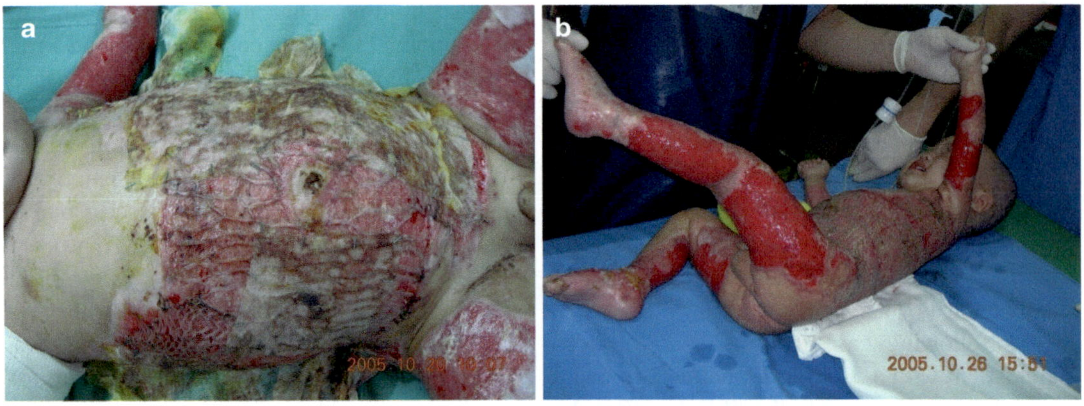

Fig. 4.25 (**a**) After wound closure of trunk area, (**b**) the second operation was performed on extremities using CEAs and AlloDerm® with (**c**) 1:4 meshed skin graft to preserve joint functions. (**d**) postoperative 21 days, all wound completely closed

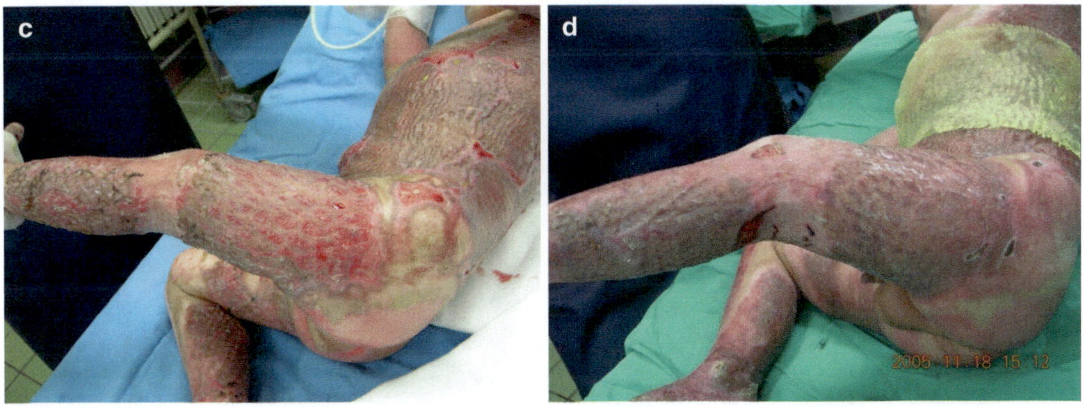

Fig. 4.25 (continued)

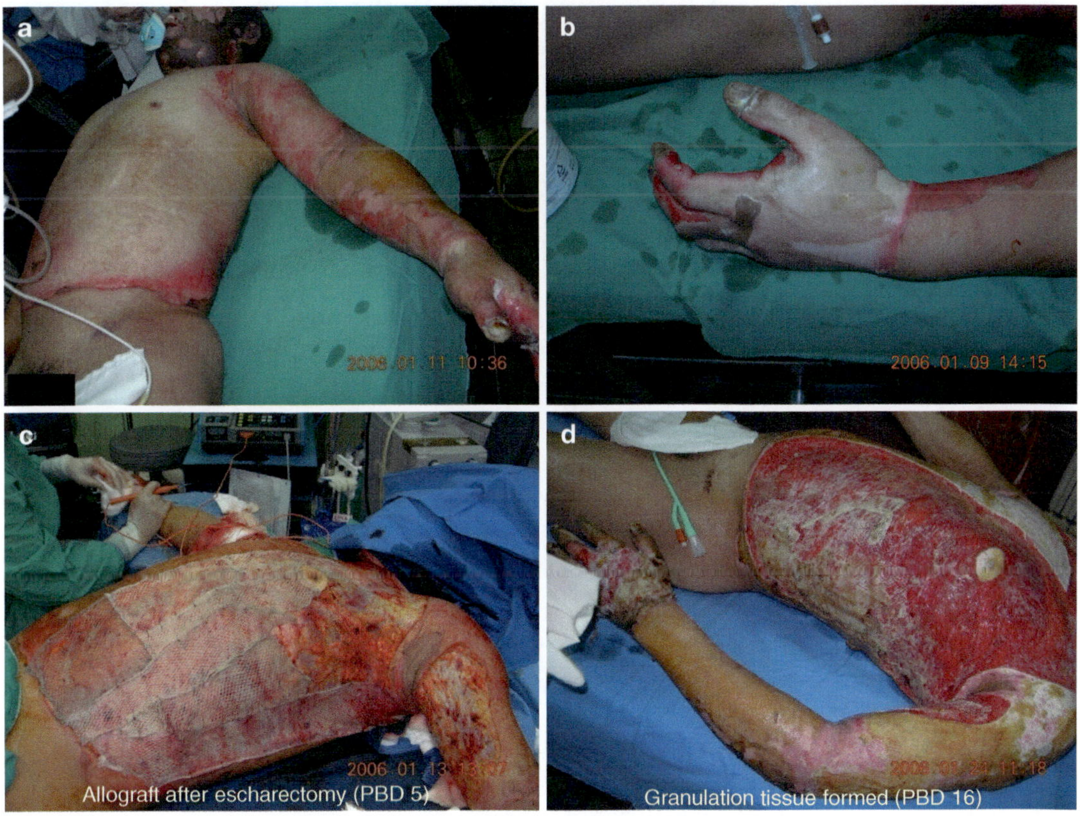

Fig. 4.26 (**a**, **b**) 51% TBSA by flame burn. (**c**) Post-burn day 5, escharectomy and allograft (**d**) Post-burn day 16, the skin allograft was removed

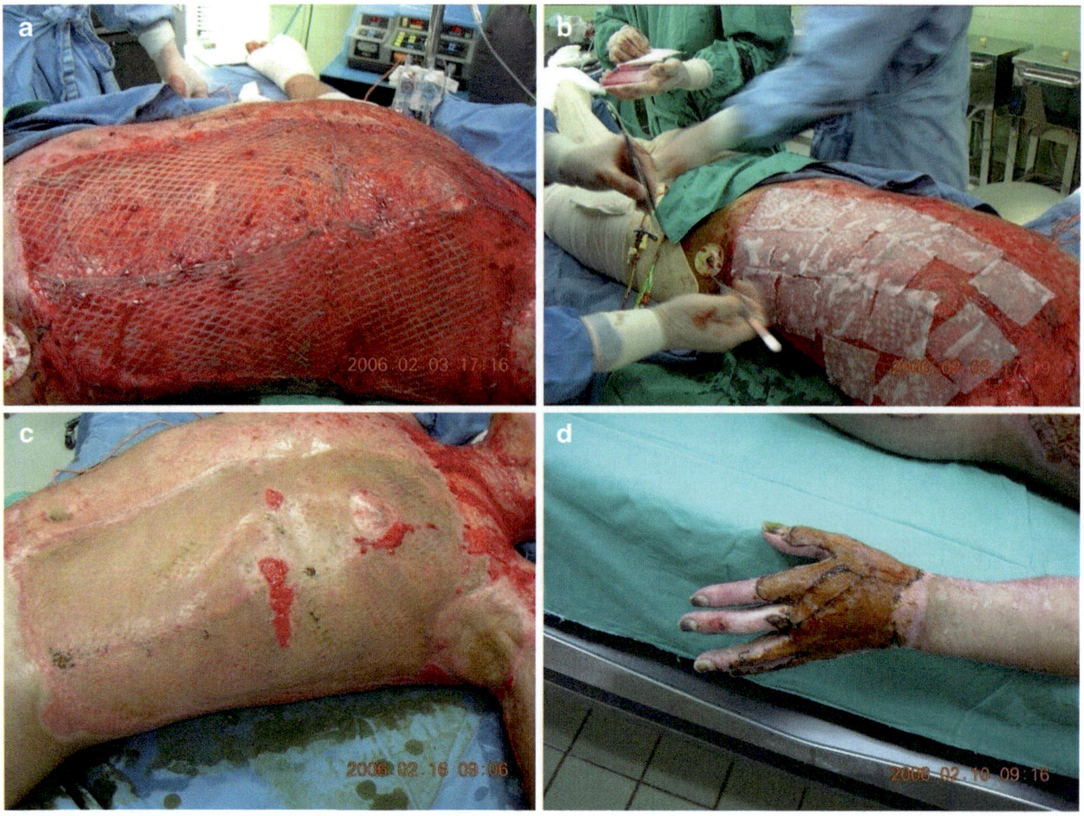

Fig. 4.27 (**a**) On day 16 after 1:5 meshed autograft with (**b**) CEAs was applied on the granulation tissue formed wound bed. (**c**) First skin graft day 11, noted good healing process on anterior chest area, (**d**) sheet STSG was performed on left dorsum of hand to save hand function

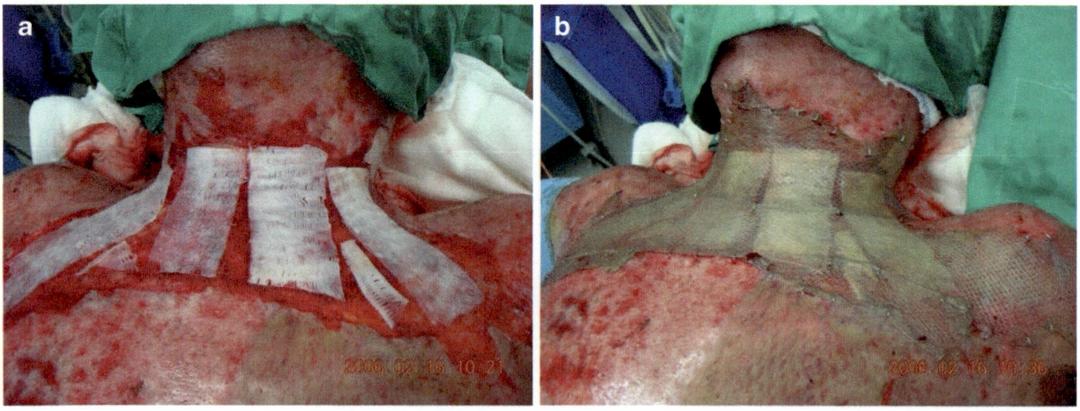

Fig. 4.28 (**a**, **b**) After wound closure of trunk area, the neck area was performed with 1 to 1 meshed autograft with AlloDerm® without CEA to minimize contractures of neck area. (**c**) Note completely healed on first operation and (**d**) second skin graft day 11, completely healed noted on anterior neck area

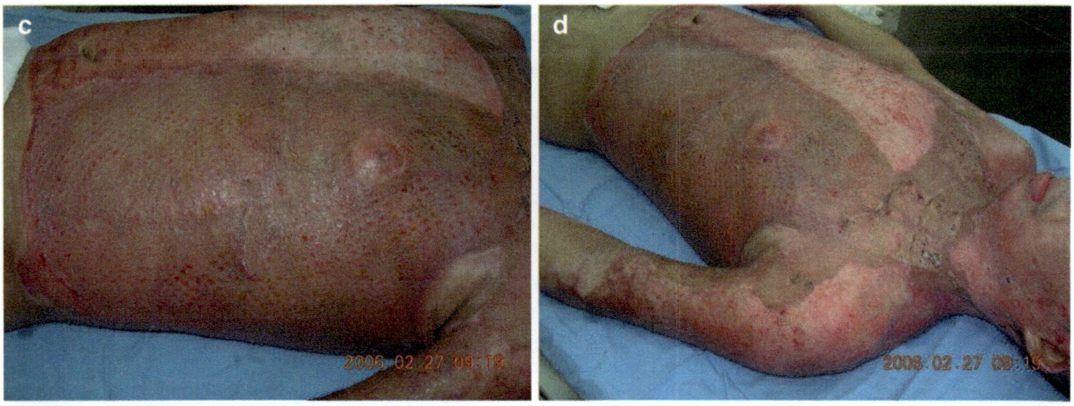

Fig. 4.28 (continued)

Table 4.1 Age/sex, burn, mode, and the burn percentage of TBSA were calculated for 16 subjects

		n	(%)
Sex	Male	10	(62.50)
	Female	6	(37.50)
Age	Mean ± SD (years) (min, max)	18.31 ± 14.36 (0, 42)	
	0–9 (person)	6	(37.50)
	10–19 (person)	2	(12.50)
	20–29	4	(25.00)
	30–39	3	(18.75)
	40 or older	1	(6.25)
Causes of burns			
	Scalding burn	3	(18.75)
	Electrical burn	2	(12.50)
	Flame burn	11	(68.75)
Total burn area	% (TBSA)	46.13	±18.7
	cm^2	5902.9	±210.66
Third-degree burn area	% (TBSA)	33.91	±21.83
	cm^2	4165.7	±881.59

Table 4.2 Data and CEA area used in early excision and graft

	cm^2 (mean ± *SD*)
The size of the test area	1420 ± 827.36
The size of applied CEA	1423.8 ± 824.98
The size of biopsy	3.25 ± 2.23

ered successful in all 16 patients (100%). However, although the take rate in one patient was 92.50%, the investigator judged that additional surgery was clinically required regardless of the take rate in the subject because "there was a partial loss in the graft site of the right upper arm, and necrosis occurred in the scar tissue flap of the chest area." Therefore, it can be stated that the final clinical success rate of engraftment was 93.75%, or 15 subjects out of 16.

Table 4.3 Summary of results

	Visiting day	
Success rate of engraftment (%)	Day 28	93.75
Take rate (%, mean ± *SD*)	Day 14	86.69 ± 13.48
	Day 28	90.21 ± 13.66
	Last visit	91.38 ± 13.81

4.7 Various Application Techniques of CEA

4.7.1 Cell Suspension Type: Cell Spray Technique

Clinical trials for various applications besides grafts with CEA sheets were tested. A cultured epithelial cell spray technique was tested to reduce operative time for CEA grafts by shortening the standard CEA-sheet production time of a minimum of 2–3 weeks to the shortest time possible and by the removal of a complex process in the production of sheets [40]. Additionally, a clinical trial was conducted to provide information for the development of artificial skin at a future date by combining a few attempts to

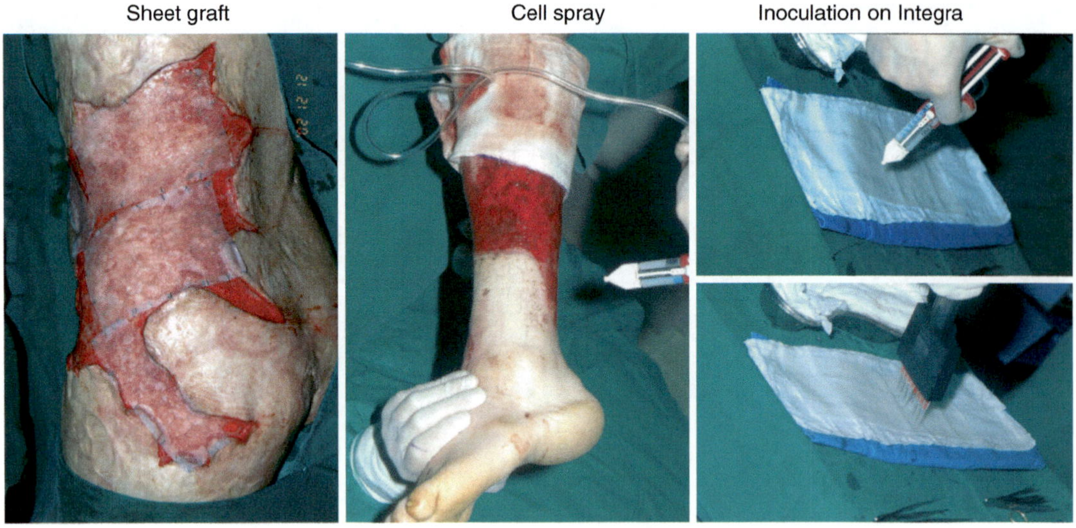

Fig. 4.29 CEA can be available in various types: in sheet type, cell spray type, and cell inoculation on artificial dermis. As artificial and collagen matrix developed, the conjunction usage of CEA and dermal substitute together improved the take rate of CEA as high as 90%. But cell inoculation technique is not recommendable in my experience and needs more experimental studies

induce a connection between epithelial cells and dermal substitutes which are needed for the production of the artificial skin being developed by several laboratories. These results have been described below. CEA is available in several forms, including sheet, cell spray, and cell inoculation on artificial dermis. After the development of human dermal matrix and collagen matrix, the use of CEA and dermal substitute together improved the take rate of CEA by up to 90%. However, in my experience, the cell inoculation technique is not recommended, and more experimental studies are needed because it is still less effective and has a low take rate for clinical adaptation (Fig. 4.29).

A clinical trial was conducted to expand the range of applications for the cell spray technique and make it more accessible and to be widely used in culture epithelial cell therapy and accordingly obtain significant results, which will be delineated below.

When utilizing a cell spray technique, cell suspension should be prepared prior to spraying. In cell suspension, cells grow to approximately 200 times in number of the original cell number in approximately 2 weeks after skin biopsy, and the number of cells in a 1 cc suspension is approximately 10×10^7. The cell spray method is as follows: using a Tissomat spray machine (Baxter, Illinois, USA), spray fibrin glue and cell suspension in two connected syringes, 20–30 cm away from the wound, and then apply wet gauze dressing to prevent the sprayed area from drying. Open the dressing to check after nearly 5 days, and if there is no infection, among other parameters, maintain the dressing for 7–10 days by which epithelialization will be nearly complete. After epithelialization is complete, carefully remove the gauze (Fig. 4.30).

The advantages of a cell spray technique include the following:

- It reduces the normal time of 2–3 weeks for cell culturing to approximately 16 days on average, allowing for faster application in clinical practice.
- For biopsies, split-thickness skin can be used for culturing, thus not requiring full-thickness skin larger than 1 cm^2, thus allowing for easier culture biopsies when necessary.
- Cells are sprayed along with fibrin, reducing cell injury. Wound healing and CEA take rates can be increased because of connections between fibrin and cells.
- Ease of handling facilitates quicker and easier application to wide areas and reduces opera-

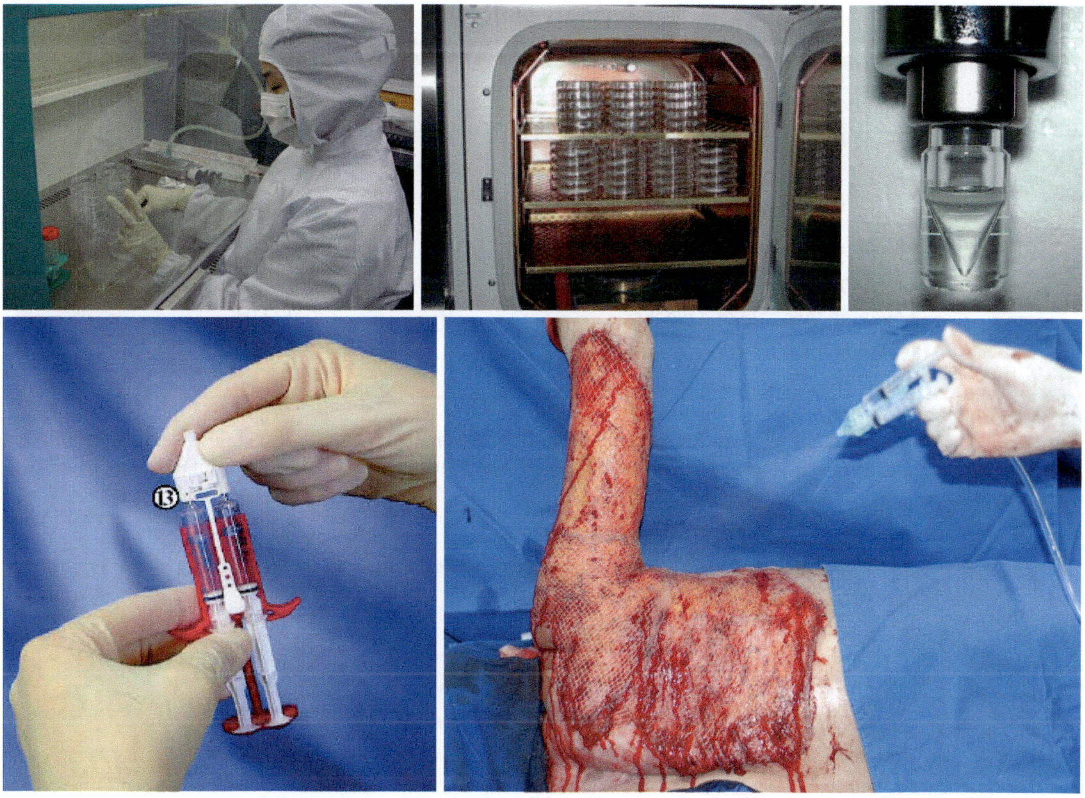

Fig. 4.30 Keraheal® is processed under GMP certified lab and it can increase up to 200 folds within 2 weeks. It can be sprayed directly over wide wound area and very effective to spray over massive burned surface area

tive time, aiding in saving lives in major burn patients.

- It is cost-effective because production costs for sheets, among other materials, are reduced.

Next, the author describes the results and clinical findings of specific clinical trials.

4.8 Cell Suspension: Keraheal®

A clinical trial for major burn treatment was conducted using Keraheal® (MCTT, Seoul, Korea), an autologous epithelial cell suspension, from February 2007 to October 2008, with 22 subjects. The results are as presented below.

A total of 22 subjects were examined, with TBSA burn areas ranging from 33% to 66% (Fig. 4.31).

The mean TBSA burned area was 52%, and the mean size of Keraheal used was 1135 cm^2. The average take rate at 2 and 4 weeks was 95% and 99%, respectively. The overall take rate on wide-mesh autograft with AlloDerm was over 90%. Currently, the suspension type of CEA is awaiting KFDA approval (Fig. 4.32).

In this clinical example, a 25-year-old male patient suffered flame burns to both thigh areas with third-degree burns. A cell spray technique was planned for the patient. On day 2 after the burn, a full-thickness skin biopsy of 1 cm^2 was performed, and on day 10 after the burn, a total escharectomy was performed. On day 17, after the wound surface had stabilized and the granulation tissue had formed, three vials of 1 cc of cell suspension each were prepared. Following a 1:3 mesh skin autograft, cell suspension and fibrin glue was sprayed using a Tissomat spray machine. On postoperative day 3, the wound was opened, and on day 6, it was confirmed that epithelialization was nearly complete. On day 16 after surgery, the findings revealed a good state of healing,

Summary of Result

(February, 2007 – October, 2008)

• Number of Patients	22
• Mean Age (yrs)	37.8
• Mean TBSA burned (%)	52.3
• Mean TBSA full-thickness burns (%)	40.95
• Mean size of Keraheal used (cm^2)	1135.7
• Average take rate at 2weeks	95.48%
• Average take rate at 4 weeks	99.50%
• Average take rate on wide meshed autograft with AlloDerm	Over 90%

Fig. 4.31 The mean TBSA burned was 52% and the mean size of Keraheal used was 1135 cm^2. Average take rate at 2 weeks was 95% and 99% at 4 weeks. The overall take rate on wide meshed autograft with AlloDerm was over 90%

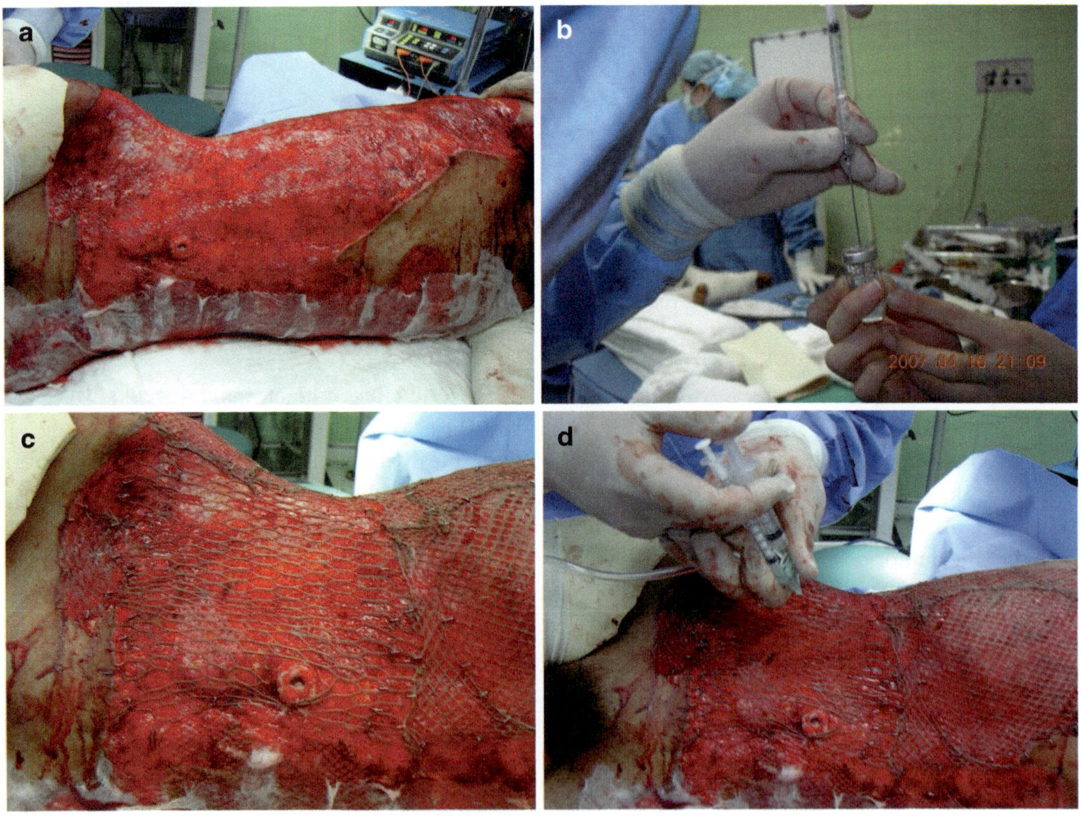

Fig. 4.32 (**a**) After removal of cadaver skin allograft, wide meshed autograft was applied on the newly formed granulation tissues. (**b**) Cultured spray type of keratinocyte, (**c**, **d**) Keraheal, was simply inoculated over wide meshed autograft using Tissomat and followed by Tissucol® (fibrin glue) spray to prevent hematoma and seroma collection which enhances wound healing process on the chest and back area

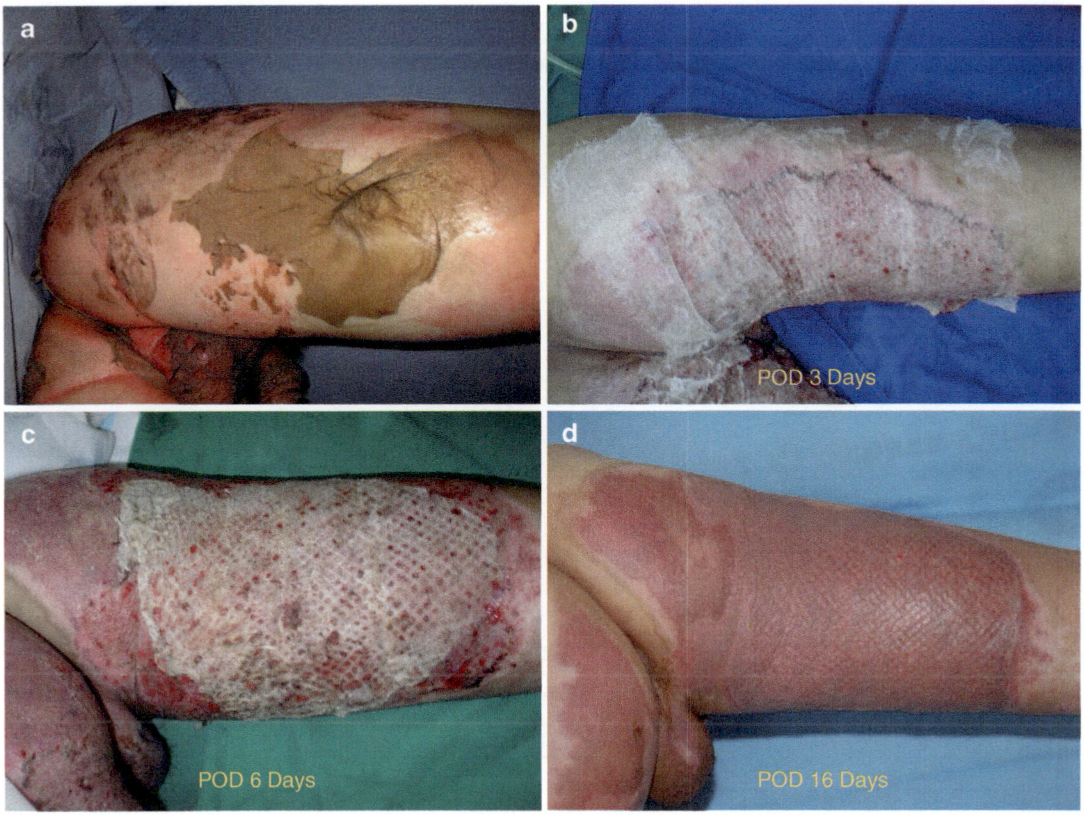

Fig. 4.33 (**a**) third-degree burn on both thigh area. Post-burn day 10, escharectomy and removal of separated necrotic tissue. (**b**) On day 17, three vials of 1 cc suspension was sprayed on the 1:3 mesh auto-skin graft areas. On postoperative day 3, rapidly started epithelialization, (**c**) On day 6 almost healing state was noted. (**d**) On day 16, more compactly epithelialization was noted

confirming that the wound healing process progressed faster than expected (Fig. 4.33).

The following case involved a 37-year-old male patient who suffered flame burns on his left back and flank areas as well as third-degree burns of 55% TBSA. On days 4–6 after the burn, escharectomy was performed, and a cadaveric allograft was applied to the excised burn wound, and a full-thickness skin biopsy of 1 cm^2 was performed for a keratinocyte cell suspension (Fig. 4.34). Burn wound excision was performed after 18–21 days, followed by the removal of the allograft. Then, a 1:3–6 wide-mesh autograft was applied on the back and flank areas, and six vials of 6 cc cell suspension were sprayed on the total mesh-engrafted area (Fig. 4.35). For the large joint axilla area, human dermal matrix was applied to minimize scar contracture. After the application of a meshed autograft using a sandwich technique, cell spray was sprayed (Fig. 4.36). Scarring was evaluated in some areas using the

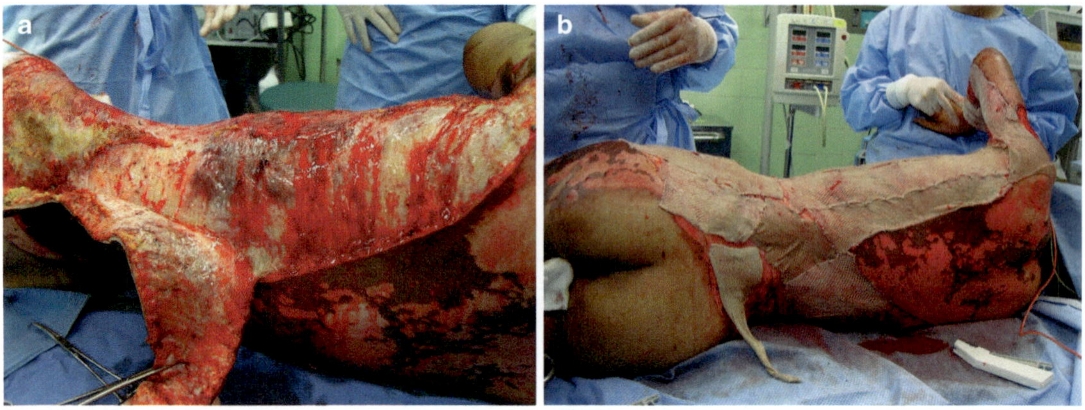

Fig. 4.34 (**a**) On days 4–6 after the burn staged escharectomy, (**b**) cadaver skin allograft was applied and skin biopsy of 1 square centimeters was obtained for culturing. At the lab, keratinocytes were isolated from the skin biopsy by magnetic cell isolation method and cultured using serum free medium under the GMP facility for 16 days

Subjects

Case	Age/Sex	Mode	Burn % of TBSA (3rd degree %)	Keraheal spray area (cm2)
1	47/F	FB	45(40)	200
2	26/M	CB	66(40)	400
3	39/M	FB	35(25)	900
4	15/M	FB	41(30)	1287
5	47/M	EB	**56(50)**	**1644**
6	30/M	SB	**58(40)**	**750**
7	30/M	FB	33(28)	996.6
8	37/M	FB	**55(55)**	**775**
9	51/M	CB	**58(48)**	**532.8**
10	56/M	CB	62(46)	300.6
11	39/M	FB	**51(40)**	**200**
12	24/M	FB	60(41)	300
13	54/M	FB	50(40)	300
14	33/M	FB	**55(55)**	**3300**
15	18/F	FB	**60(40)**	**1600**
16	11/M	EB	60(45)	1800
17	41/F	FB	49(47)	200
18	47/M	FB	51(31)	200
19	19/M	EB	45(32)	2700
20	47/M	EB	47(35)	1500
21	48/M	EB	66(58)	3500
22	46/M	FB	43(35)	1600

Fig. 4.35 Total of 22 subjects were studied and the range of TBSA burned area is from 33% to 66%

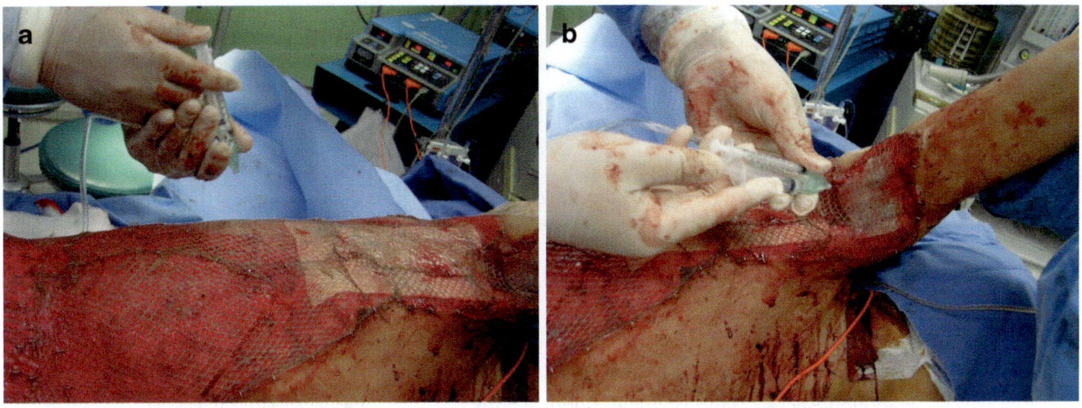

Fig. 4.36 (**a**, **b**) On joint areas, acellular dermal matrix was concurrently used with wide meshed autograft to minimize post-scar contractures. Keraheal® was sprayed on these areas also

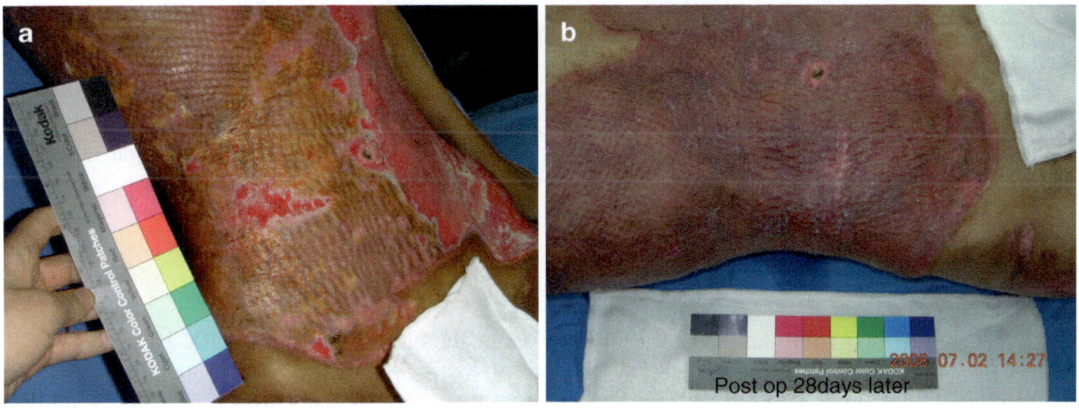

Fig. 4.37 (**a**, **b**) The take rate was estimated at 2 and 4 weeks by naked eye examinations of two certified burn surgeons and digital imaging. The status of scar formation was analyzed based on Vancouver scar scale at 8, 12, and 24 weeks respectively

Vancouver scar scale by date for scar tissue evaluation [41] (Fig. 4.37).

4.9 Cell Suspension Type: TPX-103(TEGO Science, Inc., Seoul, Korea)

Next, to popularize the spray technique, minimize the culture time which is an obstacle to its convenient use, and to prepare methods for its applications in deep second-degree burns, laser therapy, dermabrasion, and cosmetic surgery, among others, a phase III clinical trial of TPX-103 (TEGO Science, Inc.) evaluating its efficacy and safety on second-degree burns was conducted from November 2012 to June 2013. The feature of TPX-103 is its ability to reduce culture time for autologous keratinocyte single cell suspension to 8–14 days. Therefore, the trial aimed to apply this quickly to clinical practice by reducing culture times and was designed for effective treatment of cosmetic lesions or laser therapy, as well as second-degree burns. The following table shows the clinical results of 13 patients with second-degree burns (Fig. 4.38). TPX-103 is an autologous keratinocyte suspension for which a phase II open-label clinical trial was conducted on patients with

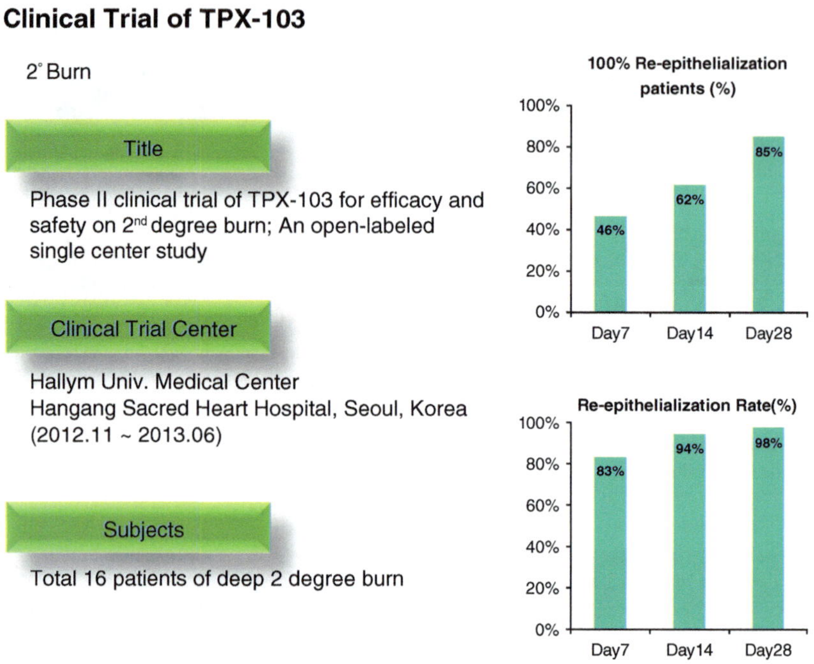

Fig. 4.38 TPX-103 is an autologous keratinocyte suspension for which a phase II open-label clinical trial was conducted on patients with second-degree burns with the approval of the MFDS from November 15, 2012 to June 24, 2013. TPX-103 spray was applied to all 13 subjects enrolled in the trial with 1 mL of TPX-103 on each wound site up to 500 cm^2

second-degree burns with the approval of the MFDS from November 15, 2012 to June 24, 2013. TPX-103 spray was applied to all 13 subjects enrolled in the trial with 1 mL of TPX-103 on each wound site up to 500 cm^2. The trial was completed without any dropouts. As a result of the clinical trial, 100% re-epithelialization was confirmed in 61.54% (8/13 people) of the subjects at 14 days after the administration of TPX-103 and 84.62% (11/13 people) of the subjects after 28 days. Additionally, 14 days after the administration of TPX-103, the re-epithelialization rate was 93.69 ± 11.32% and 97.69 ± 5.63% after 24 days. This technique requires further evaluation and more clinical trials and studies for establishing it as a cell suspension technique (Fig. 4.38).

4.10 Clinical Application of CEA in Reconstructive Surgery

4.10.1 CEA Combined with Dermal Substitutes

It is not easy to make an application of CEA to reconstructive surgery [42]. This is because there is no dermal layer which is fundamental to reconstruction, therefore it is not possible to make satisfactory corrections of scar contracture. However, it appears that for patients with nearly full body burns, a good result can be expected by combining CEA and dermal substitutes which can replace the dermal layer. This concept is well explained for cases involving the combined use of human dermal matrix which can be done with a single-step operation, as described above.

A 23-year-old male patient suffered flame burn with TBSA of 35%. Excisional and incisional releases were performed for severe scar contracture, and then a dermal matrix and 1:4 ratio wide-mesh graft were used in conjunction with CEA that had been cultured 3 weeks prior to reconstructive surgery (Fig. 4.39). This yielded reasonable results, with correction effects visible in the majority of severe scar contracture areas in the anterior chest (Fig. 4.40).

The following case involved a 10-year-old male patient who underwent dermal substitute AlloDerm® and a 1:6 auto-mesh skin graft for the reconstruction of severe scar contractures in the chest and abdomen caused by flame burns on 67% of the entire body surface was performed. To improve graft survival and accelerate recovery, a CEA was performed simultaneously using a 1:6 auto-mesh skin graft. By 19 days after the procedure, the dermal substitute and CEA had been engrafted, and most of the wound had healed. Three weeks prior, a skin biopsy was prepared to make CEA sheets, and then 1:6 wide-mesh skin grafts with CEA sheets were applied, yielding significant results although not fully satisfactory (Fig. 4.41).

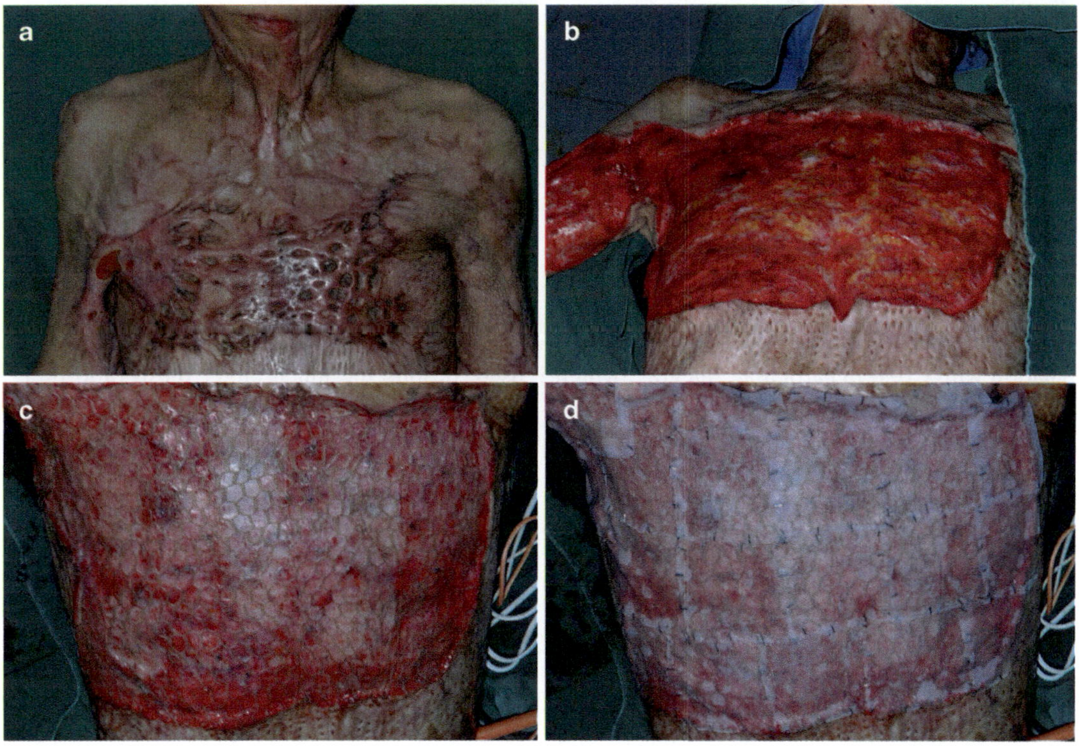

Fig. 4.39 (**a**) Severe scar contracture noted on anterior neck and entire chest. (**b**) Excisional release on anterior chest right axilla area. (**c**, **d**) Human dermal matrix and 1:4 ratio wide-mesh graft were used in conjunction with CEA sheets

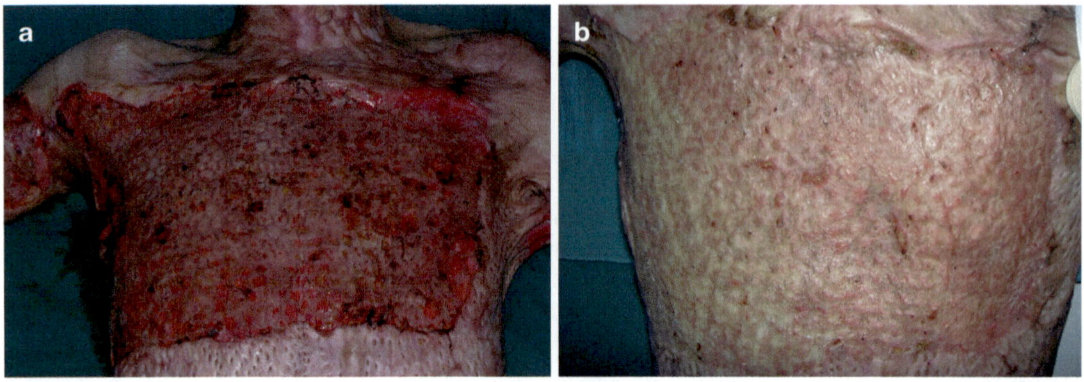

Fig. 4.40 (**a**) 10 days after operation, epithelialization was noted completely. (**b**) Postoperative 1 month later operative wound was healed completely without any complication and effective operation outcome

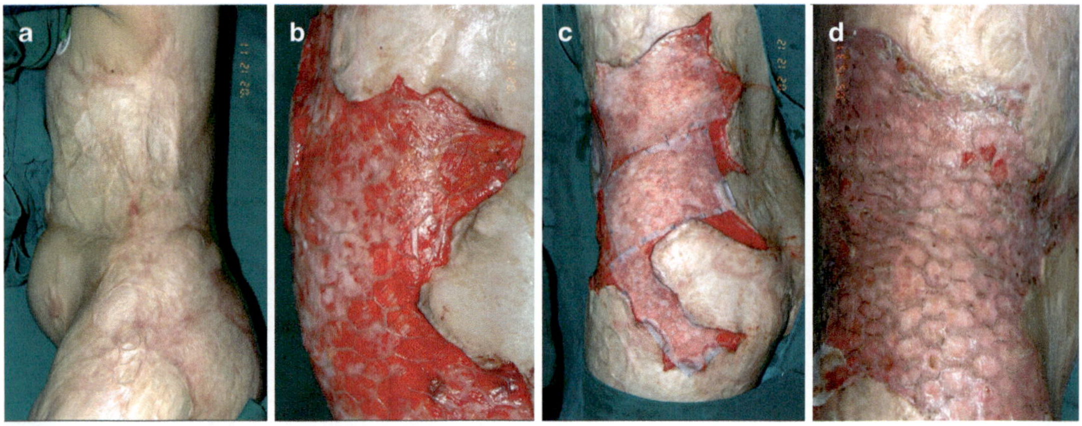

Fig. 4.41 (**a**) Severe scar contracture noted on the chest and abdomen. (**b**) Human dermal substitute and 1:6 automesh skin graft were performed and (**c**) CEA sheets were covered simultaneously. (**d**) 19 days after the procedure, the dermal substitute and CEA had been engrafted and most of the wound had healed

Other dermal substitutes can be used in combination with CEA. In particular, Integra®, which requires a two-step operation, is also available because there is sufficient time to produce CEA sheets while forming neodermis for 2–3 weeks. The 10-year-old male patient developed severe scar contractures in the entire anterior chest and abdomen after flame burn treatment. A full-thickness skin biopsy and full release were performed, and dermal substitute Integra® was engrafted. Then, on day 24 after surgery, when the neodermis had been formed, a 1:9 maximized-size mesh skin graft using CEA sheets was applied. In this case, it appeared that contracture developed further than the human dermal matrix, but clinical findings indicate that Integra® can be used, despite the much larger mesh ratio of 1:9 and individual differences. Therefore, further clinical studies are needed in this area (Fig. 4.42).

In the next section, the author introduces a clinical trial of wide-mesh skin grafts and CEA-sheet grafts, in addition to the findings of early experimental clinical trials involving the combined use of dermal substitutes. Significant findings were obtained from this clinical trial which provided the valuable experience and basis of clinical applications for many cases introduced previously. The following case involves a 32-year-old female patient with deep second- and third-degree burns on the anterior chest and neck

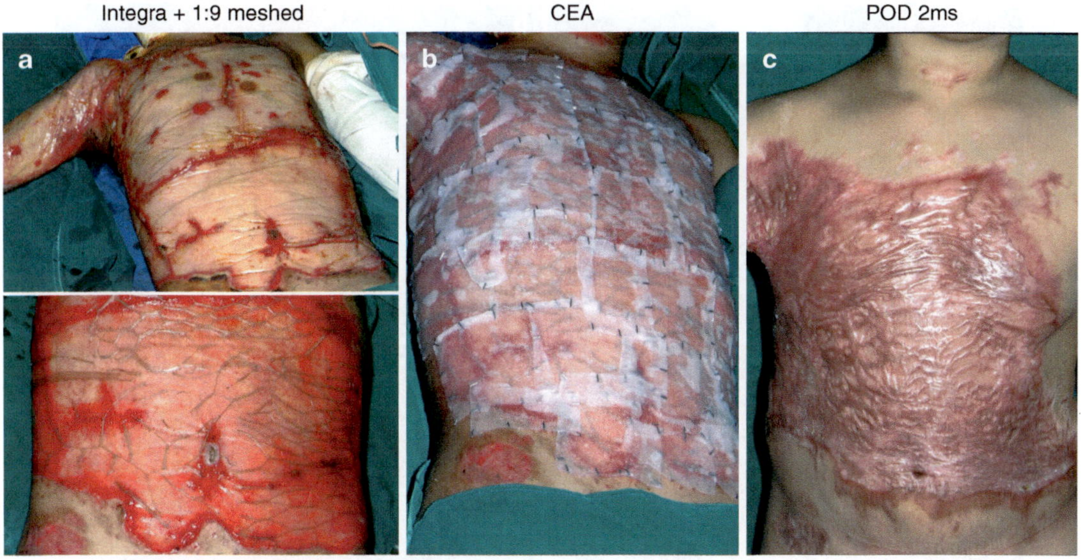

Fig. 4.42 (**a**, **b**) On day 24 days after the Integra application, wide 1:9 meshed autografts and CEA sheets were applied (**c**) At post op 2 months, unfortunately, contracture has marked development. For this reason, our aim is developing cultured epithelial cells combined with artificial dermis that is close to natural human skin

areas as a result of flame burns. Eschar separation and wound management, along with necrotic tissue removal, were performed. Furthermore, a dermal matrix AlloDerm® and 1:6 wide-mesh skin graft with CEA-sheet graft were performed in the right axilla and shoulder areas 21 days after a culture biopsy was performed during an earlier period of burn. For comparative observation, only CEA sheets were grafted without mesh skin grafting on the left anterior chest. As a result, on day 16 after surgery, the healing process was much faster in the wide-mesh autograft area with human dermal matrix but much slower on the left side where only CEA sheets were grafted (Fig. 4.43). The left side showed signs of healing after 40 days, and hypopigmentation was observed a year after surgery. However, there was no significant difference in scar contracture. This clinical trial shows that the presence of even very small auto-skin (over 1:9 ratio very wide-mesh auto-skin) is crucial to the healing process of CEA-sheet grafts in burn wound management and that CEA-sheet grafts alone do not play a huge role in skin pigmentation. Because CEA lacks the ability to control skin pigmentation on its own, we are researching skin pigmentation control with the proper ratio of melanocytes and keratinocytes. However, it was demonstrated that the combined use of dermal substitutes with an auto-mesh skin graft and covering with a CEA sheet is a good alternative technique for reducing scar contracture rates and hypopigmentation (Fig. 4.44).

4.10.2 CEA from Palm and Sole Area

The author believes that cells maintain the nature of the area where they exist, even among cultured cells, and they keep their unique properties within the cultured state. This is just an established theory and has not been firmly validated. Unfortunately, there are only a few relatable cases, and the results of completed clinical trials could not be introduced. Despite this, the author wants to introduce some results believing that a few cases have been observed which are worth mentioning.

The author obtained satisfactory results from a one-stage correction with FTSG for fingers and palm flexor contractures in early childhood; however, a color mismatch between the skin color of the original palm and the engrafted skin can be a serious psychological problem for highly sensi-

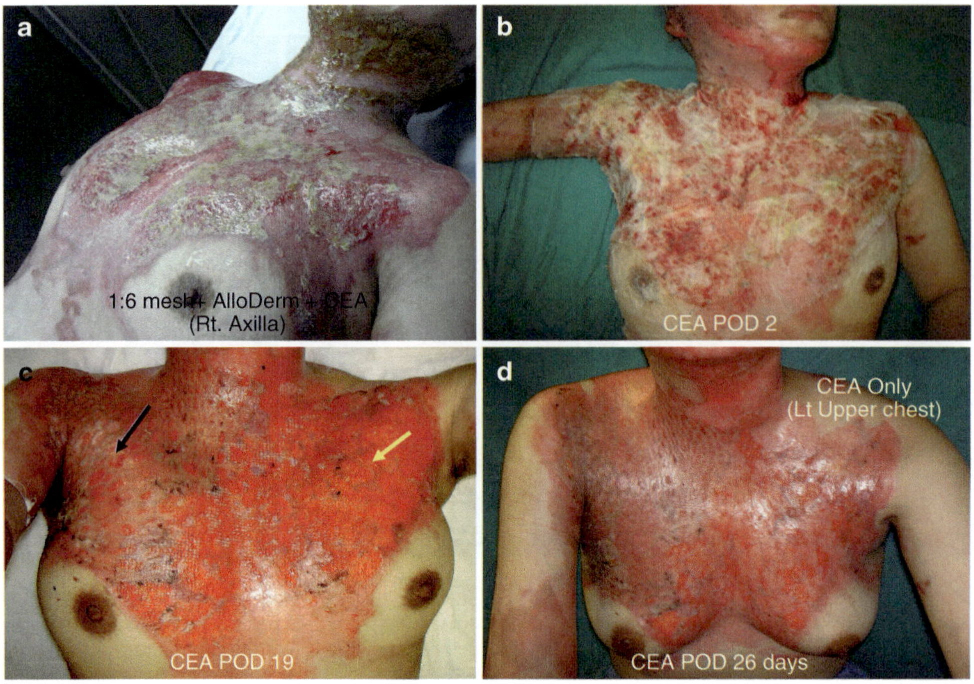

Fig. 4.43 (**a**) Deep second- and third-degree burn on anterior chest and neck area. 21 days after the burn, human dermal matrix with 1:6 auto-mesh graft was covered with CEA on right axilla area (black arrow) and CEA alone on left upper chest (yellow arrow) area. (**b**) Postoperative 2 days' view, (**c**) 19 and (**d**) 26 days, shows that left upper chest area is not yet completely healed

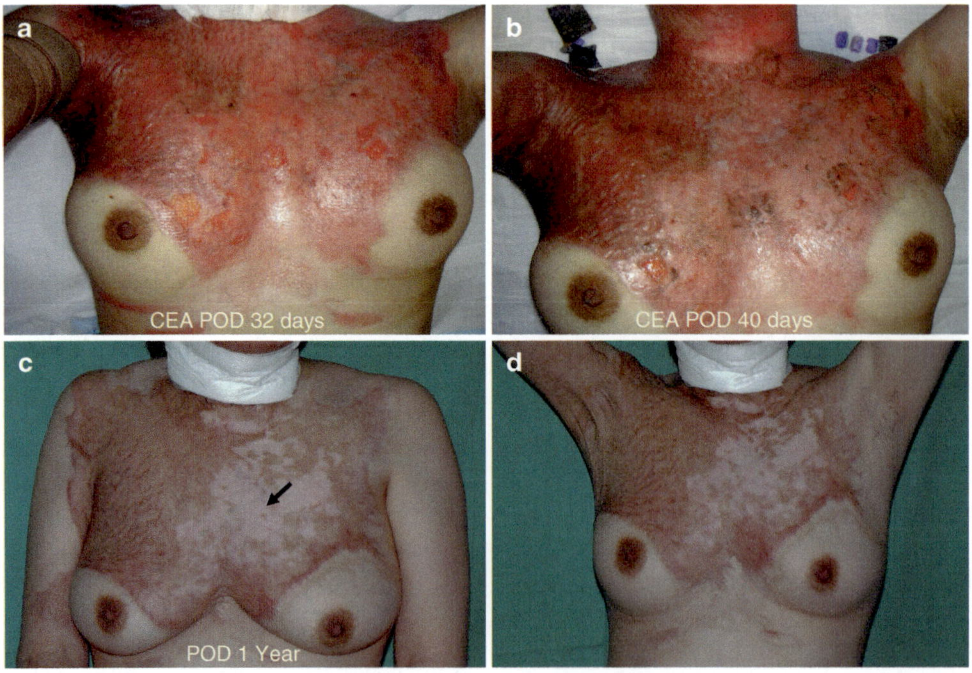

Fig. 4.44 (**a**, **b**) Postoperative 32, 40 days, CEA only applied left side area healed finally. (**c**, **d**) Postoperative 1 year after, CEA applied area showed similarities to the artificial dermis applied area except hypopigmentation disorder (black arrow)

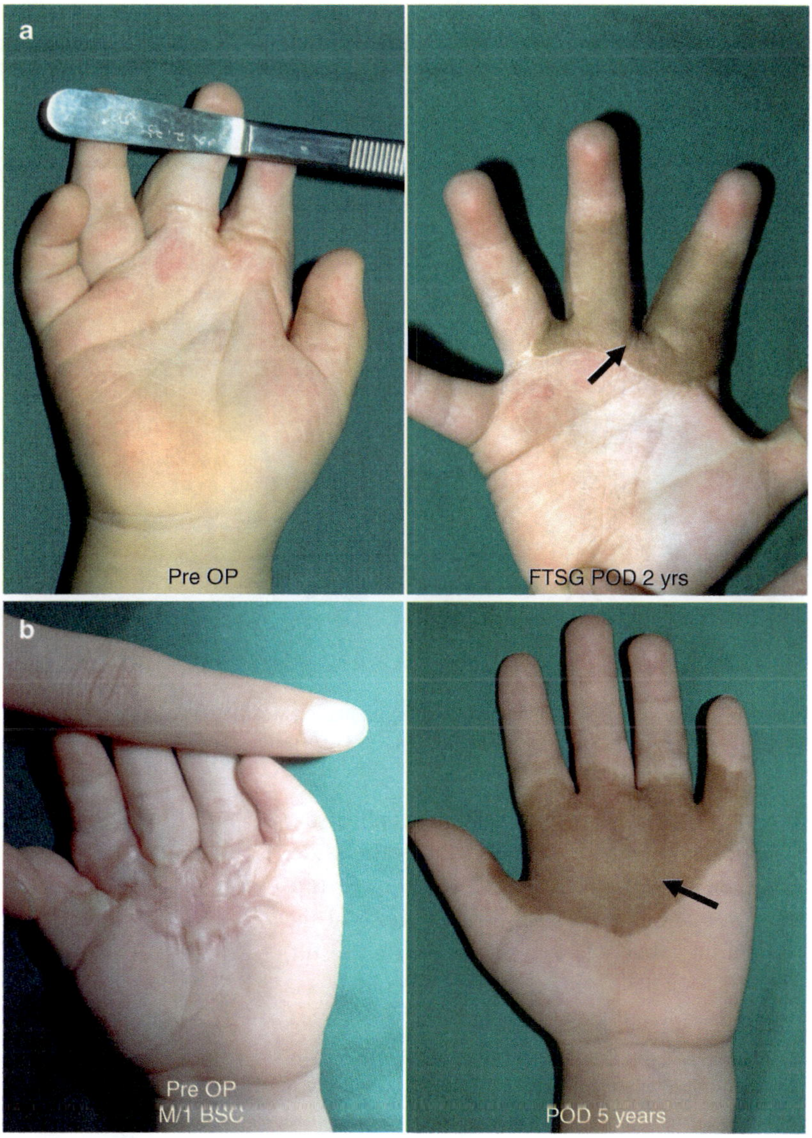

Fig. 4.45 (**a**, **b**) Full-thickness skin graft to palm area often gives unsatisfactory aesthetical results. This full-thickness engrafted region of the pigmentation tends to darken (black arrows) with coarse skin texture due to repeating minor scratches and exposure to sun

tive children (Fig. 4.45). In such cases, a dermal over graft technique with STSG in the instep side of the sole is used to treat the problem (Refer: Chap. 5 Figs. 5.52 and 5.53). A clinical trial was conducted to resolve using improved cell culture techniques, and the results are presented below.

An 8-year-old male patient sustained an electric rice cooker steam injury at the age of 1. At the age of 2, he underwent corrective surgery for severe scar contracture, including release and FTSG, and showed good functional recovery. However, as he grew, hyperpigmentation developed on the operation site, necessitating the use of a cell culture technique to alleviate psychiatric stress caused by the hyperpigmentation. For the cell culture, 2 × 3 cm cells were collected at 12/1000-in. thickness from the stratum lucidum layer of the inside step area of the sole and were cultured for 10 days to produce CEA sheets. Only the very thin epidermal layer was removed by dermabrasion procedure, removing only hyperpigmentaion. CEA-sheet graft was performed, followed by wet dressing for 10 days (Fig. 4.46). After complete healing, follow-up checks were

CEA from sole epidermal keratinocyte

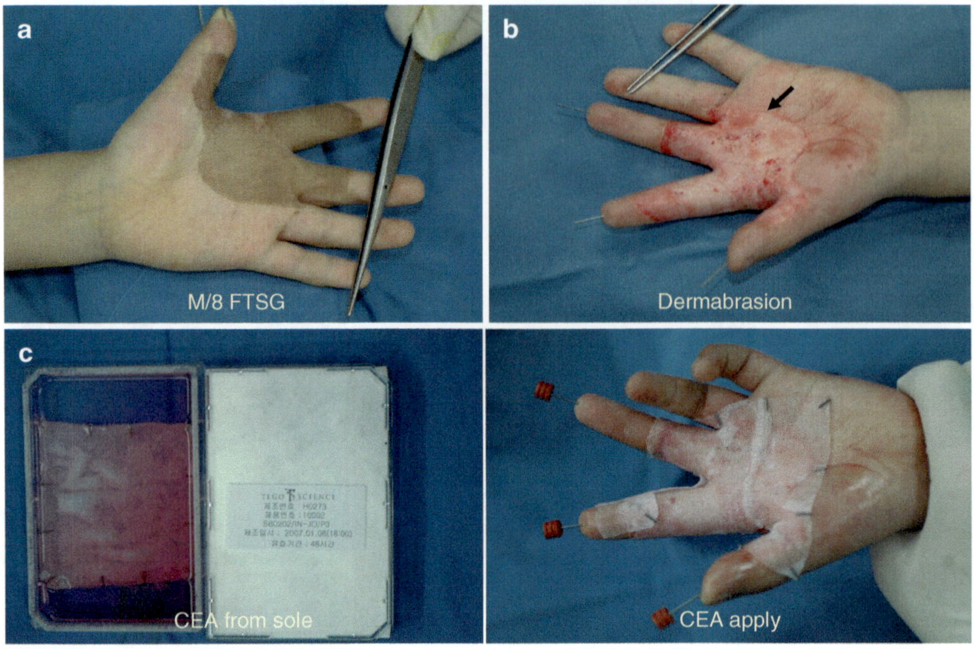

Fig. 4.46 (**a**) Preoperative view, darkened pigmentation was noted on the left palm. (**b**) After dermabrasion of epidermal portion of full-thickness engrafted region, (**c**) CEA processed from sole skin was applied

observed. After 3 months, a hypertrophic scar was observed in an area of the palm side. However, in some finger sites, the skin texture and color of the palm side matched those of the surrounding skin, which was a significant result, implying that the transfer of cell characteristics is possible (Fig. 4.47).

The following case involves a 4-year-old male patient who was given extra care. Cell biopsy was performed on the opposite side of the palm, and more extensive attempts were made, but improvement was observed when compared to the first case. It was confirmed once more that hypertrophic scarring only developed after dermabrasion with a CEA-sheet graft lacking the epidermal and dermal layers and that the formation of a stable epidermal layer was essential. This is an issue that has not been completely addressed. However, the results provided some support for the theory that cultured cells retain their natural cell characteristics (Figs. 4.48 and 4.49). This reminded the author that it was crucial to find cultured epidermal cells that are of appropriate match for the cultivated epidermal and dermal layers for producing normal skin. For the author, the purpose of writing this is

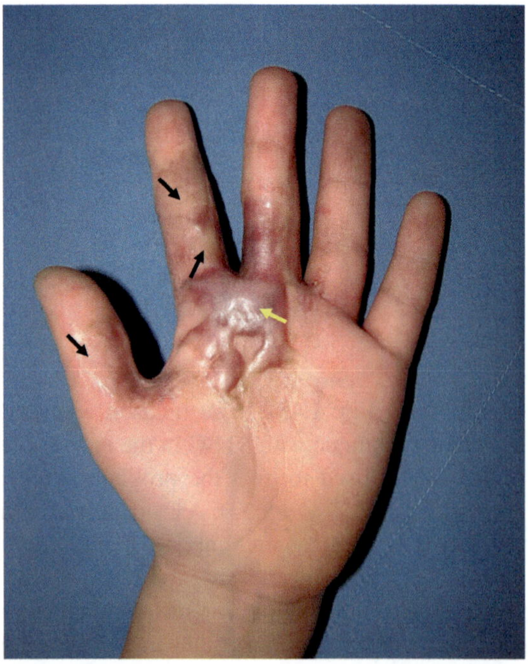

Fig. 4.47 3 months after the procedure, interestingly, some regions developed hypertrophic scars even though only epidermis portion was dermabraded (yellow arrow). And some regions showed good result with color and texture match to the surrounding normal palm area (black arrows)

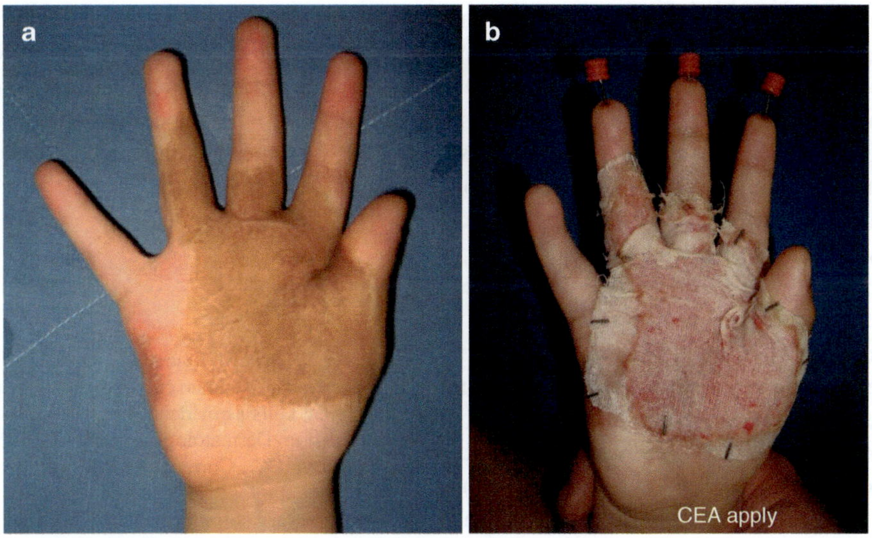

Fig. 4.48 (**a**) Preoperative view, (**b**) CEA derived from opposite palm biopsy

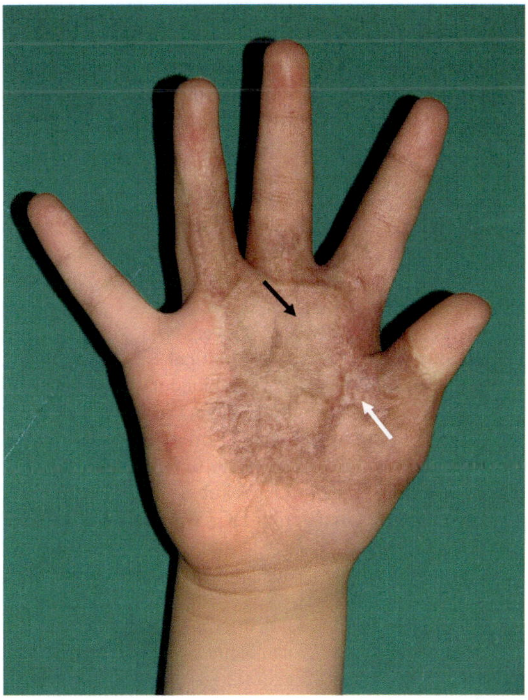

Fig. 4.49 2 months after the procedure, some regions developed hypertrophic scars when only epidermis portion was dermabraded (yellow arrow). Some regions showed color and texture match to the surrounding palm area (black arrow)

his passion and desire to provide valuable information for the development and production of the real artificial skin in the future. In the final chapter, the authors looks forward to achieving additional advanced outcomes in the future.

4.11 Conclusion

Beginning with a human clinical study of CEA in 1981, keratinocyte cell therapy has remarkably improved with take rate up to >90% compared to the disappointing rates seen during earlier stages of development. Because of advanced culture techniques, we can create sufficient areas of cultured cells as needed for clinical practice. However, there is a considerable disadvantage related to the culture time of at least 2 weeks to use CEA, and thus it is not available quickly. Moreover, in order to produce sufficient area amount to cover the human body surface, a minimum of 2–3 weeks are needed; thus, for patients with massive burns requiring immediate treatment, the reduction of sheet production and culture time requires further development. Therefore, the author produced cell suspensions to reduce production times for cultured epithelial sheets and to shorten the complex process. Furthermore, it has been verified that in harvesting donor skin, split-thickness skin is effective for culturing, thereby not necessitating full-thickness skin. Cell suspension spray technique can be applied in clinical practice easily and quickly; this method reduces production time and a easy, direct wide wound area coverage. It shows adequate results for major burn management. Currently, the concept of wound healing via cultured cell therapy primarily focuses on epithelialization, and there is still much more development needed for it to function as skin in the full sense of the word. The author supplemented the dermal layer using human dermal matrix and obtained a supplemental effect for the dermal layer in some areas by using a sandwich technique with wide-mesh skin and CEA. Furthermore, targeting reduced culture time in CEA, the TPX-103 project was carried out, which focused on the development of combined techniques for cell suspension and an expansion of the range of its applications and obtained promising results. Additionally, a study on the expansion of clinical applications of CEA validated a hypothesis that all cells in the human body maintain their own nature, even though they are cultured, and the author regrets only partial results could be achieved from a clinical trial of the skin on the palm and sole involving the stratum lucidum that other skin areas do not have. There are aims of continuing and elevating this research in the future, working with the next generation of surgeons, the author aims to contribute to a wide range of areas of treatments and techniques in various wound management sectors, could be developed including second-degree burns, traumatic wounds, laser therapy, chronic wounds, and DM foot, by preparing a standard protocol for CEH, which went through a clinical trial prior to CEA. Additionally, it was meaningful to the author that this contribution was made to the application of National Health Insurance to ensure that people can benefit from wider treatment areas. The author has worked on cell therapy for the last 20 years, understanding the immense potential for additional research in this field. He hopes that this study motivates readers and looks forward to the development of the "True artificial skin." Regardless of incomplete results, it is imperative for the author to provide information that can be referred to various clinical courses.

References

1. Gielen V, Faure M, Mauduit G, Thivolet J. Progressive replacement of human cultured epithelial allografts by recipient cells as evidenced by HLA class I antigens expression. Dermatologica. 1987;175(4):166–70.
2. Compton CC. Current concepts in pediatric burn care: the biology of cultured epithelial autografts: an eight-year study in pediatric burn patients. Eur J Pediatr Surg. 1992;2(4):216–22.
3. Leigh IM, Purkis PE, Navsaria HA, Phillips TJ. Treatment of chronic venous ulcers with sheets of cultured allogenic keratinocytes. Br J Dermatol. 1987;117(5):591–7. https://doi.org/10.1111/j.1365-2133.1987.tb07491.x.
4. Rue LW 3rd, Cioffi WG, McManus WF, Pruitt BA Jr. Wound closure and outcome in extensively burned patients treated with cultured autologous keratinocytes. J Trauma. 1993;34(5):662–7; discussion 667-8.
5. Boyce ST, Goretsky MJ, Greenhalgh DG, Kagan RJ, Rieman MT, Warden GD. Comparative assessment of cultured skin substitutes and native skin autograft for treatment of full-thickness burns. Ann Surg. 1995;222(6):743–52.
6. Boyce ST, Kagan RJ, Meyer NA, Yakuboff KP, Warden GD. The 1999 clinical research award. Cultured skin substitutes combined with Integra artificial skin to replace native skin autograft and allograft for the closure of excised full-thickness burns. J Burn Care Rehabil. 1999;20(6):453–61.
7. Boyce ST, Kagan RJ, Yakuboff KP, Meyer NA, Rieman MT, Greenhalgh DG, Warden GD. Cultured skin substitutes reduce donor skin harvesting for closure of excised, full-thickness burns. Ann Surg. 2002;235(2):269–79.
8. Boyce ST, Warden GD. Principles and practices for treatment of cutaneous wounds with cultured skin substitutes. Am J Surg. 2002;183(4):445–56.
9. Sheridan R. Closure of the excised burn wound: autografts, semipermanent skin substitutes, and permanent skin substitutes. Clin Plast Surg. 2009;36(4):643–51.
10. Choi JH, Ko JH, Seo DK, Lee JW, Jeon S, Oh SJ, Jang YC. Treatment of partial thickness burn wounds with cultured epidermal homografts. J Korean Soc Plast Reconstr Surg. 2006;33(5):587–91.
11. Phillips TJ, Gilchrest BA. Clinical applications of cultured epithelium. Epithelial Cell Biol. 1992;1(1):39–46.

12. Pye RJ. Cultured keratinocytes as biological wound dressings. Eye (Lond). 1988;2(Pt 2):172–8.
13. Phillips TJ, Gilchrest BA. Cultured epidermal allografts as biological wound dressings. Prog Clin Biol Res. 1991;365:77–94.
14. Iuchi S, Dabelsteen S, Easley K, Rheinwald JG, Green H. Immortalized keratinocyte lines derived from human embryonic stem cells. Proc Natl Acad Sci U S A. 2006;103(6):1792–7.
15. Lo CH, Akbarzadeh S, McLean C, Ives A, Paul E, Brown WA, Cleland H. Wound healing after cultured epithelial autografting in patients with massive burn injury: a cohort study. J Plast Reconstr Aesthet Surg. 2019;72(3):427–37.
16. Lo CH, Chong E, Akbarzadeh S, Brown WA, Cleland H. A systematic review: current trends and take rates of cultured epithelial autografts in the treatment of patients with burn injuries. Wound Repair Regen. 2019;27(6):693–701.
17. Phillips TJ, Provan A, Colbert D, Easley KW. A randomized single-blind controlled study of cultured epidermal allografts in the treatment of split-thickness skin graft donor sites. Arch Dermatol. 1993;129(7):879–82.
18. Dhennin C. Skin substitutes and skin culture. Rev Prat. 2002;52(20):2249–52.
19. Lataillade JJ, Bey E, Thepenier C, Prat M, Leclerc T, Bargues L. Skin engineering for burns treatment bull. Acad Natl Med. 2010;194(7):1339–51.
20. Dreifke MB, Jayasuriya AA, Jayasuriya AC. Current wound healing procedures and potential care. Mater Sci Eng C Mater Biol Appl. 2015;48:651–62.
21. Bargues L, Prat M, Leclerc T, Bey E, Lataillade JJ. Present and future of cell therapy in burns. Pathol Biol (Paris). 2011;59(3):e49–56.
22. Hynds RE, Bonfanti P, Janes SM. Regenerating human epithelia with cultured stem cells: feeder cells, organoids and beyond. EMBO Mol Med. 2018;10(2):139–50.
23. Muehleman C, Wise RD. Epidermal culture and grafting. A brief review. J Am Podiatr Med Assoc. 1993;83(8):462–5.
24. Rowan MP, Cancio LC, Elster EA, Burmeister DM, Rose LF, Natesan S, Chan RK, Christy RJ, Chung KK. Burn wound healing and treatment: review and advancements. Crit Care. 2015;19:243.
25. Teepe RG, Burger A, Ponec M. Immunohistochemical studies on regeneration in cultured epidermal autografts used to treat full-thickness burn wounds. Clin Exp Dermatol. 1994;19(1):16–22.
26. Han S. Innovations and advances in wound healing. Berlin, Heidelberg: Springer; 2016. p. 223–5.
27. Fratianne R, Papay F, Housini I, Lang C, Schafer IA. Keratinocyte allografts accelerate healing of split-thickness donor sites: applications for improved treatment of burns. J Burn Care Rehabil. 1993;14(2 Pt 1):148–54.
28. Isik FF, Gibran NS, Jang YC, Sandell L, Schwartz SM. Vitronectin decrease microvascular endothelial cell apoptosis. J Cell Physiol. 1998;175(2):149–55.
29. Jang YC, Arumugam S, Ferguson M, Gibran NS, Isik FF. Changes in matrix composition during the growth and regression of human hemangiomas. J Surg Res. 1998;80(1):9–15.
30. Arumugam S, Jang YC, Chen-Jensen C, Gibran NS, Isik FF. Temporal activity of plasminogen activators and matrix metalloproteinases during cutaneous wound repair. Surgery. 1999;125(6):587–93.
31. Jang Y-C, Arumugam S, Gibran N, Isik F. Role of alpha(v) integrins and angiogenesis during wound repair. Wound Repair Regen. 1999;7(5):375–80.
32. Jang YC, Tsou R, Gibran NS, Isik FF. Vitronectin deficiency is associated with increased wound fibrinolysis and decreased microvascular angiogenesis in mice. Surgery. 2000;127(6):696–704.
33. Jang YC, Isik FF, Gibran NS. Nerve distribution in hemangiomas depends on the proliferative state of the microvasculature. J Surg Res. 2000;93(1):144–8.
34. Gibran NS, Jang YC, Isik FF, Greenhalgh DG, Muffley LA, Underwood RA, Usui ML, Larson J, Smith DG, Ansel JC, Olerud JE. Diminished neuropeptide levels contribute to the impaired cutaneous healing response associated with diabetes mellitus. J Surg Res. 2002;108(1):122–8.
35. Gauglitz GG, Zedler S, von Spiegel F, Fuhr J, von Donnersmarck GH, Faist E. Functional characterization of cultured keratinocytes after acute cutaneous burn injury. PLoS One. 2012;7(2):e29942.
36. Atiyeh BS, Costagliola M. Cultured epithelial autograft (CEA) in burn treatment: three decades later. Burns. 2007;33(4):405–13.
37. Woodroof EA, Phipps RP, Greenwood JE, Hickerson W, Herndon D. The search for an ideal temporary skin substitute: AWBAT plus, a combination product wound dressing medical device. Eplasty. 2010;10:e60.
38. Boyce ST, Glafkides MC, Foreman TJ, Hansbrough JF. Reduced wound contraction after grafting of full-thickness burns with a collagen and chondroitin-6-sulfate (GAG) dermal skin substitute and coverage with biobrane. J Burn Care Rehabil. 1988;9(4):364–70.
39. Herzog SR, Meyer A, Woodley D, Peterson HD. Wound coverage with cultured autologous keratinocytes: use after burn wound excision, including biopsy followup. J Trauma. 1988;28(2):195–8.
40. Munster AM. Cultured skin for massive burns. A prospective, controlled trial. Ann Surg. 1996;224(3):372–5; discussion 375-7.
41. Ha TS, Cho YS, Kim DH, Hur J, Chun W, Kim JH, Kim YY, Son YS. Clinical study of autologous cultured keratinocyte cell spray "Keraheal™"on severe burn wound. J Korean Burn Soc. 2007;10(2):112–7.
42. Hayashi M, Yoshitake K, Tokunaka R, Yoshida Y, Oshima M, Tatsuta S, Hamada T, Kamitomo A, Hamajima A. Combination of meshed dermis graft and cultured epithelial autograft for massive burns: three case reports. Medicine (Baltimore). 2018;97(48):e13313.

Esthetic Skin Graft

5

5.1 Introduction

This chapter will introduce dermabrasion and dermal resurfacing (overgraft) technique for new aspect concept of esthetic skin grafting. Firstly, it will introduce the different points of skin thickness for each graft site of the body based on the engrafted skin thickness, which is the most important aspect of consequential surgical outcomes, and long-term follow-up results. The key point is finely adjusting the skin thickness depending on the site of the dermal resurfacing, on either parts of the face or forearm and hand. The surgical outcomes of the selection of these sites and the long-term follow-up results will also be introduced. Next, the instruments required for the preparation of the surgery and the manner of their use will be introduced. The dermabrasion skills and engrafting techniques essential for performing the surgery will be described, and the postoperative wound dressing methods, complications, postoperative long-term management, and a laser therapy supported with various examples. The outcomes of dermal resurfacing performed on artificial dermis, these results indicates a vast applicability range of this surgical technique as it proved that dermal over skin graft (dermal resurfacing) acceptance is possible even when the graft is from a different environment or consists of various materials such as dermal substitute. In application part, the infinite possibilities and outcomes of dermabrasion and dermal resurfacing with full-thickness skin grafts (FTSG) and not thin STSG will be introduced, maximizing the final esthetic effects of the dermal resurfacing. FTSG is a useful grafting method in concurrently achieving excellent functional and esthetic effects in the emaciated area where unstable bone and skin regions occur due to soft tissue defects. Additionally, it is effective for regions requiring soft tissue repair and reinforcement augmentation for widely depressed deformities and the joint areas. The author performed dermabrasion and dermal overgraft using only thin split-thickness skin graft for simple esthetic purposes in earlier periods but gradually increased the thickness of the skin graft owing to further clinical experience, which ultimately led to the successful result by FTSG. Additionally, it was observed from clinical experiences that overgraft was possible even when performing full-thickness skin graft with attached subcutaneous fat layer. This will also be described.

Y.-C. Jang, *The Art of Skin Graft*, https://doi.org/10.1007/978-981-97-0017-2_5

5.2 Esthetic Skin Graft: Dermabrasion and Dermal Resurfacing (Overgraft) Technique

5.2.1 The Concept of Esthetic Skin Graft Using Dermabrasion and Dermal Overgraft Technique

Generally, skin graft is considered as one of the prompt treatment measures to cover a burn or trauma wound [1], but it is not esthetically appealing, primarily because the skin graft site is distinct from its surrounding tissue in terms of color and texture and is usually accompanied by a considerable deformity of the surrounding tissues. Therefore, a prejudice has prevailed regarding skin graft being a chiefly surgical treatment, which leaves behind unsightly dysmorphia [2, 3]. In this chapter, the author has attempted to emphasize on and develop an esthetic concept of the dermabrasion and dermal overgraft techniques to address some of these prejudices. This esthetic-based technique was described by Webster, J. P. in 1954 and Erol, O. in 1990, who attempted thin STSG at approximately 0.3 mm on an irregular burn scar and hypopigmentation site [4]. Additionally, there were other cases reporting attempts at very thin STSG (0.15 mm) in vitiligo [5–10] or depigmented burn scars [11–13], but it was not applied more actively for esthetic purposes. Hence, universal and practical surgical techniques to obtain a definite esthetic outcome for wide burn or traumatic scars are yet to be introduced [14–16]. The author aimed to correct wide, unsightly scars or pigmentation disorders in the areas under constant external exposure, including the face, neck, forearm, and dorsum of the hand, by performing esthetic corrective skin graft and expanding its range of applications. Usually, several difficult limitations are associated with correcting a wide burn or traumatic scar and fully achieving acceptable esthetic results. The author actively attempted the skin graft technique, where dermabrasion is conducted on the scar bed using a dermabrader and a thin split skin is grafted over the site. This method is extremely useful in sites where the tissue expander technique, serial excision, local flap, or FTSG cannot be applied due to the wide range of the scars. Typically, these techniques are used as conventional methods to correct wide burn or traumatic scars; however, the limitations of these methods include their restricted excision amount and unsightly color mismatch or conspicuous graft or flap margin and disfigurement of surrounding structures. The direct removal of scar tissues causes disfigurements in the surrounding tissues, such as those of the eyes, nose, mouth, and three-dimensional curved surfaces and a long linear surgical scar line and dog ear deformity, which are the drawbacks of these procedures as they create further unesthetic surgical scars. The author suggests various simple and easy methods to resolve such drawbacks, among which is the thin STSG technique.

Before this technique is performed, the choice of operable surgical indication is an important component.

5.2.1.1 Surgical Indications

The operative indicators of scar beds include the following:

The operation indication of dermal overgraft is influenced by whether or not the operation results are excellent. Because this technique is delicate, it has an impact on the surrounding tissue and scar bed. The indications include an irregular scar surface, hyperpigmentation, hypopigmentation, vitiligo, and a conspicuous graft surface area (black arrows). A typical surgical indication of a pigmentation lesion without scar irregularities or disfigurement is shown in Fig. 5.1.

1. The regions with no tissue deformities around a scar contracture. If present, the procedure should be considered after all the deformities are corrected and eventual maturation of the scar bed.
2. The regions with matured, wide, and flattened irregular surfaces and simple unsightly pigmentation disorders such as vitiligo, burn hypopigmentation [17].
3. The regions where the conspicuous graft margin and discoloration sites are distinct from

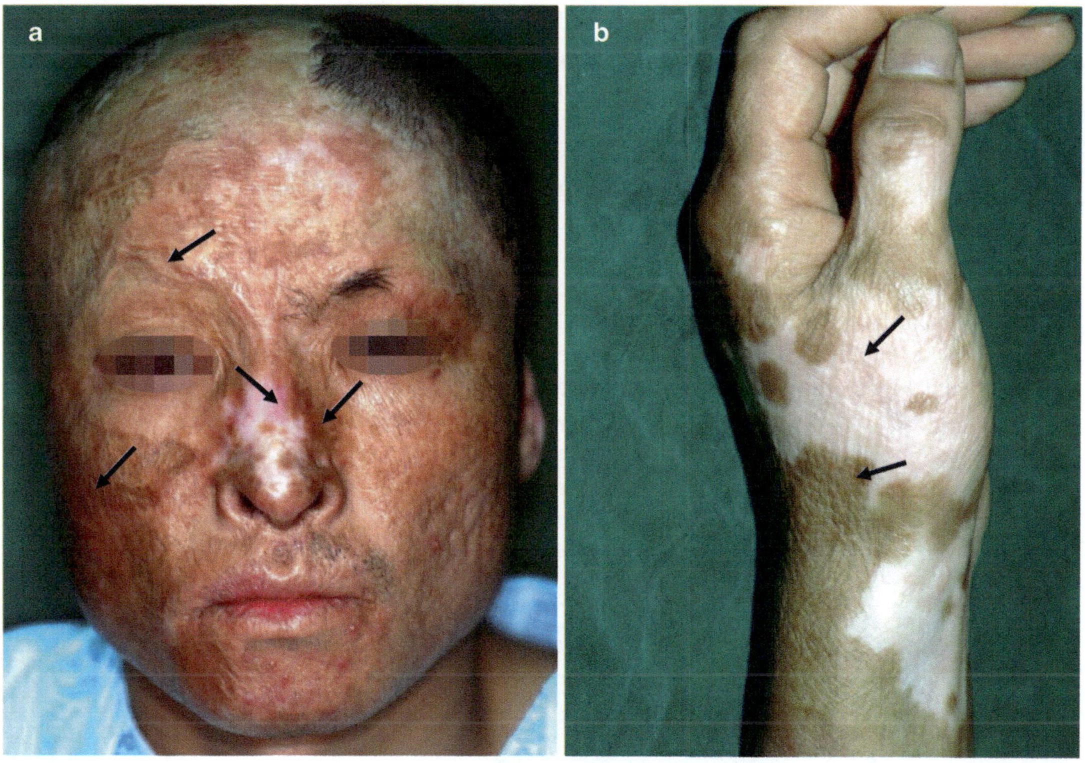

Fig. 5.1 (**a**) The indications of irregular scar surface, hyper- and hypopigmentation disorder, and conspicuous graft surface area (black arrows); (**b**) typical surgical indication of pigmentation lesion without scar irregularity and disfigurement

the surrounding tissues of the skin graft site, conducted for wound coverage due to trauma or burn.

4. The regions where wide and unsightly scars remain without surrounding tissue deformities and do not cause functional joint movement disturbances, including the dorsum of the hand, wrist, and neck area.

The key point of the procedure is patient selection, which substantially affects the surgical results. Therefore, thoroughly checking the patient conditions is important, including whether the scar bed is fully matured, tension-free, and absence of scar contracture, immature hypertrophic scars, and depressed scar bed. These factors need to meet the satisfactory condition levels prior to the surgery. It is very likely a patient with a unsightly scar on their forearm would hesitate to wear short sleeves in public, promoting patient's desire for complete scar removal. This is another factor to be considered. The limitations include visible, mildly engrafted margins or elevated skin; not quite the same skin color and texture as surrounding normal skin; and a slightly different skin color with hyperpigmented skin. However, these undesirable aspects can be improved further. Scar maturation takes a year or more, and some additional procedures such as silastic gel sheets, pressure garment wear, and Fraxel™ laser therapy are used.

5.2.1.2 Operative Procedure

Preparation

The surgical tools include electric dermabrader (Osada, Inc., Los Angeles, CA, USA) and diamond fraise wheels of various sizes.

(a, b) The dermabrader instrument is composed of an electric handpiece, a dermabrader engine, and (c) a variable-size diamond-tipped fraise wheel. If you have a surgical drill Stryker (Stryker, Inc., USA) or a dental drill [18], you can also use instruments such as a dermabrader. (d) If a thick, irregular, elevated scar bed is placed, I would like to recommend razor shaving as a method for easily removal and flattening the surface while reducing operation time (Fig. 5.2).

Electric or N_2O air dermatome: I prefer the N_2O air-driven dermatome as it is more powerful and has a lower malfunction rate. A dermatome must be handled carefully, and even pressure should be applied from all directions. The quality of the dermal overgraft skin is critical for the esthetic outcome, so donor skin must be a fine single sheet that is even in thickness (Fig. 5.3).

Irrigation syringe, 1:200,000–1:300,000 diluted epinephrine solution for hemostasis, Steri-Strip™ (3 M Health Care Conway Ave. St. Paul, MN, USA), and fine 6–0 nylon.

Although general anesthesia is typically required, local anesthesia is sufficient for cases involving a small area.

Dermabrasion

For this technique, a dermabrader is set to not exceed 20,000 rpm to avoid bending the neck of the diamond fraise wheel; if the neck does bend due to high rpm, the pivot consequently weakens. Due to this, the dermabraded surface is irregularly abraded, and the boundary surface is not precisely abraded. The key to skillful dermabrasion is to constantly move in a reciprocating

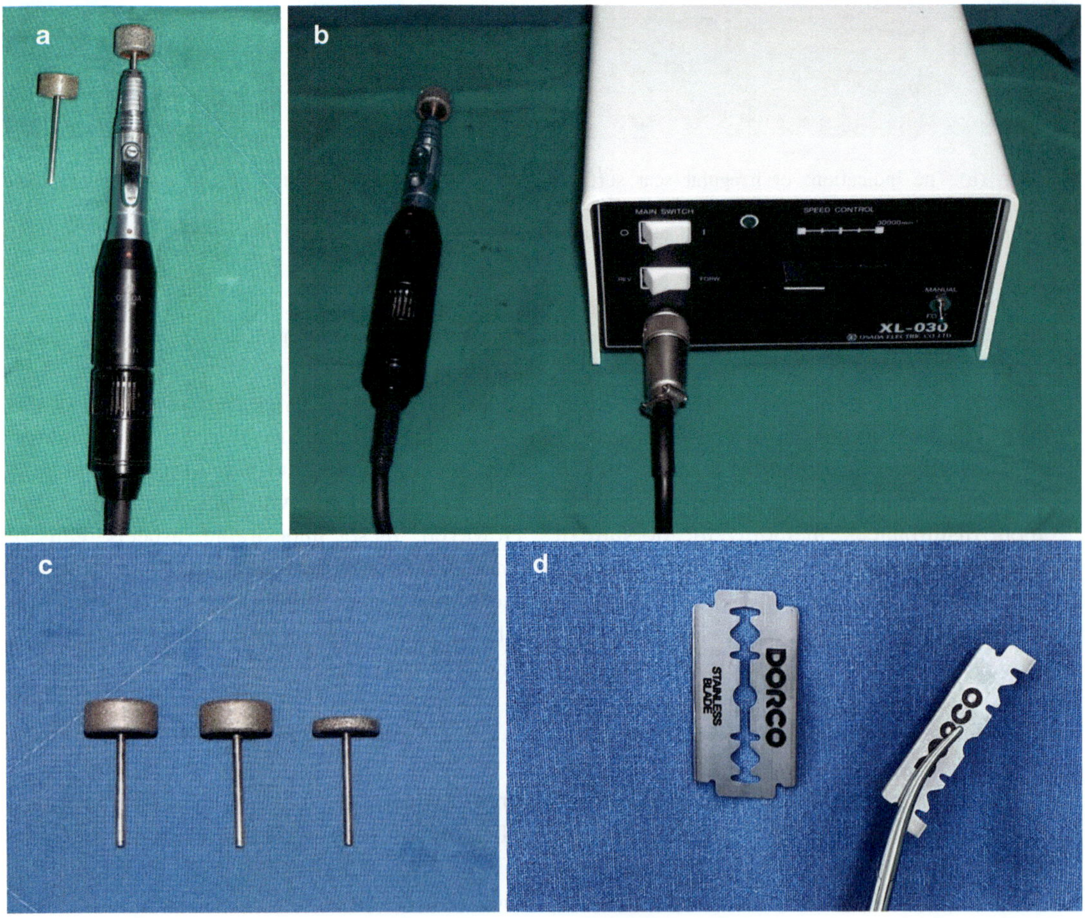

Fig. 5.2 Dermabrader instrument comprises the following: (**a**) handpiece, (**b**) dermabrader, (**c**) variable sizes of diamond-tipped fraise wheel, (**d**) razor blade

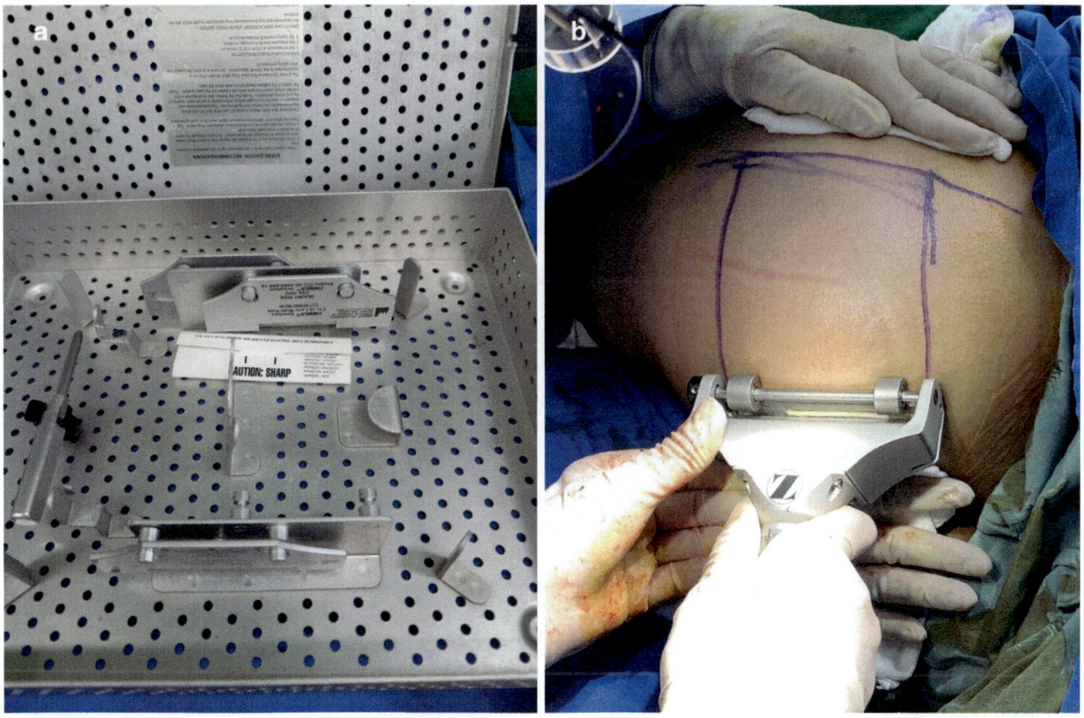

Air driven Zimmer Dermatom photo

Fig. 5.3 (**a**) N_2O air-driven dermatome; (**b**) dermatome handling must be dealt carefully with even pressure in all directions

manner in a vertical direction and abrade in a light tapping motion to ensure precise abrasion of the boundary surface.

Pinpointing the bleeding pattern is critical for determining the depth as well as whether or not epidermal islands are present. Razor shaving is a simple and effective technique for flattening thick and irregular scar surfaces. I prefer to use this technique in a variable scar condition.

In the dermabrasion technique [19–21], (a) remove the entire epidermis and the superficial layer of the irregular scar surface with a diamond-tipped fraise wheel until there are signs of capillary or slight pinpoint bleeding on the scar bed. The pinpoint bleeding pattern is critical for determining the depth as well as whether or not epidermal islands are present. (b) The dermabrader motion should be reciprocating movement rather than oscillating. (c) Razor shaving is a simple and effective technique for flattening thick and irregular scar surfaces (Fig. 5.4).

The surgical sites should be frequently wet with saline soaks beforehand to ensure it remains moist and avoid burns caused by the friction induced during dermabrasion. When the skin is abraded, the whole layer of the epidermis and superficial upper regions of the dermal layer are exposed, which causes capillary bleeding. To control this bleeding, compressive dressing should be repeatedly performed with prepared epinephrine-soaked gauze (1 to 200,000–400,000 epinephrine solution). Following dermabrasion, the abraded surface is thoroughly examined to remove even the smallest epidermal islands. This is necessary because the remaining epidermal islands may grow and epithelialize under the engrafted skin and cause partial graft loss, resulting in small and uneven depressed skin defects that reduce the esthetic effect. The boundary of the abrasion is approximately 0.5–1 cm wider than that of the original engraft site, so the graft slightly overlaps the original lesions before

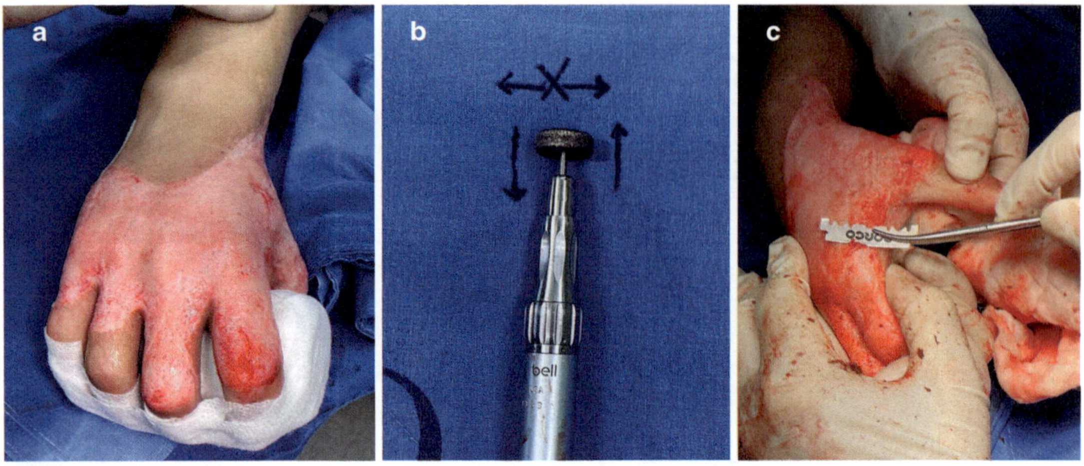

Fig. 5.4 (**a**) Very fine pinpoint bleeding on the dorsum of the hand scar bed; (**b**) dermabrader marked with directions where the motion is reciprocating and not oscillating; (**c**) razor shaving

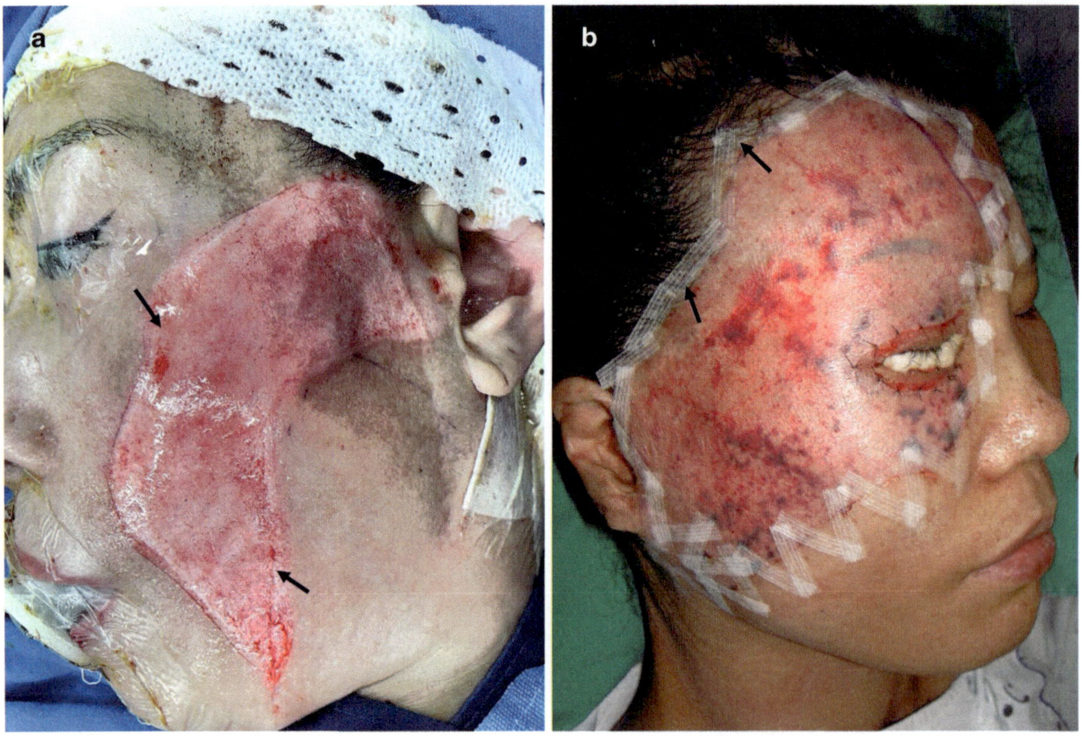

Fig. 5.5 (**a**) The boundary of the abrasion is 0.5–1 cm wider than the scar (black arrow); (**b**) regarding the boundary between the forehead and hairline, an abrasion is made approximately 1 cm inside the hairline (black arrow)

connecting naturally with the surrounding tissues (Fig. 5.5a). Regarding the boundary between the forehead and hairline, an abrasion is made approximately 1 cm inside the hairline, ensuring that the borderline graft margin is placed inside the hairline in order to create a more natural-looking hairline. The hair will grow eventually piercing the thin skin graft without skin loss in few days, and there will be no concerns regarding hair loss as no damage was done to the hair follicles (Fig. 5.5b). The same applies to the eyebrows. Even if the entire eyebrow is removed during total dermabrasion, the hair regrows in few days. This method is recommended as a natural revision method for visible eyebrow inner scars or pigmentation disorders.

Graft and Donor Skin Harvest

The skin harvesting instruments of the N_2O air-driven Zimmer dermatome are shown. Engrafting thickness is a critical factor in determining esthetic outcomes. This image depicts that up to 0.2-mm-thick skin could be collected; remember the contained dermal thickness rate; however, this rate varies depending on individual and instrument factors. The PAS stain was used to confirm whether or not the basement membrane and fine upper part of the papillary dermis were preserved in the 0.125-mm-thick donor skin. As seen in this image, almost the entire epidermal layer is preserved, along with the basement membrane of the epidermis and the upper part of the papillary dermis. However, partial epidermal papillae were also severed (Fig. 5.6).

One advantage of the dermal overgraft technique is that it has fewer donor-site morbidities than the traditional skin graft technique because the engrafting skin thickness in the latter technique is not greater than 0.2 mm.

The figure shows the findings of the donor site on the right upper thigh postoperatively after 2 years and 7 months. The skin thickness of the donor site was 0.2 mm, resulting in less visible donor-site morbidity. Recently, the buttock area has been my first choice of donor site rather than the most used donor site, the thigh area, because the thigh area is visible to others and oneself. Striae alba (multiple whitish linea lines) have no

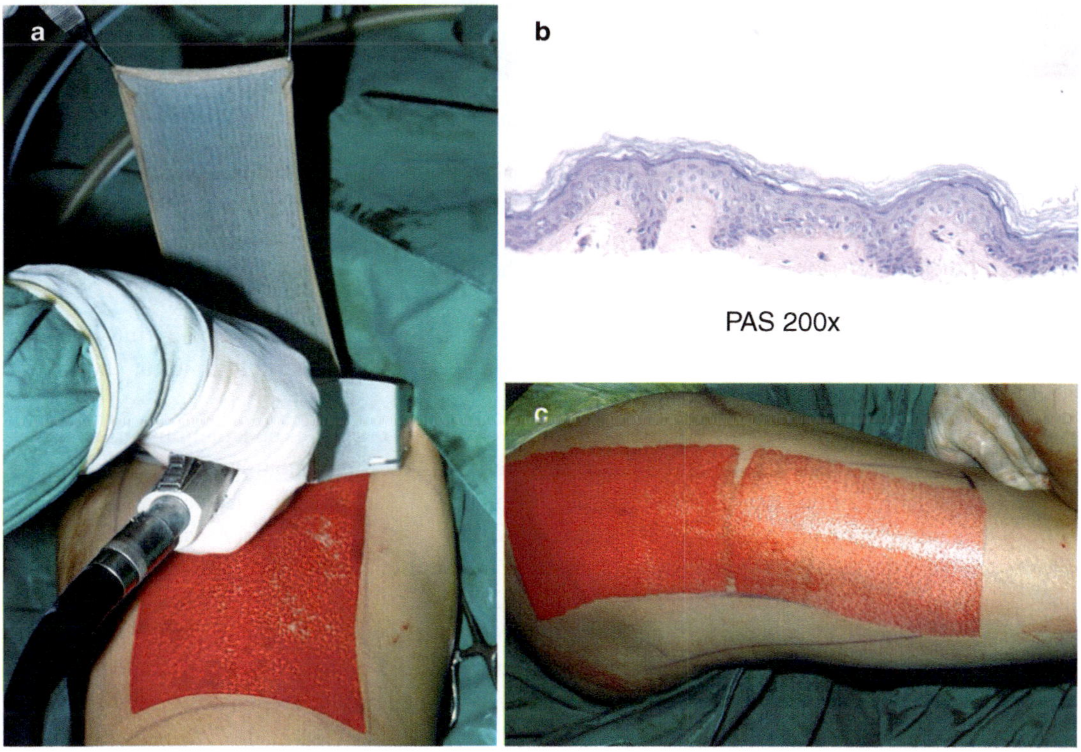

Fig. 5.6 (**a**) Harvesting instruments of N_2O-driven Zimmer dermatome. This image depicts collecting skin thickness set up to 0.2 mm; (**b**) 0.125 mm thickness of donor skin was examined with a PAS stain; (**c**) 0.125-mm-thickness skin donor site on a right lateral thigh

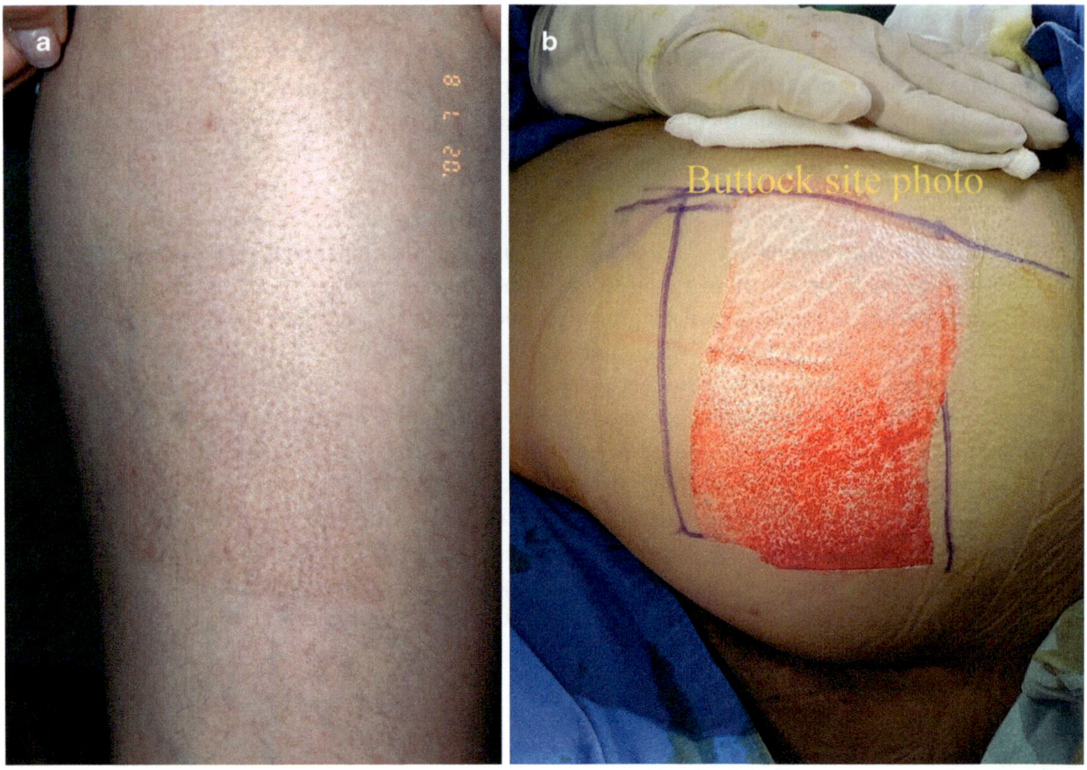

Fig. 5.7 (**a**) Postoperative 2 years and 7 months view of the donor site on the right upper thigh; the skin thickness of the donor site was 0.2 mm, resulting in less visible donor-site morbidity. (**b**) recently, I prefer the buttock area rather than the thigh area, but recently, I prefer buttock site as this donor-site morbidity is easier to cover by wearing undergarments, making it less visible; this helps to reduce emotional stress of scar visibility, especially in women

effect on the engrafted skin because the harvested skin is too thin (Fig. 5.7).

Calculating the precise area of the skin to be harvested and collecting the skin in single sheet, if possible, reduce consuming operation time. I strongly recommend, when you harvest STSG donor skin, to accurately estimate and collect as soon as possible skillfully. I am reluctance to perform STSG surgery on patients as STSG donor site scaring is usally the largest and uncorrectable and futher esthetic corrective surgery may be needed [22]. Generally, the maximum width of a harvestable skin section is restricted to 10 cm, which is the maximum width of a dermatome. Therefore, it is preferable to avoid making a graft seam line by correctly calculating the length and width of the graft area. Nevertheless, when the dermabraded wound site is larger than the collected skin and cannot be covered with a single sheet, Steri-Strip™ is used efficiently by sticking them together without engraft gaps.

This male patient received a full-thickness skin graft to correct an anterior neck scar contracture. A year later, he received a dermal overgraft to correct a conspicuous graft area as well as hyperpigmentation and hypopigmentation lesions. Dermabrasion was performed, and bleeding was effectively controlled using 1:200,000 epinephrine-soaked gauze. Skin of 0.2-mm thickness (9.5 × 19 cm × 2 sheets) was horizontally covered and secured with Steri-Strip™ (3 M Health Care, MN, USA) and 6–0 nylon suture. The center of the engrafted area was easily secured with Steri-Strip™ (black arrow). Because of the extremely thin skin graft, the engrafted seam line is not overly visible and thus does not detract from the esthetic effect (Fig. 5.8).

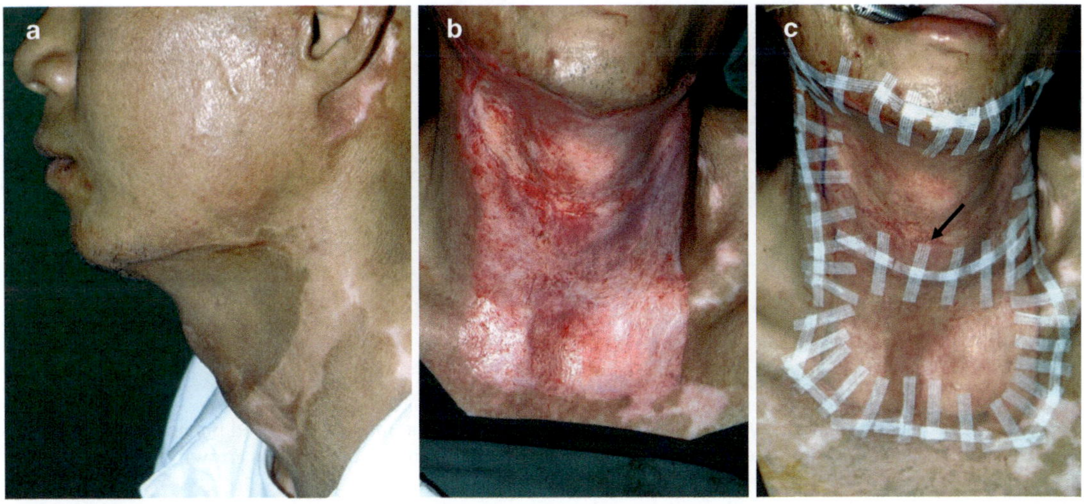

Fig. 5.8 (**a**) Preoperative lateral view: he received full thickness skin graft for the correction of anterior neck scar contracture. Note the well reconstructed cervicomental angle; (**b**) dermabrasion; (**c**) 8/1000 in. thickness skin (9.5 × 19 cm × 2 sheets) were horizontally covered and secured with Steri-Strip™ (black arrow)

In the preoperative anterior view, there was a conspicuous, engrafted, marginal pigmentation disorder with an irregular, matured scar surface. Four months after the operation, the pigmentation lesion had noticeably improved, but there was a slight difference in texture between the FTSG bed (black arrow) and the burn scar bed (yellow arrow). In the author's experience, when a dermabrasion site is present before the FTSG bed, the dermal overgraft effect has a slightly different color and texture compared to a typical scar bed. There was no visible seam line (yellow arrow), so each graft on the midline was extended (Fig. 5.9).

The decision-making of the skin graft thickness is crucial for the final result of the operation. Generally, the thickness does not exceed a maximum of 0.3 mm in case of hand and rarely exceeds 0.2 mm in cases involving the face, remaining in the 0.1–0.0.2 mm range.

A 31-year-old male patient suffered a flame burn. Three years after the burn, dermabrasion and a dermal overgraft were performed on the forehead. The entire forehead had a mature and irregular scarring surface, hypo- and hyperpigmented lesions, and 0.15-mm-thick engrafted skin. Notice the 0.15-mm thickness, especially in the dermal component with transparent thickness, which has a full layer of epidermis and a partial upper dermis (black arrow) (Fig. 5.10).

Immediately after the operation, removal of the entire epidermis and irregular scar bed, donor skin was applied in a single-sheet graft and secured with a Steri-Strip™ or 6–0 nylon suture. Five months after the operation, the irregular surface, hypopigmented lesions, skin texture, and pigmentation disorder were noticeably improved and the irregular scar had been corrected (Fig. 5.11).

One year later, this patient received two dermal overgrafts: on the first lower half of her full face and her forehead. Two years after the operation, the nose was still hyperpigmented and had a partial loss area because of poor patient care. This indicates that skin loss impairs the esthetic results in the dermal overgraft site; therefore, patients must be cautious until the graft is taken completely (Fig. 5.12).

Specifically, the thickness of the dermal overgraft in the facial area is very crucial as it is thinner than 0.125 mm, the engrafted skin color becomes lighter due to low pigmentation, and if the graft is thicker than 0.2 mm, the engrafted skin color turns darker due to the trend of little high pigmentation, but instead the texture is improved. Therefore, when performing an overgraft in the

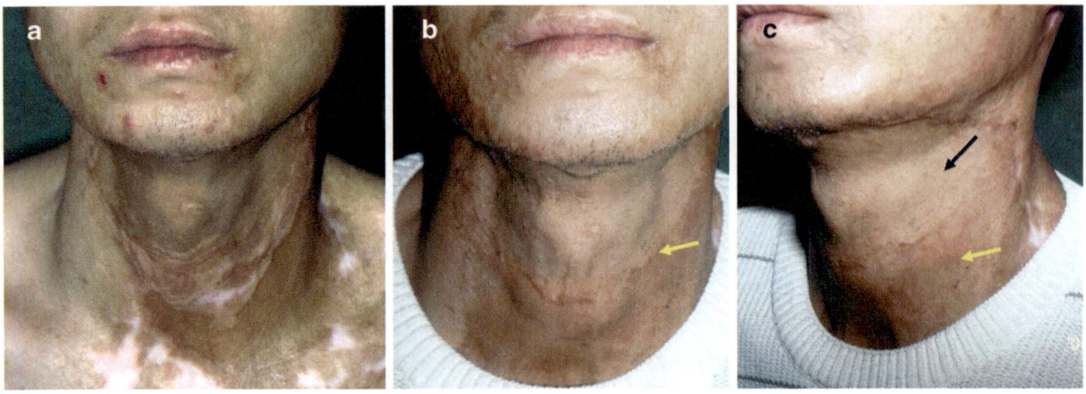

Fig. 5.9 (**a**) Preoperative anterior view; (**b**) 4 months after the operation, marked improved pigmentation lesion was noted; (**c**) difference in texture between FTSG bed (black arrow) and burn scar bed (yellow arrow)

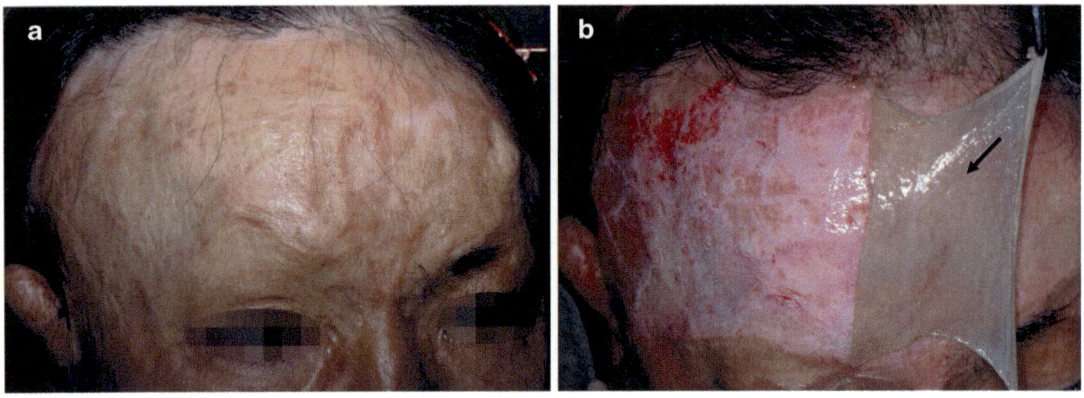

Fig. 5.10 (**a**) Matured irregular surface and hypo- or hyperpigmented lesion were noted on the entire forehead; (**b**) notice the 0.15 mm thickness, especially dermal component of transparent thickness

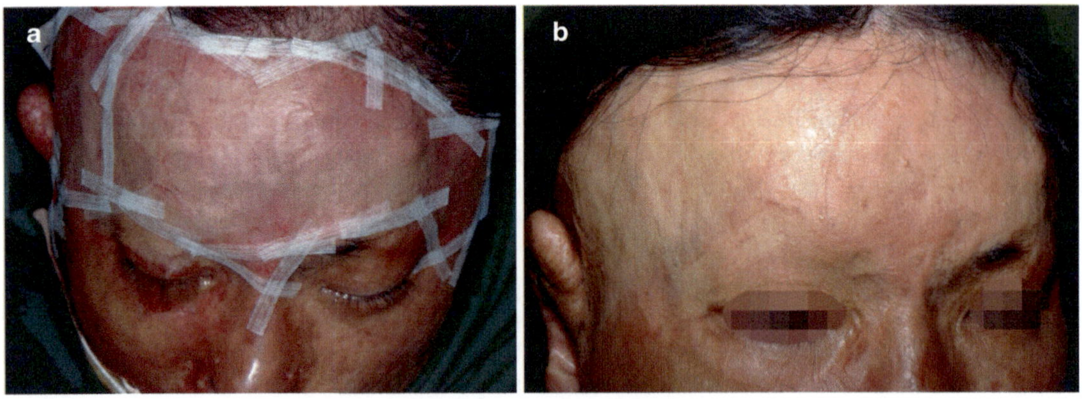

Fig. 5.11 (**a**) A postoperative view; (**b**) postoperative 5 months view

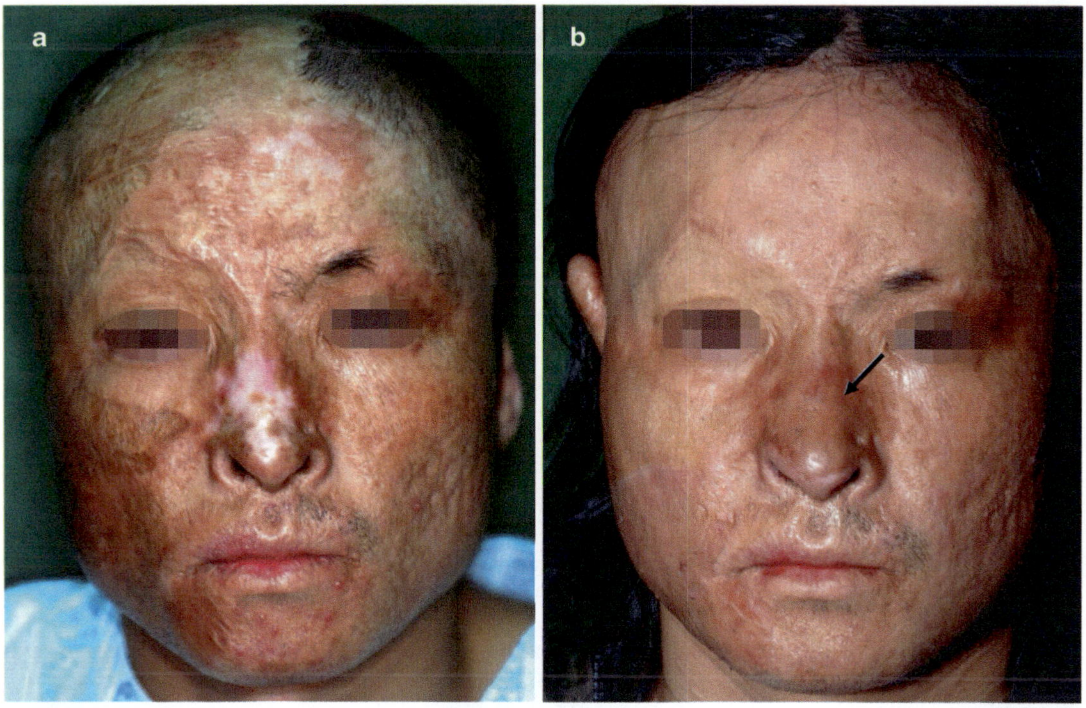

Fig. 5.12 (**a**) The same patient received two dermal overgrafts: first on the lower half of the full face and second on the forehead one year later, (preoperative view); (**b**) post-operative 2 years view; hyperpigmented nose with partial loss area remained

facial area, it is advised to carefully review the graft thickness to be able to finely control the color matching of the graft with the surrounding tissues; this ability to judge and make choices increases as surgeons get more experienced.

Recently, the author recommended 0.125-mm thickness under engraft thickness for the facial area, especially for the forehead and both cheeks and mentum area because this area is the part that actively moves. As a result, if too much thin skin is engrafted to that area, it causes unsightly fine wrinkle, reducing the esthetic effect. Therefore, for these areas, I would like to recommend 0.2-mm thickness or thicker for better skin texture.

For more clarification of thickness on the facial area, the recommended thickness for the upper and lower lids is less than 0.125 mm, and to avoid simple pigmentation disorders, it is better to not exceed 0.125 mm, if possible. I will introduce several cases for correction of lid area where thinnest skin was applied.

Initially, the range of dermabrasion on the upper and lower lid areas was limited owing to the thin skin of the lid area and the fear of developing scar contracture (black arrow). One year after the operation, an unsightly difference in color and texture was observed around the lid area (Fig. 5.13). Many plastic surgeons are hesitant to perform skin grafts on the face, especially in the eyelid region. A high level of experience with the dermal overgraft technique will solve this problem. The author attempted engraftment on a total lid area with 0.125-mm thickness and obtained acceptable results [23, 24].

A 35-year-old female patient suffered a flame burn and, preoperatively, hyperpigmented discoloration was noted on both the upper and lower lid areas, as well as an irregular scar surface on the lower cheek area. For correction of these prob-

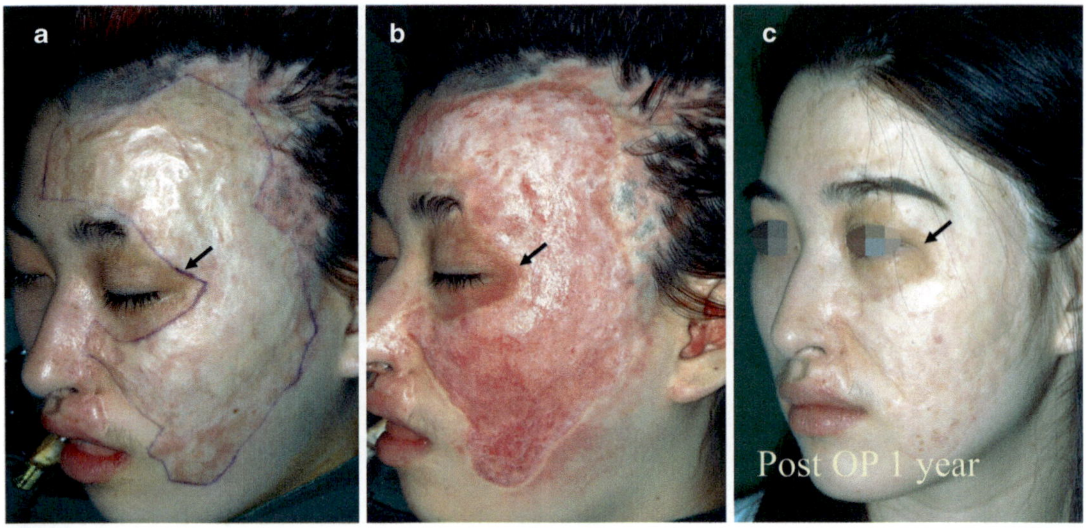

Fig. 5.13 (**a**, **b**) In the early period, range of dermabrasion on the upper and lower lid areas was limited (black arrow); (**c**) postoperative 1 year after, unsightly different color and texture were noted around the lid area

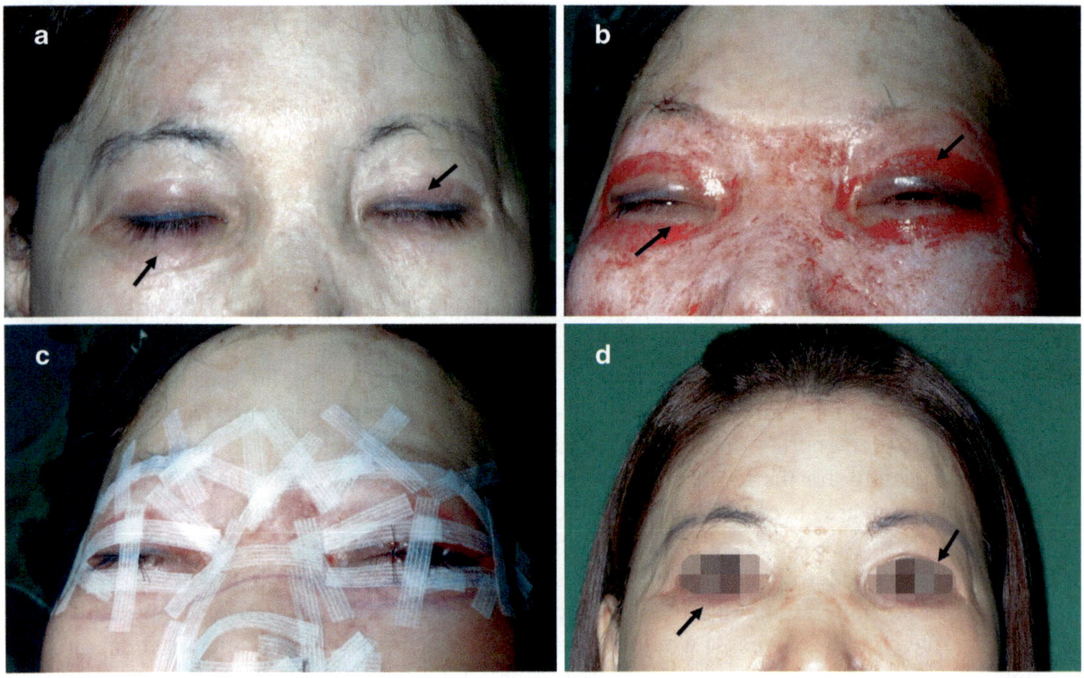

Fig. 5.14 (**a**) Note the hyperpigmentation on both upper and lower lid areas (black arrow); (**b**, **c**) 0.125-mm-thickness dermal over engraft underwent near the double fold line on the upper lid (black arrows); (**d**) postoperative 7 months later, esthetic outcome of the engrafted area was noted (black arrows)

lems, 0.125-mm thickness auto-skin graft underwent just above the double fold line on the upper lids and 0.5 cm apart from the lower lid margin (black arrows). Seven months after the operation, the engrafted upper and lower lid areas had a better esthetic outcome (black arrows) (Fig. 5.14).

According to increasing experience, dermabrasion and dermal overgraft are performed on the full surface of the upper and lower lid areas for more natural appearance. The tip of dermabrasion is giving stretched tension to the thin skin around the eyelids in the top and bottom directions and performing abrasion carefully, using a diamond-tipped fraise wheel with the narrow width while gripping a handpiece lightly and repeatedly touching the skin lightly in the up and down directions. The thickness of the graft skin is 0.1–0.125 mm, and after performing upper and lower lid tarsorrhaphy, it is important to maintain it at least for 3–4 days for hematoma prevention or engraftment will be stable.

In the preoperative, open-eye observation of this case, a spotty hyperpigmented burn scar was noted in the right upper and lower eyelids. She underwent a 0.125-mm-thick dermal overgraft without tarsorrhaphy and observed that the engrafted skin was fixed with only Steri strips, and not skin sutures (Fig. 5.15). Postoperative 1- and 2-month observations revealed that there was no disfigurement, and reasonable results were obtained (Fig. 5.16).

Hand and Forearm Area

For the dorsum of the hand, forearm, foot, lower extremity, or other body sites, a thickness of 0.3 mm or little more is recommended, which is thicker than the grafts preferred in other sites; this is suitable for better skin texture and color matching with the surrounding tissues.

Note the 0.38-mm medium-thickness harvested skin and the opacity of the skin thickness. A scattered, pinpoint bleeding pattern was observed in the donor site. Notice how well the bleeding was controlled with only 1:200,000 epinephrine-soaked gauze and no tourniquet. Dermal overgraft skin appears thicker than the

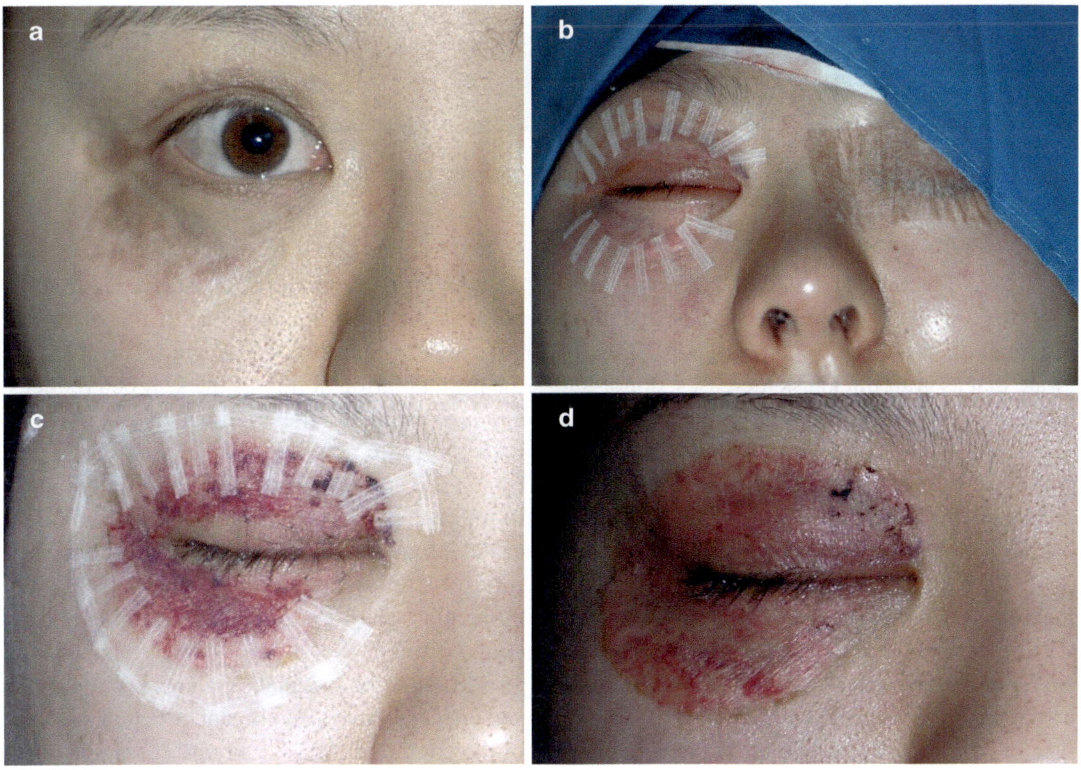

Fig. 5.15 (**a**) Preoperative open eye view: spotty hyper pigmented burn scar noted on the right upper and lower eye lid areas; (**b**) 0.125-mm-thickness dermal overgraft underwent without tarsorrhaphy; (**c**) postoperative 4 days view; (**d**) postoperative 7 days view: the engrafted skin was taken completely

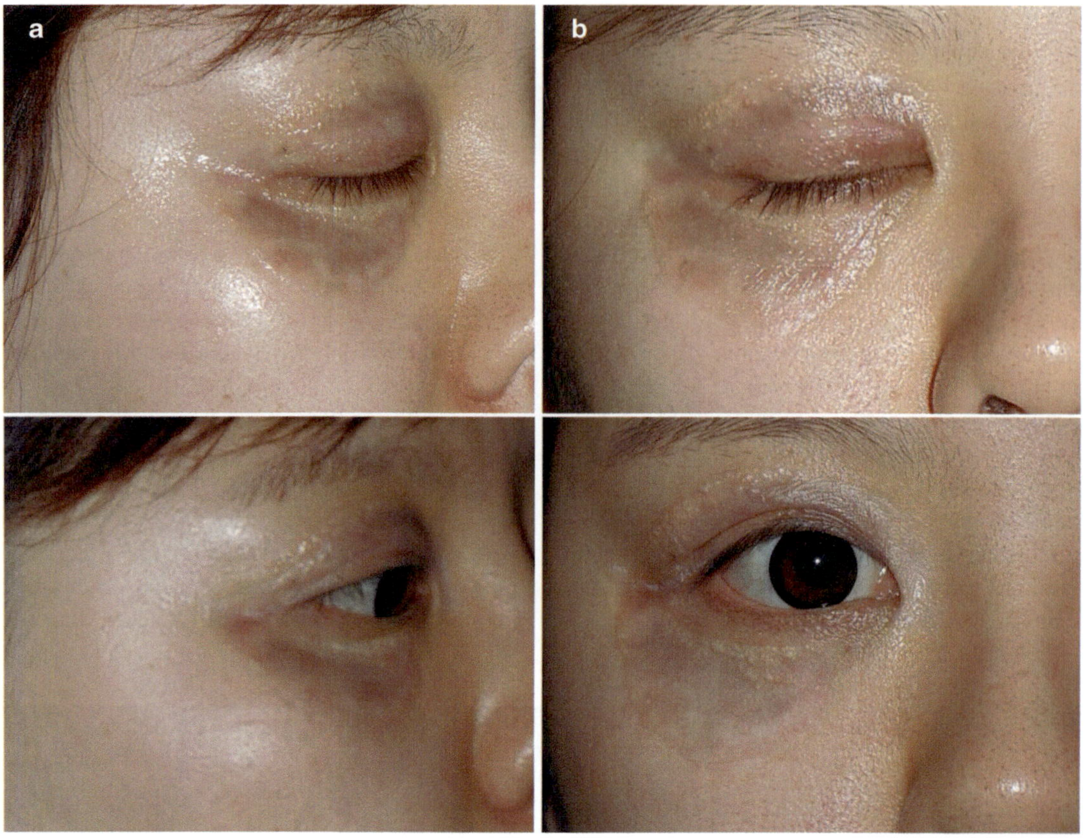

Fig. 5.16 (**a**) Postoperative 1 month view; (**b**) postoperative 2 months view: skin texture and spotty discoloration were improved without any disfigurements

facial area; I recommend at least ≥0.3-mm thickness for the best texture and color matching results (Fig. 5.17). However, surgeons must be aware that as graft thickness increases, donor-site morbidity and scarring also increase [25, 26].

Donor-Site Selection

Although the selection of the skin donor site has long been a matter of concern, the author does not consider it essential. This is because the selected donor site matches appropriately with the surrounding tissues regardless of the skin color of the original donor site. According to the author's experience, skin grafts for the face have also been mostly collected from the buttocks which are covered with undergarments to avoid donor-site morbidity. This has not significantly affected the color matching of the grafts with the surrounding tissues, which is the desired surgical outcome. It is assumed that the color of the graft matches that of the surrounding tissues regardless of its site of origin since the pigmentation ability of the scar bed reduces, and according to the findings of microscopic PAS (periodic acid-Schiff) HE staining, a portion of the epidermal papillae is partially cut off in a graft of 0.125-mm thickness, which might affect its melanocyte population. Accordingly, future studies, including histological and molecular biological studies, are needed (Fig. 5.6b).

Although the original skin color of the donor site does not have a significant effect on the color of the engrafted skin, but in rare cases, the lower extremity or dorsum of the foot engrafted skin changes to darker hyperpigmentation than the surrounding skin color. Therefore, the author does not positively recommend the application of

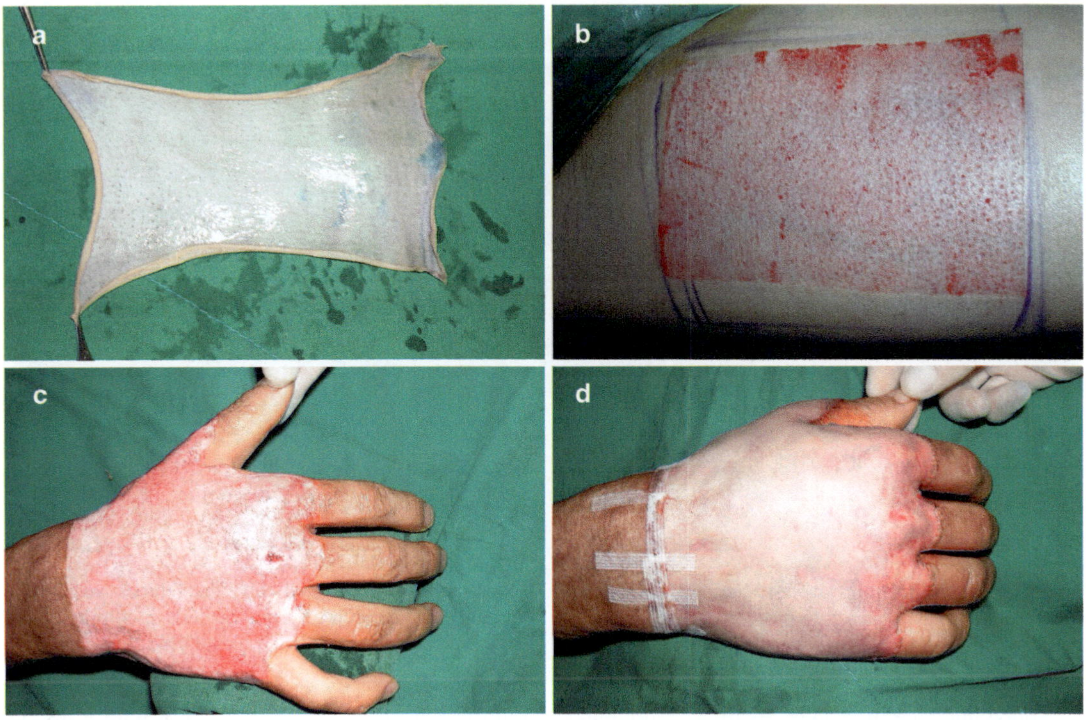

Fig. 5.17 (**a**) Example of 0.38 mm thickness and note the opacity of the harvested donor skin thickness; (**b**) note scattered pinpoint bleeding pattern; (**c**) dermabrasion; (**d**) dermal over engrafted skin looks thicker than facial area

dermal overgraft technique in these lower extremity areas.

This is an unfavorable case based on my experience with dermal overgrafts. There is a mild, flattened scar bed and a hyperpigmented lesion without any contracture or deformity. A dermal overgraft of 0.25-mm thickness was performed. Six months after the operation, an intense, dark skin color and texture on the entire engrafted skin were noted. Unfortunately, due to a lack of experience, I cannot provide a more detailed explanation of this complication. However, in the case of the lower extremities, they are slightly darker than the upper extremities, face, and other body parts. Therefore, I would advise against using this technique on the lower extremity area, especially the ankle and foot, because it has a lower effect on these sites than on other dermal overgraft sites (Fig. 5.18).

During the procedure of skin graft, after bleeding has been controlled to some extent with epinephrine-soaked gauze, covering the wound bed with the graft as soon as possible facilitates bleeding control. For overgrafts, a skin graft margin is precisely fit on the wound bed margin, and if necessary, it is secured by simple interrupted suture with 6–0 nylon or fixed with Steri-Strip™ (3 M Health Care, MN, USA).

Many surgeons routinely make slit incisions in a dependent position or across the engraft area to prevent hematoma or fluid collection during STSG. However I do no make slit incision during the surgery, only after opening the engrafted wound if hematoma is present. The reason for this choice is to develop the ability to resolve such problems without blindly depending on slit incision. Another personal reason is that an unsightly incision scar is unesthetic in the long-term follow-up in the aspect of the universal concept of skin graft. But using this very thin split-thickness technique, this slit incision will not cause significant esthetic problems because it does not leave a scar.

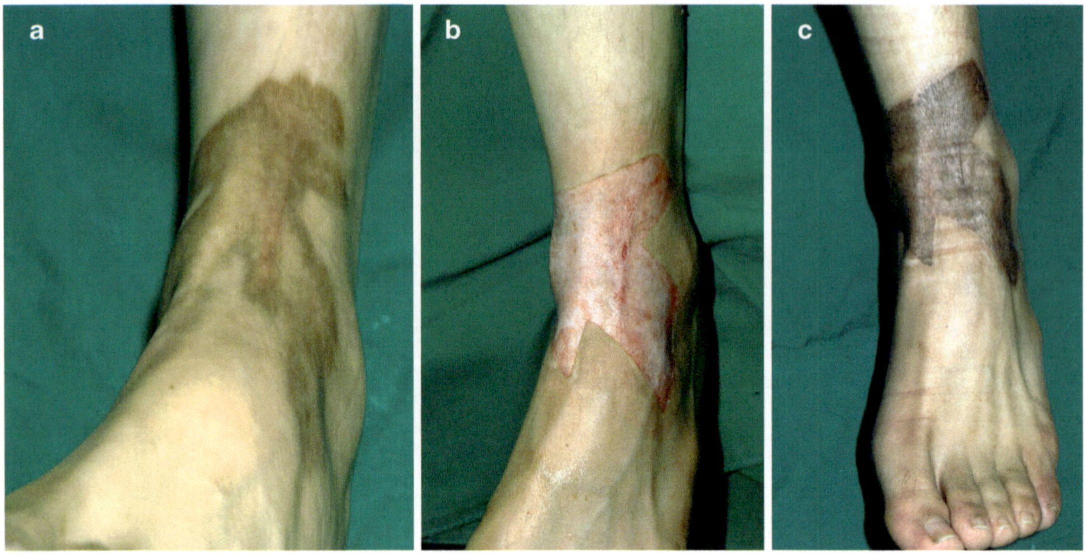

Fig. 5.18 (**a**) Notice mild scar bed and hyperpigmented lesion without any contracture or deformities; (**b**) dermabrasion and resurfacing underwent with 0.25 mm thickness which was collected from the buttock area; (**c**) 6 months after operation, an intense dark discoloration and texture were noted on the entire engrafted skin

Following engrafted skin fixation, mild bulky compressive dressing with saline chip gauze pads and 4 × 4 in. gauze pads is applied, and the graft is fixed with an elastic bandage. As it is possible for the facial area to be pressed while sleeping and chances of the bulky dressing being displaced, to avoid this happening to a facial graft , Barton's bandage or an elastic bandage net, SurgiNet (Won Industry Co., Gyeonggi-Do, Korea), is recommend.

Postoperative Dressing

Graft typically begins in 3–4 days in the absence of hematoma or seroma, and graft is completely taken in approximately 7–10 days. The author usually opens the dressing on the fourth postoperative day, and on the occurrence of hematoma or seroma beneath the graft, evacuation is performed by making a small slit incision with a no. 11 knife. The saline-soaked dressing is changed daily until the graft is completely taken and the mildly bloodstained site gradually recovers to the color of the original grafted skin, which continues to change for the next 3–4 weeks.

The most concerning complication is the occurrence of a hematoma. If it has not been controlled earlier, the hematoma can be consistently removed by making a slit incision with a no. 11 knife, followed by continued compressive saline-soaked dressing twice a day for 1 week or longer without giving up until the hematoma is fully removed. The goal of the dermal overgraft is a 100% take rate, and this must be achieved with sustained efforts because if the graft is not taken, it will not be possible to achieve an esthetic outcome, which is the primary purpose of this surgery. Despite such cases, the engrafted skin takes without a significant problem in most cases, which should be considered when planning skin graft. Normally, graft take gradually stabilizes within 2 weeks after surgery, and the color of the engrafted skin bed starts to change to a lighter shade. The overlapped skin at the graft margin sloughs off naturally. Because the engrafted skin is very thin, slight overlapping of a few mm is not visible in the engrafted margin. Therefore, this does not greatly affect surgical outcomes.

After completing the engraft procedure prior to the application of a compressive dressing, the dressing was removed 3 days later, and a small hematoma on the mentum area was observed. This hematoma was evacuated using a saline-soaked dressing through a small slit incision.

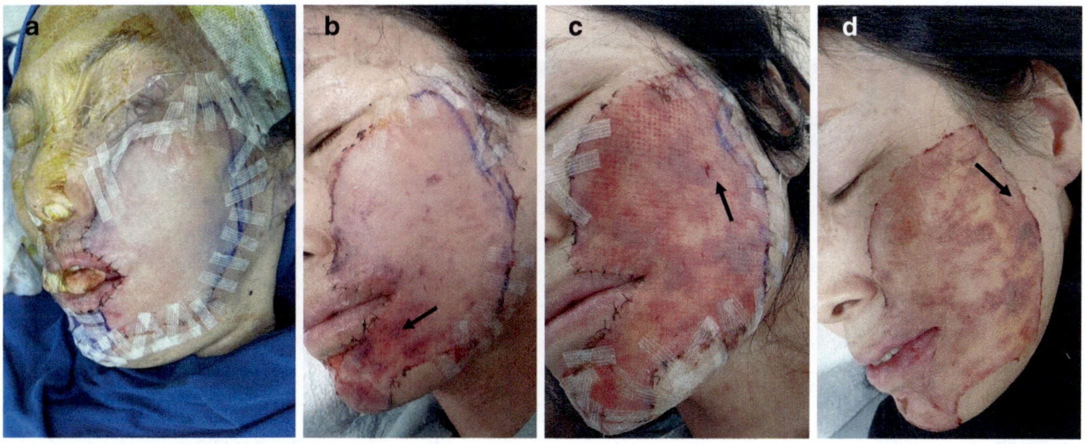

Fig. 5.19 (**a**) After complete engraft procedure before compressive dressing; (**b**) postoperative 3 days, a small hematoma was noted on the mentum area. This was evacuated using saline-soaked dressing through the small slit incision (black arrow); (**c**) postoperative 5 days, small hematoma was noted on the malar area, which was also evacuate through the slit incision (black arrow); (**d**) postoperative 10 days, engraft was taken almost completely

Five days after the procedure, a small hematoma was noted in the malar area, which was also easily evacuated through the slit incisions (black arrow). Ten days after the procedure, the entire engraft was taken almost completely. Notice the visible engrafted marginal layer, but this layer will recover slowly due to a long scar maturation period (Fig. 5.19).

Postoperative Management

It is possible for the patient to return to normal life approximately 2 weeks after surgery. However, it is recommended to use protective dressing and cream or highly moisturizing lotions, such as the lotion Emu Care (Almeca BV Adourlaan 10, 5691 RC Son en Breugel, Holland), on the surgical site. Although the engrafted skin is very thin and less visible than other usual skin graft margins, the engrafted wound margin mostly offends the eye site. During author's past, these problems were solved with pressure garment or silicone gel sheet for approximately 1 month following the surgery to maximize graft stabilization and for several months until marginal scar maturation. If the scar margin is visible even after a particular period, Fraxel laser (NAF laser-Fraxel® XENA SR 1500) can be used every 3 weeks or 1 month and 3 weeks after surgery to yield favorable results. Laser beams do not damage the stratum corneum. It is a biological barrier, and the tissue is coagulated rather than vaporized. Multiple 70–150 micron microthermal zones of dead tissue islands are created per cm^2, which are surrounded by many healthy tissues and allow for 24-h reepithelialization (Fig. 5.20).

Now days when I have been performing LASER therapy, it is combined with silastic gel sheet therapy or patient wearing a pressure garment. Postoperative one month later, laser therapy is performed once a month for at least 6 months or longer; this helps to enhance the surgical outcomes.

Small, white papules appear on the engrafted surface especially on the face and forearm area until approximately 3 weeks to 2–3 months postoperatively. This is a natural occurrence as the engrafted skin blocks the openings of the sweat glands, sebaceous glands, and hair follicles, and the secretions produced by their normal activity collect beneath the skin graft. If the number or size of these papules increases, they are stabbed and punctured with a sterilized needle and squeezed, causing their natural and uneventful disappearance. Tiny hair can grow out of the grafted skin on the face or forearm, where a large

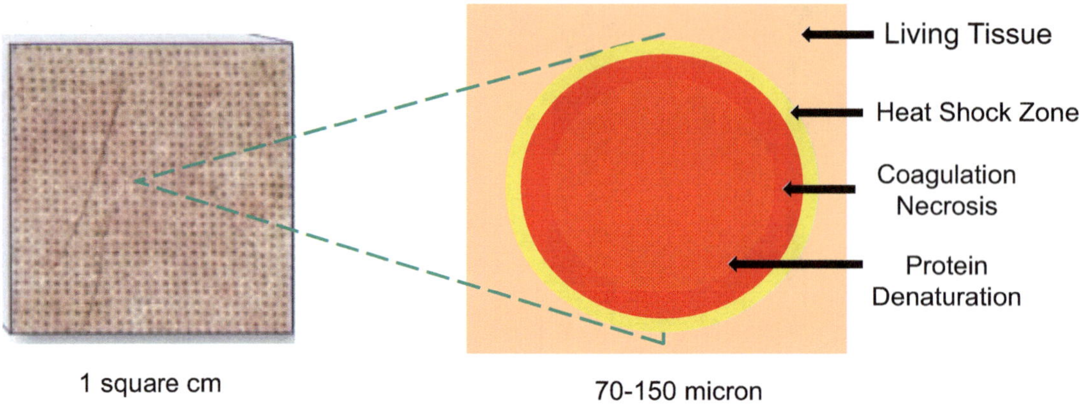

Fig. 5.20 Laser beam does not disrupt the stratum corneum which remains intact. It remains as a biological barrier; tissue is coagulated, not vaporized. Multiple 70–150 micron Micro Thermal Zone (MTZs) of islands of dead tissue are created per sq cm which are surrounded by many healthy tissues and enable re-epithelialization in 24 h

population of hair follicles is distributed. This is a natural occurrence as downy hair grows from the underneath grafted skin that has been taken. But this rarely occurs in skin engrafted scar bed area because there were already destroyed or due to the loss of pilosebaceous organs.

A mild, irregular scar surface and black, spotted pigmentation were observed on the right forearm and elbow-joint areas. For esthetic purposes, dermabrasion and dermal resurfacing were performed with 0.25-mm thickness of auto sheet skin. Two months later, clinical observations revealed multiple tiny papules (black arrow), which faded with time and downy hair pierced through the engrafted thin skin without any issue. If some papules increase in quantity and enlarge, I recommend puncturing them with a sharp injection needle tip and squeezing them out. This was the cause of partial skin loss, and an unsightly irregular scar remained. Nine months after the operation, all papules disappeared, the texture improved, and the color matching was good (Fig. 5.21).

From the author's experience, it can be said that the basic dermal overgraft methods introduced above are applicable in several situations. The author intends to describe the clinical cases of each area and modified cases of dermal overgraft based on various cases.

5.2.2 Cases of Facial Lesion

5.2.2.1 Full-Face Dermal Overgraft

Few considerations need to be addressed before a full-face dermal overgraft [27].

Prior to esthetic dermal overgraft surgery, for the preconditioning procedure, I performed total facial reconstruction over a 2-year period, with the first operation focusing on both lower lids and ectropion deformities, the dorsum of the nose, and both cheeks and upper lip areas with thick STSG (0.5-mm thickness). The second corrective surgery was performed on the lower lip and mentum as well as the anterior neck area; thick STSG (peri-oral area) and FTSG (mento-cervical area) were used in combination. The dermal overgraft technique is the final surgery; these procedures must correct all deformities, and surgeons should wait until the operation sites have fully matured between each procedure (Fig. 5.22).

Full-face dermabrasion and dermal overgraft were planned for correction of forehead pigmented lesion and previous operation site on lower lid, nose and both cheeks, and mentum and anterior neck area.

First, for adult male patients, a maximum of 10 × 25 cm (250 cm^2) × 3 pieces are needed, and sufficient donor side space is required. Such areas are needed for all the three parts of the upper, mid, and lower face horizontally. If the

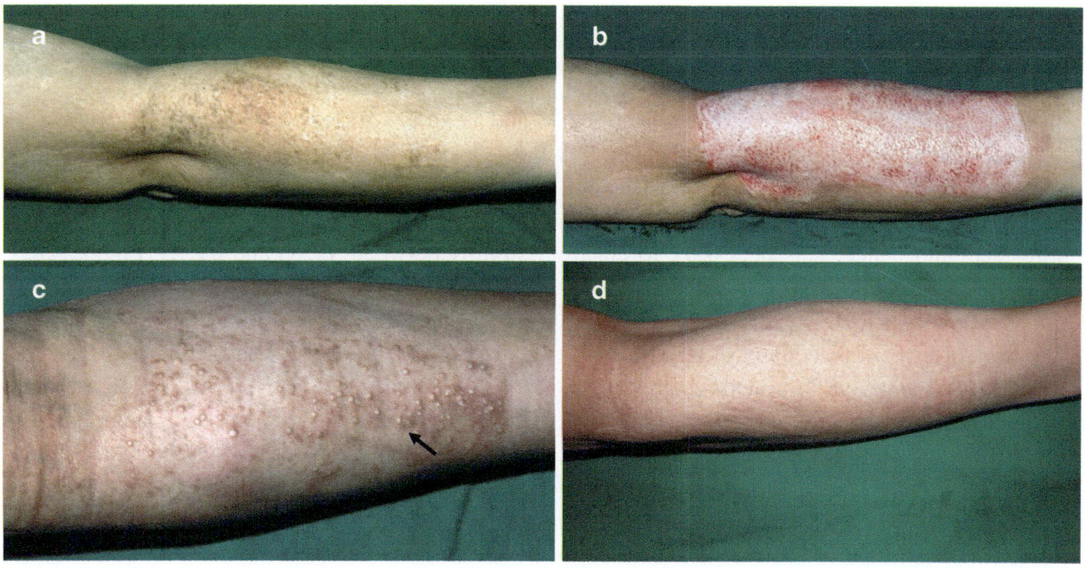

Fig. 5.21 (**a**) Spotted pigmentation on the right forearm and elbow joint area; (**b**) dermabrasion and dermal resurfacing underwent with 0.25 mm thickness; (**c**) postoperative 2 months later, multiple tiny papules revealed (black arrow) and these regions faded with time and downy hair pierced through engrafted thin skin; (**d**) postoperative 9 months, all papules have disappeared

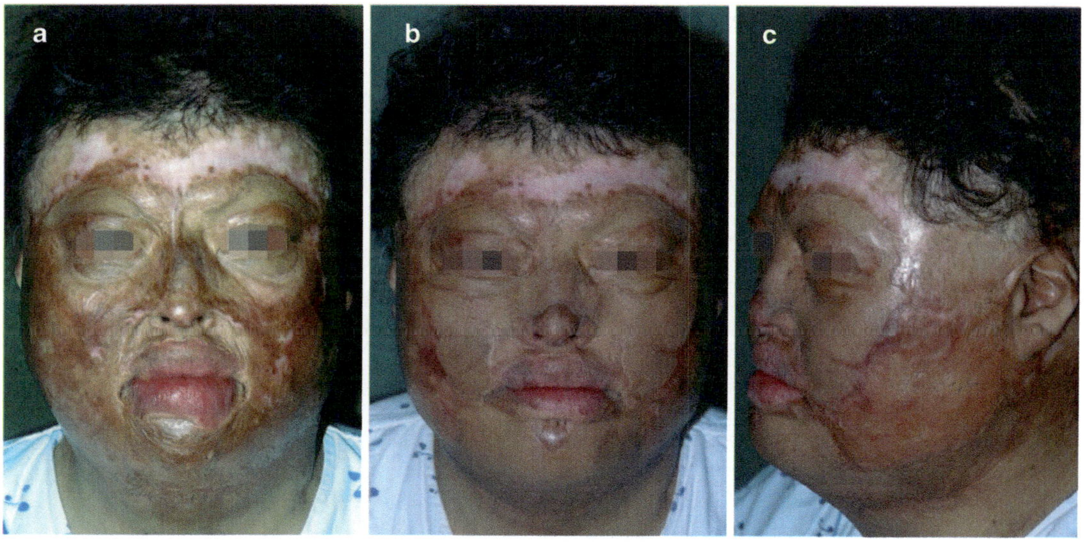

Fig. 5.22 (**a**) Preoperative view; (**b**, **c**) first operation was performed on both the lower lid and ectropion deformities, dorsum of nose and both cheeks, and upper lip area with thick STSG (0.5 mm thickness). Second corrective surgery was performed on lower lip and mentum, and anterior neck area with FTSG

donor site is large enough to be harvested as a single sheet, the operation time will be reduced and surgery will be performed more straightforwardly. As I have already mentioned in (Fig. 1.12), also in this case I have not divided esthetic unit on the forhead and both cheeks as it was very thin STSG.

Second, for the benefit of grafting, only the nose and upper lip areas can be divided into separate simple esthetic units as convenience required, which will lead to favorable outcomes.

Third, when the entire upper and lower lids are grafted, tarsorrhaphy is needed and a compressive dressing needs to be performed for the entire face, and hence, it is necessary to ensure that the eyes are securely immobilized after covering them with a delicate dressing technique. For even and straight placement of the extremely thin grafted skin, even compressive dressing is required, and there is a high risk of displacement of the engrafted skin when opening and closing of the eyes, along with hematoma. Therefore, tarsorrhaphy is an important preventive procedure.

A full-face dermabrasion was performed on the forehead, both cheeks, and the anterior neck area, except the upper and lower lips. The entire surface of the upper and lower lids was also dermabraded. The thickness of the engrafted skin was 0.2 mm, and (c, d) three pieces of skin (25 × 10 cm, 27 × 9 cm, and 20 × 10 cm) were collected from the anterior chest (Fig. 5.23) and abdomen. This was because of improper donor-site selection due to burn skin injury on the back, buttocks, and both upper thighs. Note the color and texture difference of the engrafted skin (0.25 mm) on the lower third mentum and anterior neck areas (yellow arrow). The reason for this is that the engrafted bed conditions differ slightly between STSG and FTSG (Fig. 5.24).

The key point is to cover the entire face with an even compressive elastic bandage to ensure that the graft does not wrinkle due to tightening of the bandage. If any wrinkled area is found and on opening of the dressing, hematoma or seroma should be removed by making a slit incision on the day. Simultaneously, repositioning of the graft can be attempted to smooth out the wrinkles, but such interventions should be minimized if the engrafted skin has already been taken to some extent. If the wrinkles are trimmed with sharp scissors approximately 2 weeks after the graft was taken, the wound will heal without any issues, without much affect on the esthetic effect.

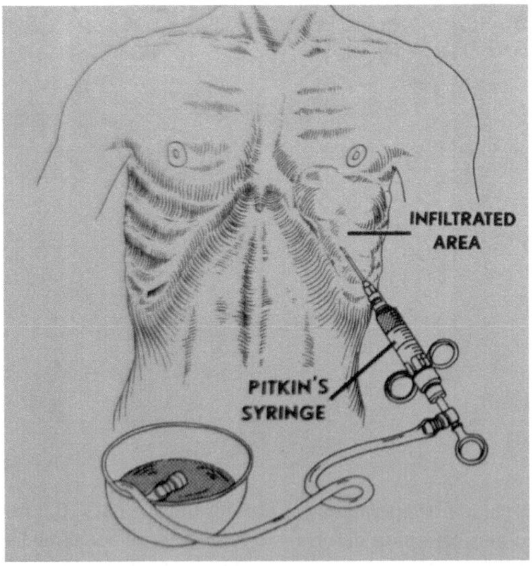

Fig. 5.23 When the donor site must be taken from anterior chest irregular area (or scalp area) with Zimmer dermatome, infiltration of the areas with saline provides a smooth surface for the graft. The saline is conveniently infiltrated using Pitkin's syringe

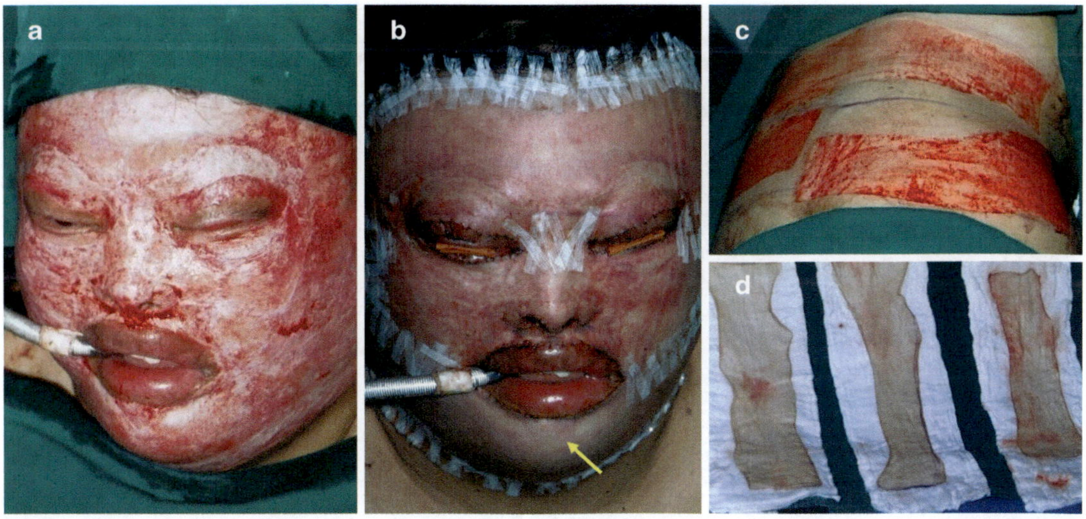

Fig. 5.24 (**a**) Full-face dermabrasion was performed. Note the full-surface upper and lower lid was also dermabraded; (**b**) the thickness of the engrafted skin was 0.2 mm and (**c**, **d**) 3 pieces of skin (25 × 10, 27 × 9, 20 × 10 cm) were collected from the anterior chest (Fig. 5.23) and abdomen area

Ten days after the procedure, blood-stained spots and multiple small papules were noted on the entire face, but there was no skin loss or defect. Ten months after the procedure, the skin color and texture had noticeably improved, but mild ectropion had developed, especially on the right lower lid. In my opinion, mild ectropion developed because the split-thickness engrafted skin shrank or contractured over time. This could be one of the points to consider before attempting a dermal overgraft on the lower lid area. The other viewpoint is that the skin color and texture on the mentum area at the FTSG site (black arrow) differ slightly from the other upper face area at the thick STSG site (Fig. 5.25).

Thirteen months after the procedure, there was a significant improvement in skin color and texture, with a more natural appearance. Postoperative 2-year and 8-month observations revealed almost no change in scarring or pigmentation disorders, except for mild ectropion, which was more slightly developed. In the postoperative 14-year (April 6, 2016) follow-up, there was almost no change in the skin color and texture of the entire face, but more ectropion developed, requiring corrective surgery (Fig. 5.26).

5.2.2.2 Regional Scar on the Face

Localized Depressed Scar on Face

Although it is considered that a partial dermal facial overgraft has a limited area and is a simple procedure, it can be rather complex because the color matching with the surrounding normal tissues and the skin texture should be concurrently ensured. Therefore, the thickness of the engrafted skin needs to be decided more carefully after identifying the condition of the scar bed, whether it is depressed or elevated. If there is a difference in the thickness between the engrafted and normal skin, the following method can be attempted: a very superficial incision is made on the normal skin along the engrafted margin; after fine dermabrasion was performed along the superficial incision line the engraft skin margin is precisely fit for the incision, making the graft margin less visible.

This female patient had a depressed, glossy, hypopigmented irregular scar on her left cheek area (black arrows). The operation was performed with a 0.2-mm thickness of auto sheet skin for a minor augmentation effect on the depressed margin taken from the buttock of the donor (Fig. 5.27). Four months after the procedure, the

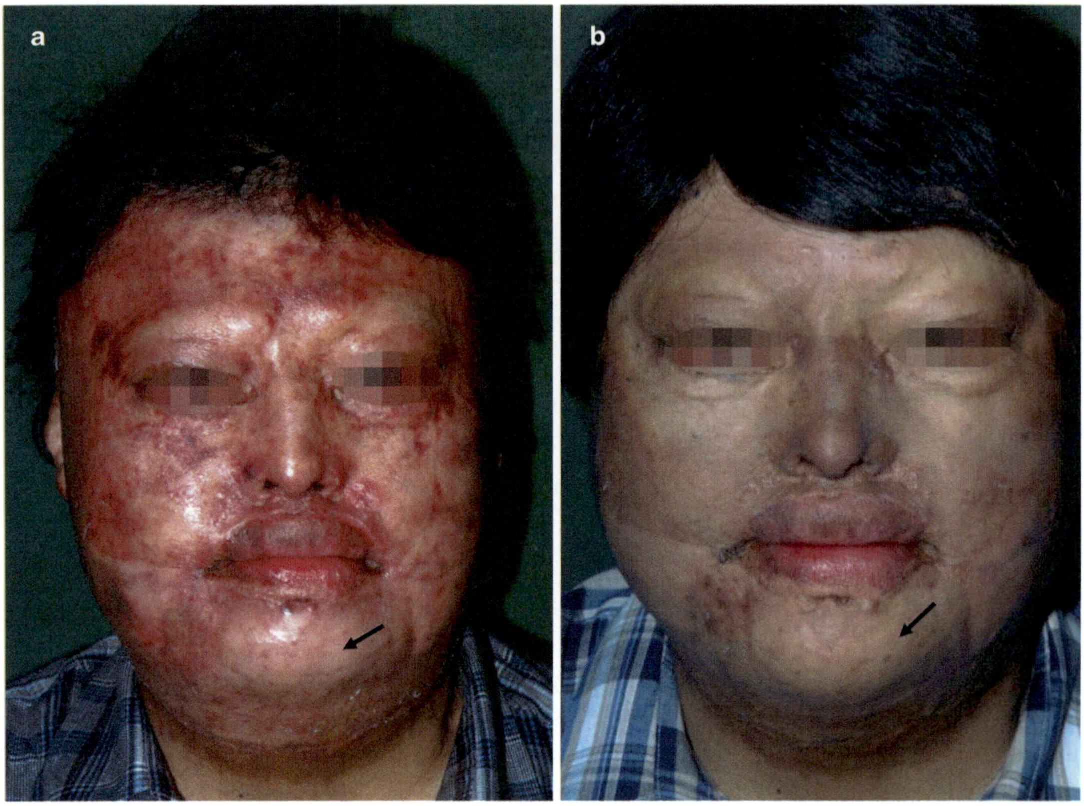

Fig. 5.25 (**a**) Postoperative 10 days, blood-stained spots and small multiple papules were noted; (**b**) postoperative 10 months later, marked improved skin color and texture were noted

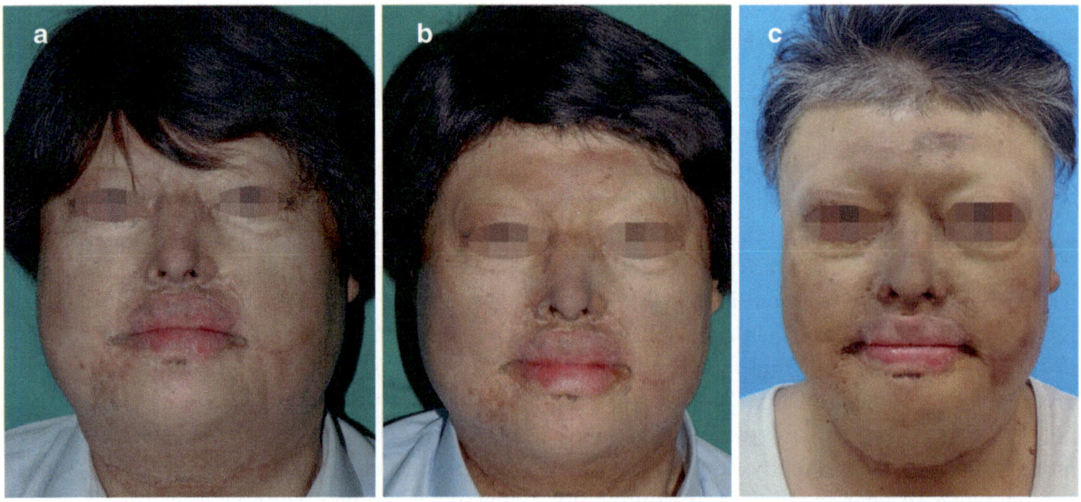

Fig. 5.26 (**a**) Postoperative 13 months view; (**b**) postoperative 2 years and 8 months view; (**c**) postoperative 14 years after, long period follow-up view, almost no change of skin color and texture on entire face

visible overgrafted lesion was still present in the front and three-quarter views (black arrows). Eight months after the procedure, the engrafted skin texture and depressed margin had noticeably improved (black arrows) (Fig. 5.28). One year after the procedure, the depressed and glossy scar

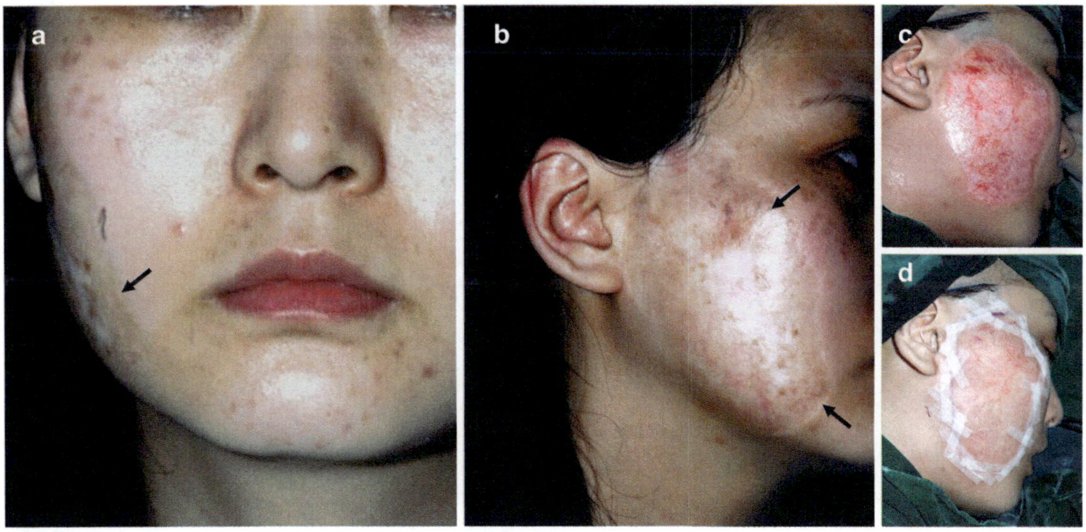

Fig. 5.27 (**a**, **b**) Old depressed, glossy, and hypopigmented irregular scar on the left cheek (black arrows); (**c**, **d**) 0.2 mm thickness for minor augmentation effect

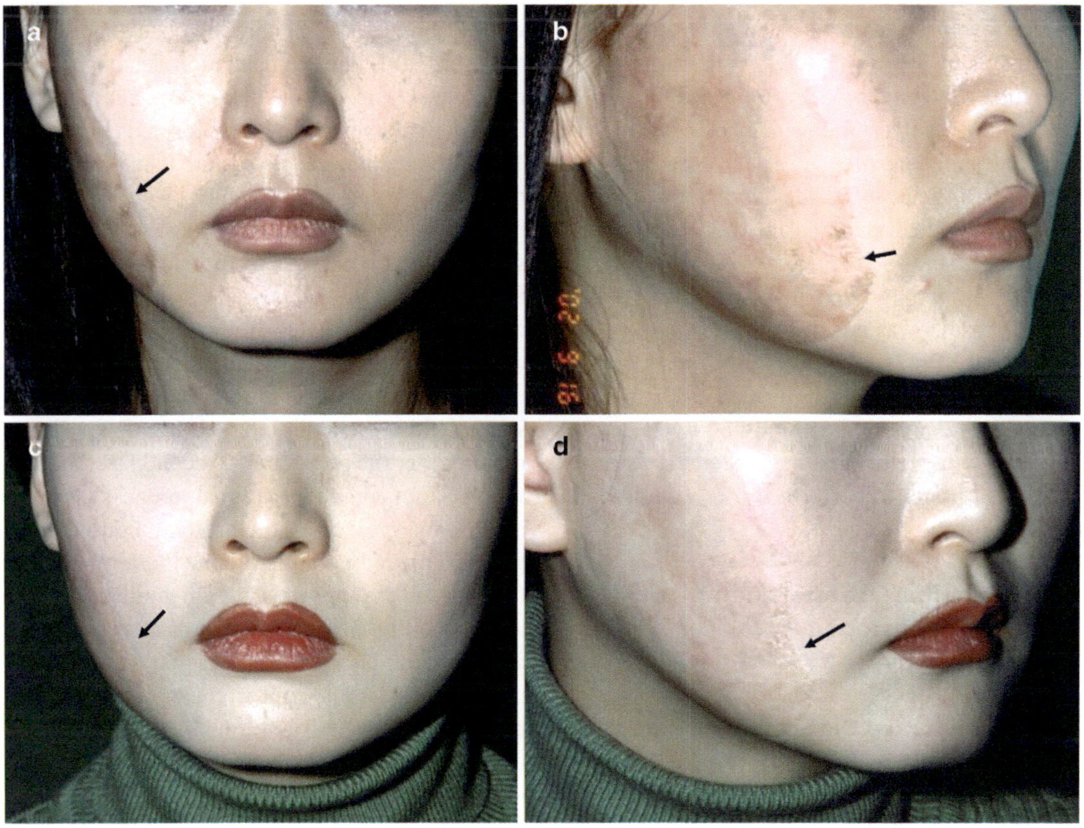

Fig. 5.28 (**a**, **b**) Postoperative 4 month later, front and three quarter view (black arrows); (**c**, **d**) postoperative 8 months later, the engrafted skin texture and depressed margin were corrected noticeably (black arrows)

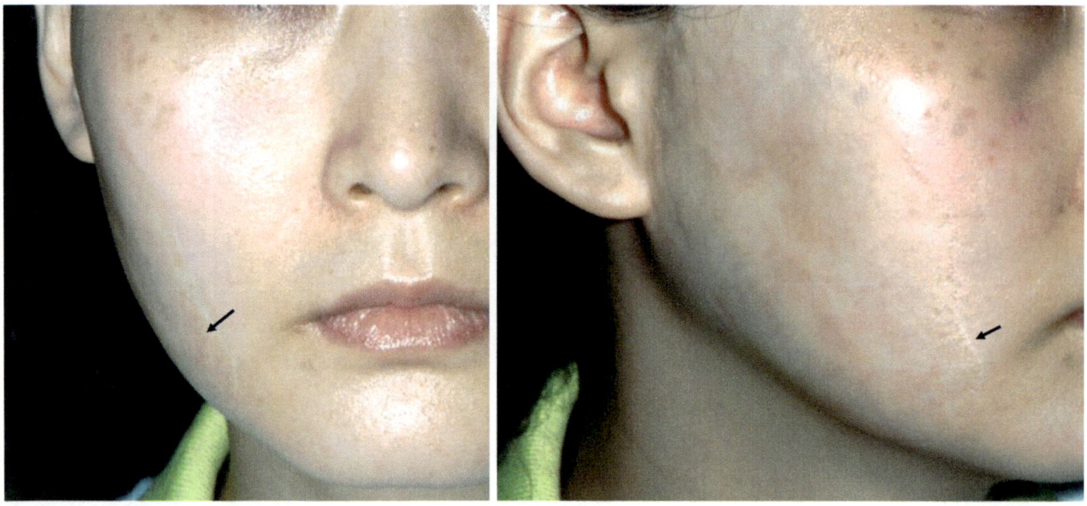

Fig. 5.29 Postoperative 1 year later, the depressed and glossy scar area was remarkably less visible by the dermal overgraft with augmentation effect (black arrow)

area was remarkably less visible as a result of the dermal overgraft with augmentation effect and improvement of skin texture. At the time of the operation (September 16, 2002), Fraxel laser was not used. To solve the problem of covering the very fine step deformity, a very shallow marginal incision was made along the depressed boundary, and the engrafted skin margin was covered with 6–0 nylon and Steri-Strip.™ As a result, an inconspicuous engrafted margin with excellent esthetic results was noted (Fig. 5.29).

Recently, Fraxel SR 1500 XENA laser combination therapy has been performed more than five times every 3 weeks, beginning 3–4 weeks after surgery, with perfect results expected. However, recently, I prefer to perform it for ≥6 months or up to a year.

5.2.2.3 Dermal Overgraft Combined with Postoperative Laser Therapy

Multiple Engrafted Old Scar on the Face

This 35-year-old male patient received multiple corrective surgeries with FTSG and STSG during his childhood. An irregular discoloration was noted on the left cheek area, and an FTSG scar was observed at the corner of the mouth. Dermabrasion was performed on the entire left cheek and on two oval-shaped island pigmentation lesions on the right cheek and mouth corner area. A 0.2-mm-thick dermal overgraft was performed (Fig. 5.30). Three days after the procedure, small areas of hematoma were noted, which were evacuated through a small slit incision, and a continuous saline-soaked compressive dressing was applied. Seven days after the procedure, the hematomas were almost completely removed, and the graft was taken completely. Two months after the procedure, Fraxel laser therapy (1550 nm 60 jl) was started with a 1-month interval (Fig. 5.31). Three months after the procedure, a second laser therapy was performed, and marginal redness and the engraft margin were still present. Four months after the procedure, a third laser therapy was performed, and the engrafted margin gradually started to change (Fig. 5.32). Five months after the procedure, a fourth laser therapy was performed, resulting in a considerable improvement of the engrafted margin (Fig. 5.33). Eight months after the procedure, an interval of 3 months, a fifth laser therapy was performed, resulting in significant improvement of the engrafted region. Thereafter, laser therapy was performed without a resting interval

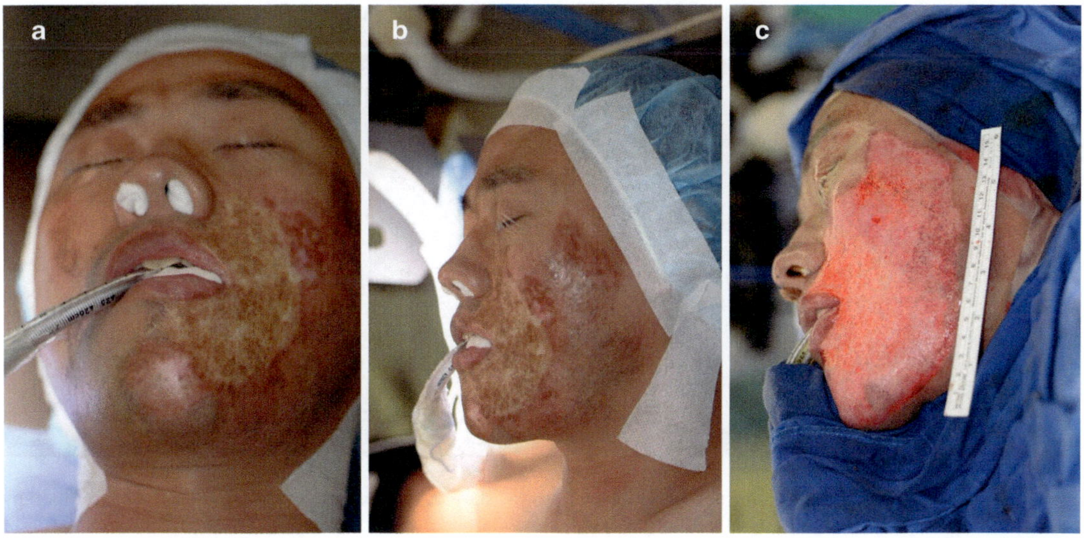

Fig. 5.30 (**a**, **b**) Preoperative view; (**c**) dermabrasion was performed on the left entire cheek and on two oval-shaped island pigmentation lesions

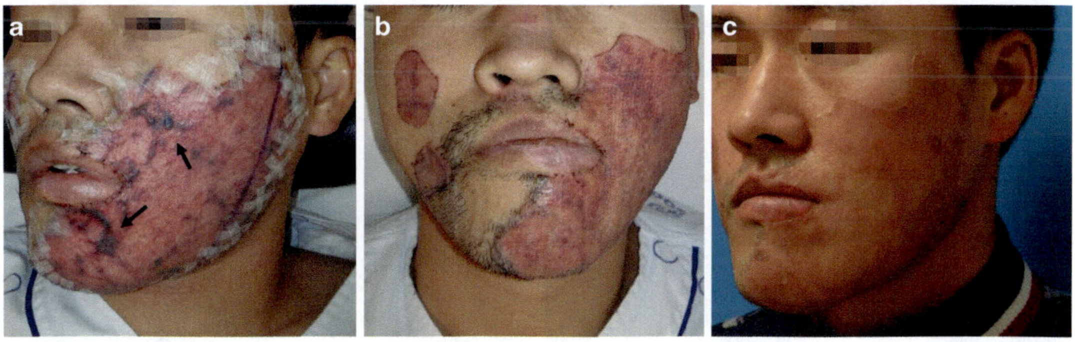

Fig. 5.31 (**a**) Postoperative 3 days, small areas of hematomas were noted; (**b**) postoperative 7 days, almost all hematomas were removed and graft taken; (**c**) postoperative 2 months, Fraxel laser therapy (1550 nm 60 jl) was started with a 1-month interval

(Fig. 5.34). Ten months after the procedure, a final laser therapy was performed, and the patient was satisfied with the results. Two islands of a round, oval scar on the right cheek were disappearing with excellent esthetic results (Fig. 5.35).

Multiple Local Flap Scars and an Engrafted Skin Lesion

A 51-year-old female patient underwent corrective surgery with various local flaps on the mentum and mouth corner area and received STSG on the left cheek 10 years ago. We noted a hyperpigmented depressed scar on the malar area (black arrow), a previous skin graft region with conspicuous engrafted margin on the cheek, and an irregular scar surface on the mentum and commissure. Dermabrasion was performed 1 cm or more wider than the original scar surface to camouflage and conceal the unsightly scar and engrafted margin (Fig. 5.36). The immediate operative observations showed that the engrafted skin thickness was 0.2 mm. The small localized hematoma was evac-

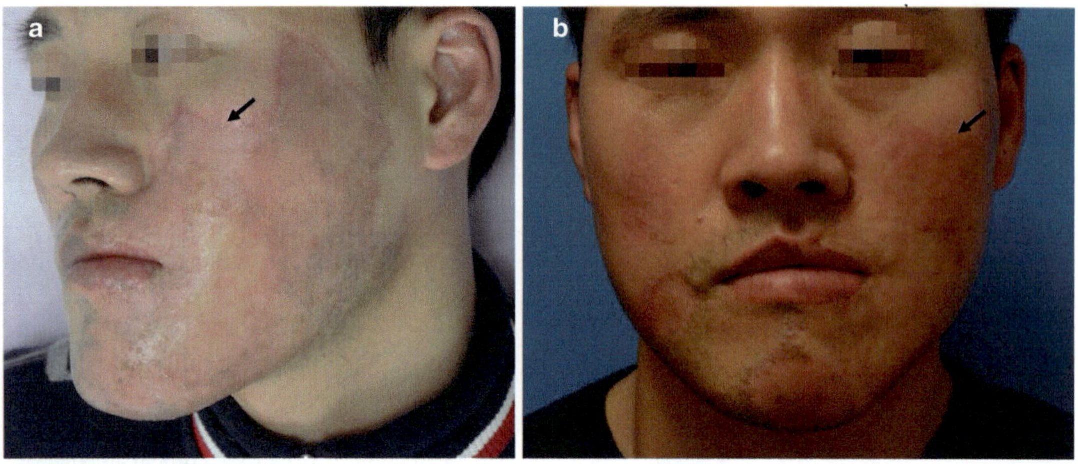

Fig. 5.32 (**a**) Postoperative 3 months, second laser therapy was started; (**b**) postoperative 4 months, third laser therapy was started, and slowly changed engrafted margin

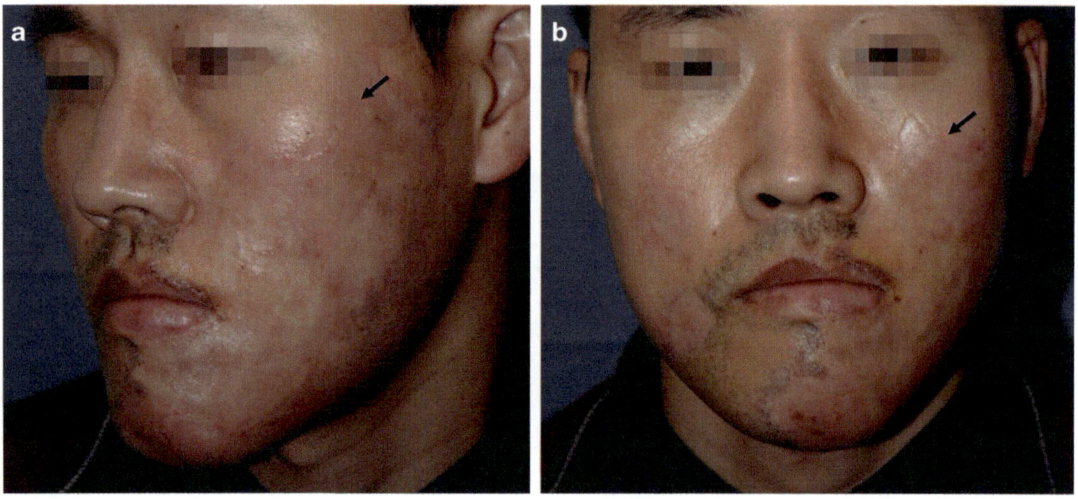

Fig. 5.33 (**a**) Postoperative 5 months view; (**b**) laser therapy fourth time

uated with a continuous saline-soaked dressing. Three weeks after the procedure, the skin was completely removed, the ecchymosis disappeared, and the engrafted overlapping skin margin was almost completely removed (Fig. 5.37). Three weeks after the procedure, we started Fraxel™ laser therapy. Five months after the procedure, the engrafted margin had a better appearance, and Fraxel™ laser therapy was performed every 3 weeks for 6 months (Fig. 5.38).

Pigmented Lesion on the Face [28, 29]

A 51-year-old female patient sustained a scalding burn 15 years ago on the right forehead and malar area. A mild, irregular burn scar on the forehead as well as hyperpigmentation and hypopigmentation were noted on the right cheek and upper and lower lids. Her main complaint was pigmentation and discoloration on the right cheek. We performed a dermal overgraft to correct the irregular scars on the forehead and pigmentation of the

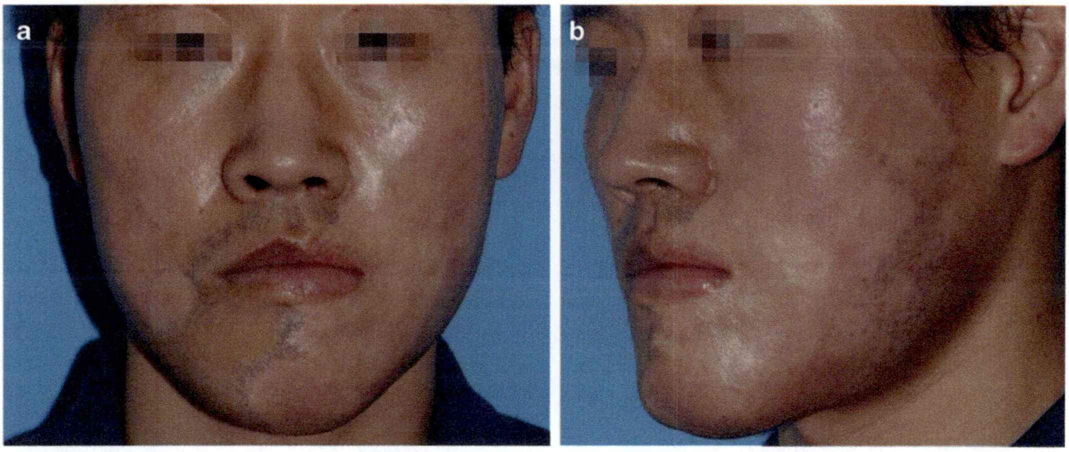

Fig. 5.34 (**a**) Postoperative 8 months, with laser therapy after 3 months interval resting time

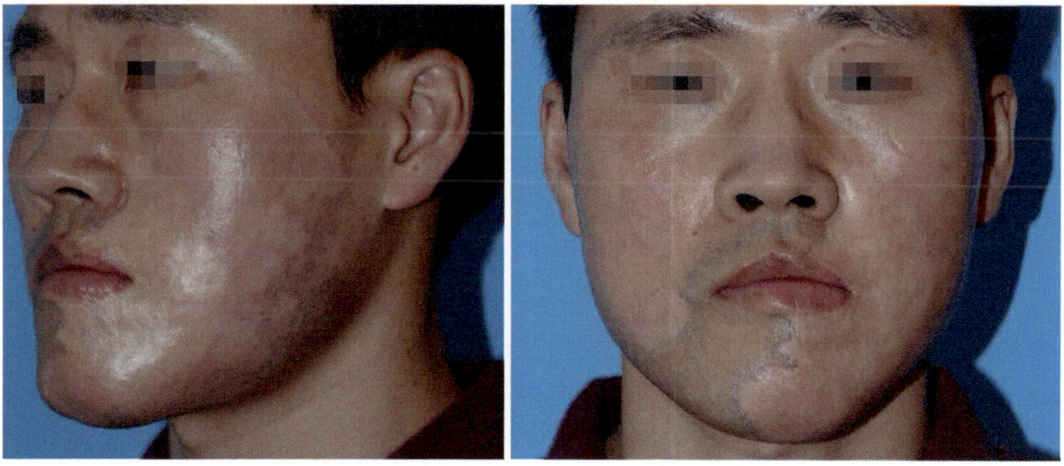

Fig. 5.35 Postoperative 10 months final laser therapy was performed

upper and lower lids and right malar area. This is a typical matured mild irregular scar and pigmentation disorder with a good surgical indication and outcome (Fig. 5.39). (a) Take note of the black arrow, which indicates where the right temple and forehead hairline were involved about 1 or 2 cm from the inner side in order to achieve a more natural hairline (black arrow). Upper and lower lid areas were dermabraded, and a 0.15-mm-thick overgraft was applied to almost the entire area, followed by tarsorrhaphy (white arrow). (b) Six days after the procedure, the engrafted skin was taken completely. The tarsorrhaphy was removed the next day for a more secure graft (Fig. 5.40). This figure depicts the postoperative observations at 1 year and 9 months: She received Fraxel laser therapy 2 months after the graft was taken completely. Laser therapy was performed every 1 month each during 5 months (Fig. 5.41).

5.2.3 Dorsum of the Hand and Forearm

Since the hands, forearms, and face are regularly exposed in everyday life, people with an unsightly big scar in these areas are vulnerable to both psy-

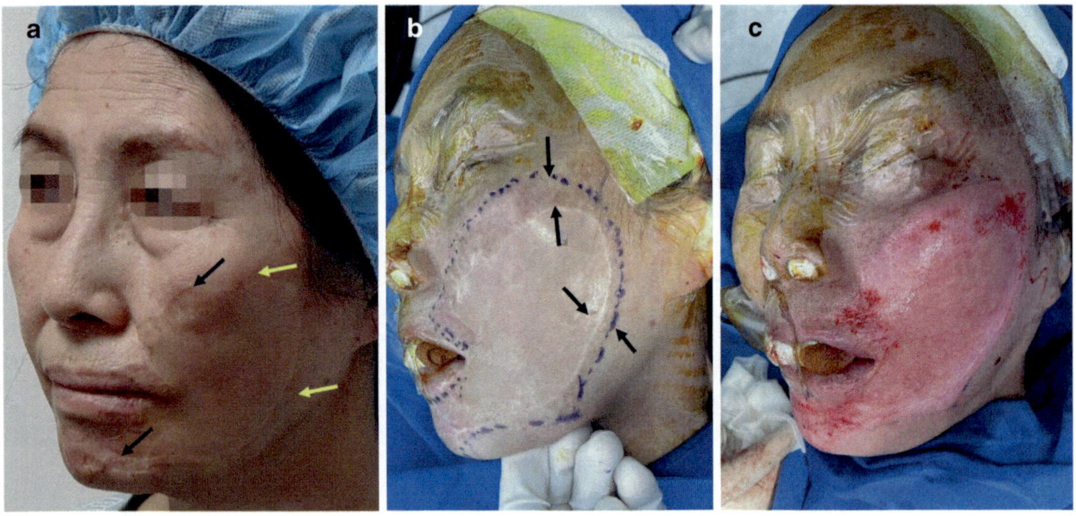

Fig. 5.36 (**a**) The hyperpigmented depressed scar on malar area (black arrow); previous skin graft region with conspicuous engrafted margin (yellow arrows) and irregular scar surface on mentum area (black arrow); (**b**, **c**) the dermabrasion was performed 1 cm or more wider than the original scar surface

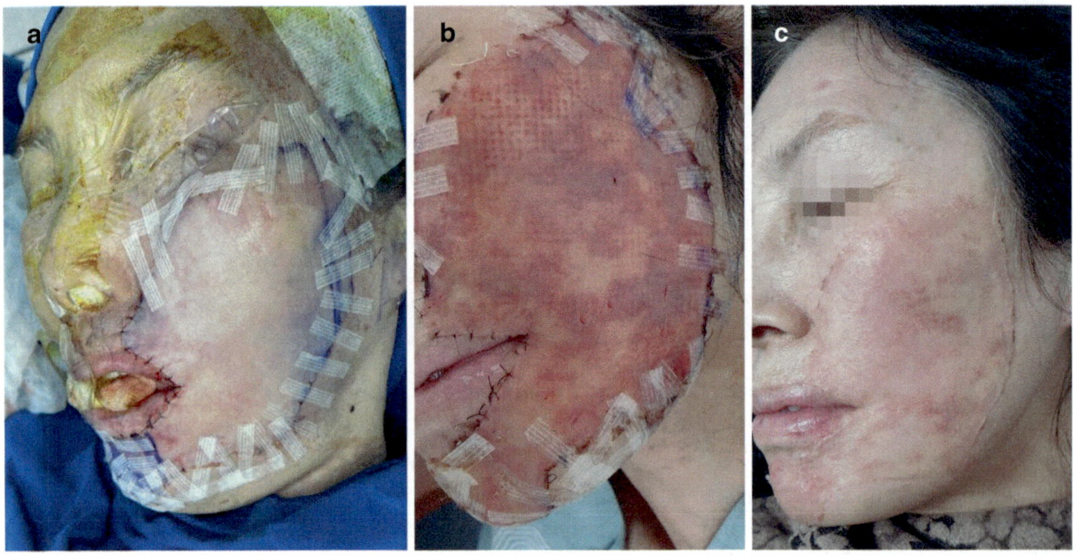

Fig. 5.37 (**a**) Immediate operative view; (**b**) postoperative 6 days view; (**c**) postoperative 3 weeks view

chological and social trauma. Therefore, dermal overgraft as an esthetic technique will be a very useful method for the correction of these scars and in the prevention of such psychiatric trauma in individuals [30]. The hands and arms have thick skin, unlike the face, and have a wide active motion range. The skin graft thickness of 0.3 mm is appropriate and esthetically suitable.

5.2.4 Unsightly Mesh Pattern on the Dorsum of the Hands

A 32-year-old female patient received a mesh skin graft on both hands for a flame burn injury. Before applying the esthetic dermal overgraft, I performed double-opposing Z-plasty on the second, third, and fourth web spaces to correct func-

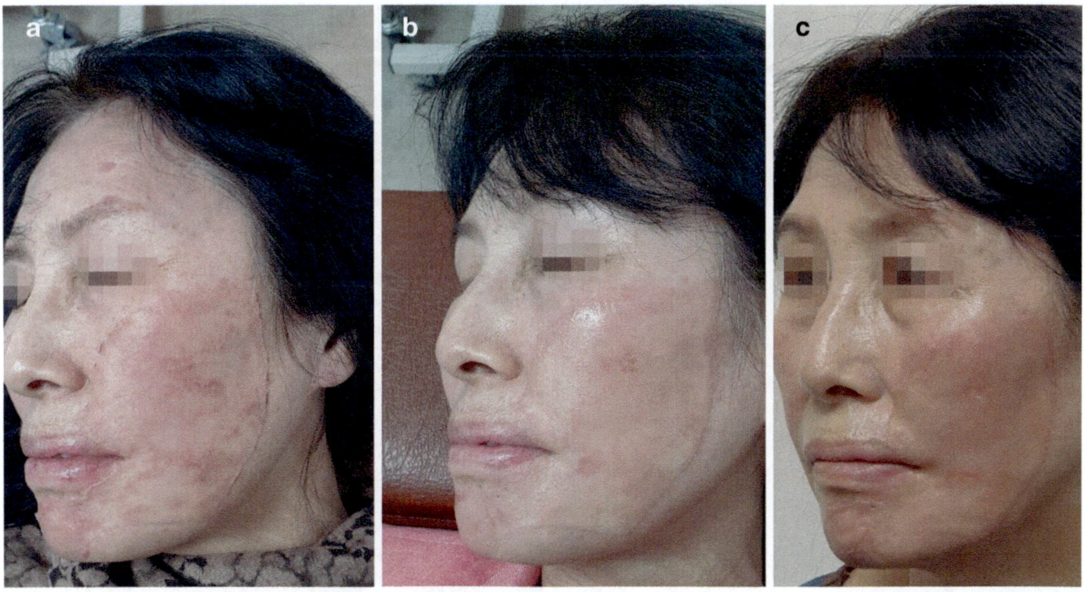

Fig. 5.38 (**a**) Three weeks after the operation, Fraxel™ laser therapy was started; (**b**) postoperative 4 months view; (**c**) postoperative 5 months view, the engrafted margin had a better appearance

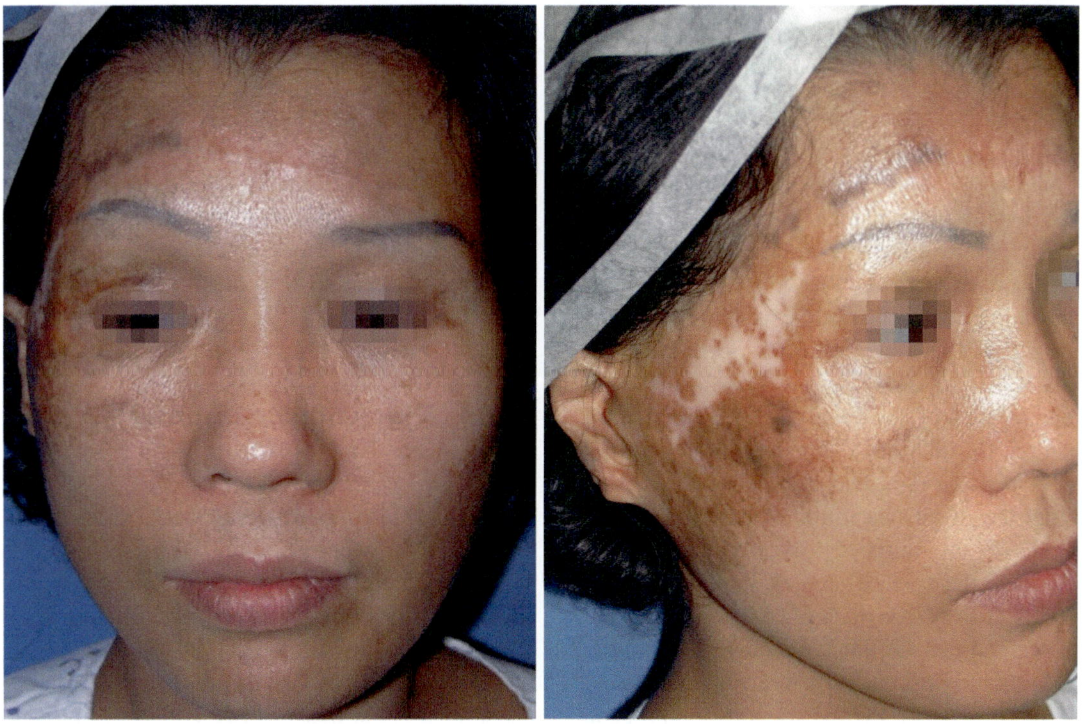

Fig. 5.39 Mild irregular burn scar on the forehead and hyper- and hypopigmentation disorder

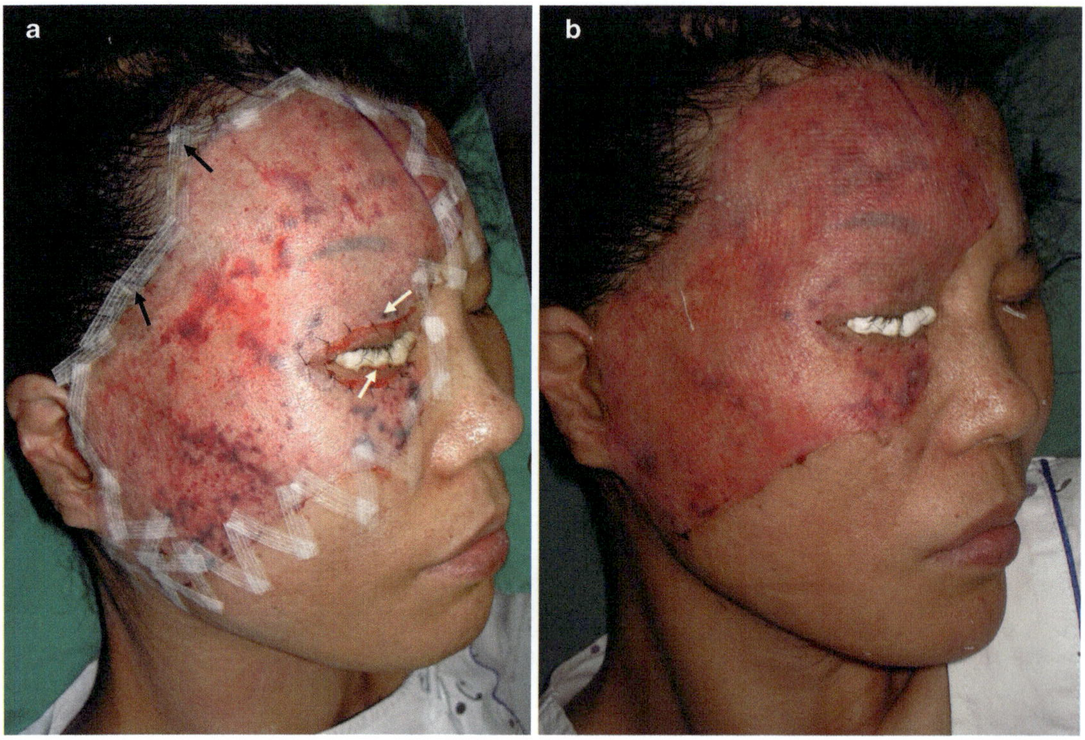

Fig. 5.40 (**a**) Right temple and forehead hairline were involved about 1 or 2 cm inner side for trying more natural hairline look (black arrow). Engraft with 0.125 mm thickness and tarsorrhaphy were performed (white arrow); (**b**) postoperative 6 days engrafted skin was taken completely

tional and esthetic problems (black arrow). For the dorsum of the hand, it is advised to perform a final corrective esthetic resurfacing dermal overgraft after the correction of all the deformities, including contractures and webbing deformities (Fig. 5.42). One year after the operation for scar maturation, dermabrasion was performed on both the dorsum of the hands. The unsightly mesh pattern is still visible. The engrafted skin thickness was 0.3 mm, and the graft was performed from the distal two-thirds of the dorsum of the hands to one-third of the proximal phalanges. Because the surface area of the dorsum of the hands differs considerably between the functional and fist positions, the maximum engrafted area should be secured by referring to the hand as a fist (Fig. 5.43). Five years after the procedure, the dorsal areas of the hands had noticeably improved in skin texture and color, and the unsightly mesh pattern had faded (Fig. 5.44). In author's experience, the unsightly mesh pattern can be easily corrected with this dermal overgraft technique; the point is you do not have to remove out the mesh pattern completely; just dermabrasion and overgraft will fade as time goes by according to engrafted scar maturation.

5.2.5 Pigmentation Disorder on the Hand

Pigmentation without scaring on the surface, dermal overgraft techique with 0.125 mm thickness can be adapted for treatment. Some surgeons have proposed suction blister epidermal graft for the treatment of vitiligo [31].

In my experience, a fine upper dermal component with epidermal papillae is more stable and has better color-matching outcomes than an epidermal graft alone. Blister epidermal grafts have fewer donor-site morbidities than dermal overgraft techniques, but they require longer opera-

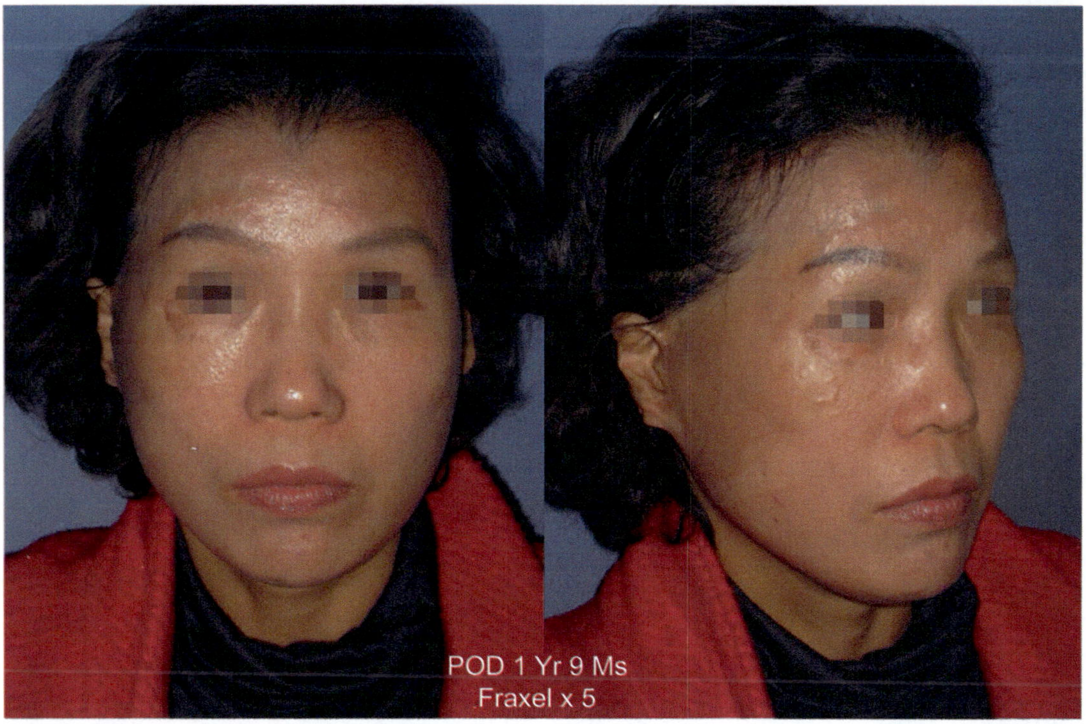

Fig. 5.41 POD 1 year and 9 months view

tion time, do not have a wide area, are unstable, and are less effective. Six months after the procedure, the hypopigmented lesion and skin texture were corrected. Ten months after the procedure, the color lightened and the texture improved (Fig. 5.45).

5.2.5.1 Forearm

Wide Burn Scar on the Forearm

A 31-year-old patient visited the clinic for the correction of an irregular scar surface on the left forearm and elbow-joint area, which had been injured due to a scaling burn during childhood. Dermabrasion and dermal overgraft were performed, and 0.25-mm-thick skin was harvested from the left buttock (I used to harvest the donor skin from the thigh area, but recently, I have been harvesting the donor skin from the buttock or back area). Three months after the procedure, irregular surfaces and texture had improved (Fig. 5.46).

Matured Shiny Burn Scar on the Forearm

A non-hypertrophic, mature glossy burn scar is also a good surgical indication of a very good effective outcome, especially if it is a wide, diffuse scar on the forearm. A 0.25-mm-thick dermal overgraft was performed (Fig. 5.47). Five months after the procedure, the skin texture had improved, and the color of the graft matched the color of the surrounding normal skin, with an inconspicuous graft margin. Postoperative findings after 2 years and 7 months revealed that the skin color and texture had not changed much over the period of 2 years (Fig. 5.48). In this case, the donor skin was harvested from the lateral thigh, but the original donor skin color had little influence on the recipient's engrafted skin color.

Tattoo Removal Using Dermal Overgraft Technique

The dermal overgraft procedure can cover partial or wide-sighted scars and professional or amateur artificial tattoos. However, if the depth or thickness of a scar or tattoo is irregular or uneven, par-

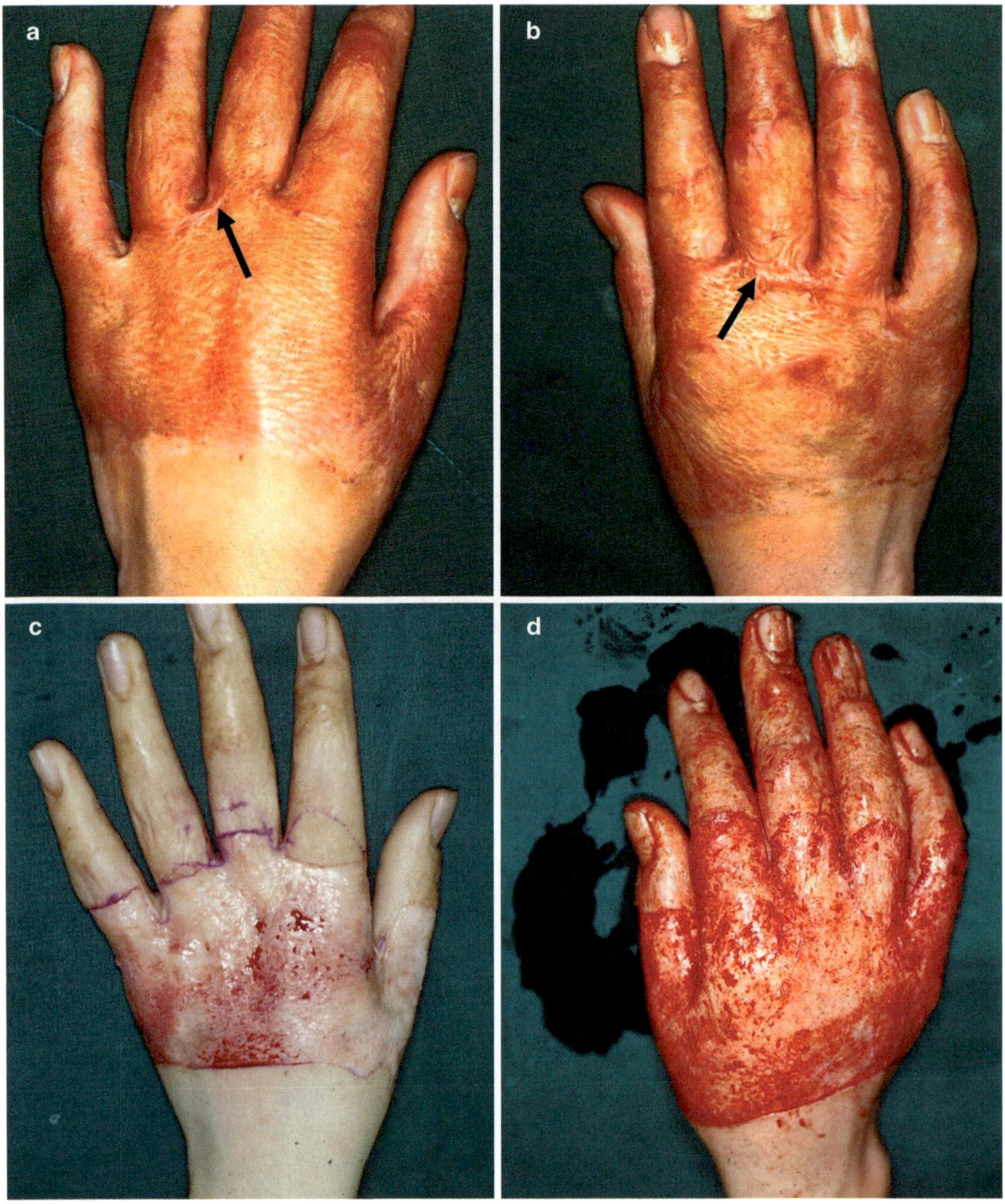

Fig. 5.42 (**a**) Preoperative view. Note minor webbing deformities (black arrows); (**b**) author performed double-opposing Z plasty on the second, third and fourth web spaces before surgery; (**c**, **d**) 1 year after, dermabrasion was performed on both dorsum of hands

tial excision via razor shaving is also required. The abrasion depth of a dermabrader is limited and very shallow; thus, regions with a thick scar or deep dermis are not easily abraded, with the fibers sticking together and making it difficult for the skin to peel neatly and time-consuming. Therefore, a razor allows for the simple and easy flattening of the region. Proper thickness of skin

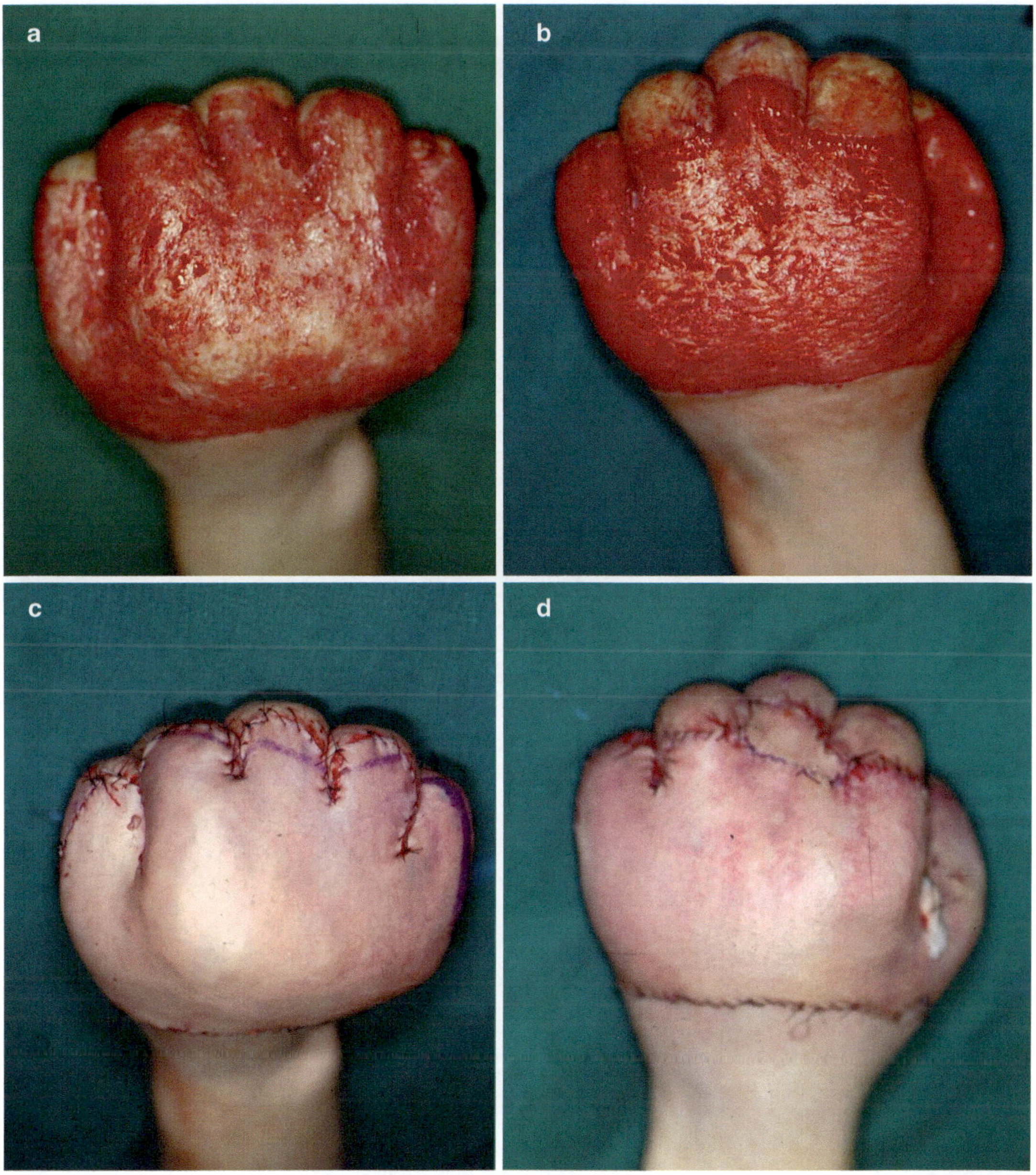

Fig. 5.43 (**a**, **b**) Dermabrasion on both hands; (**c**, **d**) engrafted skin was 0.3 mm and graft was performed from the distal two-thirds of the dorsum of the hands to one-third of the proximal phalanges. Fist position is given more expanded area to preserve for maximal engraft area on the dorsum of the hands

graft after the tattoo removal, at least a minimum thickness of 0.3 mm, is required and postoperative pressure garment and laser therapy are needed.

(a) A 31-year-old male patient got a professional tattoo on his right forearm several years ago. However, the tattoo depth was uneven, with some areas deeply inked on full layers of the skin. These areas were removed by razor shaving. The deep tattooed area was shaved with a razor (black arrows). The raw surface was covered with a 0.25-mm-thick skin (Fig. 5.49). Four days after the procedure, the dressing was open, and a

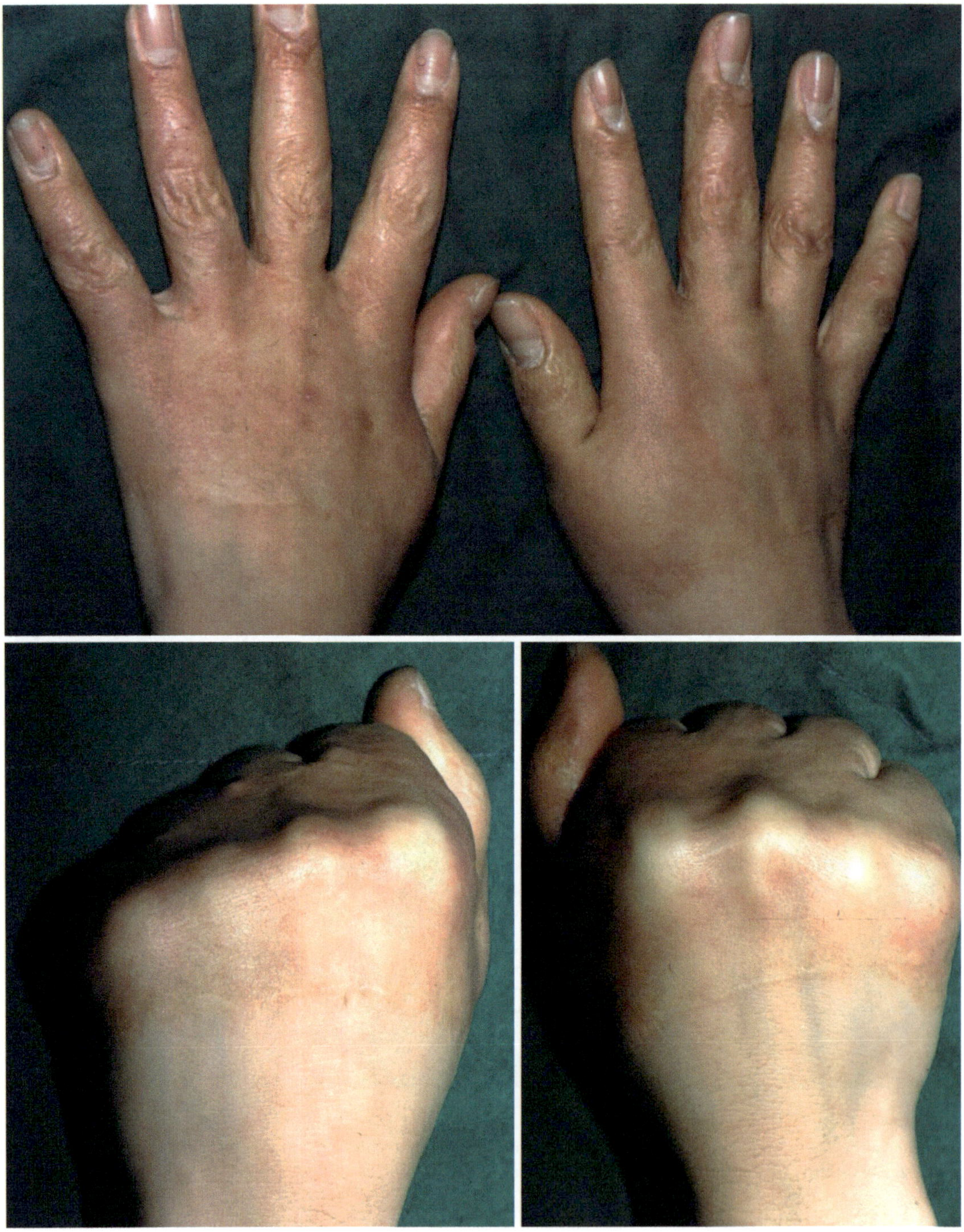

Fig. 5.44 Postoperative 5 years view, with the dorsum of the hand area greatly improved in skin texture and color and fading of the unsightly mesh pattern

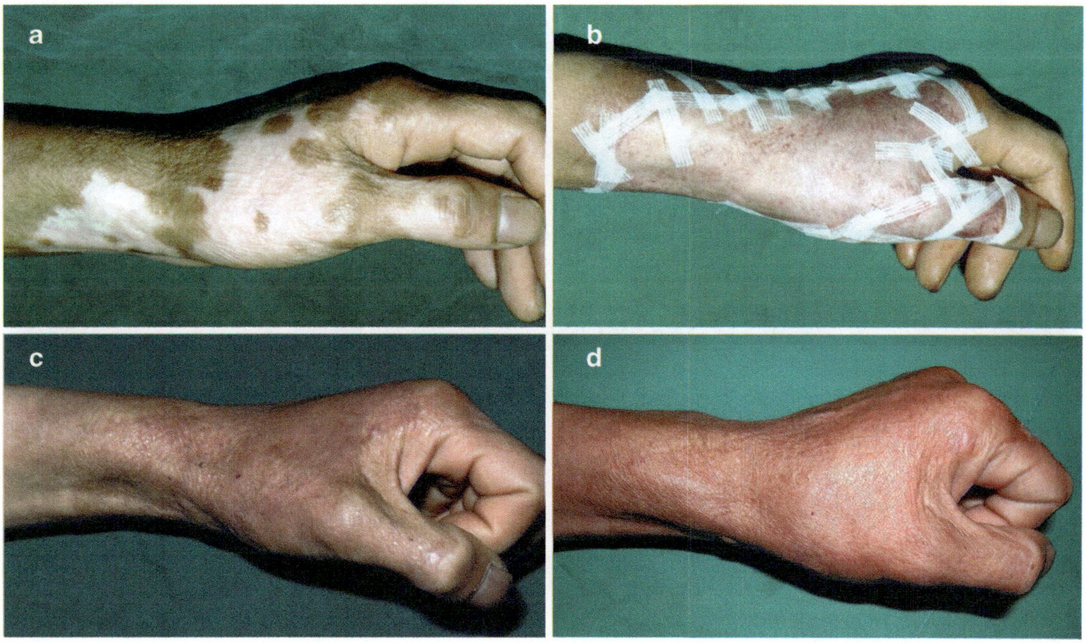

Fig. 5.45 (**a**) Pigmentation disorder without scarring bed case can also adapt dermal overgraft technique; (**b**) the engrafted skin thickness was 0.125 mm was examed with PAS stain (Refer Fig. 5.6b) shown skin thickness Is show small fine amount upper dermis with full layer of epidermis containing basement membrane in PAS stain. (**c**) postoperative 6 months view; (**d**) 10 months after operation view

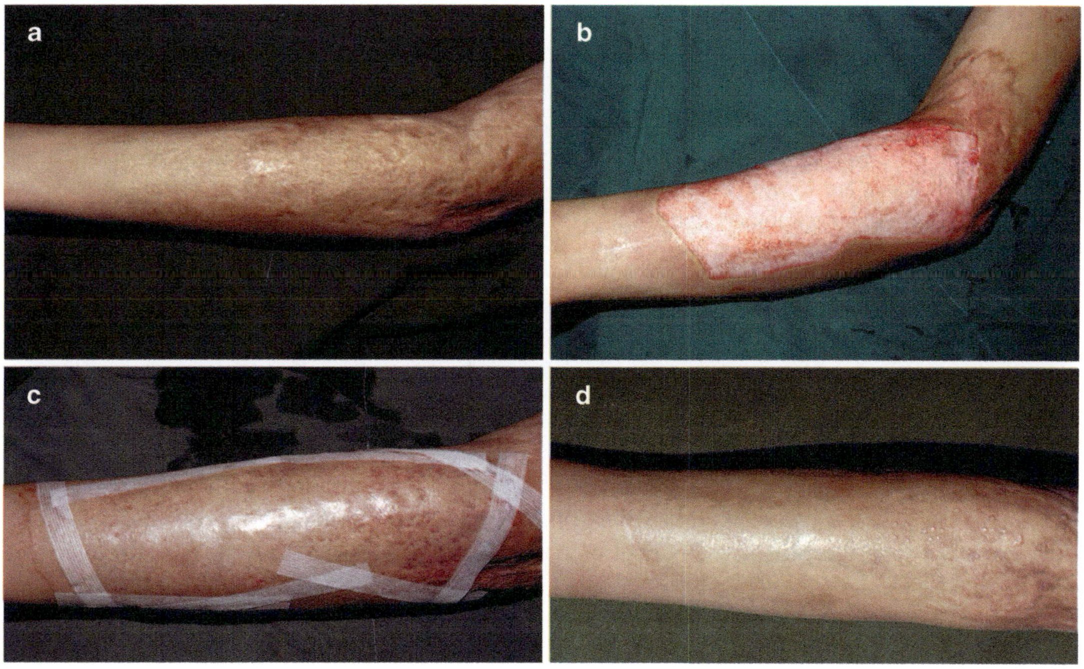

Fig. 5.46 (**a**) Irregular mild hypertrophic scar was noted on the left forearm; (**b**) dermabrasion was performed; (**c**) dermal overgraft was performed with 0.25-mm-thickness skin; (**d**) postoperative 3 months view

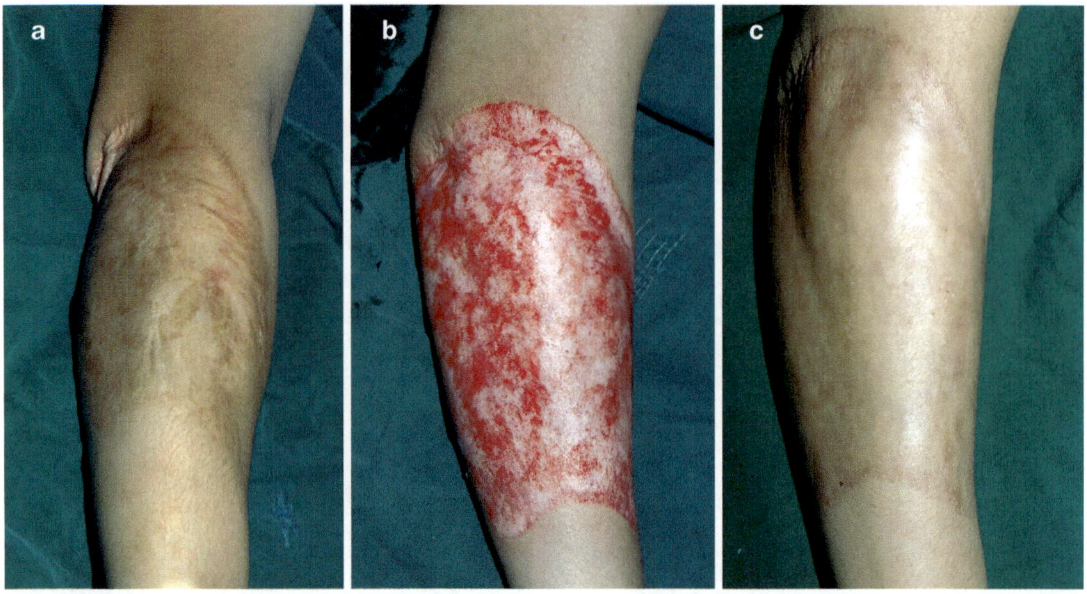

Fig. 5.47 (**a**) Matured glossy burn scar case in elbow joint and forearm area; (**b**) dermabrasion and dermal overgraft were performed with 0.25-mm-thickness skin; (**c**) Postoperative 3 months view

hematoma was noticed on the central full-layer skin defect area. (b, c) Postoperative findings after 6 and 8 days revealed a more stable appearance. (d) Postoperative findings after 2 weeks revealed that the engrafted skin was completely removed (Fig. 5.50). After 1 month postoperatively, the patient began wearing pressure garments for at least 1 year, and we planned Fraxel laser therapy (Fig. 5.51).

If scars or tattoos are located encircled on the entire forearm, considerations regarding skin harvesting and meticulous postoperative dressing care are required. Since this region also requires encircling elastic compressive dressing, which are extremely tight, and bulky dressing causes multiple large linea wrinkles due to forced encircling pressure, it results in the detachment of the engrafted skin from beneath and causes hematoma. Therefore, special caution should be taken to avoid this. In terms of dressing following the surgery, the engrafted skin is secured by spreading fine Vaseline gauze over it in one layer and applying bulky and crumpled 4 × 4 saline-soaked gauze on the engrafted skin. Then, the surgical site is covered with dry surgical pads and compressively bandaged with an elastic bandage (Fig. 5.51). This should be done cautiously since there is a risk of seroma or hematoma formation beneath the engrafted skin due to the sliding action of the muscles and tendons caused by the movement of the fingers, wrist, or elbow joints. To prevent this, fixing both the wrist and elbow joints with an immobilization splint is advised.

To reduce the chances of failure in case an encircling dermal overgraft is required, it is recommended to perform the graft in two parts, by dividing it into pronator and supinator in the maximum vertical width of not over 10 cm, rather than performing the graft at once.

5.2.5.2 Lower Extremity

According to the author's experience, dermal overgraft from the lower extremity is not recommended because the skin texture and colors are not ideal along with the occurrence of hyperpigmentation, which reduces the esthetic effect. However, simple local anesthesia can lead to a suitable esthetic effect on the scars in small areas of the lower leg.

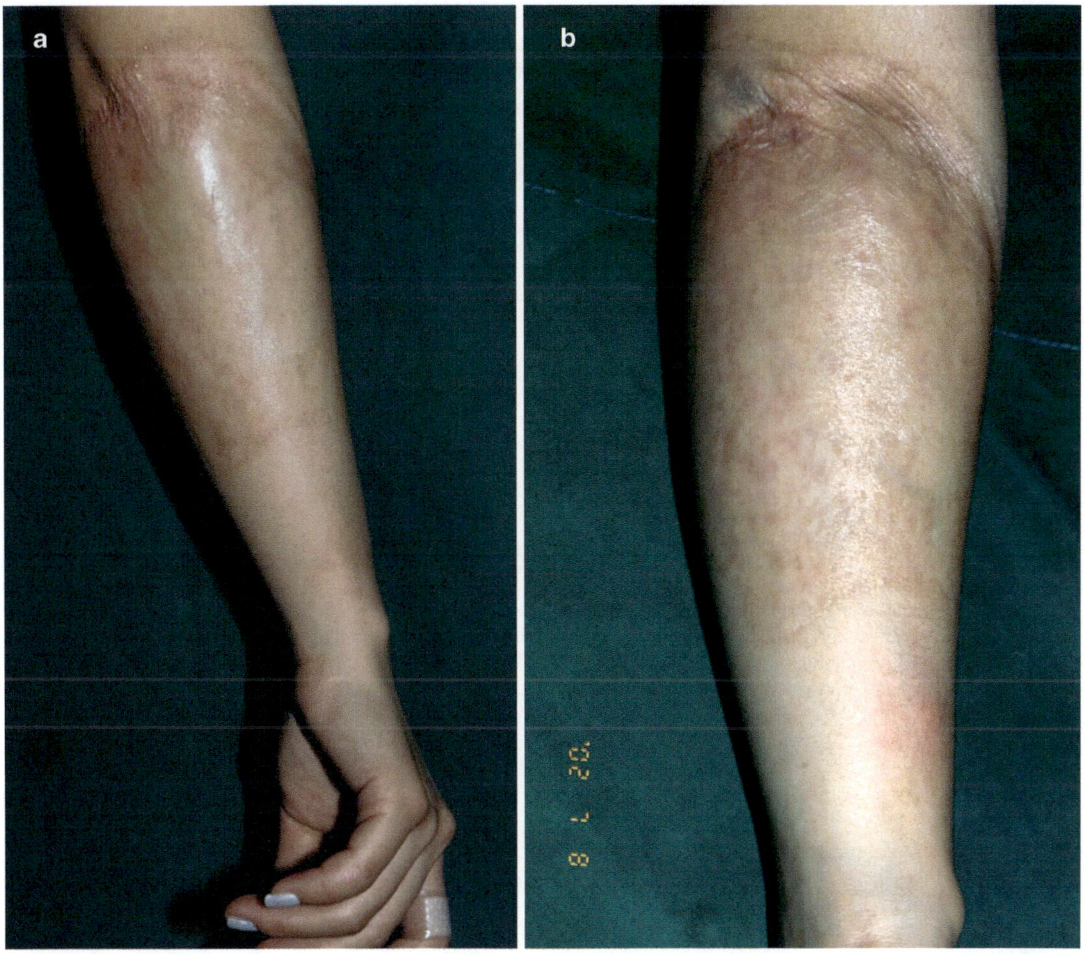

Fig. 5.48 (**a**) Postoperative 5 month view; (**b**) postoperative 2 years and 7 months view, there is no change in skin color and texture

A 13-year-old female suffered a scalding burn. A wide, glossy scar and an irregular hypopigmented lesion on the right leg area were noticed. We horizontally placed two pieces of graft of 0.2-mm thickness, which is thinner than the usual graft thickness, on the lower extremities because the patient was young and to reduce donor-site morbidity. Postoperative findings after 2 months revealed a corrected pigmented lesion and improved skin texture, with no conspicuous engraft margin on the seam line (Fig. 5.52). As mentioned previously, I do not recommend using this technique on the lower extremities because they are more prone to hyperpigmentation than other sites.

5.2.6 Special Dermal Overgraft

5.2.6.1 Palm-to-Sole Overgraft

Generally, inguinal full-thickness skin is used to correct scar contracture in the flexor part of the hand in children. FTSG in this region is very useful for functional recovery; however, there is a big difference in the color and texture of the palm since the skin of the palms and soles has stratum lucidum, which does not exist in other areas of the body. The skin texture of the engrafted full-thickness skin is thick and prone to hyperpigmentation due to external exposure, leading to sunburns and injuries because of continuous minor friction. Such unsightly grafted scars and

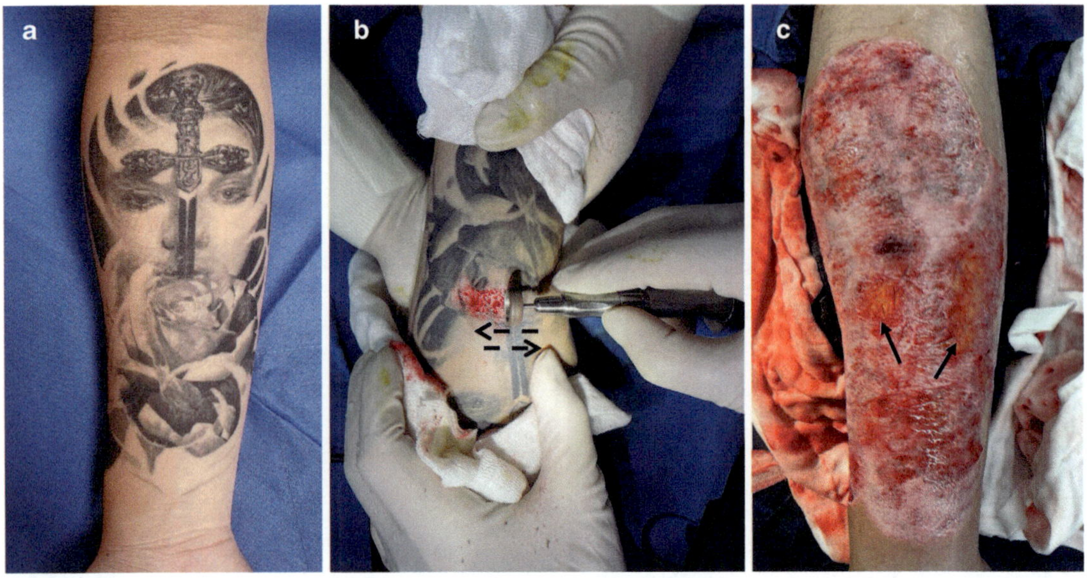

Fig. 5.49 (**a**) Dermal overgraft technique is also a useful method for the removal of artificial tattoos, especially amateur tattoos; (**b**) dermabrasion skill showing reciprocating motion (dashed arrows); (**c**) because amateur tattooing is irregular in depth, razor shaving is a good instrument for effective removal of tattoos (black arrows). This case has an unevenly inked tattoo, therefore some deeper areas required full layer skin removal

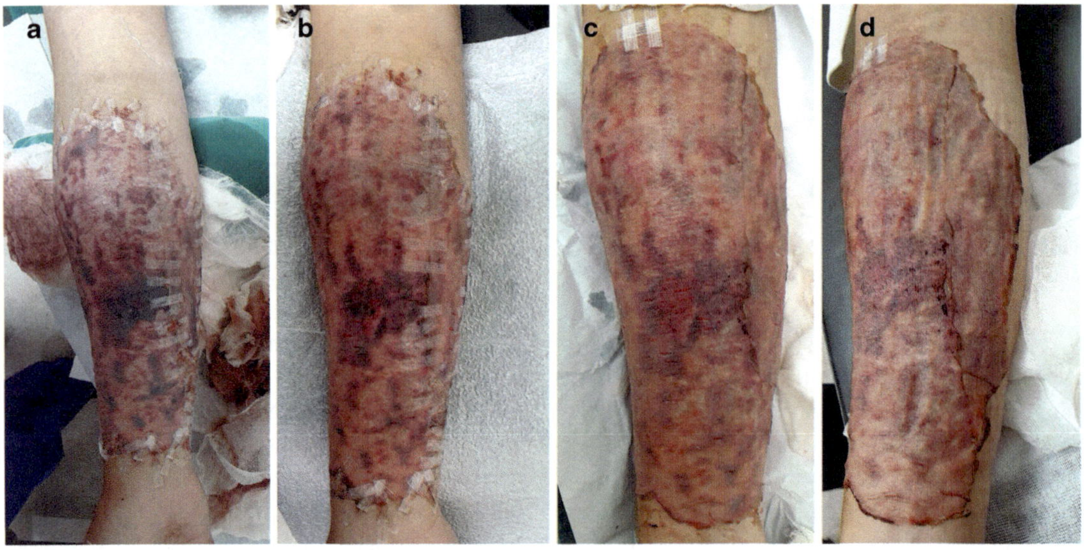

Fig. 5.50 (**a**) Postoperative 4 days, dressing was opened and hematoma was noted on the central full-layer skin defect area; (**b**, **c**) postoperative 6 days and 8 days view, hematoma lesions were slowly changing to a more stable appearance; (**d**) postoperative 2 weeks view, the engrafted skin was completely taken

pigmentation disorders that are constantly exposed are particularly stressful for children and may lead to psychological trauma. The corresponding correctional method followed by the author includes using 0.3–0.4 mm of split-thickness skin on the instep of the sole, minimally affecting weight-bearing.

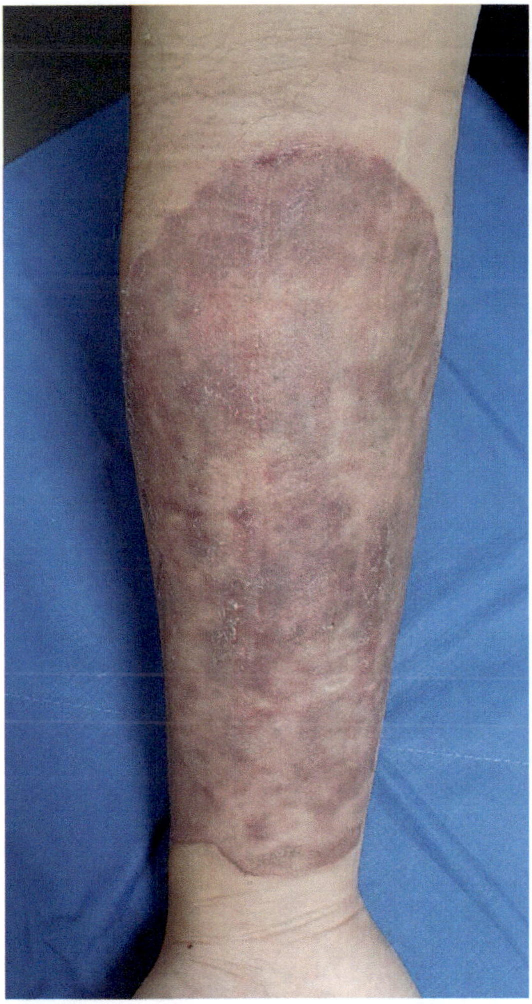

Fig. 5.51 PPostoperative 1 month after view, with stable results, however recommendation of wearing pressure garment for a year, with Fraxel laser theraphy every 3 weeks. Since this region also requires encircling elastic compressive dressing, which is extremely tight, and bulky dressing causes multiple large linea wrinkles due to forced encircling pressure, it results in the detachment of the engrafted skin from beneath and causes hematoma. Therefore, special caution should be taken to avoid this. In terms of dressing following the surgery, the engrafted skin is secured by spreading fine Vaseline gauze over it in one layer and applying bulky and crumpled 4 × 4 saline-soaked gauze on the engrafted skin. Then, only the surgical site is covered with dry surgical pads and compressively bandaged with an elastic bandage. This should be done cautiously since there is a risk of seroma or hematoma formation beneath the engrafted skin due to the sliding action of the muscles and tendons caused by the movement of the fingers, wrist, or elbow joints. Therefore, to prevent this, fixing both the wrist and elbow joints with an immobilization splint is advised

(a) A 10-year-old boy sustained a steam burn caused by an electric rice cooker at the age of 10 months. After being injured for a year, FTSG was performed for the functional recovery of the contracted index finger and palm. At the age of 10 years, a different skin texture with a marked hyperpigmented engrafted skin was noted with no functional disturbance. He was psychologically stressed caused by the dark discoloration on the right palm. (b) After removing the pigmented lesion with a dermabrader, (c) 0.3-mm-thick donor skin was obtained from the non-weight-bearing instep area of the right sole (Fig. 5.53). (a) Intraoperative view, note the texture of engrafted split sole skin after finishing dermal over engraft procedure. (b) Four months after the procedure, the skin texture and hyperpigmented lesion had significantly improved, with a different skin texture of the palm and sole (Fig. 5.54). According to the author's experience, when dermabrasion is performed on the engrafted skin following FTSG, it is advised to cautiously remove the only epidermal layer of the skin as a slightly deeper removal of the dermal layer poses a high risk of hypertrophic scarring or recurrent scar contracture in the palm, fingers, and web space.

The dermal overgraft technique can be used to improve the texture and color of the previous graft with artificial dermis such as Integra®, Pelnac®, and AlloDerm®.

As observed from the author's experience, although significant results were obtained from using the dermabrasion and dermal overgraft technique on the site where Integra® or Pelnac® was grafted, which are 100% biologically synthesized artificial dermis with animal collagen, they are not strongly recommended because the outcomes are less esthetically appealing compared to grafting on the normal scar bed.

The right forearm and the dorsum of the hand received Integra® for the treatment of an acute flame burn. Two years later, dermabrasion was performed for the correction of an irregular scar bed and poor skin texture. A 0.2-mm-thick skin was engrafted and secured with Steri-Strip™. Six months after the procedure, the irregular surface of the scar and skin texture had improved but to a lesser extent than the usual burn scar bed (Fig. 5.55).

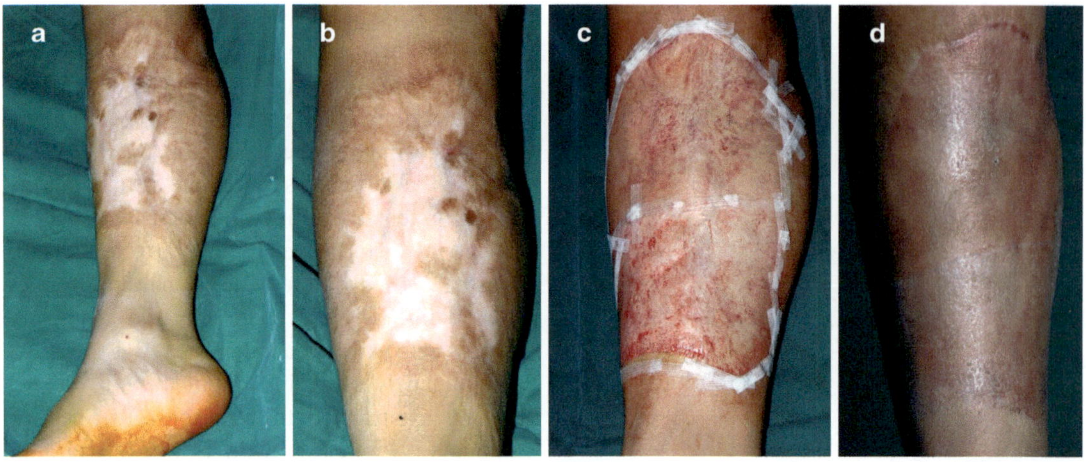

Fig. 5.52 (**a**, **b**) Glossy burn scar with hypopigmented lesion was noted on the right anterior shin; (**c**) horizontally two pieces of the engraft with 0.2-mm-thickness skin were used; (**d**) postoperative 2 months view, correction of pigmented lesion and improved skin texture were noted

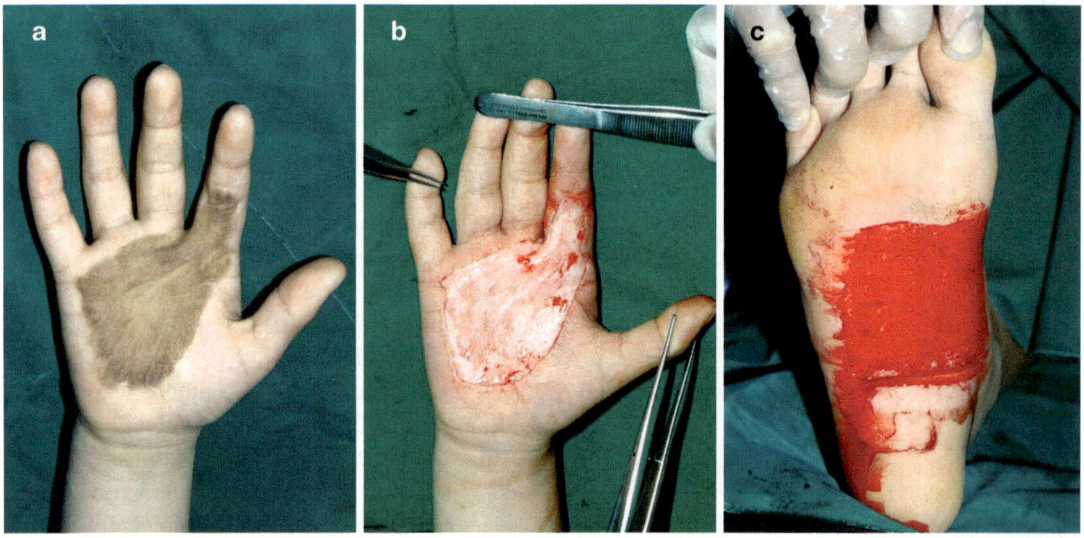

Fig. 5.53 (**a**) At age 10 years, different texture of skin with noticeable hyperpigmented engrafted skin is noted without functional disturbance; (**b**) dermabrasion was performed; (**c**) the 12/1000 in. thickness donor skin was obtained from the non-weight-bearing instep area of the right sole

A 5-year-old female patient complained of severe itching on the previous mesh-grafted lesion on the lower leg. Integra® artificial dermis was engrafted. Observations were made immediately and after 2 weeks revealed the formation of an orange-colored elapsed neodermis. Postoperative findings after 1 year and 2 months revealed that the outcome was not acceptable because of hyperpigmentation and an irregular surface. I performed a 0.15-mm-thick dermal overgraft for the improvement of the pigmented and irregular surface. Eight months after the procedure, the skin color and texture had improved, but these results were less acceptable than usual dermal overgraft on the burn scar or trauma scar bed. One of the reasons could be that the young girl's skin is thin

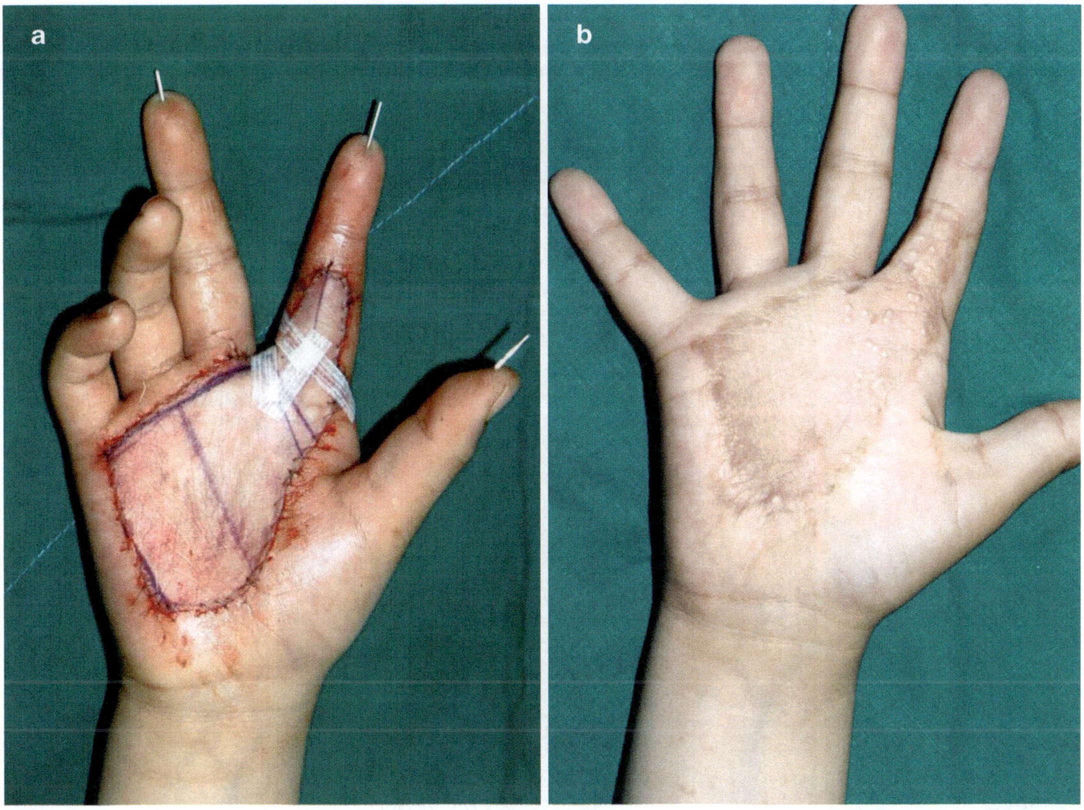

Fig. 5.54 (**a**) Note the texture of sole skin with thick appearance, different to the other usual skin; (**b**) postoperative 4 months view, skin texture and hyperpigmented lesion were noticeably improved on the skins of the palm and sole

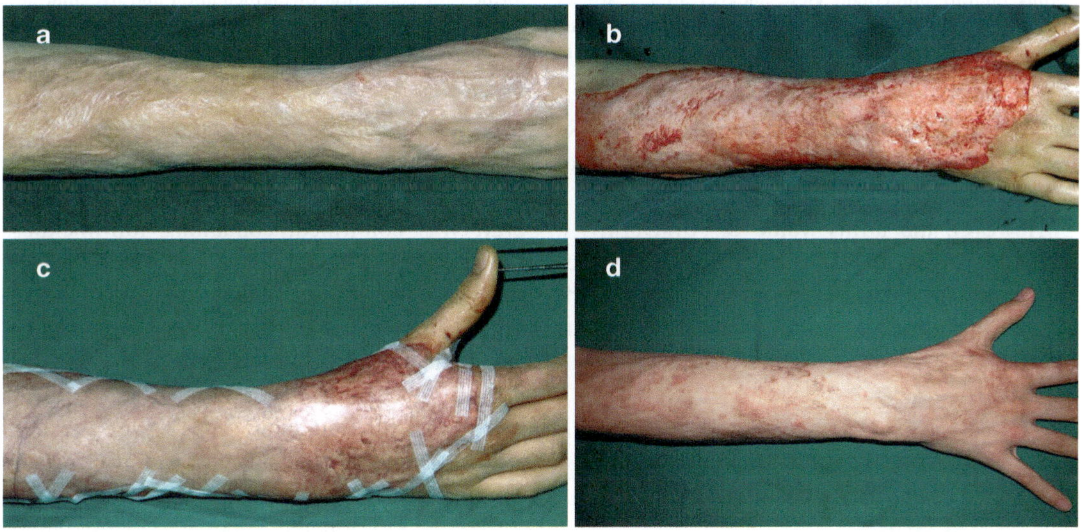

Fig. 5.55 (**a**) Two years ago, right forearm and dorsum of the hand were treated using Integra®; (**b**) dermabrasion was performed; (**c**) 0.2-mm-thickness skin was engrafted and secured with Steri-Strip™; (**d**) 6 months after the procedure, improvement on scar irregular surface and skin texture was observed

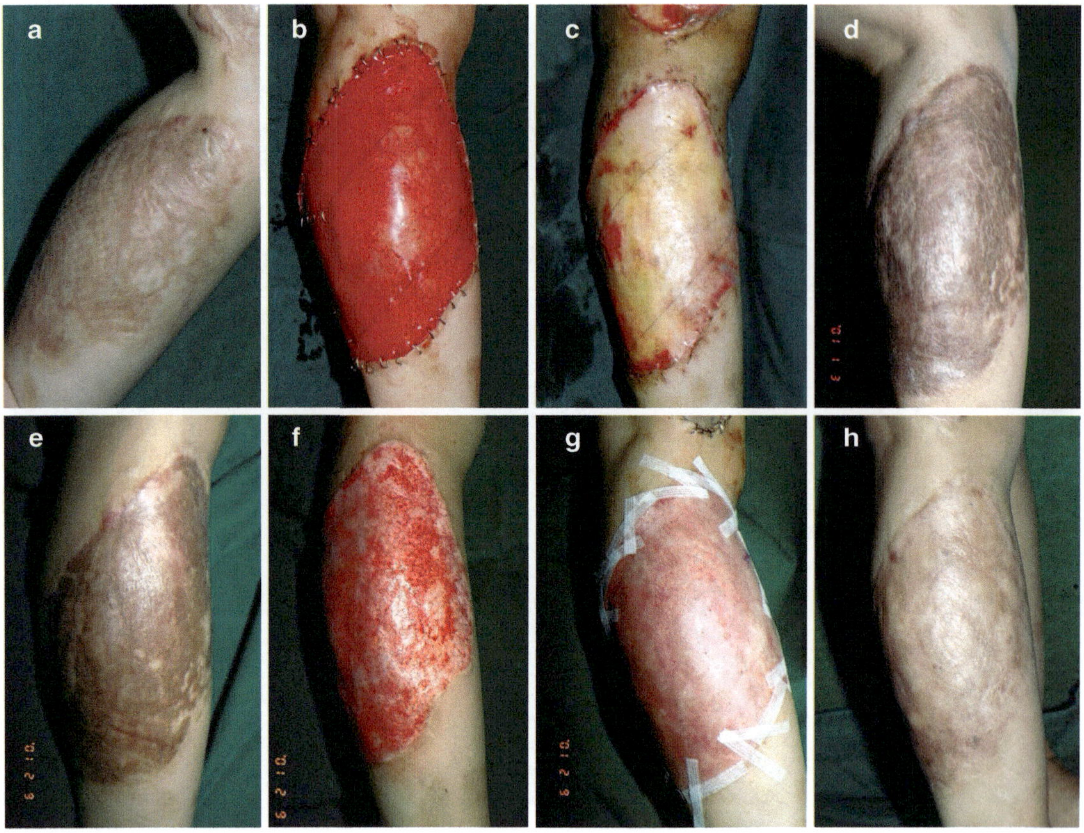

Fig. 5.56 (**a**) Severe itching on the previous mesh-grafted lesion on the right lower leg; (**b**) Integra® artificial dermis engraft immediate view and (**c**) after 2 weeks orange-colored elapsed neodermis was well formed; (**d**) postoperative 1.2 years view, the result was not acceptable because of hyperpigmentation and irregular surface; (**e**, **f**, **g**) dermal resurfacing with 0.15 mm thickness was performed for correction of pigmentation and irregular surface; (**h**) 8 months after the operation skin color and texture were improved, but less acceptable than usual

and rapidly growing and the engrafted skin thickness of ≥0.15 mm may be too thin in the initial period (Fig. 5.56).

However, the utility value of AlloDerm®, a human dermal matrix, is very high and very useful for adaptation using dermal overgraft technique. This is described along with clinical cases in Chap. 3.

5.3 Dermabrasion and Dermal Over FTSG with Composite Fat Graft

Recently, the application range of dermal overgraft has been expanded. As the author gains more experience with the mentioned dermal overgraft technique, novel attempts have been made for the gradual increase of the engrafting skin thickness, and the availability of composite graft was confirmed, containing full-thickness skin and subcutaneous fat layer, which was the final goal of the clinical trials.

This female patient sustained an injury on her left ankle after a traffic accident, resulting in an open tibia and fibular fracture. At that time, she received a titanium plate and K-wire fixation, with a rotational pedicle flap for wound coverage. Three years later, there was a noticeable unsightly depressed scar on the upper part caused by a STSG used to cover a donor flap defect, and a white, bulky flap coverage site was noted as well (Fig. 5.57). To correct the depressed, unsightly scar, incisional release was performed for the

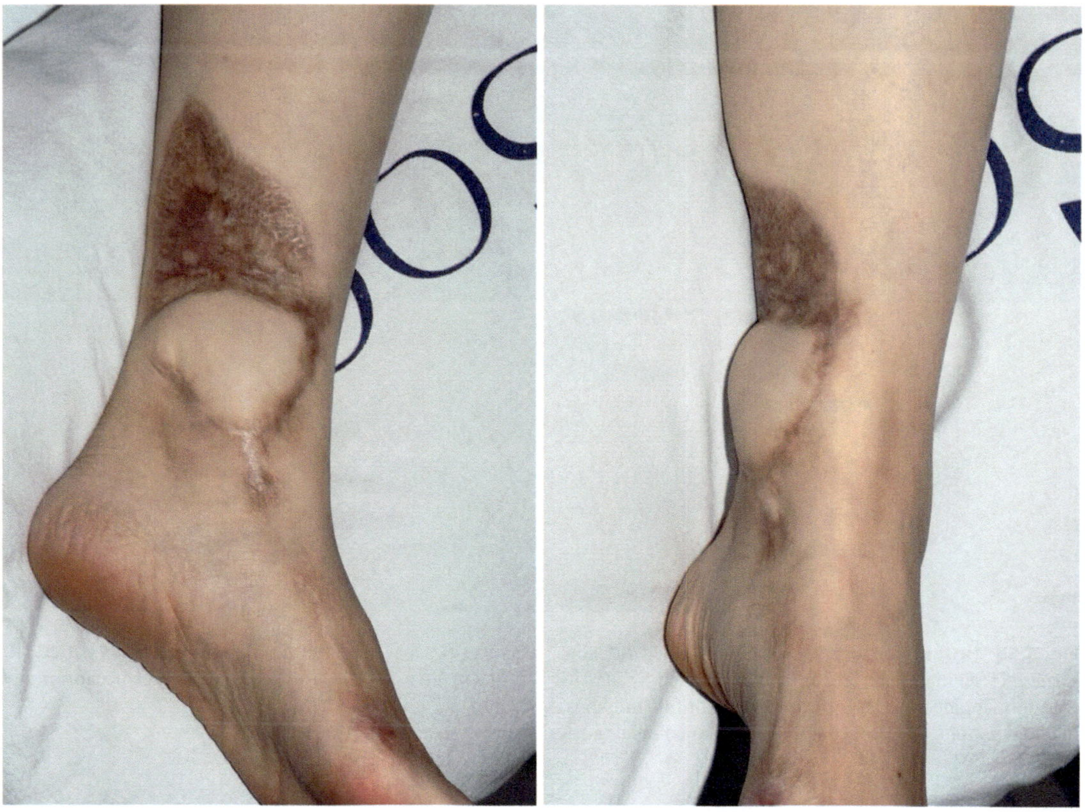

Fig. 5.57 She received titanium plate and K-wire fixation with rotational pedicle flap for wound coverage. Three years after the surgery, unsightly depressed scar was noted on the upper part caused by split-thickness skin graft for coverage of pedicle donor flap defect and a white, bulky flap coverage site was noted

previously contracted STSG margin. Notice the fully released margin, which is over 2–3 cm wide, and the corrected depressed scar on the upper border (black arrow). Lateral flap bulkiness was undermined, and partial fat (red arrow) was removed to conduct the debulking process at the flap margin. The pigmented, depressed STSG site was dermabraded and covered with a 6.5 × 14-cm full-thickness inguinal donor skin, with an attached dense subcutaneous fat layer. Tie-over dressing was performed, although four-directional flaps were undermined. Note that there was no slit incision on the entire engrafted full-thickness skin. The tie-over dressing was removed 6 days later; there was no hematoma or marginal necrosis. The engrafted FTSG skin color had changed to a slight purple color, which is a sign of good processing of FTSG composite fat graft. The engrafted skin had a more stable color and mild, edematous skin texture at postoperative 9 days (Fig. 5.58). At 12 days postoperatively, the edematous skin texture had almost disappeared, and by postoperative week 2, the edematous condition had almost subsided. At postoperative weeks 3 and 6, the process of improving skin color and texture will continue for a long time. The engrafted skin texture matured rapidly and softened relative to the surrounding normal skin tissue (Fig. 5.59). At postoperative month 10, the depressed defect margin was elevated and corrected with FTSG and fat augmentation, but it was slightly undercorrected (Fig. 5.60). Thereafter, a debulking procedure was performed, and the other pedicle area (black arrow) will undergo this procedure later (Fig. 5.61). This is one of the main reasons why I do not prefer flap surgeries such as local, rotational, reverse, and free flap, which require

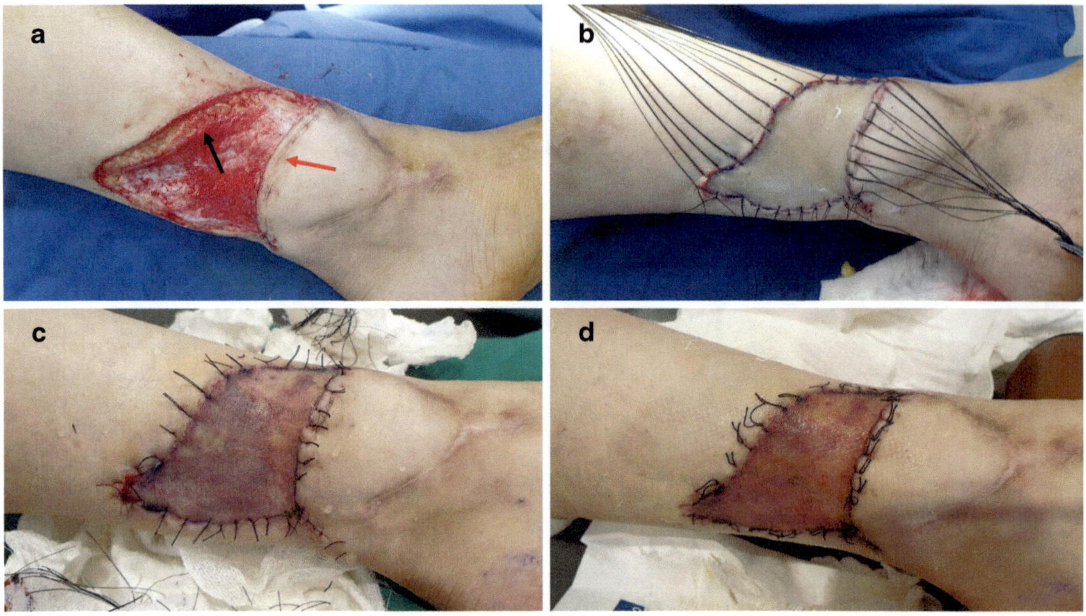

Fig. 5.58 (**a**) Incisional release was performed for contracted STSG marginal release. The pigmented STSG site was dermabraded out and (**b**) covered with full-thickness inguinal donor skin attached to the subcutaneous fat tissue layer; (**c**) tie-over dressing was removed 6 days after; (**d**) postoperative 9 days after engrafted skin became more stable

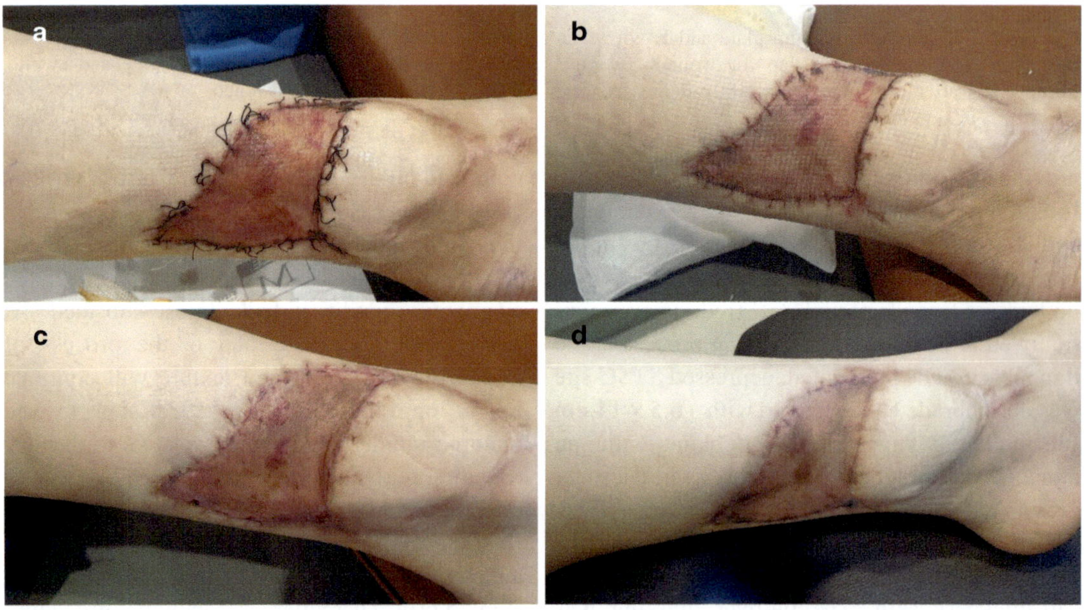

Fig. 5.59 (**a**) Postoperative 12 days after, edematous skin texture almost disappeared and (**b**) postoperative 2 weeks the edematous condition almost subsided; (**c**) postoperative 3 weeks view; (**d**) postoperative 6 weeks, process of improving skin color and texture will continue for a year or more

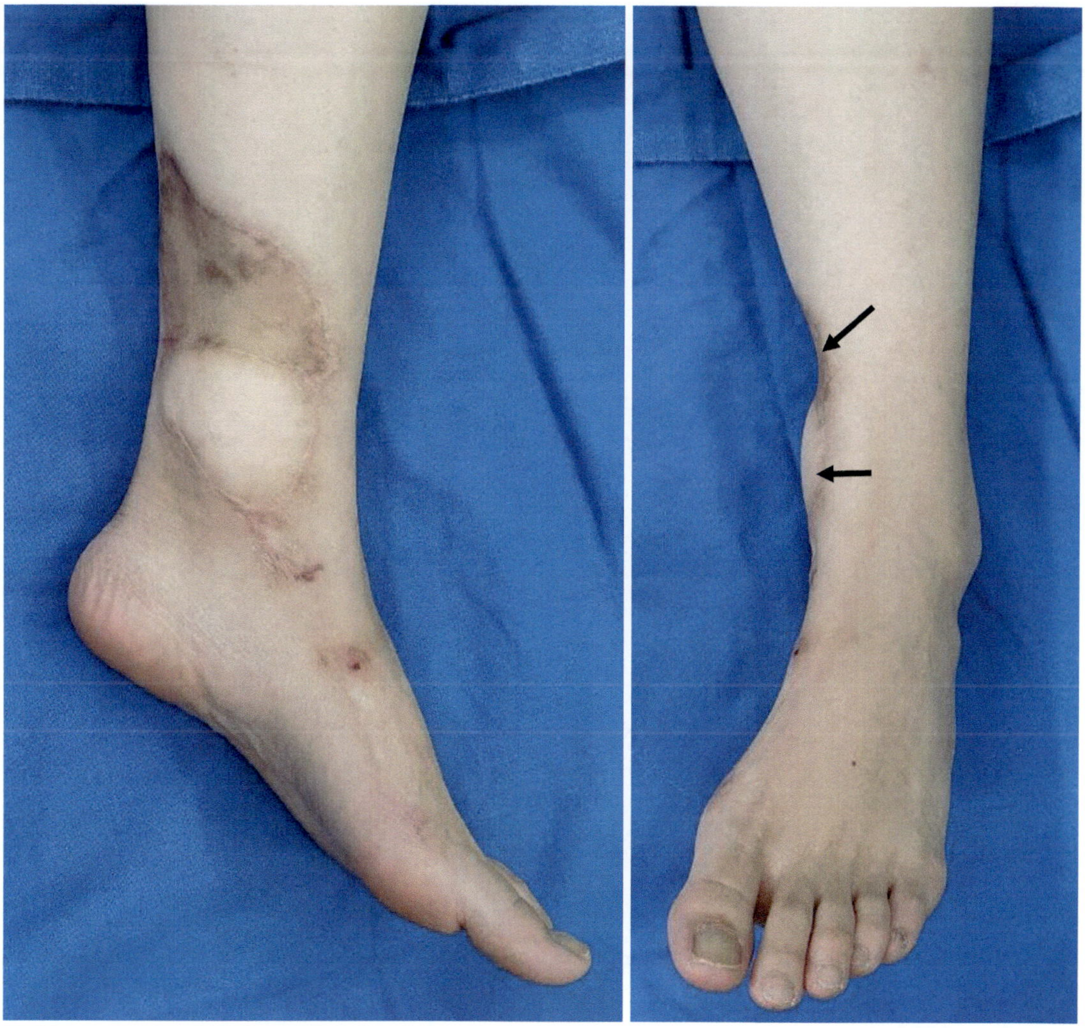

Fig. 5.60 Postoperative 10 months view, depressed defect margin was elevated and corrected with FTSG and fat augmentation, but little bit undercorrected. Flap bulkiness will be corrected with the debulking process in the future

repeated debulking procedures to correct an unnatural appearance.

Since this technique has functional and esthetic advantages and is useful for augmentation supplement, it can be used to repair soft tissue defects induced by severe trauma or burns. This technique was already introduced in some cases and illustration in Chaps. 2 and 3.

Lastly, a patient with the total loss of facial skin due to flame burn, who made a special impact on the author, will be introduced. The patient endured an arduous journey undergoing numerous surgical procedures for a period of 3 years and 6 months (October 05, 1999, to May, 21, 2003).

This female patient was transferred to our department 1 month after sustaining a severe injury from a flame burn and presented with a raw surface over her entire face. Split-thickness skin grafting was performed using 0.3-mm-thick donor skin, which was taken from the scalp (Fig. 5.62). Lower lid ectropion was corrected with 0.5-mm STSGs covering a large area (black arrows). Perioral microstomia was corrected via

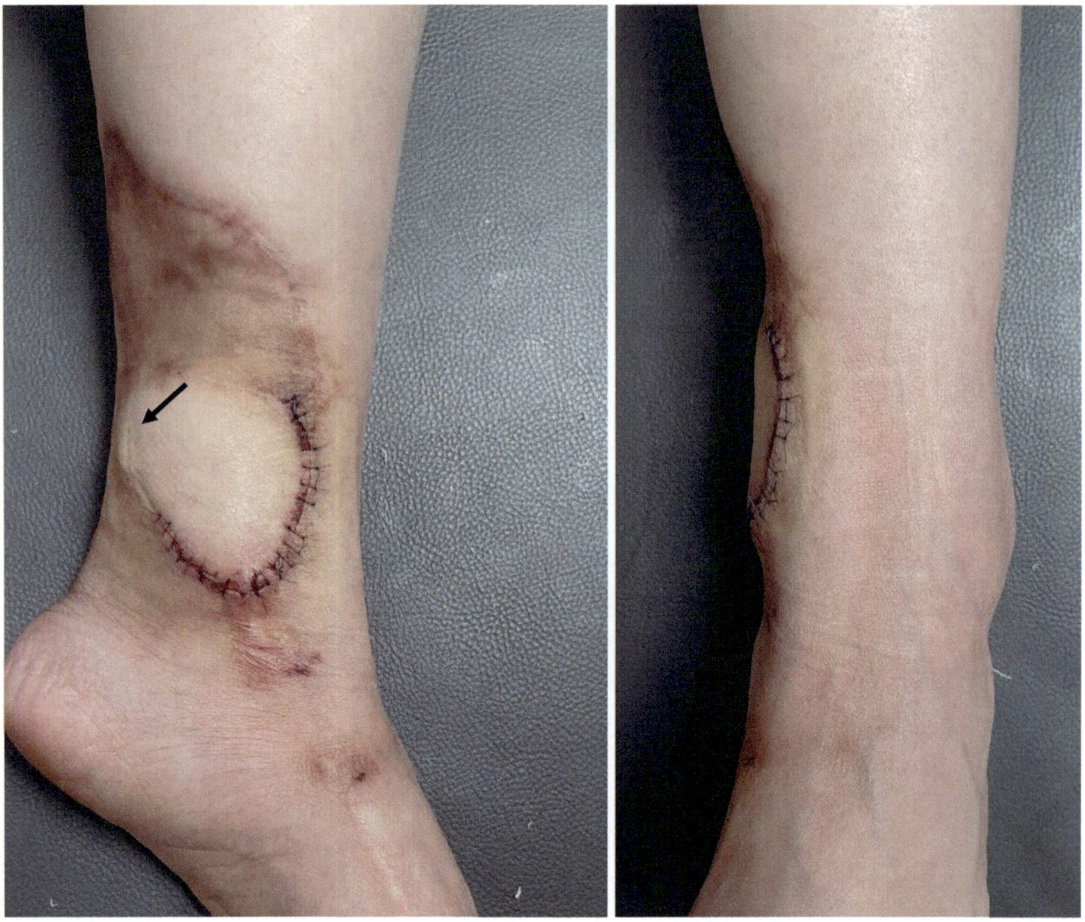

Fig. 5.61 Postoperative 10 months view, debulking operation was performed on the right and lower margins. Engrafted FTSG skin color lightened

local flap with a dermal resurfacing on the chin to release the lower lip and commissure with a medium-thickness skin graft (Fig. 5.63).

One year after the prior procedure, the patient's chin showed a marked improvement following overgraft (arrow). However, she also had a notable philtrum defect as well as irregularities of the upper eyelids and left nostril. Seven months after the procedure, philtrum reconstruction using a composite graft from the triangular fossa of the ear (black arrow) was performed. A postoperative view of the entire face 21 months after the initial split-thickness graft is shown in Fig. 5.64.

A previous image has been shown for comparison. The preoperative image shows eyelid and nasal defects. Postoperative observations after 2 months revealed an upper eyelid correction with blepharoplasty and alar reconstruction with a rotational local flap. Right alar nasi and philtrum were noted with a more natural appearance 1 year and 9 months later (Fig. 5.65).

However, the patient was dissatisfied with deep grief because she could not regain her original face. Faced with these practical impossibilities, and frustrations of the limitations of my own ability, has made me realize the very importance of burn prevention education (Fig. 5.66).

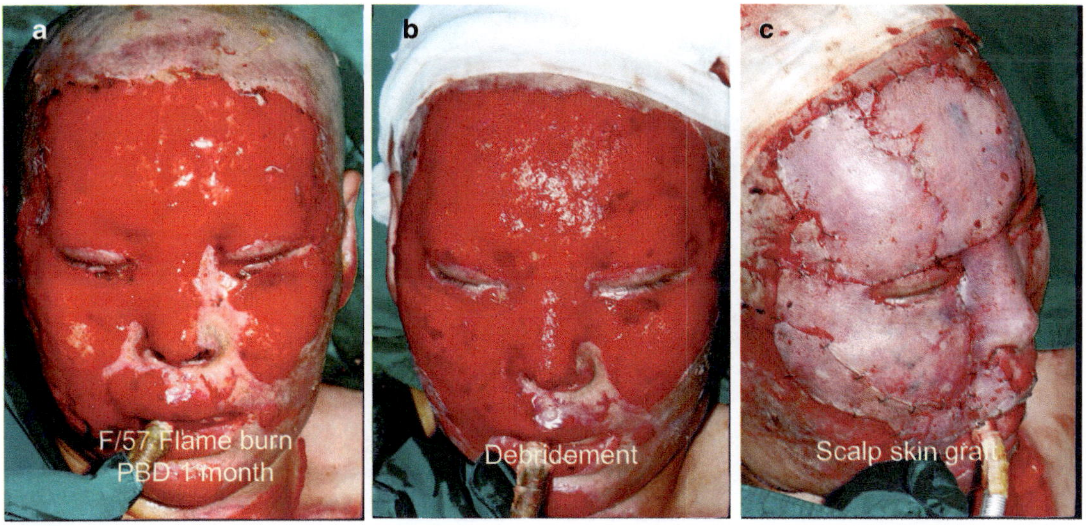

Fig. 5.62 Finally, I would like to introduce one memorable patient who had a prolonged suffering journey; she underwent reconstruction of her burned face for over three and a half years (Oct./05/1999–May/21/2003). (**a**, **b**) Injury by a flame burn and presented with a raw surface over her entire face; (**c**) STSG was performed using 0.3-mm-thick donor skin taken from the scalp

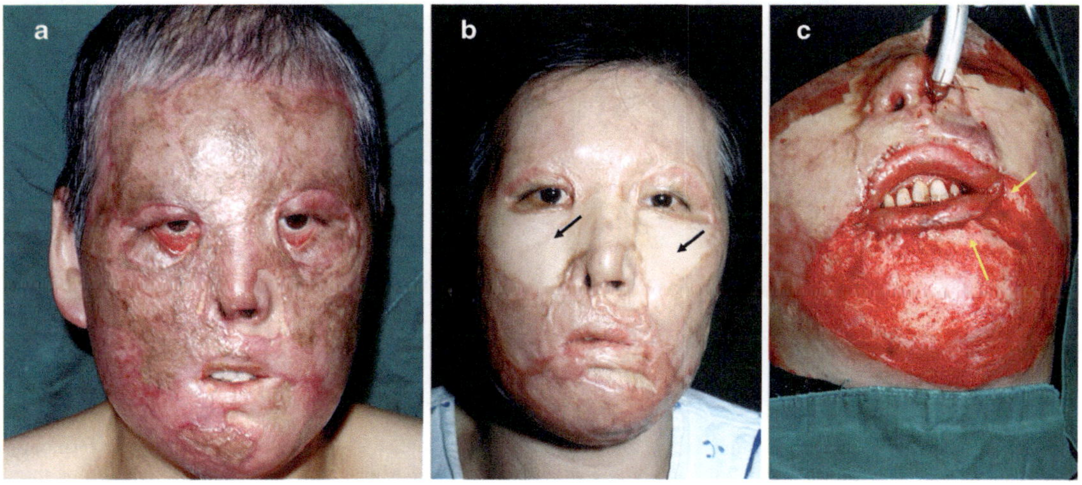

Fig. 5.63 (**a**) Postoperative 6 weeks view; (**b**) lower lid ectropion was corrected with 0.5-mm split-thickness skin (black arrows); (**c**) perioral microstomia was corrected via local flap, with a dermal resurfacing on the chin (yellow arrow) to release the lower lip and commissure

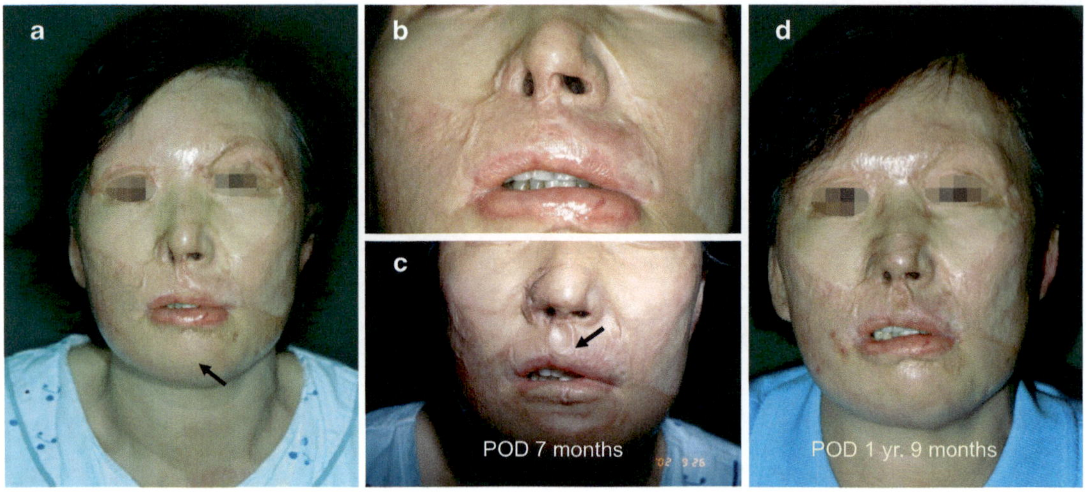

Fig. 5.64 (**a**) Postoperative one year, the patient's chin and lower lip showed significant improvement following dermal resurfacing procedure and local flap (black arrow); (**b**) she also had a notable philtrum defect as well as irregularities of the upper eyelids and left nostril defect; (**c**) postoperative view 7 months after philtrum reconstruction (black arrow); (**d**) postoperative view of the entire face 21 months after the initial split-thickness graft

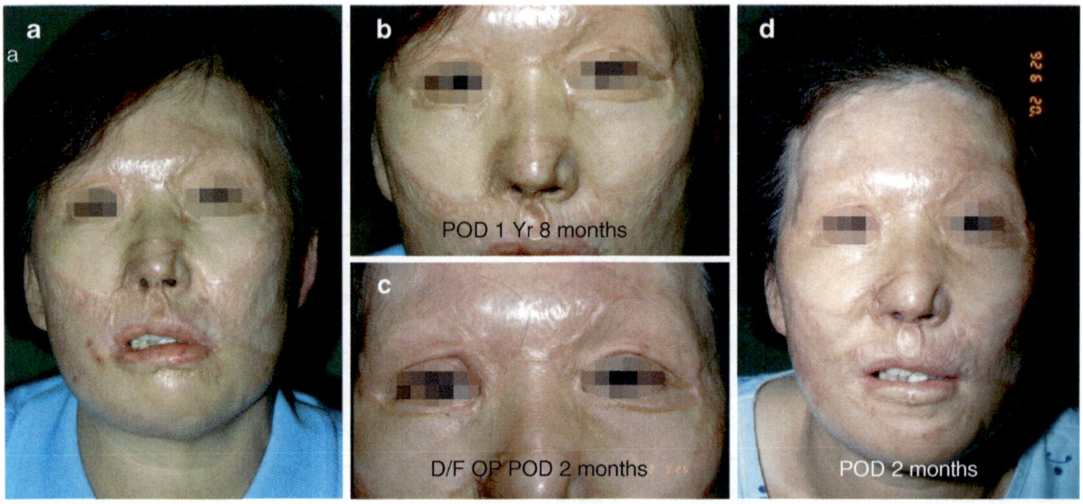

Fig. 5.65 (**a**) Previous photo for comparison; (**b**) preoperative photo showing eyelid and nasal defects and (**c**) postoperative 2 months view showing upper eyelid correction with blepharoplasty and alar reconstruction with rotational local flap; (**d**) postoperative 1 year and 9 months later, right alar nasi and philtrum were noted to be more natural in appearance

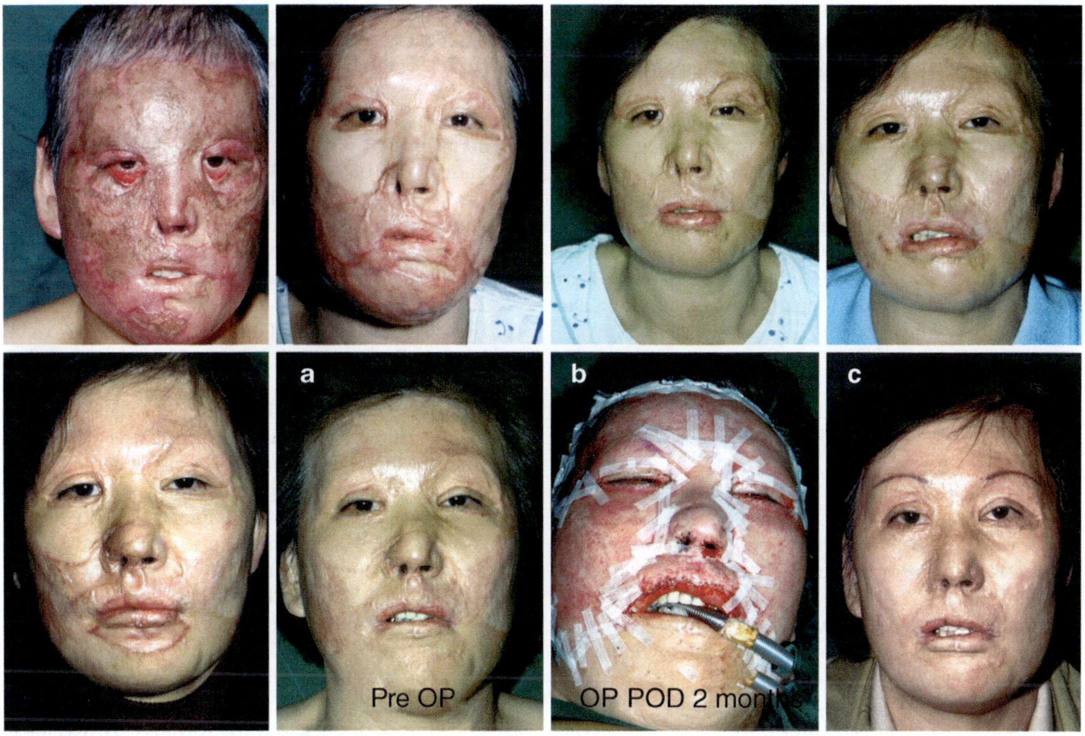

Fig. 5.66 These sequence of photos shows past serial change to present. (**a**, **b**) Finally, a full-face dermal resurfacing operation was performed; (**c**) postoperative 2 years, final result of dermal resurfacing surgery

5.4 Conclusion

The variable techniques of dermabrasion and dermal overgraft described above are the summary and introduction of the various trials and long-term follow-up results that the author has experienced to date. The author expanded on the range of overgraft applications on the various thicknesses of skin and even in FTSG and STSG, based on the concept of its basic principle and methods, which were verified through several clinical experiences. Recently, as reported by the article "Skin-Fat Composite Grafts for Reconstructing Large Full-Thickness Skin Defects" published in the *Journal of Plastic and Reconstructive Surgery*, the author introduced numerous advantages of grafts from various aspects, including full-thickness skin with subcutaneous fat layer. Additionally, overgraft is possible with any skin thickness, even in the wound bed where artificial dermis is grafted, including Integra®, Pelnac®, and Terudermis®, made of bovine or porcine collagen, and AlloDerm®, made of human dermal matrix from cadaver skin, which are different from the raw surface created by dermabrasion of the existing skin graft site or scar bed. This suggests that skin graft from the perspective of esthetic and reconstructive surgery can lead to excellent results, indicating its significance. Therefore, the range of utility of dermal overgraft is so extensive that it is applicable from simple pigmentation disorder to the skin graft of different thicknesses. Furthermore, FTSG demonstrates the possibility that it will be very useful in the future. Dermabrasion and dermal over FTSG are elaborated in Chap. 3 about full-thickness skin graft and Chap. 4 about artificial dermis, in terms of techniques along with examples of various cases.

Acknowledgments In closing, I would like to express my sincerest gratitude to the friends and family who contributed to the creation of this book, Diane Heajih Jang, Jiwon Jahng, and John Kim.

I am also thankful to the Springer medical publishing company and its staff for supporting the publication of this book. In particular, I would like to appreciate Lauren Kim, whose assistance was critical in coordinating this book.

I would like to dedicate this book to President Dae Won Yoon of Hallym University, where I worked for 25 years with the professor in Hangang Sacred Heart Hospital, Burn Center, Department of Plastic and Reconstructive Surgery.

References

1. Shimizu R, Kishi K. Skin graft. Plast Surg Int. 2012;2012:563493.
2. Braza ME, Fahrenkopf MP. Split-thickness skin grafts. In: StatPearls. Treasure Island (FL): StatPearls Publishing; 2022.
3. Sonthalia S, Kachhawa D. Jodhpur technique. In: StatPearls. Treasure Island (FL): StatPearls Publishing; 2022.
4. Onur Erol O, Atabay K. The treatment of burn scar hypopigmentation and surface irregularity by dermabrasion and thin skin grafting. Plast Reconstr Surg. 1990;85(5):754–8.
5. Kahn AM, MJJ C. Vitiligo: treatment by dermabrasion and epithelial sheet grafting. Am Acad Dermatol. 1995;33(4):646–8.
6. Olsson MJ, Juhlin L. Epidermal sheet grafts for repigmentation of vitiligo and piebaldism, with a review of surgical techniques. Acta Derm Venereol. 1997;77(6):463–6.
7. Agrawal K, et al. Vitiligo: repigmentation with dermabrasion and thin split-thickness skin graft. Dermatol Surg. 1995;21:295; PMID: 7728478.
8. Falabella R. Surgical approaches for stable vitiligo. Dermatol Surg. 2005;31(10):1277–84.
9. Majid I. Grafting in vitiligo: how to get better results and how to avoid complications. J Cutan Aesthet Surg. 2013;6(2):83–9.
10. Dellatorre G, Bertolini W, Castro CCS. Optimizing suction blister epidermal graft technique in the surgical treatment of vitiligo. An Bras Dermatol. 2017;92(6):888–90.
11. Harashina T, Iso R. The treatment of leukoderma after burns by a combination of dermabrasion and "chip" skin grafting. Br J Plast Surg. 1985;38(3):301–5.
12. Driscoll DN, Levy AN, Gama AR. Dermabrasion and thin epidermal grafting for treatment of large and small areas of postburn leukoderma: a case series and review of the literature. J Burn Care Res. 2016;37(4):e387–93.
13. Chen B, Xu M, Li B. The clinical experience for treating post-burn depigmentation with tiny epidermal particles graft. Int Wound J. 2017;14(1):165–71.
14. Açikel C, Ulkür E, Güler MM. Treatment of burn scar depigmentation by carbon dioxide laser-assisted dermabrasion and thin skin grafting. Plast Reconstr Surg. 2000;105(6):1973–8.
15. Ho D, Jagdeo J. Excellent aesthetic and functional outcome after fractionated carbon dioxide laser skin graft revision surgery: case report and review of laser skin graft revision techniques. J Drugs Dermatol. 2015;14(11):1285–8.
16. Herskovitz I, Hughes OB, Macquhae F, Rakosi A, Kirsner R. Epidermal skin grafting. Int wound J. 2016;13 Suppl 3(Suppl 3):52–6.
17. Hann SK, Park YK. Dermabrasion and epithelial sheet grafting. J Am Acad Dermatol. 1996;35(4):652.
18. Gupta S, Jangra RS, Gupta S. Precision dermabrasion of small areas of vitiliginous skin using dental diamond burs. J Cutan Aesthet Surg. 2021;14(2):220–1.
19. Ashique KT, Kaliyadan F, Jayasree P. Ready-to-use device for dermabrasion in vitiligo surgery. J Cutan Aesthet Surg. 2020;13(4):338–9.
20. Ashique KT, Kaliyadan F, George RR. Dermabrasion of the recipient skin in vitiligo surgery: an easier way out. Indian J Dermatol Venereol Leprol. 2018;84(4):498–9.
21. Ebrahimi A, Radmanesh M, Kavoussi H. Recipient site preparation for epidermal graft in stable vitiligo by a special fraise. An Bras Dermatol. 2015;90(1):55–60.
22. Kanapathy M, Mosahebi A. Comparative study on the donor site aesthetic outcome between epidermal graft and split-thickness skin graft. Int Wound J. 2019;16(2):354–9; (page 6).
23. Tost F. Periocular surgery and the impact of split-thickness skin grafts. Klin Monbl Augenheilkd. 2011;228(1):35–40.
24. Tost F, Kempin R. Post-surgical management of split-thickness skin grafts in oculoplastic surgery. Klin Monbl Augenheilkd. 2015;232(1):27–32.
25. Asuku M, Yu TC, Yan Q, Böing E, Hahn H, Hovland S, Donelan MB. Split-thickness skin graft donor-site morbidity: a systematic literature review. Burns. 2021;47(7):1525–46.
26. Humrich M, Goepel L, Gutknecht M, Lohrberg D, Blessmann M, Bruning G, Diener H, Dissemond J, Hartmann B, Augustin M. Health-related quality of life and patient burden in patients with split-thickness skin graft donor site wounds. Int Wound J. 2018;15(2):266–73.
27. Shokri T, Smith J, Ducic Y. Paradigms in complex facial scar management. Semin Plast Surg. 2020;34(4):305–13.
28. Bedford L, Daveluy S. Skin resurfacing dermabrasion. In: StatPearls. Treasure Island (FL): StatPearls Publishing; 2022.

29. Maranda EL, Wang MX, Shareef S, Tompkins BA, Emerson C, Badiavas EV. Surgical management of leukoderma after burn: a review. Burns. 2018;44(2):256–62.
30. van Geel N, Ongenae K, Naeyaert JM. Surgical techniques for vitiligo: a review. Dermatology. 2001;202(2):162–6.
31. Kar BR, Raj C. Suction blister epidermal grafting for vitiligo involving angles of lip: experience of 112 patients. J Cutan Aesthet Surg. 2018;11(1):13–9.

GPSR Compliance

The European Union's (EU) General Product Safety Regulation (GPSR) is a set of rules that requires consumer products to be safe and our obligations to ensure this.

If you have any concerns about our products, you can contact us on ProductSafety@springernature.com

In case Publisher is established outside the EU, the EU authorized representative is:

Springer Nature Customer Service Center GmbH
Europaplatz 3
69115 Heidelberg, Germany

Batch number: 10732801

Printed by Printforce, the Netherlands